The Science of Cholesterol

Volume I

The Science of Cholesterol
Volume I

Edited by **Ashley Martin**

FOSTER ACADEMICS
New Jersey

Published by Foster Academics,
61 Van Reypen Street,
Jersey City, NJ 07306, USA
www.fosteracademics.com

The Science of Cholesterol: Volume I
Edited by Ashley Martin

International Standard Book Number: 978-1-63242-394-8 (Hardback)

Printed in China.

Contents

Preface

Cholesterol is something that is both harmful and helpful to the human body. It is a substance that is essential to our body and its normal functions, but at higher levels in the blood, it transforms into an ever present danger that elevates the risk of heart attack in a person. Cholesterol is found in each cell of the human body and has its natural functions, both manufactured in the body and found in food. It has its uses in the body including helping to manufacture vitamin D. It is when cholesterol crosses a certain limit that it becomes extremely harmful to the human system. The major factors that affect high cholesterol levels are diet and exercise and weight. Limiting the intake of fat helps lower cholesterol, though there are some who seem to have a predilection towards higher cholesterol levels. The most dangerous factor in high cholesterol is that such high levels don't have any outward symptoms, unless one is routinely screened for said levels. Unhealthy eating and lack of exercise increase the chances of increased cholesterol levels.

What cannot be emphasised more than enough is the need for healthy living and this book compiles all the statistics that point towards our need to do so. It has never before been clearer than in this age when man is slowly starting to lead a more sedentary lifestyle coupled with often unhealthy eating habits. The researches compiled in this book attempt to understand humanity's predilection towards such self-defeating and harmful lifestyle habits.

Editor

1

Predictors of Metabolic Syndrome in the Iranian Population: Waist Circumference, Body Mass Index, or Waist to Hip Ratio?

Mojgan Gharipour,[1] Nizal Sarrafzadegan,[1] Masoumeh Sadeghi,[2] Elham Andalib,[3] Mohammad Talaie,[1] Davood Shafie,[4] and Esmaiel Aghababaie[4]

[1] *Isfahan Cardiovascular Research Centre, Isfahan Cardiovascular Research Institute, Isfahan University of Medical Sciences, Isfahan, Iran*
[2] *Rehabilitation Research Center, Isfahan Cardiovascular Research Institute, Isfahan University of Medical Sciences, P.O. Box 81465-1148, Isfahan, Iran*
[3] *Hypertension Research Centre, Isfahan Cardiovascular Research Institute, Isfahan University of Medical Sciences, Isfahan, Iran*
[4] *Cardiology Department, School of Medicine, Isfahan University of Medical Sciences, Isfahan, Iran*

Correspondence should be addressed to Masoumeh Sadeghi; sadeghimasoumeh@gmail.com

Academic Editor: Gerhard M. Kostner

This study aimed to investigate whether body mass index (BMI), waist circumference (WC), or waist to hip ratio (WHR) could be a better predictor of metabolic syndrome and, if so, what would be the cutoff points for these surrogates to appropriately differentiate metabolic syndrome in different age and sex subgroups. *Methods.* The present cross-sectional study was conducted on a sample of Isfahan Cohort Study (ICS). In total, 468 individuals (194 with and 274 subjects without metabolic syndrome) according to the National Cholesterol Education Program's Adult Treatment Panel III (ATP-III) criteria were selected. Anthropometric indices were measured and plotted using receiver-operating characteristic (ROC) curves. *Results.* According to ROC curve analysis, WC and WHR parameters were better indicators of metabolic syndrome compared to BMI in women, whereas in men WHR had a lower discriminating value compared to the other two parameters. Among these three anthropometric parameters, BMI had a lower sensitivity and WC and WHR both had a higher sensitivity for predicting metabolic syndrome in women compared with in men. The cut points for WC were nearly equal in men and women, 90.3 versus 90.0, respectively. Women had higher cut points for BMI (28.5 kg/m^2) compared to men (26.0 kg/m^2). Our results showed the highest sensitivity and specificity for WC cut points specially in women. To predict metabolic syndrome, we looked into optimal age-specific cut points for BMI, WC, and WHR. The results indicated that WC had the highest discriminating value compared to other indicators in the different age subgroups. The optimal cut points for all three parameters gradually increased with age. *Conclusion.* Our results demonstrated that regardless of gender and age variables, WC could be a preferred parameter for predicting metabolic syndrome compared to BMI and WHR in Iranian population.

1. Introduction

Metabolic syndrome is known to be a cluster of variety of cardiac and metabolic-related factors such as obesity, elevated blood pressure, glucose metabolism disturbances, and raised lipid levels leading to increased risk of mortality and morbidity [1–4]. From all these risk factors, existing diagnostic criteria emphasize the importance of body fat [5]. It has been suggested that central obesity as an indicator of body fat can be easily and cost-effectively estimated by measuring body mass index (BMI) and waist circumference (WC) which might discriminate metabolic syndrome from nonmetabolic syndrome status [6, 7].

To diagnose metabolic syndrome, different cutoff points for these anthropometric parameters have been defined to diagnose central obesity and therefore metabolic syndrome. These cutoff points are mainly derived from studies conducted on western populations [8, 9]. We believe that ethnic and racial differences in our population might require different cutoff points and or use of different anthropometric parameters for diagnosis of metabolic syndrome. There are controversies on mortality and morbidity rates related to the defined cutoff points [10] and also lack of sex and age specificity. To our knowledge, no previous studies have investigated appropriate cut points for body fat indices that could have the highest value for diagnosis of metabolic syndrome neither have demonstrated the best indicators for central obesity related to different age and sex subgroups. We therefore investigated BMI, WC, or waist to hip ratio (WHR) in Iranian population to evaluate which one could better define metabolic syndrome and what cutoff points for these surrogates are more appropriate to diagnose metabolic syndrome in different age and sex subgroups.

2. Methods

This is a cross-sectional study conducted on 468 participants who were selected from those enrolled in Isfahan Cohort Study which was a population-based cohort and previously reported [11, 12]. Isfahan Cohort Study (ICS) was conducted in 2001 in three central provinces in Iran including Isfahan, Arak, and Najafabad and enrolled 6504 participants with age ≥35 years old. The primary outcomes of the cohort were detecting the incidence of cardiovascular diseases (CVDs) and mortality and morbidity resulted from it in addition to the incidence of major risk factors for CVDs. All participants underwent a complete clinical examination for cardiovascular evaluation including systolic blood pressure (SBP) and diastolic blood pressures (DBP), fasting blood sugar, and fasting serum lipid indices measurements. We excluded all subjects with history of any cardiovascular or related disorders, pregnant women, breast feeding mothers, and those subjects with serious systemic illnesses from the study. The study protocol was approved by human research ethics committee of Isfahan Cardiovascular Research Institute, a WHO collaborative center. An informed consent was obtained from all participants prior to enrolment in the study. Details of ISC study were reported previously [13]. All participants were asked to fast for 8–12 hours before attending the first visit in order to obtain demographics information, a medical history, to conduct clinical examination and venous blood samples for lab tests. We first assessed coronary artery disease risk factors as per the following definitions. Current smoking history: if patients regularly smoke a tobacco product/products one or more times per day or have smoked for 30 days prior to admission [14]; hypercholesterolemia: total cholesterol ≥ 5.0 mmol/L, HDL-cholesterol ≥ 1.0 mmol/L in men, and ≥1.1 mmol/L in women, triglycerides ≥ 2.0 mmol/L [15]; hypertension: SBP ≥ 140 mmHg and/or DBP ≥ 90 mmHg and/or use of antihypertensive treatment [16]; and diabetes mellitus: symptoms of diabetes plus presence of at least one of the following lab tests including plasma glucose concentration ≥ 11.1 mmol/L, fasting plasma glucose ≥ 7.0 mmol/L, and 2-hpp ≥ 11.1 mmol/L) [17].

Blood pressure was measured using a standard mercury sphygmomanometer on the right arm with subjects seated and after at least 10-minute resting. Measures of WC were obtained by a measure tape of horizontal plane, midway between the inferior margin of the ribs and the superior border of the iliac crest. Body weight and height were measured by using a digital scale accurate to the nearest 0.1 kg and a wall stadiometer, respectively. To measure BMI the Quetelet formula was used (weight in kilograms divided by height in meters squared). Total cholesterol, high density lipoprotein-cholesterol (HDL-C), triglyceride, and blood glucose were assessed using a spectrophotometer. The variation coefficient was <5% for all laboratory measurements. The definition of metabolic syndrome was based on the presence of three or more components out of five defined criteria for metabolic syndrome by the amended National Cholesterol Education Program's Adult Treatment Panel III (ATP-III) [18]. The ATP-III criteria include (1) fasting triglycerides > 150 mg/dL or lipid medications; (2) SBP > 130 mmHg, DBP > 85 mmHg, or use of antihypertensive medications; (3) fasting plasma glucose > 110 mg/dL or use of diabetes medications; (4) HDL cholesterol < 40 mg/dL (men) or <50 mg/dL (women); and (5) waist circumference > 102 cm (men) or >88 cm (women). Using the previous criteria we found 194 patients who were diagnosed to have metabolic syndrome and 274 patients without metabolic syndrome.

2.1. Statistical Analysis. The results were presented as absolute frequencies and percentages for categorical variables and mean ± SD for continuous variables. Categorical variables were compared using chi-square test or Fisher's exact test when more than 20% of cells with expected count of less than 5 were observed. Continuous variables were also compared using *t*-test. To compare the ability of BMI, WC, and WHR to predict presence of metabolic syndrome, these indices were plotted using receiver-operating characteristic (ROC) curves. The areas under the curve (AUC) and associated 95% confidence intervals (CIs) were compared. The larger the AUC, the more accurate the test. A P value <0.05 was considered statistically significant. To determine the best sex- and age-related cut points for BMI, WC, and WHR in relation to the subject's metabolic syndrome we looked into the shortest distance between any point on the ROC curve and the top left corner of the y axis and plotted separate ROC curves for each variable and associated AUC [5]. Intercooled STATA (version 9.1) was used to analyze data and plot curves as well as to determine sensitivity and specificity. Statistical comparisons for all variables between the two genders were also performed using SPSS software (version 19.0, SPSS Inc., Chicago, IL, USA).

3. Results

In total, 468 subjects (194 with and 247 without metabolic syndrome) were evaluated for this study. The male to female (M/F) ratio in metabolic syndrome group was 42% to 58% and in the group without metabolic syndrome was 56% to 44% (Table 1). Percentage of current smokers was similar between men with and without metabolic syndrome. None of the females were current smokers. In both sex subgroups, the overall prevalence of high blood pressure, diabetes mellitus,

TABLE 1: Baseline characteristics and clinical parameters in men and women with and without MetS.

Variables	Men			Women		
	Without MetS (N = 154)	with MetS (N = 82)	P value	Without MetS (N = 120)	with MetS (N = 112)	P value
Hypertension (%)	18 (11.7)	40 (48.8)	**<0.001**	18 (15.0)	37 (33.0)	**0.001**
Diabetes mellitus (%)	4 (2.6)	29 (35.4)	**<0.001**	3 (2.5)	39 (34.8)	**<0.001**
Dyslipidemia (%)	100 (64.9)	73 (89.0)	**<0.001**	79 (65.8)	105 (93.8)	**<0.001**
Age (years)	57.58 ± 10.22	57.68 ± 9.69	0.942	54.21/8.50	56.25/9.05	0.078
BMI (kg/m^2)	25.62 ± 3.32	29.13 ± 3.44	**<0.001**	28.41/4.61	32.26/4.53	**<0.001**
Systolic blood pressure (mm Hg)	118.47 ± 15.40	135.52 ± 16.35	**<0.001**	119.04/18.63	128.90/17.19	**<0.001**
Diastolic blood pressure (mm Hg)	77.29 ± 7.12	84.80 ± 8.05	**<0.001**	76.93/7.49	80.10/9.30	**0.005**
Fasting blood glucose (mg/dL)	83.86 ± 20.24	108.06 ± 47.16	**<0.001**	81.93/11.54	109.80/45.94	**<0.001**
Total cholesterol (mg/dL)	200.86 ± 37.52	210.85 ± 46.65	0.078	213.18/35.54	218.48/45.12	0.319
HDL cholesterol (mg/dL)	45.23 ± 11.04	38.38 ± 6.96	**<0.001**	53.80/11.56	44.79/9.31	**<0.001**
LDL cholesterol (mg/dL)	117.01 ± 25.14	117.28 ± 28.08	0.939	101.03/24.25	121.71/27.77	0.844
Triglyceride (mg/dL)	142.35/63.99	269.63/196.30	**<0.001**	134.18/60.38	232.85/123.59	**<0.001**

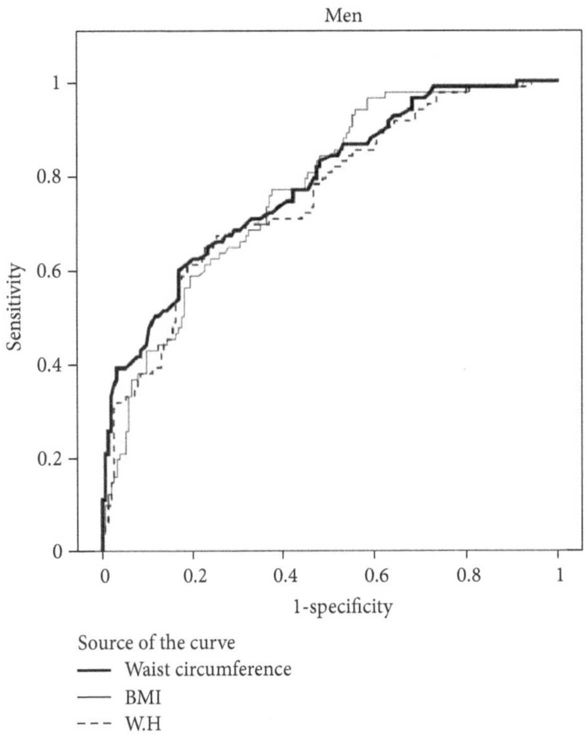

FIGURE 1

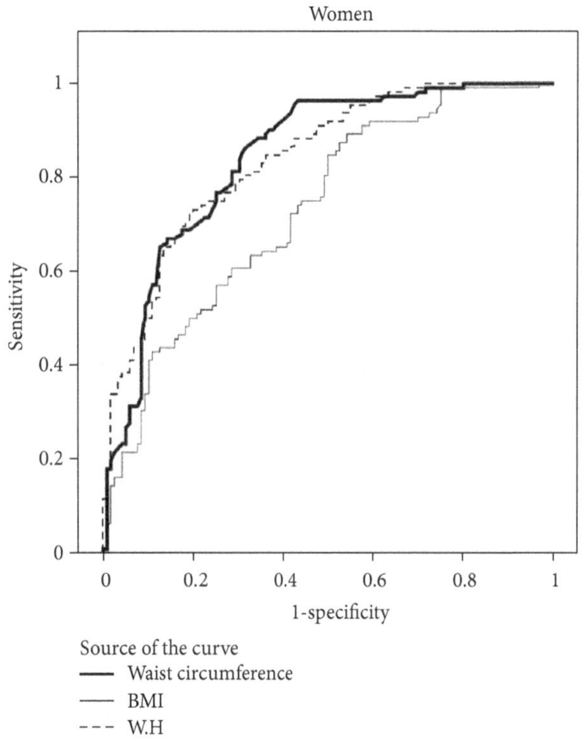

FIGURE 2

and dyslipidemia was higher in the group with metabolic syndrome. The average of BMI, SBP and DBP, blood glucose, total serum cholesterol, and serum triglycerides was significantly higher in both men and women with metabolic syndrome compared to subjects without metabolic syndrome.

The predicting values for metabolic syndrome and corresponding AUC of BMI, WC, and WHR in both genders are shown in Table 2, Figures 1 and 2.

We found that in women, WC (with the AUC of 0.85) and WHR parameters (with the AUC of 0.84) were better indicators of metabolic syndrome compared to BMI (with the AUC of 0.73), whereas in men WC (with the AUC of 0.78) and BMI (with the AUC of 0.77) were better indicators of metabolic syndromes and WHR (with the AUC of 0.75) had a lower discriminating value comparatively.

In general, from the three studied anthropometric parameters, WC and WHR had a higher sensitivity and BMI had a lower sensitivity for predicting metabolic syndrome in women compared with in men. Further ROC analysis resulted in optimal gender-specific cut points for BMI, WC,

TABLE 2: Areas under the ROC curve cutoffs, sensitivity and specificity of WC, BMI, and WHR by sex.

	AURC (95% CI)	*P* value	Cut-off	Sensitivity	Specificity
Women					
WC	0.85 (0.79–0.90)	<0.001	90.3	86.6%	68.3%
BMI	0.73 (0.67–0.79)	<0.001	28.5	79.5%	50.8%
WHR	0.84 (0.79–0.89)	<0.001	0.88	83.0%	65.0%
Men					
WC	0.78 (0.72–0.84)	<0.001	90.0	82.9%	51.9%
BMI	0.77 (0.71–0.83)	<0.001	26.0	80.5%	54.5%
WHR	0.75 (0.69–0.82)	<0.001	0.93	80.5%	50.6%

TABLE 3: Cut points for areas under the ROC curve, sensitivity and specificity of WC, BMI, and WHR by age groups.

	AURC (95% CI)	*P* value	Cut-off	Sensitivity (95% CI)	Specificity (95% CI)
Age of 40–49 years					
WC	0.78 (0.69–0.86)	<0.001	88.5	83.3%	52.5%
BMI	0.71 (0.62–0.81)	<0.001	27.5	79.2%	50.0%
WHR	0.71 (0.63–0.80)	<0.001	0.88	81.3%	57.5%
Age of 50–59 years					
WC	0.84 (0.79–0.90)	<0.001	89.0	89.5%	62.0%
BMI	0.79 (0.73–0.85)	<0.001	27.5	81.0%	62.0%
WHR	0.79 (0.73–0.86)	<0.001	0.89	85.5%	53.7%
Age of ≥60 years					
WC	0.78 (0.70–0.85)	<0.001	92.0	81.4%	55.8%
BMI	0.77 (0.70–0.84)	<0.001	28.8	80.0%	61.6%
WHR	0.76 (0.68–0.83)	<0.001	0.93	82.9%	52.3%

and WHR together along with associated sensitivity and specificity. As shown in Table 2, the cut points for WC were nearly equal in men and women (90.3 versus 90.0), respectively. Women, on the other hand, had higher cut points for BMI (28.5 kg/m^2) compared to men (26.0 kg/m^2). With regard to WHR women had lower cut points compared to men. The highest sensitivity and specificity were exhibited by the WC cut points.

The optimal age-specific cut points for BMI, WC, and WHR for predicting metabolic syndrome are presented in Table 3. Our results demonstrated that in the different age subgroups, WC had the highest AUC for discriminating metabolic syndrome compared to other indicators. All the studied anthropometric parameters had their highest sensitivity and specificity shown in the subgroup aged 50–59 years old. The optimal cut points for the three parameters gradually increased with age.

4. Discussion

The aim of the present study was determining discriminating values of common anthropometric parameters for metabolic syndrome as well as discovering age- and sex-specific cutoff points for these parameters in Iranian population. According to our findings, two indices of WC and WHR were better indicators of metabolic syndrome compared to BMI in women, while WC and BMI were more preferable than for discriminating this syndrome in men [19]. On the other hand, WC had the highest value for predicting metabolic syndrome with appropriate sensitivity and specificity. The value of WC, BMI, and WHR in differentiating metabolic syndrome from nonmetabolic syndrome has been a matter of controversy. Beydoun et al. found BMI to be inferior o WC among men in general and White men in particular for prediction of metabolic syndrome, but not women [5]. What Beydoun is suggesting is consistent with other reports by Reeder et al. [20], Moreno et al. [21], and Wang et al. [22]. However, another report suggested that WC, WHR, and BMI values were equally useful indicators to identify the presence of metabolic abnormalities in Chinese population [23]. Given different results reported by variety of population-based studies in different ethnicities from western and eastern countries on the discriminating value of WC, WHR, and BMI we believe that the selection of each parameter for diagnosis of metabolic syndrome should be specified to each ethnic population. Hence, among Iranian population, WC might be the most appropriate indicator to discriminate metabolic syndrome regardless of gender and age variables. Our study also showed superiority of WC to other indices in different age subgroups. Because of correlation between WC with abdominal fat mass and because WC is more associated with cardiovascular risk compared to BMI, currently, WC and its related values are widely used as a representative indicator of abdominal adiposity [24–26].

In our study, the cutoff values of WC for diagnosis of metabolic syndrome were partially equal in men and women, whereas the cut points of BMI were higher for women and the WHR was higher for men. One of the main findings in our study was observation of the increasing trend of the cutoff points for all anthropometric indices with age increase. In similar studies to ours, the cutoff points of BMI in men were reported to be lower than in women, but our results showed that the cut points were considerably higher compared to what has been previously revealed in other populations [23]. In fact, due to the same reason, the currently used cut points which are derived from studies on European, American, or southeastern populations may not be applicable to Iranian ethnic groups [27]. Therefore, we recommend replacing the obtained cutoff points after validation in Iranian population.

In the current study, we did not assess the value of the combination of anthropometric parameters in comparison with their use alone. However, some previous studies on other populations showed that WC together with BMI were good discriminating indices for metabolic syndrome [22]. Beydoun et al. indicated that instead of using just one of these parameters, it is possible to increase both sensitivity and specificity of diagnosis of metabolic syndrome by combining both WC and BMI to a practical clinical level [5]. Wrist circumference is reported as a significant predictor of diabetes in both genders of adult population. However, its predictability is independent of BMI or WC only among females. Because of its simple and easy-to-detect nature, wrist circumference could be considered as a new anthropometric assessment for prediction of type 2 diabetes and metabolic syndrome.

Other studies on Iranian population also showed that BMI and WC have the same power to predict metabolic syndrome [26–30]. Mirmiran et al. confirmed importance of waist circumference in risk stratification of metabolic syndrome in adulthood [31, 32].

5. Limitation

The present study is limited by its cross-sectional nature so we could not evaluate outcome measures. Consequently, the authors are mindful that differences could only be imputed from the previously documented data.

6. Conclusion

Our findings demonstrated that in Iranian women, the two indices of WC and WHR were better indicators of metabolic syndrome while in men, WC and BMI were superior indicators. We observed that WC, regardless of age subgroup or gender, had the highest predicting value for discriminating metabolic syndrome with appropriate sensitivity and specificity. The optimal cut points for metabolic syndrome for all three parameters gradually increased with age.

References

[1] Q. Qiao, J. Pitkäniemi, J. Tuomilehto et al., "Comparison of different definitions of the metabolic syndrome in relation to cardiovascular mortality in European men and women," *Diabetologia*, vol. 49, no. 12, pp. 2837–2846, 2006.

[2] G. N. Thomas, C. M. Schooling, S. M. McGhee et al., "Metabolic syndrome increases all-cause and vascular mortality: the Hong Kong cardiovascular risk factor study," *Clinical Endocrinology*, vol. 66, no. 5, pp. 666–671, 2007.

[3] A. M. J. Wassink, Y. Van Der Graaf, J. K. Olijhoek, and F. L. J. Visseren, "Metabolic syndrome and the risk of new vascular events and all-cause mortality in patients with coronary artery disease, cerebrovascular disease, peripheral arterial disease or abdominal aortic aneurysm," *European Heart Journal*, vol. 29, no. 2, pp. 213–223, 2008.

[4] M. Gharipour, R. Kelishadi, A. Khosravi, S. Shirani, M. Masjedi, and N. Sarrafzadegan, "The impact of a community trial on the pharmacological treatment in the individuals with the metabolic Program," *Archives of Medical Science*, vol. 8, no. 6, pp. 1009–1017, 2001.

[5] M. A. Beydoun, M. T. Fanelli Kuczmarski, Y. Wang, M. A. Mason, M. K. Evans, and A. B. Zonderman, "Receiver-operating characteristics of adiposity for metabolic syndrome: the healthy aging in neighborhoods of diversity across the life span (HANDLS) study," *Public Health Nutrition*, vol. 14, no. 1, pp. 77–92, 2011.

[6] M. Takahashi, K. Shimomura, P. Proks et al., "A proposal of combined evaluation of waist circumference and BMI for the diagnosis of metabolic syndrome," *Endocrine Journal*, vol. 56, no. 9, pp. 1079–1082, 2009.

[7] J. A. Al-Lawati and P. Jousilahti, "Body mass index, waist circumference and waist-to-hip ratio cut-off points for categorisation of obesity among Omani Arabs," *Public Health Nutrition*, vol. 11, no. 1, pp. 102–108, 2008.

[8] A. Misra, J. S. Wasir, and N. K. Vikram, "Waist circumference criteria for the diagnosis of abdominal obesity are not applicable uniformly to all populations and ethnic groups," *Nutrition*, vol. 21, no. 9, pp. 969–976, 2005.

[9] A. A. Tavassoli, M. Gharipour, A. Khosravi et al., "Gender differences in obesogenic behaviour, socioeconomic and metabolic factors in a population-based sample of iranians: the IHHP study," *Journal of Health, Population and Nutrition*, vol. 28, no. 6, pp. 602–609, 2010.

[10] F. Razak, S. S. Anand, H. Shannon et al., "Defining obesity cut points in a multiethnic population," *Circulation*, vol. 115, no. 16, pp. 2111–2118, 2007.

[11] N. Sarraf-Zadegan, G. Sadri, H. Malek Afzali et al., "Isfahan healthy heart programme: a comprehensive integrated community-based programme for cardiovascular disease prevention and control. Design, methods and initial experience," *Acta Cardiologica*, vol. 58, no. 4, pp. 309–320, 2003.

[12] N. Sarrafzadegan, A. Baghaei, G. Sadri et al., "Isfahan healthy heart program: evaluation of comprehensive, community-based interventions for non-communicable disease prevention," *Prevention and Control*, vol. 2, no. 2, pp. 73–84, 2006.

[13] N. Sarrafzadegan TM, M. Sadeghi, R. Kelishadi et al., "The isfahan cohort study: rationale, methods and main findings," *Journal of Human Hypertension*, vol. 25, no. 9, pp. 545–553, 2011.

[14] E. Barrett-Connor, E. G. V. Giardina, A. K. Gitt, U. Gudat, H. O. Steinberg, and D. Tschoepe, "Women and heart disease: the role of diabetes and hyperglycemia," *Archives of Internal Medicine*, vol. 164, no. 9, pp. 934–942, 2004.

[15] D. Wood, G. De Backer, O. Faergeman, I. Graham, G. Mancia, and K. Pyörälä, "Prevention of coronary heart disease in clinical practice. Recommendations of the second joint task force of European and other societies on coronary prevention," *European Heart Journal*, vol. 19, no. 10, pp. 1434–1503, 1998.

[16] J. Chalmers MS, G. Mancia, J. Whitworth et al., "World health organization-international society of hypertension guidelines for the management of hypertension. Guidelines sub-committee of the world health organization," *Clin Exp Hypertens*, vol. 21, no. 5-6, pp. 1009–1060, 1999.

[17] American Diabetes Association, "Diagnosis and classification of diabetes mellitu," *Diabetes Care*, vol. 31, supplement 1, pp. 55–60, 2008.

[18] National Cholesterol Education Program (NCEP) Expert Panel on Detection E. Treatment of High Blood Cholesterol in Adults (Adult TreatmentPanel), "Third report of the national cholesterol education program (NCEP)expert panel on detection, evaluation, and treatment of High blood cholesterol inadults (Adult Treatment Panel III) final report," *Circulation*, vol. 25, no. 106, pp. 3143–3421, 2002.

[19] R. Heidari, M. Sadeghi, M. Talaei, K. Rabiei, N. Mohammadifard, and N. Sarrafzadegan, "Metabolic syndrome in menopausal transition: isfahan healthy heart program, a population based study," *Diabetology and Metabolic Syndrome*, vol. 2, no. 1, article 59, 2010.

[20] B. A. Reeder, A. Senthilselvan, J. P. Després et al., "The association of cardiovascular disease risk factors with abdominal obesity in Canada," *CMAJ*, vol. 157, no. 1, pp. S39–S45, 1997.

[21] L. A. Moreno, I. Pìneda, G. Rodríguez, J. Fleta, A. Sarría, and M. Bueno, "Waist circumference for the screening of the metabolic syndrome in children," *Acta Paediatrica, International Journal of Paediatrics*, vol. 91, no. 12, pp. 1307–1312, 2002.

[22] Y. Wang, E. B. Rimm, M. J. Stampfer, W. C. Willett, and F. B. Hu, "Comparison of abdominal adiposity and overall obesity in predicting risk of type 2 diabetes among men," *American Journal of Clinical Nutrition*, vol. 81, no. 3, pp. 555–563, 2005.

[23] Y. Liu, G. Tong, W. Tong, L. Lu, and X. Qin, "Can body mass index, waist circumference, waist-hip ratio and waist-height ratio predict the presence of multiple metabolic risk factors in Chinese subjects?" *BMC Public Health*, vol. 11, article 35, 2011.

[24] G. N. Thomas, S. Y. Ho, K. S. L. Lam, E. D. Janus, A. J. Hedley, and H. L. Tai, "Impact of obesity and body fat distribution on cardiovascular risk factors in Hong Kong Chinese," *Obesity Research*, vol. 12, no. 11, pp. 1805–1813, 2004.

[25] S. Zhu, S. B. Heymsfield, H. Toyoshima, Z. Wang, A. Pietrobelli, and S. Heshka, "Race-ethnicity-specific waist circumference cutoffs for identifying cardiovascular disease risk factors," *American Journal of Clinical Nutrition*, vol. 81, no. 2, pp. 409–415, 2005.

[26] A. Misra, M. Madhavan, N. K. Vikram, R. M. Pandey, V. Dhingra, and K. Luthra, "Simple anthropometric measures identify fasting hyperinsulinemia and clustering of cardiovascular risk factors in Asian Indian adolescents," *Metabolism*, vol. 55, no. 12, pp. 1569–1573, 2006.

[27] WHO Organization WH, "Physical status: the use and interpretation of anthropometry," Report of a WHO Expert Committee, World Health Organization, Geneva, Switzerland, 1995.

[28] M. Barzin, F. Hosseinpanah, H. Saber, P. Sarbakhsh, NakhodaK, and F. Azizi, "Gender differences time trends for metabolic syndrome and its components among tehranian children and adolescents," *Cholesterol*, vol. 2012, Article ID 804643, 6 pages, 2012.

[29] M. Barzin, F. Hosseinpanah, S. Fekri, and F. Azizi, "Predictive value of body mass index and waist circumference for metabolic syndrome in 6-12-year-olds," *Acta Paediatrica, International Journal of Paediatrics*, vol. 100, no. 5, pp. 722–727, 2011.

[30] Y. Jahangiri Noudeh, F. Hadaegh, N. Vatankhah et al., "Wrist circumference as a novel predictor of diabetes and prediabetes: results of cross-sectional and 8. 8-year follow-up studies," *The Journal of Clinical Endocrinology & Metabolism*, vol. 2013, 2013.

[31] P. Mirmiran, N. Noori, and F. Azizi, "A prospective study of determinants of themetabolic syndrome in adults," *Nutrition, Metabolism & Cardiovascular Diseases*, vol. 18, no. 8, pp. 567–573, 2008.

[32] G. M. Haas, T. Bertsch, and P. Schwandt, "Trends of components of the metabolic syndrome in German first graders throughout 10 years: the PEP family heart study," *Cholesterol*, vol. 2012, Article ID 231962, 5 pages, 2012.

2

Trends of Components of the Metabolic Syndrome in German First Graders Throughout 10 Years: The PEP Family Heart Study

Gerda-Maria Haas,[1] Thomas Bertsch,[2] and Peter Schwandt[1,3]

[1] *Arteriosklerose-Präventions-Institut, 81477 München, Germany*
[2] *Institute of Clinical Chemistry, Klinikum Nürnberg, 90419 Nürnberg, Germany*
[3] *Ludwig-Maximilians-Universität München, 80539 München, Germany*

Correspondence should be addressed to Peter Schwandt, api.schwandt.haas@t-online.de

Academic Editor: Roya Kelishadi

Although childhood overweight and obesity are increasing worldwide, some countries report trends for stabilization. However, the trend for the potentially atherogenic components of the metabolic syndrome (MetS) in children and adolescents is not well understood. Therefore, the purpose of this study was to analyze the trend of the five components of over 10 years in 2228 first graders aged 6 years. Waist circumference (WC) remained mainly unchanged between 1994 and 2003 whereas the other four components continuously decreased. In boys and girls mean values of triglycerides (−25.9% and −28.6%, resp.), HDL cholesterol (−19.8% and −23.4%, resp.), fasting glucose (−7.3% and −9%, resp.), systolic (−3.8% and −4.1%, resp.), and diastolic (−10.2% and −9.7%, resp.) blood pressure significantly decreased. Whereas the prevalence of abdominal adiposity was stable at baseline and after 10 years (−1% in boys and +2% in girls), the prevalence of hypertension, hypertriglyceridemia, low HDL-C, and glucose was very low without any trend.

1. Introduction

Overweight, obesity, and the metabolic syndrome (MetS) are an emerging health problem in industrialized and developing countries [1, 2]. Ethnic disparities are reported regarding the prevalence of MetS, which was four times higher in Iranian than in German adolescents as well as regarding single components in terms of considerably higher prevalence of dyslipidemia in Brazilian and Iranian compared with German youths [3, 4].

Secular trends of childhood overweight and obesity in terms of increased body mass index (BMI) are heterogeneous in different countries with a large variation across countries [5–7]. However, BMI is not a component of the metabolic syndrome (MetS) according to the International Diabetes Federation (IDF) defining central obesity for children and adolescents as waist circumference (WC) at or above the 90th percentile [8]. Increasing prevalence of central adiposity indicates increasing cardiovascular risk [9, 10]. Furthermore, early elementary school years are a critical period for increases in obesity prevalence sharply increasing from 10.4% to 19.6% below and above age six years [11]. Therefore, the purpose of this study was to assess the trend of the five single components over 10 years in a large sample of six-year-old first graders.

2. Material and Methods

We investigated 2228 German first graders (1116 boys and 1112 girls, median age 6.0 years) who participated in yearly cross-sectional surveys between 1994 and 2003. Continuously trained research assistants measured waist circumference (WC), systolic and diastolic blood pressure (BP), fasting triglycerides (TG), high-density cholesterol (HDL-C), and fasting plasma glucose (FPG) as previously described [12]. We used the IDF cut-offs for the five MetS components in terms of WC $\geq$ 90th percentile, SBP $\geq$ 130 or DBP $\geq$ 85 mm Hg, TG $\geq$ 1.7 mmol/L, HDL-C $\leq$ 1.03 mmol/L and glucose $\geq$ 5.6 mmol/L [8].

TABLE 1: Characteristics and components of the metabolic syndrome in 2228 first graders between 1994 and 2003.

	1994	1995	1996	1997	1998	1999	2000	2001	2002	2003
1,116 boys; mean (SD)										
Mean age (SD)	6.4 (0.5)	6.4 (0.5)	6.4 (0.5)	6.6 (0.5)	6.5 (0.5)	6.4 (0.5)	6.4 (0.5)	6.4 (0.5)	6.4 (0.5)	6.3 (0.5)
Median	6.0	6.0	6.0	7.0	6.0	6.0	6.0	6.0	6.0	6.0
BMI (kg/m^2)	15.8 (2.4)	15.6 (1.7)	16.0 (1.8)	16.2 (2.4)	16.4 (2.3)	15.8 (1.7)	15.6 (1.7)	16.1 (1.8)	16.0 (2.1)	15.9 (2.4)
WC (cm)	56.9 (5.6)	56.0 (4.8)	58.0* (4.7)	58.6 (6.8)	58.7* (5.7)	57.4 (4.2)	56.8 (4.0)	56.3 (4.7)	56.6 (4.8)	56.3 (6.1)
SBP mmHg (SD)	105.1 (10.0)	104.2 (8.7)	104.7 (8.9)	106.2 (9.2)	104.5 (10.3)	104.0 (6.8)	103.9 (8.6)	101.8* (7.8)	102.6* (6.7)	101.1* (7.7)
DBP mmHg (SD)	70.7 (8.4)	67.1* (7.1)	70.9 (9.0)	71.1 (6.8)	71.8 (7.8)	66.2* (7.1)	67.4* (7.5)	62.1* (7.1)	63.8* (7.0)	63.5* (5.7)
Triglycerides (mmol/L) (SD)	0.85 (0.42)	0.65* (0.28)	0.64* (0.22)	0.67 (0.21)	0.63* (0.16)	0.76* (0.33)	0.67* (0.25)	0.61* (0.26)	0.62* (0.23)	0.63* (0.23)
HDL-cholesterol (mmol/L) (SD)	1.73 (0.35)	1.55* (0.40)	1.51* (0.28)	1.60 (0.34)	1.57* (0.26)	1.39* (0.31)	1.37* (0.24)	1.47* (0.28)	1.47* (0.36)	1.54* (0.26)
1,112 girls; mean (SD)										
Mean age (SD)	6.4 (0.5)	6.4 (0.5)	6.3 (0.5)	6.6 (0.5)	6.4 (0.5)	6.4 (0.5)	6.4 (0.5)	6.3 (0.4)	6.3 (0.5)	6.3 (0.5)
Median	6.0	6.0	6.0	7.0	6.0	6.0	6.0	6.0	6.0	6.0
BMI (kg/m^2)	15.6 (2.4)	15.7 (2.2)	15.7 (1.7)	16.2* (2.4)	15.8 (1.3)	15.9 (2.2)	16.2* (2.0)	15.8 (1.8)	16.3* (2.6)	15.9 (1.9)
WC (cm)	55.0 (5.4)	55.4 (5.5)	56.4* (4.4)	58.8* (5.9)	56.4 (3.9)	57.3* (6.1)	57.1* (5.8)	55.5 (4.7)	56.9* (5.5)	56.1 (4.8)
SBP mmHg (SD)	105.2 (10.0)	104.1 (9.0)	103.5 (9.2)	104.3 (9.4)	105.0 (9.6)	104.0 (10.2)	104.2 (8.2)	101.5* (7.6)	102.9 (6.9)	100.9* (7.6)
DBP mmHg (SD)	71.0 (8.5)	67.1* (6.9)	70.0 (8.4)	71.8 (9.7)	71.9 (7.6)	66.0* (8.6)	67.5* (7.5)	63.7* (7.0)	64.5* (6.7)	64.1* (7.0)
Triglycerides (mmol/L) (SD)	0.91 (0.41)	0.71* (0.26)	0.73* (0.30)	0.68* (0.07)	0.88 (0.42)	0.74* (0.21)	0.82 (0.22)	0.73* (0.30)	0.73* (0.29)	0.65* (0.21)
HDL-cholesterol (mg/dL)	1.71 (0.35)	1.38* (0.36)	1.49* (0.34)	1.50 (0.47)	1.38* (0.47)	1.41* (0.27)	1.41* (0.30)	1.28* (0.36)	1.40* (0.29)	1.31* (0.21)

$P < 0.05$ compared with baseline values.

TABLE 2: Prevalence (%) of the five components of MetS according to the IDF definition in 2228 German first graders between 1994 and 2003.

Year of enrollment of first graders	WC ≥ 90th percentile	TG ≥ 1.7 mmol/L	HDL-C ≤ 1.03 mmol/L	SBP ≥ 130 mmHg DBP ≥ 85 mmHg
		boys		
1994	9.6	4.2	1.8	0
1995	5.3	2.9	7.8	0
1996	12.1	0	5.6	0
1997	10.7	0	0	3.6
1998	19.1	0	0	2.1
1999	7.6	3.3	10.0	0
2000	6.7	0	8.3	0
2001	6.5	0	0	0
2002	6.8	0	10.8	0
2003	9.1	0	5.9	0
		girls		
1994	6.7	4.8	0.7	0
1995	5.5	0	14.0	0
1996	8.3	0	5.2	1
1997	18.8	0	20.0	6.3
1998	6.5	8.3	8.3	0
1999	12.7	0	4.8	0
2000	10.8	0	9.4	0
2001	9.5	0	26.3	1.6
2002	11.3	0	7.7	0
2003	11.4	0	18.9	0

WC indicates waist circumference, TG: triglycerides, HDL-C: high-density lipoprotein cholesterol, SBP: systolic blood pressure, DBP: diastolic blood pressure.

For statistical analyses, we used SPSS 18.0 and the Kruskal-Wallis rank test for multisample ordinal comparisons, the Wilcoxon rank-sum test for pairwise comparisons and for linear trends across time ANOVA. $P < 0.05$ was considered significant.

3. Results and Discussion

As presented in Table 1 mean values of waist circumference (−1% in boys and +2% in girls) and of body mass index (+0.6 in boys +1.9% in girls) remained stable between 1994 and 2003. This is consistent with the stabilization of BMI between 1999 and 2010 among children and adolescents in USA, UK, and Sweden [13–15]. In Stockholm, the prevalence of obesity differed in 10-year-old boys by +0.6% and in girls by −1.6% between 1999 and 2003 which is comparable with the urban area of Nuremberg [15]. "Mean WC greatly increased among US children between 1988–1994 and 1999–2004" [13]. However, among 2–5-year-old children the increase was +2.3% in boys and +1.6% in girls and among 6–11-year-old children WC increased by +4.2% in boys and +4.9% in girls. We found a slight decrease by −1% in boys respectively, a slight increase by +2% in girls from 1994 to 2003 among 6-year-old first graders. These small differences between the monocentric PEP Family Heart Study using the same staff, location, and equipment and the NHANES design, which includes different ethnicities, are remarkable though different measuring points for WC were used (midway between lowest rib and iliac crest versus high point of the iliac crest). Furthermore, periods of assessment are different as well as age (6-year olds and ages 6–11 years). Among Australian children the mean WC z-score in 2–16-year-old children increased more in girls than in boys at a faster rate than BMI between 1985 and 2007 [9]. In Spanish adolescents and in British adolescents and children aged 2–5 years WC increased significantly in both genders from 1995 to 2000–2002, respectively, from 1977 to 1997 [16–18]. A recent review compares mean values of WC in 6-year-old children from 11 countries [19].

However, the mean values of the other four components of MetS significantly decreased (Table 1). The strongest decrease was observed for mean TG (−25.9% in boys, −28.6% in girls) and HDL-C (−19.8% in boys, −23.4% in girls). DBP (−10.2% in boys, −9.7% in girls) and SBP (−3.8% in boys, −4.1% in girls) decreased less, and fasting glucose (−7.3% in boys, −9% in girls) was available only for the last 4 years. Because all measurements were performed at entry in the PEP Family Heart Study before any lifestyle advice was implemented, we suggest that the decrease of the nonanthropometric risk variables might be due to secular changes.

We registered no clear trend of the prevalence of four MetS components between 1994 and 2003 among 6-year-old children except for glucose for the last four years of the study, however unavailable values from the years before (Table 2). The prevalence of abdominal obesity decreased in boys (−0.5% from 9.6% at baseline) but increased in girls (+4.7% from 6.7% at baseline). In children with abdominal obesity the interrelationship with hypertension ($\chi^2 = 29.3$, $P < 0.001$) and hypertriglyceridemia ($\chi^2 = 4.6$, $P = 0.013$) was significant, and the interrelationship between hypertriglyceridemia and low HDL-C was ($\chi^2 = 39.8$, $P < 0.001$). In 1994 the prevalence of raised triglycerides (4.2% in boys and 4.8% in girls) and of low HDL-C (1.8% in boys and 0.7% in girls) was far less than 21.5%, respectively, 18.7% in 5–17.9-year-old obese children in European Union in 2006 [14]. The highest prevalence of hypertension in 6-year-old was 3.6% in boys and 6.3% in girls in 1997 and was considerably lower than in European Union in 2006. A very large European multicenter study in 26 008 overweight children reported that 50% had at least one cardiovascular risk factor related to the degree of overweight in terms of high BMI [20]. Since only 5.9% of the 12.6-year-old children were normal weight, the risk factor profiles cannot be compared with mainly normal-weight first graders of the current study, which however focused on WC as the major MetS component. Furthermore, studies from Germany reporting secular trends of BMI did not present nonanthropometric risk variables [21–24].

This is the first study documenting stable mean values of waist circumference and decreasing trends for the mean other four components of the metabolic syndrome over 10 years in first graders at the critical age of six years. However, it is unclear whether stable WC reflects a plateau between 1994 and 2003 and whether continuous decrease of MetS components mean values indicates leveling off in cardiovascular risk. Further strength of this monocentric study is constancy of staff, location, procedures, methods, and equipment and that all first graders lived in the same PEP families over ten years. A limitation of this study is the low prevalence of MetS components in this large cohort, which only allows a trend analysis of mean values regarding the four nonanthropometric variables. A further limitation is the relatively small sample size of 2228 first graders to detect a 10% difference between changes of prevalence [13]. Furthermore, the percentage of children with central obesity (≥90th percentile) was too small for categorizing the participants in prevalence groups of high WC (≥85th, ≥95th, ≥97th, and ≥99th percentiles) as has been done for Californian adolescents. This very large study (8.3 million multiethnic adolescents) was powered to demonstrate declining prevalence of high BMI for some groups but not for Indian and black girls [25].

4. Conclusions

This is the first study presenting ten years' trends of the mean values of the five components of the metabolic syndrome according to the definition of the International Diabetes Federation in first graders. Mean values of waist circumference as well as the prevalence of abdominal adiposity remained stable in 6-year-old children between 1994 and 2003. But the prevalence of hypertension, hypertriglyceridemia, low HDL-C, and hyperglycemia were low and inconsistent though mean values of blood pressure, triglycerides, HDL-cholesterol, and glucose decreased continuously in both genders.

Longitudinal studies are needed to confirm these disparate trends.

Conflict of Interests

None of the authors has a conflict of interest.

Acknowledgments

The authors thank the families participating in this project for their outstanding cooperation and dedication. For their excellent work and engagement, they thank the study staff and the many physicians and nurses for blood collection. All authors read and approved the final paper. This paper is funded by Foundation for the Prevention of Atherosclerosis, Nuremberg, Germany; Ludwig Maximilian University, Munich, Germany; Bavarian Ministry of Health, Munich; City of Nuremberg.

References

[1] C. L. Ogden, S. Z. Yanovski, M. D. Carroll, and K. M. Flegal, "The epidemiology of obesity," *Gastroenterology*, vol. 132, no. 6, pp. 2087–2102, 2007.

[2] R. Kelishadi, "Childhood overweight, obesity, and the metabolic syndrome in developing countries," *Epidemiologic Reviews*, vol. 29, no. 1, pp. 62–76, 2007.

[3] P. Schwandt, R. Kelishadi, and G. M. Haas, "Ethnic disparities of the metabolic syndrome in population-based samples of German and Iranian adolescents," *Metabolic Syndrome and Related Disorders*, vol. 8, no. 2, pp. 189–192, 2010.

[4] P. Schwandt, R. Kelishadi, R. Q. C. Ribeiro, G. M. Haas, and P. Poursafa, "A three-country study on the components of the metabolic syndrome in youths: the BIG Study," *International Journal of Pediatric Obesity*, vol. 5, no. 4, pp. 334–341, 2010.

[5] Y. Wang and T. Lobstein, "Worldwide trends in childhood overweight and obesity," *International Journal of Pediatric Obesity*, vol. 1, no. 1, pp. 11–25, 2006.

[6] B. Rokholm, J. L. Baker, and T. I. A. Sørensen, "The levelling off of the obesity epidemic since the year 1999—a review of evidence and perspectives," *Obesity Reviews*, vol. 11, no. 12, pp. 835–846, 2010.

[7] J. C. Han, D. A. Lawlor, and S. Y. Kimm, "Childhood obesity," *The Lancet*, vol. 375, no. 9727, pp. 1737–1748, 2010.

[8] P. Zimmet, G. Alberti, F. Kaufman et al., "The metabolic syndrome in children and adolescents," *The Lancet*, vol. 369, no. 9579, pp. 2059–2061, 2007.

[9] S. P. Garnett, L. A. Baur, and C. T. Cowell, "The prevalence of increased central adiposity in Australian school children 1985 to 2007," *Obesity Reviews*, vol. 12, pp. 887–896, 2011.

[10] H. S. Kahn, G. Imperatore, and Y. J. Cheng, "A population-based comparison of BMI percentiles and waist-to-height ratio for identifying cardiovascular risk in youth," *Journal of Pediatrics*, vol. 146, no. 4, pp. 482–488, 2005.

[11] A. Datar, V. Shier, and R. Sturm, "Changes in body mass during elementary and middle school in a national cohort of Kindergarteners," *Pediatrics*, vol. 128, pp. e1411–e1417, 2011.

[12] P. Schwandt, H. C. Geiß, M. M. Ritter et al., "The Prevention Education Program (PEP). A prospective study of the efficacy

of family-oriented life style modification in the reduction of cardiovascular risk and disease: design and baseline data," *Journal of Clinical Epidemiology*, vol. 52, no. 8, pp. 791–800, 1999.
[13] C. L. Ogden, M. D. Carroll, B. K. Kit, and K. M. Flegal, "Prevalence of obesity and trends in body mass index among US children and adolescents 1999–2010," *Japan Automobile Manufacturers Association*, vol. 307, pp. 483–490, 2012.
[14] R. R. Kipping, R. Jago, and D. A. Lawlor, "Obesity in children. Part 1: epidemiology, measurement, risk factors, and screening," *British Medical Journal*, vol. 337, no. 7675, pp. 922–927, 2008.
[15] E. Sundblom, M. Petzold, F. Rasmussen, E. Callmer, and L. Lissner, "Childhood overweight and obesity prevalences levelling off in Stockholm but socioeconomic differences persist," *International Journal of Obesity*, vol. 32, no. 10, pp. 1525–1530, 2008.
[16] L. A. Moreno, A. Sarría, J. Fleta, A. Marcos, and M. Bueno, "Secular trends in waist circumference in Spanish adolescents, 1995 to 2000–02," *Archives of Disease in Childhood*, vol. 90, no. 8, pp. 818–819, 2005.
[17] H. D. McCarthy, S. M. Ellis, and T. J. Cole, "Central overweight and obesity in British youth aged 11–16 years: cross sectional surveys of waist circumference," *British Medical Journal*, vol. 326, no. 7390, pp. 624–626, 2003.
[18] H. D. McCarthy, K. V. Jarrett, P. M. Emmett, and I. Rogers, "Trends in waist circumferences in young British children: a comparative study," *International Journal of Obesity*, vol. 29, no. 2, pp. 157–162, 2005.
[19] P. Schwandt and G. M. Haas, "Waist circumference in children and adolescents from different ethnicities," in *Childhood Obesity*, Sevil Ari Yuca, Ed., chapter 4, 2012, http://www.in-techopen.com/.
[20] D. I'Allemand, S. Wiegand, T. Reinehr et al., "Cardiovascular risk in 26,008 European overweight children as established by a multicenter database," *Obesity*, vol. 16, no. 7, pp. 1672–1679, 2008.
[21] C. Meigen, A. Keller, R. Gausche et al., "Secular trends in body mass index in German children and adolescents: a cross-sectional data analysis via CrescNet between 1999 and 2006," *Metabolism*, vol. 57, no. 7, pp. 934–939, 2008.
[22] H. Kalies, J. Lenz, and R. von Kries, "Prevalence of overweight and obesity and trends in body mass index in German preschool children, 1982–1997," *International Journal of Obesity*, vol. 26, no. 9, pp. 1211–1217, 2002.
[23] K. Kromeyer-Hauschild and K. Zellner, "Trends in overweight and obesity and changes in the distribution of body mass index in schoolchildren of Jena, East Germany," *European Journal of Clinical Nutrition*, vol. 61, no. 3, pp. 404–411, 2007.
[24] A. Moss, J. Klenk, K. Simon, H. Thaiss, T. Reinehr, and M. Wabitsch, "Declining prevalence rates for overweight and obesity in German children starting school," *European Journal of Pediatrics*, vol. 171, pp. 289–299, 2011.
[25] K. A. Madsen, A. E. Weedn, and P. B. Crawford, "Disparities in peaks, plateaus, and declines in prevalence of high BMI among adolescents," *Pediatrics*, vol. 126, no. 3, pp. 434–442, 2010.

3

Cholesterol: Its Regulation and Role in Central Nervous System Disorders

Matthias Orth[1] and Stefano Bellosta[2]

[1] *Institut für Laboratoriumsmedizin, Vinzenz von Paul Kliniken gGmbH, Adlerstraße 7, Postfach 103163, 70199 Stuttgart, Germany*
[2] *Dipartimento di Scienze Farmacologiche e Biomolecolari, Facoltà di Farmacia, Università di Milano, Via Balzaretti 9, 20133 Milano, Italy*

Correspondence should be addressed to Matthias Orth, orth@vinzenz.de

Academic Editor: Gloria L. Vega

Cholesterol is a major constituent of the human brain, and the brain is the most cholesterol-rich organ. Numerous lipoprotein receptors and apolipoproteins are expressed in the brain. Cholesterol is tightly regulated between the major brain cells and is essential for normal brain development. The metabolism of brain cholesterol differs markedly from that of other tissues. Brain cholesterol is primarily derived by *de novo* synthesis and the blood brain barrier prevents the uptake of lipoprotein cholesterol from the circulation. Defects in cholesterol metabolism lead to structural and functional central nervous system diseases such as Smith-Lemli-Opitz syndrome, Niemann-Pick type C disease, and Alzheimer's disease. These diseases affect different metabolic pathways (cholesterol biosynthesis, lipid transport and lipoprotein assembly, apolipoproteins, lipoprotein receptors, and signaling molecules). We review the metabolic pathways of cholesterol in the CNS and its cell-specific and microdomain-specific interaction with other pathways such as the amyloid precursor protein and discuss potential treatment strategies as well as the effects of the widespread use of LDL cholesterol-lowering drugs on brain functions.

1. Introduction

Cholesterol is an important structural component of cellular membranes and myelin and a precursor of oxysterols, steroid hormones, and bile acids. Cholesterol is a major constituent of the human brain (with about 35 grams of cholesterol in an adult brain [1]), and the brain is the most cholesterol-rich organ [2], containing about 20% of the body's total cholesterol. Brain lipids consist of glycerophospholipids, sphingolipids, and cholesterol in roughly equimolar proportions [3]. Cholesterol is tightly regulated between the major brain cells—neurons and glia, that is, astrocytes, microglia, and oligodendrocytes—and is essential for normal brain development. Cholesterol is required for synapse and dendrite formation [4, 5], and for axonal guidance [6]. Cholesterol depletion leads to synaptic and dendritic spine degeneration, failed neurotransmission, and decreased synaptic plasticity [7]. Cholesterol is a pivotal constituent of cell membranes, steroid hormones, and for the function of the hedgehog protein [8]. Defects in cholesterol metabolism lead to structural and functional central nervous system (CNS) diseases such as Smith-Lemli-Opitz syndrome [9], Niemann-Pick type C (NPC) disease [10], Huntington's disease [11], and Alzheimer's disease [12]. These metabolic defects affect different metabolic pathways such as (1) cholesterol biosynthesis, (2) lipid transport and lipoprotein assembly, (3) receptors that mediate the cellular uptake of lipids, and (4) signaling molecules [13].

Unlike cholesterol in other organs in the periphery, brain cholesterol is primarily derived by *de novo* synthesis. The intact blood brain barrier (BBB) prevents the uptake of lipoproteins from the circulation in vertebrates [14]. In cells outside the brain, the need for cholesterol is covered by uptake of lipoprotein cholesterol by cells as well as by *de novo* synthesis [15]. The importance of this isolated cholesterol pool in the CNS has been described as early as 1834 when Couerbe called cholesterol "un element principal" (a key element) of the CNS [16]. Cholesterol is synthesized via the isoprenoid biosynthetic pathway (for further details see [17]). Isoprenoid biosynthesis starts with acetyl-CoA as a substrate, which by means of 6 subsequent enzyme reactions is converted into isopentenyl-pyrophosphate, the basic C_5 isoprene unit used for synthesis of all subsequent isoprenoids. In total, at least 20 enzymes are involved for the generation of cholesterol [17]. The 3-hydroxy-3-methylglutaryl-coenzyme A reductase (*Hmgcr*; EC 2.3.3.10) is the rate limiting enzyme in cholesterol biosynthesis and the target of statin pharmacotherapy [18]. Besides cholesterol, the cholesterologenic pathway forms other important intermediates such as mevalonate, farnesyl pyrophosphate, squalene, and lanosterol [19]. The first enzymes of the isoprenoid/cholesterol biosynthetic pathway, that is, the conversion of acetyl-CoA to farnesyl pyrophosphate, are localized in the cytosol except for *Hmgcr* which, together with most enzymes involved in cholesterol synthesis, is localized in the endoplasmatic reticulum [20, 21].

In contrast to the distribution in plasma lipoproteins, essentially all (>99.5%) cholesterol in the CNS is present in an unesterified, free form [2]. There are two major pools of CNS cholesterol: one pool (containing up to 70% of the CNS cholesterol) consists of the myelin sheaths of oligodendroglia; the other pool is made up by plasma membranes of astrocytes and neurons. The lipid-protein composition of myelin differs from that of other cell membranes; myelin dry weight consists of about 70% lipids and 30% proteins, in other cell membranes the distribution is about 30% lipids and about 70% proteins [2]. Major lipid constituents of myelin are cholesterol, phospholipids, and glycosphingolipids in molar ratios of about 4 : 4 : 2. The lipid composition, in particular the cholesterol composition of myelin, is believed to have a pivotal role in membrane morphology and function such as the transmission of nerve impulses. In neurons (which are composed of cell body and axon), electrical impulses are transmitted rapidly along the axon. The axon is wrapped by myelin made up from the membranes of several oligodendrocytes, separated by periodic gaps in the myelin sheath—called nodes of Ranvier. This discontinuous insulation allows the saltatory conduction of the action potential. Due to its reduced permeability to ions, the cholesterol enrichment of the myelin sheath propagates the transmission of current along the axon rather than across the membranes of oligodendrocytes [22].

2. Brain Cholesterol

Brain cholesterol is considered to be a distinct pool from body cholesterol. Unlike cholesterol in other organs, there is only minute exchange of cholesterol towards other organs (2). The majority of brain cholesterol accumulates between the perinatal period and adolescence when neurons are encircled by specialized plasma membranes termed myelin. After myelination, the metabolism of cholesterol in the adult brain is characterized by a very low turnover and minimal losses [23]. However, recent results indicate that both cholesterol synthesis and degradation are active in the adult brain as well and that alteration in these mechanisms profoundly influences higher-order brain functions [24].

Several levels of evidence indicate a distinct metabolism of CNS cholesterol. The brain does not respond to many control mechanisms operative in maintaining cholesterol homeostasis in the whole organism. The half-life of brain cholesterol in the adult organism is between 6 months and 5 years [25, 26], the half-life of plasma cholesterol, in contrast, is only a few days [27]. In the 1940s, administration of deuterated water into rats led to an incorporation of the label into the unsaponifiable lipids of the brain [28]. Similar findings were observed in unrelated studies employing deuterated cholesterol in dogs [29]. From the current level of knowledge, in the CNS of mammals such as mice, rats, and humans, >95% of cholesterol is synthesized *de novo* from acetate and exchange between plasma lipoprotein cholesterol and brain cholesterol has only very little impact [1, 30–33]. However, some studies could demonstrate the transfer of small amounts of cholesterol from the periphery through the BBB to the CNS. In humans, after administration of 4-^{14}C-labelled cholesterol, on average 3.2% of the serum label was detected in the CNS cholesterol [34]. A drawback of this study is the fact that all patients were terminally ill (most of them with malignancies) and a defective BBB could not be excluded. No label was detected within the first days after injection and the authors described the cholesterol exchange as negligible. The accumulation of minute amounts of cholesterol was also observed in adult guinea pigs after administration of hexadeuterium-labelled cholesterol with an accumulation of 1.23% and 0.93% in the cerebrum and cerebellum, respectively [35], and in mice and rats after feeding a diet containing hexadeuterium-labelled cholesterol with an accumulation of less than 1% [36].

Recent data indicate that besides being an important constituent of the brain cell membranes, cholesterol as well as the receptors for cholesterol-containing molecules are pivotal signaling molecules for brain morphology during embryonic development. During embryonic development and in the early postnatal period, the central nervous system undergoes an enormous cellular expansion. A sufficient availability of cholesterol as well as a correct ratio of cholesterol and phospholipids is crucial for the physicochemical properties of cells within the CNS. It is conceivable that during evolution a checkpoint was established that determines which sufficient cholesterol is available to proceed with the expansion of the brain or whether cell division and growth are slowed down [37]. The highest rate of cholesterol synthesis in humans and rodents occurs during the first postnatal weeks [30, 38, 39]. This time window corresponds with the peak of the myelination process and the myelination process is delayed when cholesterol biosynthesis is deficient [40].

3. Sterol Flux between CNS Cells

A sufficient availability of cholesterol is necessary for normal neuronal function and morphology, and both a lack and surplus of cholesterol impair these features [41, 42]. Cholesterol in neurons can be synthesized by neurons themselves [43, 44] and can also be taken up from other cells within the CNS, namely, from oligodendrocytes [45]. Oligodendrocytes have a central role in cholesterol synthesis in the CNS.

On the contrary, the role of neurons and glial cells in cholesterol biosynthesis is still poorly understood [46]. Data indicate that neurons (in particular regions of the brain and/or under certain conditions) synthesize and take up cholesterol from circumjacent oligodendrocytes. Enzymes such as *Hmgcr* and 7-dehydrocholesterol reductase (*Dhcr7; EC 1.3.1.21*) are expressed with high transcript levels in cortical, cholinergic, and hippocampal neurons [47]. The expression of cholesterol-synthesizing enzymes as well as sterol-sensing factors, intracellular transporters, cholesterol shuttle proteins, and lipoprotein receptors is different within regions of the brain [13, 48]. Consequently, different regions of the brain differ markedly in their cholesterol content [49].

During maturation of neurons, the endogenous synthesis of cholesterol is impaired and the neurons depend on cholesterol provided by astrocytes [50]. Brain-derived neurotrophic factor (BDNF) is an important stimulus for *de novo* synthesis of cholesterol in neurons [51]. The significant transfer and uptake of oligodendrocytes-derived cholesterol by neurons could be demonstrated by conditional ablation of cholesterol synthesis in mice neurons. The conditional gene inactivation of the squalene synthase gene (*fdft1*) in neurons revealed a normal phenotype and function [45]. This supports the hypothesis that significant amounts of cholesterol are transferred between different cell types in the CNS.

The transfer of cholesterol between different cells is influenced by the fluidity of cell membranes and the distribution of microdomains such as lipid rafts (also known as detergent-resistant membrane fraction (DRM)). One example for a disease with altered composition of cell membranes is the deficiency of *Dhcr7*. Total or partial deficiency of *Dhcr7* causes Smith-Lemli-Opitz syndrome with the clinical triad developmental deformities, incomplete myelination, and mental retardation [52]. Tissue cholesterol and total sterol levels are markedly reduced, and 7-dehydrocholesterol levels are highly elevated [53]. High concentration of 7-dehydrocholesterol inhibits *Hmgcr* which exacerbates the cellular cholesterol deficit [54]. The altered membrane composition, in particular the increased 7-dehydrocholesterol levels, increases membrane fluidity [55] and decreases the intermolecular packing of phospholipid fatty acyl chains [56, 57]. The altered membrane composition leads to functional changes. The depletion of cholesterol, followed by replacement by 7-dehydrocholesterol in hippocampal membranes, does not restore the ligand-binding of the serotonin 1A receptor [58].

Abnormalities in cholesterol homeostasis have been also observed in Huntington's disease [59] and stress the necessity of cholesterol transfer within cells of the CNS (i.e., between the major site of cholesterol biosynthesis—oligodendroglia cells—and neurons). Transcription of genes in the cholesterol and fatty acid biosynthetic pathways are downregulated in human postmortem Huntington's disease striatal and cortical tissues as well as in murine models of Huntington's disease [60]. The hallmark of Huntington's disease, the accumulation of mutant huntingtin protein within neurons, is affected by the inefficient palmitoylation of huntingtin. This palmitoylation is crucial for the normal function since this process enhances the hydrophobicity of this protein and determines the membrane association and the subcellular trafficking between membrane domains [11, 61]. The accumulation of cytoplasmic and nuclear inclusions leads to neuronal dysfunction and later to neuropathological changes such as cell loss and atrophy in the putamen and neostriatum.

4. Net Sterol Flux of CNS Cholesterol

Most of the CNS cholesterol is recycled. However, mechanisms to export cholesterol into the circulation are mandatory to maintain homeostasis. Two different pathways for exporting cholesterol have been identified so far. Similar to other cells such as macrophages, cells of the CNS, in particular astrocytes, shed cholesterol associated with apolipoprotein (apo) E into the cerebrospinal fluid (CSF). Despite lipoproteins in the brain are secreted predominantly by glia cells, neurons are also capable of synthesizing lipoproteins under certain conditions [62, 63]. However, the capacity of the shedding pathway is very limited and can export only 1-2 mg cholesterol per day [14]. The second, quantitatively more important mechanism is the export of cholesterol as 24(S)-hydroxycholesterol. Unlike nonoxydized cholesterol, oxysterols such as 24(S)-hydroxycholesterol can cross lipophilic membranes such as the BBB at a much faster rate than cholesterol itself [64, 65]. The introduction of a hydroxyl group into the side chain of cholesterol leads to a local reordering of membrane phospholipids that is energetically more favorable and allows a transfer of oxidized cholesterol through the membrane several orders of magnitude greater than that of nonoxidized cholesterol [66] (Figure 1).

The flux of 24(S)-hydroxycholesterol through the BBB is limited to about 6-7 mg per day [64, 67].

In the circulation and in most tissues, cholesterol is always present in a great excess compared to oxysterols with the ratio of cholesterol to any oxysterol being 1.000 : 1 to 100.000 : 1 [68]. In the brain, however, the ratio is much lower and varies between 500 : 1 and 1000 : 1 [67]. Oxysterols can shuttle between the membrane leaflets and can be extracted by acceptors such as lipoproteins. Plasma oxysterols are associated with membranes and in plasma are bound to lipoproteins [69], similar to other lipids present in trace amounts such as gangliosides [70, 71]. Similar to the ganglioside/cholesterol ratio [70], the ratio of 24(S)-hydroxycholesterol to cholesterol in plasma is rather constant and patients with hypercholesterolemia show higher plasma concentration of 24(S)-hydroxycholesterol [68].

While in the brain the oxidation of the steroid side chain at position 24 is the primary mechanism for the elimination of cholesterol, outside the brain the oxidation occurs at position 27. The enzyme responsible for this reaction is sterol 27-hydroxylase (27-OHC, CYP27A1) and macrophages have particularly high activities of CYP27A1 [68]. 27-hydroxycholesterol is able to pass the BBB [65] and the daily influx of 27-hydroxycholesterol into the brain has been estimated to be 5 mg. This flux is dependent on the concentration in the

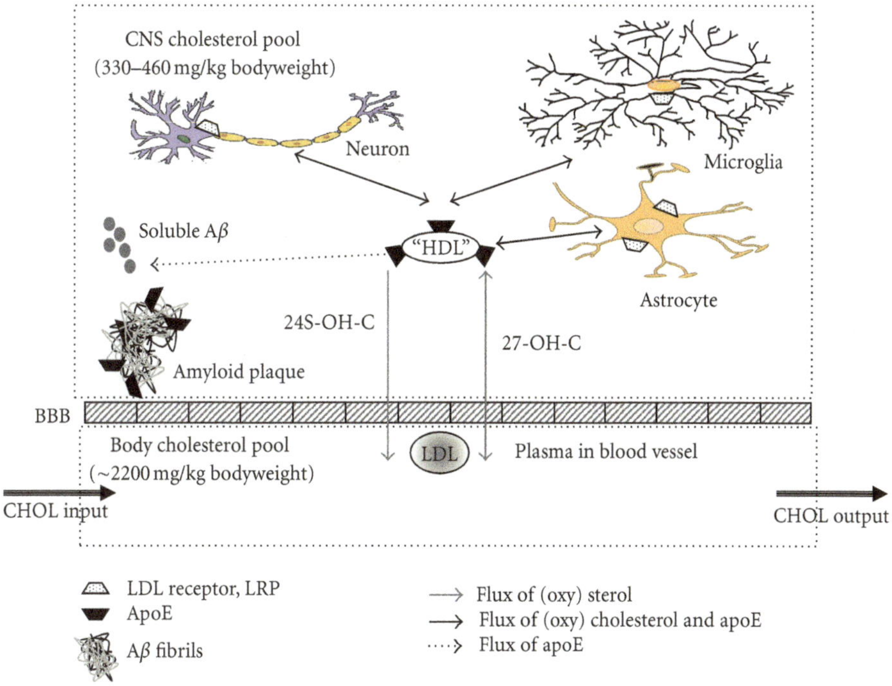

Figure 1: Major cholesterol and apoE pathways in the CNS. Cholesterol is synthesized de novo in brain cells (neurons, astrocytes, microglial cells). Efflux of CNS cholesterol through the BBB occurs as 24(S)-hydroxycholesterol (24S-OH-C) and 27-hydroxycholesterol (27-OH-C). 24S-OH-C is produced exclusively in the CNS, 27-OH-C is produced in most organs. Unlike cholesterol, 24-S-OH-C and 27-OH-C can cross the BBB because of the hydroxylated side chains. Primarily astrocytes and microglia secrete HDL-like lipoproteins composed of cholesterol and phospholipids and apoE as the major apoprotein. ApoE is the ligand of these lipoproteins to the receptors of the LDL receptor family such as the LDL-receptor and LRP. Exchange of cholesterol and apos between CNS cells occurs via these lipoproteins. In plasma, 24S-OH-C and 27-OH-C are transported on lipoproteins such as LDL and HDL. *De novo* cholesterol synthesis in CNS cells can be regulated by the apoE-mediated uptake of lipoproteins via the LDL receptor family. ApoE is produced within the CNS and interacts with Aβ. The availability of cholesterol and of apoE are thought to affect amyloidogenesis and apoE (in particular the isoform apoE4) promoting the formation of amyloid fibrils from soluble Aβ in the CNS. The data for the steady state cholesterol pool have been determined from studies in healthy adults. The flux of cholesterol across the whole body is ~700 mg/day (CHOL INPUT/OUTPUT). The flux across the CNS is only 0.9% of whole body (~12 mg/day). The efflux of 24(S)-hydroxycholesterol through the BBB is limited to ~6-7 mg per day [64, 67], the daily influx of 27-hydroxycholesterol into the brain has been estimated to be ~5 mg [1]. Please note that the brain per kg organ contains 10 times more cholesterol than the rest of the body.

circulation and on the integrity of the BBB [72]. The rate limiting step in bile acid synthesis is 7α-hydroxylation [73]. In the liver, 7α-hydroxylation of cholesterols is mediated by CYP7A and CYP39A1 while in brain and other tissues, both sterols and some steroids including dehydroepiandrosterone are prominently 7α-hydroxylated by CYP7B [73]. In human plasma, 7-hydroxycholesterol is the quantitatively most prevailing oxysterol [69].

In the total organism, the pool of cholesterol is about 2200 mg/kg body weight and similar in most species. However, the cholesterol pool in the CNS varies from about 330 mg/kg body weight in the mouse up to 460 mg/kg body weight in primates [27]. In humans, the flux of cholesterol across the whole body is about 10 mg/day per kg body weight while the flux across the CNS is 0.09 mg/day per kg body weight only [64] (Figure 1). In smaller animals such as the mouse and the baboon, the rates are several folds higher. It is remarkable that in all species studied so far, the percentage of the rate of cholesterol flux across the CNS is about 0.09% of the flux across the rest of the body [74, 75].

In humans, this efflux of 24(S)-hydroxycholesterol corresponds to the uptake of a similar amount of 24(S)-hydroxycholesterol by the liver, which indicates the exclusive production of 24(S)-hydroxycholesterol in the brain [64]. CYP46, the cytochrome responsible for the 24S-hydroxylation of cholesterol, is localized in neurons indicating that neurons have a distinct role in the excretion of cholesterol from the brain [76] and in the retina [77]. In mice, 24S-hydroxylation of cholesterol also takes place in the liver. However, 24S-hydroxylase knockout experiments in mice revealed similar steady-state levels of cholesterol in the knockout mice and in the wild-types. In contrast to the liver, the synthesis of new cholesterol in the brain was reduced by approximately 40% in knockout animals. These data suggest that the synthesis of new cholesterol and the secretion of 24(S)-hydroxycholesterol are closely linked and that at least 40% of cholesterol turnover in the brain is dependent on the action of cholesterol 24-hydroxylase [78].

Liver X-receptors (LXR) LXRα and LXRβ are important regulators of cholesterol homeostasis in the body. LXRs are expressed in most tissues and organs and are activated by a number of oxysterols, including 24(S)-hydroxycholesterol [79–81]. LXRs regulate their target genes including ABCA1 and ABCG1, which mediate the efflux of phospholipids and cholesterol from a number of cells including astrocytes [82], and LXR agonists have marked effects on gene expression in murine brain in a cell-specific manner. LXR agonists markedly enhance cholesterol efflux in astrocytes in culture and have only a limited effect on neuronal cultures [82]. The binding of oxysterols to LXR in the presence of large excesses of cholesterol has been questioned [83]. In the brain with a much lower ratio of oxysterols to cholesterol [67] it was postulated that a net export of cholesterol is feedback-regulated by LXRβ, ABCA1, CYP46, and 24(S)-hydroxycholesterol [46]. LXR-dependent ABC transporters are also involved in the influx of cholesterol from (perivascular) astrocytes into the CNS [84]. Many other nuclear receptor (with ligands such as fatty acids, oxysterols, and other lipids) are also expressed in the brain. However, for most of them we still have insufficient knowledge on their role in brain development and function [85]. Also apoE, the major apo present in the CNS, is transcriptionally regulated by the ligand-activated nuclear receptors, peroxisome proliferator-activated receptor γ(PPARγ) and LXRs [86], which form obligate heterodimers with retinoid X receptors. PPARγ: retinoid X receptors and LXR: retinoid X receptors induce the expression of apoE, its lipid transporters ABCA1 and ABCG1, and the nuclear receptors itself [87].

5. Regulation of CNS Sterol Flux by the Blood-Brain Barrier

The BBB formed by tight junctions between capillary endothelial cells, separates circulating blood from the extracellular fluid in CNS. The BBB is distinct from the blood-cerebrospinal-fluid barrier, a function of the choroidal cells of the choroid plexus.

The cells of the BBB have the potential to take up low-density lipoprotein (LDL) cholesterol through luminal endothelial receptors followed by a translocation across the endothelial cell. This uptake, however, is not relevant under physiological conditions and the lipoprotein receptor-mediated uptake of cholesterol from the plasma does not regulate brain cholesterol [88].

This finding is supported by the normal brain phenotype of humans with LDL-receptor mutations that do not express functional LDL-receptors [89]. Most of the studies, performed on patients with pharmacological downregulation of *Hmgcr* and overexpression of LDL receptors, showed no clear effect on brain cholesterol turnover [90–92] except for one study with 18 study subjects that revealed a reduced brain cholesterol turnover [93].

6. Cholesterol and the Signaling Pathway of Hedgehog

Lipoprotein receptor (i.e., LRP2 [94]) knockout mice and holoprosencephaly caused by defects in sonic hedgehog (SHH) [95] have a very similar phenotype. Cholesterol has a pivotal role in the signaling pathway of hedgehog. SHH participates in signaling in vertebrates and avertebrates [95] and is the best studied hedgehog homologue of the 3 mammalian proteins sonic (SHH), desert (DHH), and indian (IHH). SHH consists of a ~45 kDa precursor protein and undergoes autocatalytic processing to produce an ~20 kDa N-terminal signaling domain (referred to as SHH-N) and a ~25 kDa C-terminal domain with no known signaling function. During cleavage, a cholesterol molecule is appended to the carboxyl terminus. With cholesterol attached, SHH signals in an autocrine fashion. Hedgehog signaling requires the participation of dispatched protein. When SHH has reached its target cell, it binds to the Patched (PTCH1) receptor. In the absence of a ligand, PTCH1 inhibits smoothened (SMO). SMO is regulated by a small molecule, the cellular localization of which is controlled by PTCH. An anticancer drug, vismodegib, has already been developed which interferes with SMO and has the potential to inhibit constitutively active SHH signaling pathways such as in medulloblastomas [96]. PTCH1 has homology to Niemann-Pick disease type C1 protein (NPCD1), a protein involved in the transport of lipophilic molecules across membranes. PTCH1 has a sterol sensing domain (SSD), which has been shown to be essential for the suppression of SMO activity. PTCH1 regulates SMO by removing oxysterols from SMO. For this regulation, PTCH functions like a sterol pump and removes oxysterols created by 7-dehydrocholesterol reductase. After binding to SHH protein or to the SSD of PTCH, the pump is turned off allowing the accumulation of oxysterols around SMO. The interpretation of these findings is complicated by the fact that mammals, unlike drosophila melanogaster, possess more than one hedgehog (these are SHH, DHH, and IHH) with tissue specific expression [97]. Recent data show that SHH favors the integrity during maturation of the BBB, thus providing a barrier-promoting effect and an endogenous anti-inflammatory balance to CNS-directed immune attacks [98].

When embryonic development is studied in mice models, the differences of the lipoprotein uptake between species has to be accounted for as well as the maturation of the BBB during embryonic development [99]. In embryonic development, cholesterol derived in the maternal organism has to cross the yolk sac endoderm to be available for the embryo. In humans, fetuses rely on maternal cholesterol supply because the endogenous synthesis is only low. Therefore, maternal cholesterol can be crucial in fetal development [100]. The contribution of maternal cholesterol to fetal cholesterol homeostasis is more prominent in rodents [101] and appears to be essential for early embryonic development in rodents, as is also evident from the lethal fetal phenotype of mice with defects in placental cholesterol transport [102]. Unlike humans, in rodents apoB and microsomal transfer protein [103] are essential for normal embryonic development. In mice, partial or total apoB deficiency limits the uptake of apoB-containing lipoproteins at the placenta and, as a consequence, these mice suffer from apparent neural tube defects [102]. Humans with apoB deficiency do not suffer from neural tube defects [8].

7. Cholesterol Synthesis Inhibitors

Cholesterol synthesis inhibitors (CSIs) (also known as statins) are widely administered for reducing LDL cholesterol [104]. The main effect is the inhibition of *Hmgcr* but an array of pleiotropic effects of statin therapy has been observed [18, 105, 106]. Given the widespread use of statins, it is of particular interest whether CSI affect the metabolism of CNS cholesterol or not and whether an effect of (certain) CSI has any clinical impact on the CNS morphology or on neurological function [107–110]. Retrospective cohort studies have suggested that statin users have a lower prevalence of dementia. On the other hand, a randomized controlled study failed to show beneficial effects on the cognitive decline in AD [111].

This topic is rather complex due to several open issues. First, the CSIs used for the treatment of hypercholesterolemia (such as simvastatin, lovastatin, atorvastatin, fluvastatin, pravastatin, rosuvastatin, and pitavastatin) differ in their lipophilicity. A higher hydrophilicity/lower lipophilicity of a pharmaceutical compound and its active metabolites will, in the absence of specific transporters, lead to only very low concentrations within the CNS. Second, the very efficient mode of action of these substances, namely, the induced overexpression of LDL receptors, is not effective in the CNS since these receptors are not expressed within the CNS [89, 112]. Third, studies such as the 24S-hydroxylase knockout experiments in mice [78] indicate a very tight, unique, and independent regulation of cholesterol synthesis and efflux within and from the CNS. Finally, other effects of CSI—described as pleiotropic effects—such as effects on vascular injury, on cytokine production, and on nitric oxide production [18] might influence the integrity of the BBB [113] and any effects observed on cholesterol metabolism might be only indirect. In fact, it has been shown that simvastatin may reduce posttraumatic edema by preventing damage to tight junctions and neutrophil infiltration into the parenchyma, thus preserving BBB integrity [114].

Differences in BBB permeability coefficients might be a clue to the higher incidence of neurological adverse events of some statins. BBB permeability was studied using bovine brain microvessels or by analyzing brain extracts of statin-fed rats. Lovastatin and simvastatin had much higher BBB permeability coefficients than did fluvastatin, pravastatin, or rosuvastatin [115–117]. The results with atorvastatin and cerivastatin (the latter not available in the market anymore) are ambiguous. Some researchers report high BBB permeability coefficients for atorvastatin [118], others for cerivastatin [119]. Transfer of the lipophilic compounds lovastatin and simvastatin across the BBB occurs via passive diffusion, whereas pravastatin is taken up by an active, low affinity system [120]. The negative charge of fluvastatin affects the uptake by repulsion from the anionic microdomains in the plasma membrane of BBB endothelial cells [115]. Interesting results were obtained in the short-term treatment comparing the lipophilic simvastatin with the hydrophilic pravastatin in mice. Brain cholesterol synthesis in mice is significantly affected by simvastatin while whole-brain cholesterol turnover is not disturbed. Pravastatin can cross the BBB but does not affect intracellular cholesterol synthesis [107].

In a mechanistic approach, the effects of CSI on brain cholesterol could occur by forming a cholesterol gradient across the BBB which facilitates the efflux of cholesterol as 24(S)-hydroxycholesterol [121]. However, current knowledge is not sufficient to quantify the effect of CSI treatment on brain cholesterol. High doses (80 mg per day) of simvastatin did reduce the synthesis of CNS cholesterol *in vivo* (as analyzed by the efflux of 24(S)-hydroxycholesterol) [93] and the highly lipophilic lovastatin inhibited cholesterol synthesis and synaptogenesis *in vitro* [122]. The analysis of the ratio of plasma 24(S)-hydroxycholesterol to cholesterol after treatment of patients with high doses of CSI, however, revealed a decreased ratio and it was postulated that this was caused by a diminished substrate supply for CYP46A1 in the brain [93]. Conflicting data have been obtained from the treatment of patients with NPC disease. In NPC disease—a lysosomal lipidosis due to defective lipid transport [10]—the accumulation of tissue lipids in neuronal cells such as Purkinje cells cannot be treated by aggressive cholesterol lowering pharmaceutical approaches, neither in humans [123] nor in a mouse model [124], despite CSI therapy lowered whole body cholesterol very efficiently. When NPC disease was treated with allopregnanolone, a strong benefit was observed but it could have come solely from the vector, cyclodextrin. Cyclodextrin, a cyclical oligosaccharid with a hydrophilic exterior and a lipophilic interior is an ideal chelator for sterols and is the most effective treatment option for NPC disease in the mouse model [10].

Cholesterol is vital to normal brain functions including learning and memory but that involvement is as complex as cholesterol synthesis, metabolism, and excretion. Dietary cholesterol influences learning tasks in mice and rats in different experiments such as water maze and fear conditioning even though cholesterol does not cross the BBB [125, 126]. Excess cholesterol in the brain can lead to many signaling events via cholesterol metabolites, proinflammatory mediators, and antioxidant processes [126]. Correlations of cholesterol levels with cognitive function have been found to be positive, negative, or to have no relationship at all. An important confounder is patient age. High plasma cholesterol had detrimental effects in middle-aged persons [127–131] but had positive effects in the very elderly [132] and no effects in the young [133]. Cholesterol reduction by statin therapy improves memory in some cases but not others. Numerous reports as well as small trials have suggested that statin therapy causes cognitive impairment, although the true extent of this effect remains under study. The postmarketing adverse event reports generally described individuals over the age of 50 years who experienced notable but ill-defined memory loss or impairment that was reversible upon discontinuation of statin therapy. Time to onset of the event was highly variable, ranging from one day to years after statin exposure [105]. Muldoon et al. [134] observed minor decrements in cognitive functioning with statins. On the other end, treatment with lovastatin or pravastatin did not cause any psychological distress or substantially alter cognitive function [135, 136]. Data from the observational studies and clinical trials did not suggest that cognitive changes associated with statin use are common or that statin use leads to clinically significant cognitive decline. In any case, the FDA has recently updated the recommendation for statins in order to reduce the risk of cognitive adverse effects and to provide the public with more information about the safe and effective use of statins [137]. Although epidemiology and preclinical statin research have generally supported an adverse role of high cholesterol levels regarding Alzheimer's disease (AD), human studies of statins show highly variable outcomes, making it difficult to draw firm conclusions [105].

The difference in the lipophilicity of different statins studied was not suited to explain their fitness for use in the statin treatment of dementia or AD [138–140]. However, of particular interest are drug-specific effects obtained in gene expression studies when comparing different CSI [141]. Interesting results were also observed when studying the effects of statins in the presence and absence of mevalonate. Despite cholesterol synthesis was blocked by the inhibition of *Hmgcr*, as expected, the isoprenylation continued unimpeded [142]. From the current knowledge, the differing effects of different statins on brain functions might be modulated by their effects on metabolic pathways other than the cholesterol pathway.

Hypercholesteremia can induce τ-hyperphosphorylation and Aβ production in rat brain. Atorvastatin inhibited τ-hyperphosphorylation and decreased Aβ generation, thus playing a protective role in the pathogenesis of hypercholesteremia-induced neurodegeneration in the brain [143]. In mice, early treatment with both atorvastatin and pitavastatin prevented subsequent worsening of cognitive function and the amyloidogenic process, probably due to pleiotropic effects, suggesting a therapeutic potential for AD patients [144]. In AD patients, simvastatin treatment caused a modest but significant inhibition of brain cholesterol biosynthesis, as measured by a decrease of cerebrospinal fluid lathosterol and plasma 24(S)-hydroxycholesterol. Despite these effects, there were no changes in AD biomarkers [145]. In another study, atorvastatin was not associated with significant clinical benefit [146]. One possible interpretation might be that statins prevent or delay the onset of AD, but cannot slow the cognitive decline once the disease process has started.

Higher levels of isoprenoids favor APP-processing by α-secretase and less amyloid β (Aβ) is being secreted. Low concentrations of isoprenoids inhibit the metabolism of APP through the secretory pathway and lead to the intracellular accumulation of Aβ. Low intracellular cholesterol levels inhibit receptor-mediated endocytosis of APP. In mice, the inhibition of protein isoprenylation by fluvastatin, at a clinically relevant dose, reduced brain Aβ levels by increasing the trafficking of APP carboxyl terminal fragments and by enhancing Aβ clearance mediated by upregulation of low-density lipoprotein receptor-related protein 1 (LRP-1) expression [147].

Other protective effects of statins besides their plasma cholesterol lowering without alteration of the isoprenoid levels [142] were obtained in studies with stroke patients and in prospective studies. In observational studies, patients under CSI treatment had lower likelihoods of mortality as well as of poor functional outcome [148] and the discontinuation of CSI after ischemic stroke has been associated with worse outcomes [149]. Studies with very high doses (up to 8 mg/kg body weight) of lovastatin are under way and have indicated an acceptable safety profile [150]. The use of CSI, however, has been shown to increase the risk of bleeding after ischemic stroke, irrespective of plasma cholesterol concentration. Studies show no clear positive effects for CSI on cerebral hemorrhage, although atorvastatin has been shown to significantly relieve brain edema, to decrease the brain injury caused by matrix metalloproteinase-9, and to protect neurons in rats with intracerebral hemorrhage [151].

Other important confounding factors of the human epidemiological studies performed so far are the stage of Alzheimer's disease in the patients studied, the drug dose, the duration of therapy and the adherence to the prescribed drug, and the overlap of Alzheimer's disease with other forms of dementia and vascular disease [105]. While *in vitro* effects are fairly well understood, the results from *in vivo* studies in humans are conflicting and additional research work is urgently needed with highly standardized study designs to address the impact of CSI on brain cholesterol metabolism and Alzheimer's disease. Currently, routine use of CSI in CNS disease cannot be recommended except for lowering LDL cholesterol in cerebrovascular disease [106].

8. Cerebrospinal Fluid Lipoproteins

Essentially all cholesterol within the CNS is associated with cell membranes and only tiny amounts are located within the intercellular space and in the CSF under physiological conditions. Cholesterol within the intercellular space and in the CSF is associated with apos, in particular with apoE. A very high expression of apoE was observed during regeneration of peripheral nerves after damage [152] and apoE—associated with lipids—was the most abundant protein in the intracellular fluid. ApoE is also expressed within the CNS and astrocytes secrete lipoprotein particles composed of apoE, apoAI, and lipids (Figure 1). ApoE in the CNS has a higher apparent molecular weight due to a higher sialylation and is exclusively lipid-bound [14, 153]. The role of apoE-containing lipoproteins is postulated to redistribute lipids and to regulate cholesterol homeostasis within the brain.

The concentration of lipoproteins in the CSF is low. Compared to plasma, in CSF the concentration of apoE is about 5%, of cholesterol about 1%, and of phospholipids about 2% only. Triglycerides are present in trace amounts and apoB is absent. The concentration of lipids in the CSF does not correlate with the plasma lipid concentration [154]. CSF lipoproteins are bigger in size than plasma HDL and smaller than LDL, their density is between LDL and HDL [14]. Their composition with esterified cholesterol as core lipid, their size, and density is very similar to lipoproteins secreted from macrophages [155] or from transfected neuro2a cells [156]. However, nascent apoE/lipid particles secreted by cultured astrocytes are primarily discoid and contain only small amounts of lipids such as cholesterol and phospholipids [157]. Besides small amounts of apoA-I, CSF lipoproteins contain trace amounts of apoA-II, apoC-I, and apoC-III. These small, lipophilic apos are derived from the plasma and have leaked through the blood brain barrier. ApoE and apoB cannot cross the BBB [158], however, in case of a BBB breakdown, plasma components can spill into the CSF and apoB can be detected in the CSF.

9. LDL Receptor Family in the CNS

Numerous lipoprotein receptors of the LDL receptor family have been detected in the CNS by biochemical and molecular methods (LDL receptor, VLDL-receptor, apoER2/LRP8, LRP4, LRP, LRP2 (formerly known as gp330 or megalin), LRP1B, LRP5/LRP6, and LRP11/SORL1) [13, 159]. Ligands for these receptors are apoE-containing lipoproteins, lipids and other macromolecules [14, 153, 160]. However, the spatial expression in different cells such as neurons, astrocytes and microglia—even different for cell lines within different regions of the brain—and the different temporal expression with a particular high expression postnatally suggest important functions during embryogenesis and for the functioning of the CNS. In fact, these multifunctional and evolutionary ancient receptors have been shown to be intercellular signal transducers and signal modulators [13].

The differential roles of these receptors in the CNS are impeded by their redundant functions, similar or even identical specificity for certain ligands, and the coexpression in certain organs or even in one cell. Transgenic animal models are of very limited use because of relevant interspecies differences in particular in regard of structural differences of the placenta and the necessity of certain lipoproteins and lipoprotein receptors for the lipid transfer from the maternal organism during embryogenesis. The requirement for the same receptor at two stages of lipid transport into the embryo makes it difficult to unequivocally determine the participation of these molecules at a certain step, that is, on the yolk sac surface or at the neuroepithelium [37].

The study of the evolutionary highly conserved signaling pathways by mouse genetics revealed critical functions for the receptors of the apoE-receptor family. Both knockout mice lacking LRP2 [161] and double knockout mice lacking both apoER2/LRP8 and the VLDL-receptor [162] show severe defects in brain development. The latter are phenotypically indistinguishable from mice lacking the signaling protein Reelin and from mice with mutations in the cytoplasmic adapter protein Disabled-1 (*Dab1*) [163]. This phenotype suggested that apoER2/LRP8, as well as the VLDL-receptor, functions in a linear signaling pathway that is dependent on the extracellular ligand Reelin and the intracellular adaptor Dab1 for initiating a signaling cascade that regulates the migration and positioning of neurons during development [163]. Further studies revealed a signaling through the Src family tyrosine kinase through proximity triggered phosphorylation [164]. Other signaling pathways are also active in microglia and neurons as indicated by the interaction of the ATP-binding cassette transporter ABCA1 (the member 1 of human transporter subfamily ABCA), also known as cholesterol efflux regulatory protein (CERP), with the MAP-kinase-system [165].

The novel downstream interactions are partly dependent upon unique interaction motifs within the cytoplasmic domain of the receptors which helps to explain the specific and nonredundant roles of ER2/LRP8 and VLDL-receptor in shaping brain regions in response to binding of the same ligand. For instance, the specific topography of the Purkinje cell layer is regulated by the ER2/LRP8 and the VLDL-receptor and in the neocortex [166], the VLDL-receptor provides a stop signal for migrating neurons while apoER2/LRP8 regulates the migration of later-borne neurons essential for the proper lamination of neocortex and hippocampus [162]. In the peripheral neurons, LRP4 is essential for the function of the neuromuscular junction. LRP4-deficient mice are stillborn. LRP4 is an obligate coreceptor for the muscle specific tyrosine kinase MUSK and the neuronally produced ligand agrin. Only in the presence of LRP4, agrin leads to clustering and transphosphorylation of MUSK. In the absence of LRP4, MUSK transphosphorylation cannot occur and acetylcholine receptors fail to form postsynaptic clusters [167].

Despite all genes of the LDL receptor family have been disrupted in the mouse, human mutations besides the LDL receptor have been identified so far only in LRP2 and in the VLDL receptor. Defects in LRP2 cause Donnai-Barrrow syndrome, congenital agenesis of the corpus callosum, diaphragmatic hernia, facial dysmorphology, ocular anomalies, sensorineural hearing loss, and development delay [168]. The defects in patients are similar but not identical to those seen in LRP2 knockout C57bl/6X129 hybrid mice [168].This indicates genetic modifiers among species and even within different mice strains. VLDL-receptor deficiency, a fully autosomal recessive trait, leads to a similar but more severe phenotype in humans compared to mice [169]. In humans, distinct mutations have been observed in the Canadian Hutterite population [170] and in Middle Eastern populations [171]. Neuroanatomically, these mutations are indistinguishable but considerable variations exist in regard of motor development. Several, but not all, affected individuals are quadrupedal and it has been suggested that the VLDL receptor is the critical gene for the evolution of the bipedal gait [171]. Other human autosomal recessive diseases with virtually identical phenotypes to VLDL receptor deficiency are caused by mutations of chromosome 17 [172]. Crk, a downstream component of the Reelin signaling pathway, is located in this chromosome region [169].

10. Apolipoproteins (apoE and apoJ) within the CNS

The pivotal role of apoE for cholesterol recycling in the regenerating peripheral nerve has been long recognized [173]. ApoE, a 39 kD protein, is the major apo in the CNS. Three major alleles of *Apoe* (ε2, ε3, ε4) are expressed codominantly and lead to common phenotypes E22, E23, E24, E33, E34, and E44. ε3 is the most common allele (about 77%) and ε2 is the least common (about 8%) of these major alleles [174]. ApoE2 has a defective binding to the LDL-receptor and is responsible for type III hyperlipidemia. ApoE3 as well as apoE4 are high affinity ligands for the LDL-receptor [175]. ApoE consists of two domains (the N- and C-terminal domains) separated by a protease-sensitive hinge region. The differences between apoE isoforms are arginine-to-cysteine changes in the N-terminal domain. ApoE4 contains arginines at positions 112 and 158, whereas apoE3 has a Cys112 [175].

The functions of apoE in the CNS are heterogeneous and range from participation in cholesterol homeostasis and in nonlipid activities such as protein chaperoning and signal transduction [176]. ApoE is expressed in the brain in high concentrations, such that the brain is the organ with the second highest apoE expression after the liver [177]. Astrocytes are the major source of apoE followed by oligodendrocytes, microglia, and ependymal layer cells [178]. The significance of apoE expression in neurons has not been resolved yet. Some CNS neurons may express apoE under certain condition such as after excitotoxic injury [179] and apoE expression was observed in primary cultures of human hippocampal neurons and in mice expressing human apoE under the control of the human apoE promoter [176]. The stability of apoE in the brain requires the association with lipids. In knockout mice for Abca1—a gene necessary for the lipidation of apoE—the amount of apoE in the brain is reduced [180, 181]. The LDL-receptor and LRP1 are the main receptors for the uptake of apoE containing lipoprotein particles in the brain. LDL-receptor knockout mice have increased levels of apoE in brain parenchyma and in CSF [182] which suggests impaired metabolism of apoE. A conditional deletion of *Lrp1* gene in mouse brain decreases brain parenchyma apoE [182]. ApoE is the major apo of CSF lipoproteins [14, 157, 158]. Similar to lipoprotein cholesterol, apoE does not cross the BBB. This was demonstrated by the analysis of apoE phenotypes after liver transplantation when no donor apoE can be found in the CSF of the recipient [177]. Whether apoE has a major role in supporting synaptogenesis and maintenance of synaptic connections *in vivo* in the uninjured brain is unclear. In apoE knockout mice, brain morphology and behavior are not altered in the absence of injury [183, 184] and no overt cognitive defects have been reported in humans with genetic apoE deficiency [185]. It has been suggested that there is a dynamic exchange of apoE among brain cells, that apoE is the major transport protein for extracellular cholesterol and other lipids, and that apoE-mediated cholesterol exchange occurs between neuronal and nonneuronal cells of the CNS [176].

Several lines of evidence link apoE with late-onset Alzheimer's disease, the most common cause of dementia in the elderly. Epidemiological studies highlighted the ε4 allele of *Apoe* as the most common risk factor for late-onset Alzheimer's disease [186], and *in vitro* studies showed a colocalization of apoE with amyloid plaques [187] and a positive correlation between plaque density and number of ε4 alleles in Alzheimer' patients at autopsy [188].

ApoE is a risk factor with relatively low penetrance but with high prevalence [189]. Individuals with one ε4 allele are 3 to 4 times more likely than those without ε4 alleles to develop late-onset Alzheimer's disease [189] and suffer from Alzheimer's disease at a younger age [190]. Individuals with the ε2 allele have a lower risk of late-onset Alzheimer's disease compared to the ε3 allele ([186], for results of meta-analyses see http://www.alzgene.org/). However, most homozygotes for ε4 will not suffer from Alzheimer's disease and most patients with Alzheimer's disease are not homozygous for ε4 [189].

The search for the molecular mechanisms of apoE4 promoting Alzheimer's disease is still ongoing despite 20 years of intense research. These molecular mechanisms would be attractive pharmaceutical targets for the prevention and treatment of Alzheimer's disease [176]. One hypothesis proposes a "toxic" mechanism of apoE4, the other hypothesis is a failure of apoE4 to slow down the disease process as effectively as apoE3 and apoE2 do. These hypotheses have direct implications in devising therapeutic strategies. In the first hypothesis, the treatment would have to block apoE4, in the second hypothesis the treatment has to potentiate or to mimic apoE3 [191].

Biochemical studies elucidated isoform-specific differences between different apoE isoforms, in particular between apoE3 and apoE4. The design of these studies is hindered by the lack of apoE isoforms in animals. Different apoE isoforms are only present in humans; all animal apoEs studied so far contain Thr at the equivalence to the position Arg61 in human apoE4. Therefore, irrespective of the amino acid at position 112, animal apoE behaves like human apoE3 [192].

ApoE4 binds to large lipoprotein particles, attributable to the presence of Arg112, which affects the conformation of the side chain of Arg61 in the N-terminal domain resulting in domain interaction between Arg61 and Glu255 in the C-terminal domain [193]. Unlike apoE3, apoE4 is assumed to produce an unstable "molten globule" state that is responsible for the pathogenic role in Alzheimer's disease [194]. Molten globule domains interact with different target molecules, typically with high-affinity and low specificity [195]. Since the isoform-specific differences between apoE3 and apoE4 are outside the receptor-binding region, studies have evaluated the molecular interaction of apoE with proteins present in the neuritic plaque. Lipid-bound (i.e., physiologic) as well as artificially delipidated apoE forms complexes with Aβ. However, the order of stability of the complexes dependent on apoE isoform was not uniform [196, 197]. Data from *in vitro* studies indicate that apoE enhances cellular Aβ uptake and degradation [196, 198, 199] but *in vivo* studies revealed that apoE retards Aβ clearance [200, 201], possibly via an effect at the BBB [202]. Until now, the whole wild type apoE could not be crystallized and all crystallographic studies could only be performed on fragments of the protein or after site directed mutagenesis [203]. Another challenge results from self-aggregation of the protein and from the formation of oligomers. When lipids are added to the delipidated protein, the protein undergoes large structural changes [204], and it is not clear whether differences observed with the delipidated protein are retained after lipidation [203]. The structure of the N-terminal domain (i.e., the receptor binding domain) of apoE3 and apoE4 has been determined using both X-ray and NMR methods [205, 206]. The isolated C-terminal domain—responsible for lipid binding, for oligomerization and probably for Aβ binding—is known to aggregate which prevents structure determination by standard methods [192]. Studies performed with transgenic animals only expressing apoE 3 or apoE4 either in neurons or in astrocytes showed a detrimental effect of apoE4 on all subunits of mitochondrial respiratory complexes assessed and treatment of these cells with a compound disrupting apoE4 domain interaction restored mitochondrial respiratory complex IV levels. Mutant apoE4 (apoE4-Thr-61) lacking domain interaction did not induce mitochondrial dysfunction [207].

Recently, results of the first pharmacological interventions with apoE as target performed in mice have been reported. One study has targeted at the apoE isoform-specific effects on the BBB. In the absence of murine apoE, human apoE4 but not apoE3 or apoE2 leads to BBB breakdown by activating the proinflammatory cyclophilin A in pericytes [208]. Another study overexpressed (murine) apoE in the brain by the oral application of the FDA-approved RXR agonist bexarotene. This study demonstrated a beneficial effect of CNS apoE overexpression [209], and it was concluded that apoE overexpression might be able to decrease the progression of Aβ deposition. The proposed mechanism consists in the absorption of Aβ by the CNS-derived lipoproteins followed by the clearance of these particles from the brain. However, only murine apoE was tested and no apoE isoform-specific effects have been reported so far [191]. Another study employed an apoE-mimetic peptide called ApoE-(133-149) which was administered intraperitoneally, has optimized BBB penetration, and showed neuroprotection [210]. Previous studies with this peptide in mice with targeted replacement of apoE indicate human apoE isoform-specific effects on immune reactions with an increase in proinflammatory cytokines in apoE4-expressing mice [211]. Unlike native apoE, ApoE-(133-149) lacks the lipid binding region and will not be exclusively lipid-bound. Besides its immunomodulatory effects on microglia in the CNS and macrophages outside the CNS, the peptide may affect cholesterol metabolism as well as LRP expression and LRP receptor binding [211].

Apolipoprotein J (also known as clusterin) is also present in lipoprotein particles and regulates cholesterol and brain lipid metabolism [212]. Similar to apoE, the expression of clusterin in the brain changes significantly during development [213] and during different kinds of neuronal injuries [214] and increases in Alzheimer's disease [212]. Clusterin is a versatile chaperone molecule which contains several amphipathic and coiled-coil alpha-helices, typical characteristics of small heat shock proteins. Clusterin was originally identified in Sertoli cells but very early, the high expression of clusterin in the brain [215] and its role in cholesterol trafficking has been established [212]. The secondary structure of clusterin contains molten globule domains [216]. Of particular interest is the role of clusterin in the clearance of Aβ peptides. Secreted Aβ peptides bind avidly to apoE and to clusterin/apoJ, which prevents the oligomerization of these Aβ peptides. A minor part of this complex is endocytosed by microglia and astrocytes and degraded by insulin degrading enzyme and neprilysin but the major part is endocytosed without degradation. The major receptors for the uptake at the blood-brain barrier are LRP and LRP2 [94, 217]. The third clearance pathway, besides the proteolytic degradation and the endocytic uptake by microglia and astrocytes, is the efflux of Aβ peptides through the blood-brain barrier. This efflux is mediated by LRP1 [218] and by LRP2 [219]. A downregulation of LRP1 is correlated with regional Aβ accumulation in Alzheimer's disease [218]. For the clearance of Aβ in the brain, apoE and clusterin/apoJ have a comparable and interchangeable function.

In summary, the function of the apoE receptors in neurons is distinct but with similar molecular mechanisms, in particular in intra- and intercellular signaling. These receptors are critical for the formation and the function of central and of peripheral synapses. Cholesterol and apoE play a particular role as constituents of the ligands to these receptors.

11. Amyloid Precursor Protein and Cholesterol

The accumulation, oligomerization, and deposition of Aβ (a cleavage product of amyloid precursor protein APP) are hallmark of Alzheimer's pathogenesis. Aβ is a intrinsically disordered protein, which can self-aggregate and form an array of supramolecular assemblies with different morphology including oligomers, amorphous aggregates, and amyloid like fibrils. Cholesterol is involved in several steps of Aβ processing. The elimination products, the oxysterols such as the brain-specific 24(S)-hydroxycholesterol, as well as 27-hydroxycholesterol increase sAPP production and contribute to amyloidogenesis [220] with 24(S)-hydroxycholesterol having more pronounced effects than 27-hydroxycholesterol [81]. Plasma 27-hydroxycholesterol concentration was associated with CSF sAPP levels [221].

The selective expression of CYP46A1 around neuritic plaques and the potent inhibition of APP processing in neurons by 24(S)-hydroxycholesterol suggest that CYP46A1 affects the pathophysiology of Alzheimer's disease [81]. ApoE and its receptors are closely involved in these processes. ApoE as well as LRP1 are present in amyloid plaques [187] and apoE regulates isoform-specifically APP processing to Aβ by mechanisms dependent on LRP1 function. ApoE4 increases Aβ production in neuronal cells overexpressing APP to a greater extent than apoE3. After incubation with the LRP1 receptor antagonist RAP or by RNA interference, this isoform-specific effect was blunted [222]. Three other apoE receptors (LRP1B, APOER2, LRP11/SORL1) also interact with APP and regulate its trafficking and processing to Aβ [223]. All these receptors reduce Aβ processing due to their slow rate of endocytosis. In the absence of common ligands, however, APOER2 increases the distribution of APP into special cholesterol-rich membrane subdomains (also known as detergent-resistant membrane fraction (DRM) or lipid rafts) and the processing of APP to Aβ [224]. DRMs are abundant on the cell surface and are enriched in cholesterol and sphingolipids and a variety of proteins. Sorting signals that target proteins to DRMs include binding to cholesterol, sphingolipids and GPI-anchors, and other lipid modifications such as palmitoylation and myristoylation [3]. Lipid-lipid interactions are one of the major mechanisms to form

DRMs. DRMs are thought to represent liquid-ordered (L_O) domains, which coexist in the same membrane together with liquid-disordered (L_d) domains [3]. L_O domains are formed due to the preferential interaction of sphingolipids and/or phospholipids containing saturated acyl chains with cholesterol [225]. Cholesterol has been shown to be a critical regulator of DRM formation and the local regulation of cholesterol levels by cholesterol biosynthesis, compartmentalization and secretion of cholesterol is a powerful mechanism to control DRM-dependent events.

Aβ is cleared from the brain by two pathways. First, through receptor-mediated endocytosis by cells in brain parenchyma and along the interstitial fluid or through the BBB and second, through endopeptidase-mediated proteolytic degradation. The receptor-mediated endocytosis by members of the LDL-receptor family on astrocytes [226] and microglia [227] can be an efficient way to reduce brain Aβ. Most Aβ internalized by apoE receptors is degraded in lysosomes or is transcytosed into the plasma. However, Aβ can escape from degradation or transcytosis, accumulates in neurons, and exerts its toxicity on the neuronal function [228]. Opposite to murine studies in which apoE overexpression decreased Aβ deposition [208–210], in mice overexpressing Aβ under control of the PDGF promoter, the lack of apoE markedly diminished Aβ deposition [229].

Aβ generation is localized in DRMs or rafts. The enzyme responsible for the enzymatic cleavage of APP called β-secretase, or β-site APP cleaving enzyme (BACE), is found in DRMs in primary hippocampal neurons [230]. The other proteins necessary for the processing of APP have been located in the DRMs of the late Golgi and endosomes, the organelles where BACE is thought to be biologically activated. The complete Aβ generating proteolytic machinery colocalizes within DRMs of the same vesicle [231]. A clue to the complex APP processing comes from studying the effects of different cholesterol concentrations [230]. In cells being cholesterol-depleted and overexpressing APP, further lowering of cholesterol inhibits amyloidogenesis [91, 232, 233]. In neurons with normal cholesterol content, a moderate reduction of cholesterol led to increased Aβ levels whereas a strong cholesterol reduction resulted in a significant drop in Aβ generation. These cholesterol dose-dependent effects can be explained by two independent cellular mechanisms [231]. First, a moderate reduction of cholesterol causes a disorganization of DRMs allowing more BACE to interact with APP and to generate Aβ. A strong reduction in cholesterol inhibits BACE/γ-secretase activities. Despite a direct contact of BACE/γ-secretase with APP, Aβ generation is blunted. In cells overexpressing APP, APP can be mislocalized in DRMs and then cleaved by BACE [230, 233].

12. Conclusion

The pivotal effects of brain cholesterol on different cellular processes in the CNS have become apparent in the last decades. Most of these studies were performed in patients with inherited defects of cholesterol biosynthesis and in transgenic animals with defined mutations. The intriguing data on the substantial role of cholesterol in the physiology and pathophysiology of DRMs has been predominantly obtained in cell culture studies.

While many studies have focused on the cholesterol metabolism of the whole CNS, late work focused on cell-specific and even microdomain-specific effects of cholesterol. Human and animal studies are complicated by different expression of genes involved during development as well as by cell specific differences. Another challenge is the role of the BBB, which also changes during development and can be regulated under certain pathological conditions. The sterol flux between CNS cells (namely neurons and oligodendrocytes) is only poorly understood. However, whole CNS cholesterol production can be very elegantly studied by analyzing the concentrations of 24(S)-hydroxycholesterol, the exclusive metabolite of CNS cholesterol. Studies of the hedgehog signaling cascade in humans were driven by the SLO syndrome and this disease could be clarified by studying the genes involved in human patients as well as in transgenic mice models. Still under discussion are the options of treatment of CNS diseases by targeting CNS cholesterol metabolism. Differences in pharmacology, as well in the selection of patients, obscure potential beneficial or detrimental effects and it is currently not recommended to treat patients with CSI for these indications outside from clinical trials.

The analysis of CSF lipoproteins revealed some data on brain cholesterol metabolism. However, no clinical applicable tests have been developed so far which employ CSF lipoproteins or apos for the clinical diagnosis or for monitoring the effects of certain therapies. Studies of the LDL receptor family in the CNS showed a very interesting redundancy as well as interaction of these lipoprotein receptors with a wide array of important signal transduction pathways. While these receptors are capable of taking up lipoproteins, this function is only one of many others involved in cell differentiation, growth, and function. Isoform-specific effects of apoE have been the bridge to the processing of APP. A great number of studies have addressed the rather complicated molecular processing and the effects of cholesterol (both in the whole organism as well as in single cells) on this processing. From current understanding, CNS cholesterol is an auspicious target for preventing or even treating Alzheimer's disease. The full understanding of these process remains a huge challenge given the increasing number of older patients, the very complex pharmacokinetics of drugs targeting the CNS, the long time course of presymptomatic disease, and many confounding factors identified so far.

Abbreviations

Aβ: Amyloid β
apo: Apolipoprotein
APP: Amyloid precursor protein
BACE: β-site APP cleaving enzyme
BBB: Blood brain barrier
CNS: Central nervous system
CSF: Cerebrospinal fluid
CSI: Cholesterol synthesis inhibitors
Dhcr7: 7-dehydrocholesterol reductase

DRM: Detergent-resistant membrane fraction
Hmgcr: 3-hydroxy-3-methylglutaryl-coenzyme A reductase
L_d: Liquid-disordered domain
LDL: Low-density lipoprotein
L_o: Liquid-ordered domain
LXR: Liver X-receptors
NPC: Niemann-Pick type C
NPC1: Niemann-Pick disease type C1 protein
PPARγ: Peroxisome proliferator-activated receptor γ
PTCH1: Patched
RAGE: Receptor for advanced glycation end products
SHH: Sonic hedgehog
SMO: Smoothened.

Acknowledgments

This work presented was supported in part by the Deutsche Forschungsgemeinschaft (DFG Or 79 1-1 and 79/4-2), VerUm, and the Interdisciplinary center for Clinical Research, University of Leipzig (IZKF TP C16) (to MO).

References

[1] J. M. Dietschy and S. D. Turley, "Cholesterol metabolism in the brain," *Current Opinion in Lipidology*, vol. 12, no. 2, pp. 105–112, 2001.

[2] I. Björkhem, S. Meaney, and A. M. Fogelman, "Brain cholesterol: long secret life behind a barrier," *Arteriosclerosis, Thrombosis, and Vascular Biology*, vol. 24, no. 5, pp. 806–815, 2004.

[3] Z. Korade and A. K. Kenworthy, "Lipid rafts, cholesterol, and the brain," *Neuropharmacology*, vol. 55, no. 8, pp. 1265–1273, 2008.

[4] L. Fester, L. Zhou, A. Bütow et al., "Cholesterol-promoted synaptogenesis requires the conversion of cholesterol to estradiol in the hippocampus," *Hippocampus*, vol. 19, no. 8, pp. 692–705, 2009.

[5] C. Goritz, D. H. Mauch, and F. W. Pfrieger, "Multiple mechanisms mediate cholesterol-induced synaptogenesis in a CNS neuron," *Molecular and Cellular Neuroscience*, vol. 29, no. 2, pp. 190–201, 2005.

[6] E. I. Posse de Chaves, A. E. Rusinol, D. E. Vance, R. B. Campenot, and J. E. Vance, "Role of lipoproteins in the delivery of lipids to axons during axonal regeneration," *The Journal of Biological Chemistry*, vol. 272, no. 49, pp. 30766–30773, 1997.

[7] A. R. Koudinov and N. V. Koudinova, "Cholesterol homeostasis failure as a unifying cause of synaptic degeneration," *Journal of the Neurological Sciences*, vol. 229-230, pp. 233–240, 2005.

[8] J. Herz and H. H. Bock, "Lipoprotein receptors in the nervous system," *Annual Review of Biochemistry*, vol. 71, pp. 405–434, 2002.

[9] A. E. DeBarber, Y. Eroglu, L. S. Merkens et al., "Smith-Lemli-Opitz syndrome," *Expert Reviews in Molecular Medicine*, vol. 13, p. e24, 2011.

[10] M. Madra and S. L. Sturley, "Niemann-Pick type C pathogenesis and treatment: from statins to sugars," *Clinical Lipidology*, vol. 5, no. 3, pp. 387–395, 2010.

[11] R. C. Block, E. R. Dorsey, C. A. Beck, J. . Brenna, and I. Shoulson, "Altered cholesterol and fatty acid metabolism in Huntington disease," *Journal of Clinical Lipidology*, vol. 4, no. 1, pp. 17–23, 2010.

[12] G. Di Paolo and T. W. Kim, "Linking lipids to Alzheimer's disease: Cholesterol and beyond," *Nature Reviews Neuroscience*, vol. 12, no. 5, pp. 284–296, 2011.

[13] J. Herz, "Apolipoprotein E receptors in the nervous system," *Current Opinion in Lipidology*, vol. 20, no. 3, pp. 190–196, 2009.

[14] R. E. Pitas, J. K. Boyles, S. H. Lee, D. Hui, and K. H. Weisgraber, "Lipoproteins and their receptors in the central nervous system. Characterization of the lipoproteins in cerebrospinal fluid and identification of apolipoprotein B,E(LDL) receptors in the brain," *The Journal of Biological Chemistry*, vol. 262, no. 29, pp. 14352–14360, 1987.

[15] M. S. Brown and J. L. Goldstein, "Lipoprotein receptors in the liver. Control signals for plasma cholesterol traffic," *Journal of Clinical Investigation*, vol. 72, no. 3, pp. 743–747, 1983.

[16] J. P. Couerbe, "Du cerveau, considéré sous le point du vue chimique et physiologique," *Annales De Chimie Ed De Physique*, vol. 56, pp. 160–193, 1834.

[17] H. R. Waterham, "Defects of cholesterol biosynthesis," *FEBS Letters*, vol. 580, no. 23, pp. 5442–5449, 2006.

[18] S. Bellosta, N. Ferri, L. Arnaboldi, F. Bernini, R. Paoletti, and A. Corsini, "Pleiotropic effects of statins in atherosclerosis and diabetes," *Diabetes Care*, vol. 23, supplement 2, pp. B72–B78, 2000.

[19] S. H. Bae, J. N. Lee, B. U. Fitzky et al., "Cholesterol biosynthesis from lanosterol. Molecular cloning, tissue distribution, expression, chromosomal localization, and regulation of rat 7-dehydrocholesterol reductase, a Smith-Lemli-Opitz syndrome-related protein," *The Journal of Biological Chemistry*, vol. 274, no. 21, pp. 14624–14631, 1999.

[20] J. L. Gaylor, "Membrane-bound enzymes of cholesterol synthesis from lanosterol," *Biochemical and Biophysical Research Communications*, vol. 292, no. 5, pp. 1139–1146, 2002.

[21] J. L. Goldstein and M. S. Brown, "Regulation of the mevalonate pathway," *Nature*, vol. 343, no. 6257, pp. 425–430, 1990.

[22] G. J. Snipes and U. Suter, "Cholesterol and myelin," *Sub-Cellular Biochemistry*, vol. 28, pp. 173–204, 1997.

[23] P. Morell and H. Jurevics, "Origin of cholesterol in myelin," *Neurochemical Research*, vol. 21, no. 4, pp. 463–470, 1996.

[24] M. Martin, C. G. Dotti, and M. D. Ledesma, "Brain cholesterol in normal and pathological aging," *Biochimica et Biophysica Acta*, vol. 1801, no. 8, pp. 934–944, 2010.

[25] M. Andersson, P. G. Elmberger, C. Edlund, K. Kristensson, and G. Dallner, "Rates of cholesterol, ubiquinone, dolichol and dolichyl-P biosynthesis in rat brain slices," *FEBS Letters*, vol. 269, no. 1, pp. 15–18, 1990.

[26] I. Björkhem, M. Heverin, V. Leoni, S. Meaney, and U. Diczfalusy, "Oxysterols and Alzheimer's disease," *Acta Neurologica Scandinavica*, vol. 114, no. 185, pp. 43–49, 2006.

[27] J. M. Dietschy and S. D. Turley, "Cholesterol metabolism in the central nervous system during early development and in the mature animal," *Journal of Lipid Research*, vol. 45, no. 8, pp. 1375–1397, 2004.

[28] H. Waelsch, W. Sperry, and V. A. Stoyanoff, "A study of the synthesis and deposition of lipids in brain and other tissues with deuterium as an indicator," *The Journal of Biological Chemistry*, vol. 135, pp. 291–296, 1940.

[29] K. Bloch, B. N. Berg, and D. Rittenberg, "The biological conversion of cholesterol to cholic acid," *The Journal of Biological Chemistry*, vol. 149, pp. 511–517, 1943.

[30] H. Jurevics and P. Morell, "Cholesterol for synthesis of myelin is made locally, not imported into brain," *Journal of Neurochemistry*, vol. 64, no. 2, pp. 895–901, 1995.

[31] S. D. Turley, D. K. Burns, C. R. Rosenfeld, and J. M. Dietschy, "Brain does not utilize low density lipoprotein-cholesterol during fetal and neonatal development in the sheep," *Journal of Lipid Research*, vol. 37, no. 9, pp. 1953–1961, 1996.

[32] J. M. Dietschy and S. D. Turley, "Control of cholesterol turnover in the mouse," *The Journal of Biological Chemistry*, vol. 277, no. 6, pp. 3801–3804, 2002.

[33] T. Vanmierlo, O. Weingärtner, S. Van der Pol et al., "Dietary intake of plant sterols stably increases plant sterol levels in the murine brain," *The Journal of Lipid Research*, vol. 53, no. 4, pp. 726–735, 2012.

[34] A. V. Chobanian and W. Hollander, "Body cholesterol metabolism in man. I. The equilibration of serum and tissue cholesterol," *The Journal of clinical investigation*, vol. 41, pp. 1732–1737, 1962.

[35] D. Lütjohann, M. Stroick, T. Bertsch et al., "High doses of simvastatin, pravastatin, and cholesterol reduce brain cholesterol synthesis in guinea pigs," *Steroids*, vol. 69, no. 6, pp. 431–438, 2004.

[36] S. Meaney, D. Lütjohann, U. Diczfalusy, and I. Björkhem, "Formation of oxysterols from different pools of cholesterol as studied by stable isotope technique: cerebral origin of most circulating 24S-hydroxycholesterol in rats, but not in mice," *Biochimica et Biophysica Acta*, vol. 1486, no. 2-3, pp. 293–298, 2000.

[37] J. Herz and R. V. Farese Jr., "The LDL receptor gene family, apolipoprotein B and cholesterol in embryonic development," *Journal of Nutrition*, vol. 129, supplement 2S, 1999.

[38] H. A. Jurevics, F. Z. Kidwai, and P. Morell, "Sources of cholesterol during development of the rat fetus and fetal organs," *Journal of Lipid Research*, vol. 38, no. 4, pp. 723–733, 1997.

[39] E. D. Muse, H. Jurevics, A. D. Toews, G. K. Matsushima, and P. Morell, "Parameters related to lipid metabolism as markers of myelination in mouse brain," *Journal of Neurochemistry*, vol. 76, no. 1, pp. 77–86, 2001.

[40] G. Saher, B. Brügger, C. Lappe-Siefke et al., "High cholesterol level is essential for myelin membrane growth," *Nature Neuroscience*, vol. 8, no. 4, pp. 468–475, 2005.

[41] M. Ko, K. Zou, H. Minagawa et al., "Cholesterol-mediated neurite outgrowth is differently regulated between cortical and hippocampal neurons," *The Journal of Biological Chemistry*, vol. 280, no. 52, pp. 42759–42765, 2005.

[42] A. M. Pooler, S. C. Xi, and R. J. Wurtman, "The 3-hydroxy-3-methylglutaryl co-enzyme A reductase inhibitor pravastatin enhances neurite outgrowth in hippocampal neurons," *Journal of Neurochemistry*, vol. 97, no. 3, pp. 716–723, 2006.

[43] M. Saito, E. P. Benson, M. Saito, and A. Rosenberg, "Metabolism of cholesterol and triacylglycerol in cultured chick neuronal cells, glial cells, and fibroblasts: accumulation of esterified cholesterol in serum-free culture," *Journal of Neuroscience Research*, vol. 18, no. 2, pp. 319–325, 1987.

[44] S. Suzuki, K. Kiyosue, S. Hazama et al., "Brain-derived neurotrophic factor regulates cholesterol metabolism for synapse development," *Journal of Neuroscience*, vol. 27, no. 24, pp. 6417–6427, 2007.

[45] U. Fünfschilling, G. Saher, L. Xiao, W. Möbius, and K. A. Nave, "Survival of adult neurons lacking cholesterol synthesis in vivo," *BMC Neuroscience*, vol. 8, p. 1, 2007.

[46] F. W. Pfrieger, "Outsourcing in the brain: do neurons depend on cholesterol delivery by astrocytes?" *BioEssays*, vol. 25, no. 1, pp. 72–78, 2003.

[47] Z. Korade, Z. Mi, C. Portugal, and N. F. Schor, "Expression and p75 neurotrophin receptor dependence of cholesterol synthetic enzymes in adult mouse brain," *Neurobiology of Aging*, vol. 28, no. 10, pp. 1522–1531, 2007.

[48] W. Y. Ong, J. H. Kim, X. He, P. Chen, A. A. Farooqui, and A. M. Jenner, "Changes in brain cholesterol metabolome after excitotoxicity," *Molecular Neurobiology*, vol. 41, no. 2-3, pp. 299–313, 2010.

[49] Y. Zhang, E. L. Appelkvist, K. Kristensson, and G. Dallner, "The lipid compositions of different regions of rat brain during development and aging," *Neurobiology of Aging*, vol. 17, no. 6, pp. 869–875, 1996.

[50] G. Quan, C. Xie, J. M. Dietschy, and S. D. Turley, "Ontogenesis and regulation of cholesterol metabolism in the central nervous system of the mouse," *Developmental Brain Research*, vol. 146, no. 1-2, pp. 87–98, 2003.

[51] T. Numakawa, S. Suzuki, E. Kumamaru, N. Adachi, M. Richards, and H. Kunugi, "BDNF function and intracellular signaling in neurons," *Histology and Histopathology*, vol. 25, no. 2, pp. 237–258, 2010.

[52] H. Yu and S. B. Patel, "Recent insights into the Smith-Lemli-Opitz syndrome," *Clinical Genetics*, vol. 68, no. 5, pp. 383–391, 2005.

[53] P. E. Jira, H. R. Waterham, R. J. A. Wanders, J. A. M. Smeitink, R. C. A. Sengers, and R. A. Wevers, "Smith-Lemli-Opitz syndrome and the DHCR7 gene," *Annals of Human Genetics*, vol. 67, part 3, pp. 269–280, 2003.

[54] B. U. Fitzky, F. F. Moebius, H. Asaoka et al., "7-Dehydrocholesterol-dependent proteolysis of HMG-CoA reductase suppresses sterol biosynthesis in a mouse model of Smith-Lemli-Opitz/RSH syndrome," *Journal of Clinical Investigation*, vol. 108, no. 6, pp. 905–915, 2001.

[55] X. Xu, R. Bittman, G. Duportail, D. Heissler, C. Vilcheze, and E. London, "Effect of the structure of natural sterols and sphingolipids on the formation of ordered sphingolipid/sterol domains (rafts). Comparison of cholesterol to plant, fungal, and disease-associated sterols and comparison of sphingomyelin, cerebrosides, and ceramide," *The Journal of Biological Chemistry*, vol. 276, no. 36, pp. 33540–33546, 2001.

[56] S. Vainio, M. Jansen, M. Koivusalo et al., "Significance of sterol structural specificity: desmosterol cannot replace cholesterol in lipid rafts," *The Journal of Biological Chemistry*, vol. 281, no. 1, pp. 348–355, 2006.

[57] S. Ollila, M. T. Hyvönen, and I. Vattulainen, "Polyunsaturation in lipid membranes: dynamic properties and lateral pressure profiles," *Journal of Physical Chemistry B*, vol. 111, no. 12, pp. 3139–3150, 2007.

[58] P. Singh, Y. D. Paila, and A. Chattopadhyay, "Differential effects of cholesterol and 7-dehydrocholesterol on the ligand binding activity of the hippocampal serotonin1A receptor: implications in SLOS," *Biochemical and Biophysical Research Communications*, vol. 358, no. 2, pp. 495–499, 2007.

[59] V. Leoni, C. Mariotti, L. Nanetti et al., "Whole body cholesterol metabolism is impaired in Huntington's disease," *Neuroscience Letters*, vol. 494, no. 3, pp. 245–249, 2011.

[60] S. Sipione, D. Rigamonti, M. Valenza et al., "Early transcriptional profiles in huntingtin-induced striatal cells by

microarray analyses," *Human Molecular Genetics*, vol. 11, no. 17, pp. 1953–1965, 2002.

[61] M. Valenza, J. B. Carroll, V. Leoni et al., "Cholesterol biosynthesis pathway is disturbed in YAC128 mice and is modulated by huntingtin mutation," *Human Molecular Genetics*, vol. 16, no. 18, pp. 2187–2198, 2007.

[62] F. M. Harris, I. Tesseur, W. J. Brecht et al., "Astroglial regulation of apolipoprotein E expression in neuronal cells: implications for Alzheimer's disease," *The Journal of Biological Chemistry*, vol. 279, no. 5, pp. 3862–3868, 2004.

[63] Q. Xu, A. Bernardo, D. Walker, T. Kanegawa, R. W. Mahley, and Y. Huang, "Profile and regulation of apolipoprotein E (ApoE) expression in the CNS in mice with targeting of green fluorescent protein gene to the ApoE locus," *Journal of Neuroscience*, vol. 26, no. 19, pp. 4985–4994, 2006.

[64] I. Björkhem, D. Lütjohann, U. Diczfalusy, L. Ståhle, G. Ahlborg, and J. Wahren, "Cholesterol homeostasis in human brain: turnover of 24S-hydroxycholesterol and evidence for a cerebral origin of most of this oxysterol in the circulation," *Journal of Lipid Research*, vol. 39, no. 8, pp. 1594–1600, 1998.

[65] M. Heverin, S. Meaney, D. Lütjohann, U. Diczfalusy, J. Wahren, and I. Björkhem, "Crossing the barrier: net flux of 27-hydroxycholesterol into the human brain," *Journal of Lipid Research*, vol. 46, no. 5, pp. 1047–1052, 2005.

[66] S. Meaney, K. Bodin, U. Diczfalusy, and I. Björkhem, "On the rate of translocation in vitro and kinetics in vivo of the major oxysterols in human circulation: critical importance of the position of the oxygen function," *Journal of Lipid Research*, vol. 43, no. 12, pp. 2130–2135, 2002.

[67] D. Lütjohann, O. Breuer, G. Ahlborg et al., "Cholesterol homeostasis in human brain: evidence for an age-dependent flux of 24S-hydroxycholesterol from the brain into the circulation," *Proceedings of the National Academy of Sciences of the United States of America*, vol. 93, no. 18, pp. 9799–9804, 1996.

[68] I. Björkhem, A. Cedazo-Minguez, V. Leoni, and S. Meaney, "Oxysterols and neurodegenerative diseases," *Molecular Aspects of Medicine*, vol. 30, no. 3, pp. 171–179, 2009.

[69] I. Björkhem and U. Diczfalusy, "Oxysterols: friends, foes, or just fellow passengers?" *Arteriosclerosis, Thrombosis, and Vascular Biology*, vol. 22, no. 5, pp. 734–742, 2002.

[70] H. J. Senn, M. Orth, E. Fitzke, W. Koster, H. Wieland, and W. Gerok, "Human serum gangliosides in hypercholesterolemia, before and after extracorporeal elimination of LDL," *Atherosclerosis*, vol. 94, no. 2-3, pp. 109–117, 1992.

[71] H. J. Senn, M. Orth, E. Fitzke, H. Wieland, and W. Gerok, "Ganglioside in normal human serum. Concentration, pattern and transport by lipoproteins," *European Journal of Biochemistry*, vol. 181, no. 3, pp. 657–662, 1989.

[72] V. Leoni, T. Masterman, P. Patel, S. Meaney, U. Diczfalusy, and I. Björkhem, "Side chain oxidized oxysterols in cerebrospinal fluid and the integrity of blood-brain and blood-cerebrospinal fluid barriers," *Journal of Lipid Research*, vol. 44, no. 4, pp. 793–799, 2003.

[73] R. Lathe, "Steroid and sterol 7-hydroxylation: ancient pathways," *Steroids*, vol. 67, no. 12, pp. 967–977, 2002.

[74] C. Xie, D. K. Burns, S. D. Turley, and J. M. Dietschy, "Cholesterol is sequestered in the brains of mice with Niemann-Pick Type C disease but turnover is increased," *Journal of Neuropathology and Experimental Neurology*, vol. 59, no. 12, pp. 1106–1117, 2000.

[75] J. D. Wilson, "The measurement of the exchangeable pools of cholesterol in the baboon," *Journal of Clinical Investigation*, vol. 49, no. 4, pp. 655–665, 1970.

[76] E. G. Lund, J. M. Guileyardo, and D. W. Russell, "cDNA cloning of cholesterol 24-hydroxylase, a mediator of cholesterol homeostasis in the brain," *Proceedings of the National Academy of Sciences of the United States of America*, vol. 96, no. 13, pp. 7238–7243, 1999.

[77] L. Bretillon, U. Diczfalusy, I. Björkhem et al., "Cholesterol-24S-hydroxylase (CYP46A1) is specifically expressed in neurons of the neural retina," *Current Eye Research*, vol. 32, no. 4, pp. 361–366, 2007.

[78] E. G. Lund, C. Xie, T. Kotti, S. D. Turley, J. M. Dietschy, and D. W. Russell, "Knockout of the cholesterol 24-hydroxylase gene in mice reveals a brain-specific mechanism of cholesterol turnover," *The Journal of Biological Chemistry*, vol. 278, no. 25, pp. 22980–22988, 2003.

[79] B. A. Janowski, P. J. Willy, T. R. Devi, J. R. Falck, and D. J. Mangelsdorf, "An oxysterol signalling pathway mediated by the nuclear receptor LXRα," *Nature*, vol. 383, no. 6602, pp. 728–731, 1996.

[80] J. M. Lehmann, S. A. Kliewer, L. B. Moore et al., "Activation of the nuclear receptor LXR by oxysterols defines a new hormone response pathway," *The Journal of Biological Chemistry*, vol. 272, no. 6, pp. 3137–3140, 1997.

[81] J. Brown, C. Theisler, S. Silberman et al., "Differential expression of cholesterol hydroxylases in Alzheimer's disease," *The Journal of Biological Chemistry*, vol. 279, no. 33, pp. 34674–34681, 2004.

[82] K. D. Whitney, M. A. Watson, J. L. Collins et al., "Regulation of cholesterol homeostasis by the liver X receptors in the central nervous system," *Molecular Endocrinology*, vol. 16, no. 6, pp. 1378–1385, 2002.

[83] I. Björkhem, "Do oxysterols control cholesterol homeostasis?" *Journal of Clinical Investigation*, vol. 110, no. 6, pp. 725–730, 2002.

[84] L. Wang, G. U. Schuster, K. Hultenby, Q. Zhang, S. Andersson, and J. Å. Gustafsson, "Liver X receptors in the central nervous system: from lipid homeostasis to neuronal degeneration," *Proceedings of the National Academy of Sciences of the United States of America*, vol. 99, no. 21, pp. 13878–13883, 2002.

[85] M. G. Hall, L. Quignodon, and B. Desvergne, "Peroxisome proliferator-activated receptor β/δ in the brain: facts and hypothesis," *PPAR Research*, vol. 2008, Article ID 780452, 10 pages, 2008.

[86] L. Yue and T. Mazzone, "Peroxisome proliferator-activated receptor γ stimulation of adipocyte ApoE gene transcription mediated by the liver receptor X pathway," *The Journal of Biological Chemistry*, vol. 284, no. 16, pp. 10453–10461, 2009.

[87] A. Chawta, J. J. Repa, R. M. Evans, and D. J. Mangelsdorf, "Nuclear receptors and lipid physiology: opening the x-files," *Science*, vol. 294, no. 5548, pp. 1866–1870, 2001.

[88] B. Dehouck, M. P. Dehouck, J. C. Fruchart, and R. Cecchelli, "Upregulation of the low density lipoprotein receptor at the blood-brain barrier: intercommunications between brain capillary endothelial cells and astrocytes," *Journal of Cell Biology*, vol. 126, no. 2, pp. 465–473, 1994.

[89] D. Zambón, M. Quintana, P. Mata et al., "Higher incidence of mild cognitive impairment in familial hypercholesterolemia," *The American journal of medicine*, vol. 123, no. 3, pp. 267–274, 2010.

[90] G. L. Vega, M. F. Weiner, A. M. Lipton et al., "Reduction in levels of 24S-hydroxycholesterol by statin treatment in patients with Alzheimer disease," *Archives of Neurology*, vol. 60, no. 4, pp. 510–515, 2003.

[91] K. Fassbender, M. Stroick, T. Bertsch et al., "Effects of statins on human cerebral cholesterol metabolism and secretion of Alzheimer amyloid peptide," *Neurology*, vol. 59, no. 8, pp. 1257–1258, 2002.

[92] M. Simons, F. Schwärzler, D. Lütjohann et al., "Treatment with simvastatin in normocholesterolemic patients with Alzheimer's disease: a 26-week randomized, placebo-controlled, double-blind trial," *Annals of Neurology*, vol. 52, no. 3, pp. 346–350, 2002.

[93] S. Locatelli, D. Lütjohann, H. H. J. Schmidt, C. Otto, U. Beisiegel, and K. Von Bergmann, "Reduction of plasma 24S-hydroxycholesterol (cerebrosterol) levels using high-dosage simvastatin in patients with hypercholesterolemia: evidence that simvastatin affects cholesterol metabolism in the human brain," *Archives of Neurology*, vol. 59, no. 2, pp. 213–216, 2002.

[94] T. E. Willnow, J. Hilpert, S. A. Armstrong et al., "Defective forebrain development in mice lacking gp330/megalin," *Proceedings of the National Academy of Sciences of the United States of America*, vol. 93, no. 16, pp. 8460–8464, 1996.

[95] E. Roessler, E. Belloni, K. Gaudenz et al., "Mutations in the human Sonic Hedgehog gene cause holoprosencephaly," *Nature genetics*, vol. 14, no. 3, pp. 357–360, 1996.

[96] P. M. Lorusso, A. Jimeno, G. Dy et al., "Pharmacokinetic dose-scheduling study of hedgehog pathway inhibitor vismodegib (GDC-0449) in patients with locally advanced or metastatic solid tumors," *Clinical Cancer Research*, vol. 17, no. 17, pp. 5774–5782, 2011.

[97] P. W. Ingham, Y. Nakano, and C. Seger, "Mechanisms and functions of Hedgehog signalling across the metazoa," *Nature Reviews Genetics*, vol. 12, no. 6, pp. 393–406, 2011.

[98] J. I. Alvarez, A. Dodelet-Devillers, H. Kebir et al., "The Hedgehog pathway promotes blood-brain barrier integrity and CNS immune quiescence," *Science*, vol. 334, no. 6063, pp. 1727–1731, 2011.

[99] J. Herz, T. E. Willnow, and R. E. Farese, "Cholesterol, hedgehog and embryogenesis," *Nature Genetics*, vol. 15, no. 2, pp. 123–124, 1997.

[100] M. E. Baardman, J. J. Erwich, R. M. Berger et al., "The origin of fetal sterols in second-trimester amniotic fluid: endogenous synthesis or maternal-fetal transport?" *American Journal of Obstetrics and Gynecology*, vol. 207, no. 3, pp. 202.e19–202.e25, 2012.

[101] L. A. Woollett, "The origins and roles of cholesterol and fatty acids in the fetus," *Current Opinion in Lipidology*, vol. 12, no. 3, pp. 305–312, 2001.

[102] M. M. Véniant, E. Kim, S. McCormick et al., "Insights into apolipoprotein B biology from transgenic and gene-targeted mice," *Journal of Nutrition*, vol. 129, supplement 2S, pp. 451S–455S, 1999.

[103] M. Raabe, L. M. Flynn, C. H. Zlot et al., "Knockout of the abetalipoproteinemia gene in mice: reduced lipoprotein secretion in heterozygotes and embryonic lethality in homozygotes," *Proceedings of the National Academy of Sciences of the United States of America*, vol. 95, no. 15, pp. 8686–8691, 1998.

[104] Cholesterol Treatment Trialists C, C. Baigent, L. Blackwell et al., "Efficacy and safety of more intensive lowering of LDL cholesterol: a meta-analysis of data from 170, 000 participants in 26 randomised trials," *The Lancet*, vol. 376, no. 9753, pp. 1670–1681, 2010.

[105] N. E. Shepardson, G. M. Shankar, and D. J. Selkoe, "Cholesterol level and statin use in Alzheimer disease: II. review of human trials and recommendations," *Archives of Neurology*, vol. 68, no. 11, pp. 1385–1392, 2011.

[106] J. Z. Willey and M. S. V. Elkind, "3-Hydroxy-3-methylglutaryl-coenzyme A reductase inhibitors in the treatment of central nervous system diseases," *Archives of Neurology*, vol. 67, no. 9, pp. 1062–1067, 2010.

[107] K. M. Thelen, K. M. Rentsch, U. Gutteck et al., "Brain cholesterol synthesis in mice is affected by high dose of simvastatin but not of pravastatin," *Journal of Pharmacology and Experimental Therapeutics*, vol. 316, no. 3, pp. 1146–1152, 2006.

[108] D. L. Sparks, D. J. Connor, P. J. Browne, J. E. Lopez, and M. N. Sabbagh, "HMG-CoA reductase inhibitors (statins) in the treatment of Alzheimer's disease and why it would be ill-advise to use one that crosses the blood-brain barrier," *Journal of Nutrition, Health and Aging*, vol. 6, no. 5, pp. 324–331, 2002.

[109] I. Serbanescu, M. A. Ryan, R. Shukla, M. A. Cortez, O. C. Snead, and S. C. Cunnane, "Lovastatin exacerbates atypical absence seizures with only minimal effects on brain sterols," *Journal of Lipid Research*, vol. 45, no. 11, pp. 2038–2043, 2004.

[110] O. Maier, J. De Jonge, A. Nomden, D. Hoekstra, and W. Baron, "Lovastatin induces the formation of abnormal myelin-like membrane sheets in primary oligodendrocytes," *GLIA*, vol. 57, no. 4, pp. 402–413, 2009.

[111] B. McGuinness, J. O'Hare, D. Craig, R. Bullock, R. Malouf, and P. Passmore, "Cochrane review on 'statins for the treatment of dementia'," *International Journal of Geriatric Psychiatry*. In press.

[112] T. Yamamoto, C. G. Davis, and M. S. Brown, "The human LDL receptor: a cysteine-rich protein with multiple Alu sequences in its mRNA," *Cell*, vol. 39, no. 1, pp. 27–38, 1984.

[113] W. A. Banks and M. A. Erickson, "The blood-brain barrier and immune function and dysfunction," *Neurobiology of Disease*, vol. 37, no. 1, pp. 26–32, 2010.

[114] T. Beziaud, X. Ru Chen, N. El Shafey et al., "Simvastatin in traumatic brain injury: effect on brain edema mechanisms," *Crit Care Med*, vol. 39, no. 10, pp. 2300–2307, 2011.

[115] F. Guillot, P. Misslin, and M. Lemaire, "Comparison of fluvastatin and lovastatin blood-brain barrier transfer using in vitro and in vivo methods," *Journal of Cardiovascular Pharmacology*, vol. 21, no. 2, pp. 339–346, 1993.

[116] A. Saheki, T. Terasaki, I. Tamai, and A. Tsuji, "In vivo and in vitro blood-brain barrier transport of 3-hydroxy-3-methylglutaryl coenzyme A (HMG-CoA) reductase inhibitors," *Pharmaceutical Research*, vol. 11, no. 2, pp. 305–311, 1994.

[117] K. I. Nezasa, K. Higaki, T. Matsumura et al., "Liver-specific distribution of rosuvastatin in rats: comparison with pravastatin and simvastatin," *Drug Metabolism and Disposition*, vol. 30, no. 11, pp. 1158–1163, 2002.

[118] N. Kandiah and H. H. Feldman, "Therapeutic potential of statins in Alzheimer's disease," *Journal of the Neurological Sciences*, vol. 283, no. 1-2, pp. 230–234, 2009.

[119] R. H. Knopp, "Drug treatment of lipid disorders," *The New England Journal of Medicine*, vol. 341, no. 7, pp. 498–511, 1999.

[120] A. Tsuji, A. Saheki, I. Tamai, and T. Terasaki, "Transport mechanism of 3-hydroxy-3-methylglutaryl coenzyme A reductase inhibitors at the blood-brain barrier," *Journal of Pharmacology and Experimental Therapeutics*, vol. 267, no. 3, pp. 1085–1090, 1993.

[121] R. M. Uranga and J. N. Keller, "Diet and age interactions with regards to cholesterol regulation and brain pathogenesis,"

Current Gerontology and Geriatrics Research, vol. 2010, Article ID 219683, 14 pages, 2010.

[122] T. Mailman, M. Hariharan, and B. Karten, "Inhibition of neuronal cholesterol biosynthesis with lovastatin leads to impaired synaptic vesicle release even in the presence of lipoproteins or geranylgeraniol," *Journal of Neurochemistry*, vol. 119, no. 5, pp. 1002–1015, 2011.

[123] M. C. Patterson, A. M. Di Bisceglie, J. J. Higgins et al., "The effect of cholesterol-lowering agents on hepatic and plasma cholesterol in Niemann-Pick disease type C," *Neurology*, vol. 43, no. 1, pp. 61–64, 1993.

[124] B. Liu, H. Li, J. J. Repa, S. D. Turley, and J. M. Dietschy, "Genetic variations and treatments that affect the lifespan of the NPC1 mouse," *Journal of Lipid Research*, vol. 49, no. 3, pp. 663–669, 2008.

[125] I. Bohr, "Hypercholesterolemic diet applied to rat dams protects their offspring against cognitive deficits. Simulated neonatal anoxia model," *Physiology and Behavior*, vol. 82, no. 4, pp. 703–711, 2004.

[126] B. G. Schreurs, "The effects of cholesterol on learning and memory," *Neuroscience and Biobehavioral Reviews*, vol. 34, no. 8, pp. 1366–1379, 2010.

[127] R. A. Whitmer, S. Sidney, J. Selby, S. Claiborne Johnston, and K. Yaffe, "Midlife cardiovascular risk factors and risk of dementia in late life," *Neurology*, vol. 64, no. 2, pp. 277–281, 2005.

[128] K. Yaffe, E. Barrett-Connor, F. Lin, and D. Grady, "Serum lipoprotein levels, statin use, and cognitive function in older women," *Archives of Neurology*, vol. 59, no. 3, pp. 378–384, 2002.

[129] A. Solomon, I. Kåreholt, T. Ngandu et al., "Serum cholesterol changes after midlife and late-life cognition: twenty-one-year follow-up study," *Neurology*, vol. 68, no. 10, pp. 751–756, 2007.

[130] J. Näslund, V. Haroutunian, R. Mohs et al., "Correlation between elevated levels of amyloid β-peptide in the brain and cognitive decline," *Journal of the American Medical Association*, vol. 283, no. 12, pp. 1571–1577, 2000.

[131] M. Kivipelto, E. L. Helkala, T. Hänninen et al., "Midlife vascular risk factors and late-life mild cognitive impairment: a population-based study," *Neurology*, vol. 56, no. 12, pp. 1683–1689, 2001.

[132] M. M. Mielke, P. P. Zandi, M. Sjögren et al., "High total cholesterol levels in late life associated with a reduced risk of dementia," *Neurology*, vol. 64, no. 10, pp. 1689–1695, 2005.

[133] L. A. Perry, C. B. Stigger, B. E. Ainsworth, and J. Zhang, "No association between cognitive achievements, academic performance and serum cholesterol concentrations among school-aged children," *Nutritional Neuroscience*, vol. 12, no. 4, pp. 160–166, 2009.

[134] M. F. Muldoon, C. M. Ryan, S. M. Sereika, J. D. Flory, and S. B. Manuck, "Randomized trial of the effects of simvastatin on cognitive functioning in hypercholesterolemic adults," *American Journal of Medicine*, vol. 117, no. 11, pp. 823–829, 2004.

[135] M. F. Muldoon, S. D. Barger, C. M. Ryan et al., "Effects of lovastatin on cognitive function and psychological well-being," *American Journal of Medicine*, vol. 108, no. 7, pp. 538–546, 2000.

[136] S. Trompet, P. Van Vliet, A. J. M. De Craen et al., "Pravastatin and cognitive function in the elderly. Results of the PROSPER study," *Journal of Neurology*, vol. 257, no. 1, pp. 85–90, 2010.

[137] FDA and US Food and Drug Administration, "FDA Drug Safety Communication: Important safety label changes to cholesterol-lowering statin drugs 2012," http://www.fda.gov/Drugs/DrugSafety/ucm293101.htm?utm_source=fdaSearch&utm_medium=website&utm_term=safety%20changes%20to%20cholesterol-lowering%20statin%20drugs&utm_content=1, 2012.

[138] Z. Arvanitakis, J. A. Schneider, R. S. Wilson et al., "Statins, incident Alzheimer disease, change in cognitive function, and neuropathology," *Neurology*, vol. 70, no. 19, part 2, pp. 1795–1802, 2008.

[139] M. D. M. Haag, A. Hofman, P. J. Koudstaal, B. H. C. Stricker, and M. M. B. Breteler, "Statins are associated with a reduced risk of Alzheimer disease regardless of lipophilicity. The Rotterdam Study," *Journal of Neurology, Neurosurgery and Psychiatry*, vol. 80, no. 1, pp. 13–17, 2009.

[140] T. D. Rea, J. C. Breitner, B. M. Psaty et al., "Statin use and the risk of incident dementia: the Cardiovascular Health Study," *Archives of Neurology*, vol. 62, no. 7, pp. 1047–1051, 2005.

[141] W. Dong, S. Vuletic, and J. J. Albers, "Differential effects of simvastatin and pravastatin on expression of Alzheimer's disease-related genes in human astrocytes and neuronal cells," *Journal of Lipid Research*, vol. 50, no. 10, pp. 2095–2102, 2009.

[142] S. L. Cole, A. Grudzien, I. O. Manhart, B. L. Kelly, H. Oakley, and R. Vassar, "Statins cause intracellular accumulation of amyloid precursor protein, β-secretase-cleaved fragments, and amyloid β-peptide via an isoprenoid-dependent mechanism," *The Journal of Biological Chemistry*, vol. 280, no. 19, pp. 18755–18770, 2005.

[143] F. Lu, X. Li, A. Q. Suo, and J. W. Zhang, "Inhibition of tau hyperphosphorylation and beta amyloid production in rat brain by oral administration of atorvastatin," *Chinese Medical Journal*, vol. 123, no. 14, pp. 1864–1870, 2010.

[144] T. Kurata, K. Miyazaki, M. Kozuki et al., "Atorvastatin and pitavastatin improve cognitive function and reduce senile plaque and phosphorylated tau in aged APP mice," *Brain Research*, vol. 1371, no. C, pp. 161–170, 2011.

[145] A. Serrano-Pozo, G. L. Vega, D. Lütjohann et al., "Effects of simvastatin on cholesterol metabolism and Alzheimer disease biomarkers," *Alzheimer Disease and Associated Disorders*, vol. 24, no. 3, pp. 220–226, 2010.

[146] H. H. Feldman, R. S. Doody, M. Kivipelto et al., "Randomized controlled trial of atorvastatin in mild to moderate Alzheimer disease: LEADe," *Neurology*, vol. 74, no. 12, pp. 956–964, 2010.

[147] N. Sato, M. Shinohara, H. Rakugi et al., "Dual effects of statins on Abeta metabolism: upregulation of the degradation of APP-CTF and Abeta clearance," *Neurodegenerative Diseases*, vol. 10, no. 1–4, pp. 305–308, 2012.

[148] M. S. V. Elkind, A. C. Flint, R. R. Sciacca, and R. L. Sacco, "Lipid-lowering agent use at ischemic stroke onset is associated with decreased mortality," *Neurology*, vol. 65, no. 2, pp. 253–258, 2005.

[149] M. Blanco, F. Nombela, M. Castellanos et al., "Statin treatment withdrawal in ischemic stroke: a controlled randomized study," *Neurology*, vol. 69, no. 9, pp. 904–910, 2007.

[150] M. S. V. Elkind, R. L. Sacco, R. B. Macarthur et al., "The Neuroprotection with Statin Therapy for Acute Recovery Trial (NeuSTART): an adaptive design phase I dose-escalation study of high-dose lovastatin in acute ischemic stroke," *International Journal of Stroke*, vol. 3, no. 3, pp. 210–218, 2008.

[151] J. J. Cui, D. Wang, F. Gao et al., "Effects of atorvastatin on pathological changes in brain tissue and plasma MMP-9 in

rats with intracerebral hemorrhage," *Cell Biochemistry and Biophysics*, vol. 62, no. 1, pp. 87–90, 2012.

[152] M. J. Ignatius, P. J. Gebicke-Harter, and J. H. P. Skene, "Expression of apolipoprotein E during nerve degeneration and regeneration," *Proceedings of the National Academy of Sciences of the United States of America*, vol. 83, no. 4, pp. 1125–1129, 1986.

[153] R. E. Pitas, J. K. Boyles, and S. H. Lee, "Astrocytes synthesize apolipoprotein E and metabolize apolipoprotein E-containing lipoproteins," *Biochimica et Biophysica Acta*, vol. 917, no. 1, pp. 148–161, 1987.

[154] B. A. Evans, J. E. Evans, S. P. Baker et al., "Long-term statin therapy and CSF cholesterol levels: implications for alzheimer's disease," *Dementia and Geriatric Cognitive Disorders*, vol. 27, no. 6, pp. 519–524, 2009.

[155] A. Von Eckardstein, Y. Huang, J. J. P. Kastelein et al., "Lipid-free apolipoprotein (apo) A-I is converted into alpha-migrating high density lipoproteins by lipoprotein-depleted plasma of normolipidemic donors and apo A-I-deficient patients but not of Tangier disease patients," *Atherosclerosis*, vol. 138, no. 1, pp. 25–34, 1998.

[156] S. Bellosta, B. P. Nathan, M. Orth, L. M. Dong, R. W. Mahley, and R. E. Pitas, "Stable expression and secretion of apolipoproteins E3 and E4 in mouse neuroblastoma cells produces differential effects on neurite outgrowth," *The Journal of Biological Chemistry*, vol. 270, no. 45, pp. 27063–27071, 1995.

[157] M. J. LaDu, S. M. Gilligan, J. R. Lukens et al., "Nascent astrocyte particles differ from lipoproteins in CSF," *Journal of Neurochemistry*, vol. 70, no. 5, pp. 2070–2081, 1998.

[158] M. Buttini, M. Orth, S. Bellosta et al., "Expression of human apolipoprotein E3 or E4 in the brains of Apoe(-/-) mice: isoform-specific effects on neurodegeneration," *Journal of Neuroscience*, vol. 19, no. 12, pp. 4867–4880, 1999.

[159] C. Pottier, D. Hannequin, S. Coutant et al., "High frequency of potentially pathogenic SORL1 mutations in autosomal dominant early-onset Alzheimer disease," *Molecular Psychiatry*, vol. 17, no. 9, pp. 875–879, 2012.

[160] M. J. Ignatius, E. M. Shooter, R. E. Pitas, and R. W. Mahley, "Lipoprotein uptake by neuronal growth cones in vitro," *Science*, vol. 236, no. 4804, pp. 950–962, 1987.

[161] R. Spoelgen, A. Hammes, U. Anzenberger et al., "LRP2/megalin is required for patterning of the ventral telencephalon," *Development*, vol. 132, no. 2, pp. 405–414, 2005.

[162] I. Hack, S. Hellwig, D. Junghans et al., "Divergent roles of ApoER2 and Vldlr in the migration of cortical neurons," *Development*, vol. 134, no. 21, pp. 3883–3891, 2007.

[163] J. Herz and Y. Chen, "Reelin, lipoprotein receptors and synaptic plasticity," *Nature Reviews Neuroscience*, vol. 7, no. 11, pp. 850–859, 2006.

[164] M. S. Durakoglugil, Y. Chen, C. L. White, E. T. Kavalali, and J. Herz, "Reelin signaling antagonizes β-amyloid at the synapse," *Proceedings of the National Academy of Sciences of the United States of America*, vol. 106, no. 37, pp. 15938–15943, 2009.

[165] T. Witzlack, T. Wenzeck, J. Thiery, and M. Orth, "cAMP-induced expression of ABCA1 is associated with MAP-kinase-pathway activation," *Biochemical and Biophysical Research Communications*, vol. 363, no. 1, pp. 89–94, 2007.

[166] M. Larouche, U. Beffert, J. Herz, and R. Hawkes, "The reelin receptors Apoer2 and Vldlr coordinate the patterning of purkinje cell topography in the developing mouse cerebellum," *PLoS ONE*, vol. 3, no. 2, Article ID e1653, 2008.

[167] Y. Zong, B. Zhang, S. Gu et al., "Structural basis of agrin-LRP4-MuSK signaling," *Genes & Development*, vol. 26, no. 3, pp. 247–258, 2012.

[168] S. Kantarci, L. Al-Gazali, R. S. Hill et al., "Mutations in LRP2, which encodes the multiligand receptor megalin, cause Donnai-Barrow and facio-oculo-acoustico-renal syndromes," *Nature Genetics*, vol. 39, no. 8, pp. 957–959, 2007.

[169] K. M. Boycott, C. Bonnemann, J. Herz et al., "Mutations in VLDLR as a cause for autosomal recessive cerebellar ataxia with mental retardation (*Dysequilibrium syndrome*)," *Journal of Child Neurology*, vol. 24, no. 10, pp. 1310–1315, 2009.

[170] K. M. Boycott, S. Flavelle, A. Bureau et al., "Homozygous deletion of the very low density lipoprotein receptor gene causes autosomal recessive cerebellar hypoplasia with cerebral gyral simplification," *American Journal of Human Genetics*, vol. 77, no. 3, pp. 477–483, 2005.

[171] T. Ozcelik, N. Akarsu, E. Uz et al., "Mutations in the very low-density lipoprotein receptor VLDLR cause cerebellar hypoplasia and quadrupedal locomotion in humans," *Proceedings of the National Academy of Sciences of the United States of America*, vol. 105, no. 11, pp. 4232–4236, 2008.

[172] T. J. Park and T. Curran, "Crk and Crk-like play essential overlapping roles downstream of disabled-1 in the reelin pathway," *Journal of Neuroscience*, vol. 28, no. 50, pp. 13551–13562, 2008.

[173] G. E. Handelmann, J. K. Boyles, K. H. Weisgraber, R. W. Mahley, and R. E. Pitas, "Effects of apolipoprotein E, β-very low density lipoproteins, and cholesterol on the extension of neurites by rabbit dorsal root ganglion neurons in vitro," *Journal of Lipid Research*, vol. 33, no. 11, pp. 1677–1688, 1992.

[174] M. Orth, W. Weng, H. Funke et al., "Effects of a frequent apolipoprotein E isoform, apoE4(Freiburg) (Leu28 → Pro), on lipoproteins and the prevalence of coronary artery disease in Whites," *Arteriosclerosis, Thrombosis, and Vascular Biology*, vol. 19, no. 5, pp. 1306–1315, 1999.

[175] R. W. Mahley, "Apolipoprotein E: Cholesterol transport protein with expanding role in cell biology," *Science*, vol. 240, no. 4852, pp. 622–630, 1988.

[176] D. K. Lahiri, "Apolipoprotein E as a target for developing new therapeutics for Alzheimer's disease based on studies from protein, RNA, and regulatory region of the gene," *Journal of Molecular Neuroscience*, vol. 23, no. 3, pp. 225–233, 2004.

[177] M. F. Linton, R. Gish, S. T. Hubl et al., "Phenotypes of apolipoprotein B and apolipoprotein E after liver transplantation," *Journal of Clinical Investigation*, vol. 88, no. 1, pp. 270–281, 1991.

[178] R. W. Mahley, K. H. Weisgraber, and Y. Huang, "Apolipoprotein E4: a causative factor and therapeutic target in neuropathology, including Alzheimer's disease," *Proceedings of the National Academy of Sciences of the United States of America*, vol. 103, no. 15, pp. 5644–5651, 2006.

[179] X. Pu-Ting, J. R. Gilbert, Q. Hui-Ling et al., "Specific regional transcription of apolipoprotein E in human brain neurons," *American Journal of Pathology*, vol. 154, no. 2, pp. 601–611, 1999.

[180] S. E. Wahrle, H. Jiang, M. Parsadanian et al., "ABCA1 is required for normal central nervous system apoE levels and for lipidation of astrocyte-secreted apoE," *The Journal of Biological Chemistry*, vol. 279, no. 39, pp. 40987–40993, 2004.

[181] V. Hirsch-Reinshagen, L. F. Maia, B. L. Burgess et al., "The absence of ABCA1 decreases soluble ApoE levels but does not diminish amyloid deposition in two murine models of Alzheimer disease," *The Journal of Biological Chemistry*, vol. 280, no. 52, pp. 43243–43256, 2005.

[182] Q. Liu, C. V. Zerbinatti, J. Zhang et al., "Amyloid precursor protein regulates brain apolipoprotein E and cholesterol metabolism through lipoprotein receptor LRP1," *Neuron*, vol. 56, no. 1, pp. 66–78, 2007.

[183] R. Anderson, J. C. Barnes, T. V. P. Bliss et al., "Behavioural, physiological and morphological analysis of a line of apolipoprotein E knockout mouse," *Neuroscience*, vol. 85, no. 1, pp. 93–110, 1998.

[184] A. M. Fagan, B. A. Murphy, S. N. Patel et al., "Evidence for normal aging of the septo-hippocampal cholinergic system in apoE (-/-) mice but impaired clearance of axonal degeneration products following injury," *Experimental Neurology*, vol. 151, no. 2, pp. 314–325, 1998.

[185] D. M. Holtzman, J. Herz, and G. Bu, "Apolipoprotein E and apolipoprotein E receptors: normal biology and roles in Alzheimer disease," *Cold Spring Harb Perspect Med*, vol. 2, no. 3, Article ID a006312, 2012.

[186] E. H. Corder, A. M. Saunders, W. J. Strittmatter et al., "Gene dose of apolipoprotein E type 4 allele and the risk of Alzheimer's disease in late onset families," *Science*, vol. 261, no. 5123, pp. 921–923, 1993.

[187] W. J. Strittmatter, A. M. Saunders, D. Schmechel et al., "Apolipoprotein E: high-avidity binding to β-amyloid and increased frequency of type 4 allele in late-onset familial Alzheimer disease," *Proceedings of the National Academy of Sciences of the United States of America*, vol. 90, no. 5, pp. 1977–1981, 1993.

[188] D. E. Schmechel, A. M. Saunders, W. J. Strittmatter et al., "Increased amyloid β-peptide deposition in cerebral cortex as a consequence of apolipoprotein E genotype in late-onset Alzheimer disease," *Proceedings of the National Academy of Sciences of the United States of America*, vol. 90, no. 20, pp. 9649–9653, 1993.

[189] A. Ward, S. Crean, C. J. Mercaldi et al., "Prevalence of apolipoprotein E4 genotype and homozygotes (APOE e4/4) among patients diagnosed with Alzheimer's disease: a systematic review and meta-analysis," *Neuroepidemiology*, vol. 38, no. 1, pp. 1–17, 2012.

[190] D. Blacker, J. L. Haines, L. Rodes et al., "ApoE-4 and age at onset of Alzheimer's disease: the NIMH genetics initiative," *Neurology*, vol. 48, no. 1, pp. 139–147, 1997.

[191] W. J. Strittmatter, "Medicine. Old drug, new hope for Alzheimer's disease," *Science*, vol. 335, no. 6075, pp. 1447–1448, 2012.

[192] D. M. Hatters, C. A. Peters-Libeu, and K. H. Weisgraber, "Apolipoprotein E structure: insights into function," *Trends in Biochemical Sciences*, vol. 31, no. 8, pp. 445–454, 2006.

[193] G. Ramaswamy, Q. Xu, Y. Huang, and K. H. Weisgraber, "Effect of domain interaction on apolipoprotein E levels in mouse brain," *Journal of Neuroscience*, vol. 25, no. 46, pp. 10658–10663, 2005.

[194] N. Zhong and K. H. Weisgraber, "Understanding the association of apolipoprotein E4 with Alzheimer disease: clues from its structure," *The Journal of Biological Chemistry*, vol. 284, no. 10, pp. 6027–6031, 2009.

[195] A. K. Dunker, C. J. Oldfield, J. Meng et al., "The unfoldomics decade: an update on intrinsically disordered proteins," *BMC Genomics*, vol. 9, supplement 2, p. S1, 2008.

[196] D. A. Sanan, K. H. Weisgraber, S. J. Russell et al., "Apolipoprotein E associates with β amyloid peptide of Alzheimer's disease to form novel monofibrils. Isoform ApoE4 associates more efficiently than ApoE3," *Journal of Clinical Investigation*, vol. 94, no. 2, pp. 860–869, 1994.

[197] M. J. LaDu, M. T. Falduto, A. M. Manelli, C. A. Reardon, G. S. Getz, and D. E. Frail, "Isoform-specific binding of apolipoprotein E to β-amyloid," *The Journal of Biological Chemistry*, vol. 269, no. 38, pp. 23403–23406, 1994.

[198] S. Aleshkov, C. R. Abraham, and V. I. Zannis, "Interaction of nascent apoe2, apoe3, and apoe4 isoforms expressed in mammalian cells with amyloid peptide β (1-40). Relevance to Alzheimer's disease," *Biochemistry*, vol. 36, no. 34, pp. 10571–10580, 1997.

[199] Q. Jiang, C. Y. D. Lee, S. Mandrekar et al., "ApoE promotes the proteolytic degradation of Aβ," *Neuron*, vol. 58, no. 5, pp. 681–693, 2008.

[200] R. B. DeMattos, J. R. Cirrito, M. Parsadanian et al., "ApoE and clusterin cooperatively suppress Aβ levels and deposition: evidence that ApoE regulates extracellular Aβ metabolism in vivo," *Neuron*, vol. 41, no. 2, pp. 193–202, 2004.

[201] R. D. Bell, A. P. Sagare, A. E. Friedman et al., "Transport pathways for clearance of human Alzheimer's amyloid β-peptide and apolipoproteins E and J in the mouse central nervous system," *Journal of Cerebral Blood Flow and Metabolism*, vol. 27, no. 5, pp. 909–918, 2007.

[202] B. V. Zlokovic, "The blood-brain barrier in health and chronic neurodegenerative disorders," *Neuron*, vol. 57, no. 2, pp. 178–201, 2008.

[203] C. Frieden and K. Garai, "Structural differences between apoE3 and apoE4 may be useful in developing therapeutic agents for Alzheimer's disease," *Proceedings of the National Academy of Sciences of the United States of America*, vol. 109, no. 23, pp. 8913–8918, 2012.

[204] C. A. Peters-Libeu, Y. Newhouse, D. M. Hatters, and K. H. Weisgraber, "Model of biologically active apolipoprotein E bound to dipalmitoylphosphatidylcholine," *The Journal of Biological Chemistry*, vol. 281, no. 2, pp. 1073–1079, 2006.

[205] C. Wilson, M. R. Wardell, K. H. Weisgraber, R. W. Mahley, and D. A. Agard, "Three-dimensional structure of the LDL receptor-binding domain of human apolipoprotein E," *Science*, vol. 252, no. 5014, pp. 1817–1822, 1991.

[206] A. Sivashanmugan and J. Wang, "A unified scheme for initiation and conformational adaptation of human apolipoprotein E N-terminal domain upon lipoprotein binding and for receptor binding activity," *The Journal of Biological Chemistry*, vol. 284, no. 21, pp. 14657–14666, 2009.

[207] H. K. Chen, Z. S. Ji, S. E. Dodson et al., "Apolipoprotein E4 domain interaction mediates detrimental effects on mitochondria and is a potential therapeutic target for alzheimer disease," *The Journal of Biological Chemistry*, vol. 286, no. 7, pp. 5215–5221, 2011.

[208] R. D. Bell, E. A. Winkler, I. Singh et al., "Apolipoprotein E controls cerebrovascular integrity via cyclophilin A," *Nature*, vol. 485, no. 7399, pp. 512–516, 2012.

[209] P. E. Cramer, J. R. Cirrito, D. W. Wesson et al., "ApoE-directed therapeutics rapidly clear beta-amyloid and reverse deficits in AD mouse models," *Science*, vol. 335, no. 6075, pp. 1503–1506, 2012.

[210] M. P. Vitek, D. J. Christensen, D. Wilcock et al., "APOE-mimetic peptides reduce behavioral deficits, plaques and tangles in Alzheimer's disease transgenics," *Neurodegenerative Diseases*, vol. 10, no. 1–4, pp. 122–126, 2012.

[211] J. R. Lynch, W. Tang, H. Wang et al., "APOE genotype and an ApoE-mimetic peptide modify the systemic and central nervous system inflammatory response," *The Journal of Biological Chemistry*, vol. 278, no. 49, pp. 48529–48533, 2003.

[212] T. Nuutinen, T. Suuronen, A. Kauppinen, and A. Salminen, "Clusterin: a forgotten player in Alzheimer's disease," *Brain Research Reviews*, vol. 61, no. 2, pp. 89–104, 2009.

[213] Y. Charnay, A. Imhof, P. G. Vallet et al., "Clusterin expression during fetal and postnatal CNS development in mouse," *Neuroscience*, vol. 155, no. 3, pp. 714–724, 2008.

[214] A. Iwata, K. D. Browne, X. H. Chen, T. Yuguchi, and D. H. Smith, "Traumatic brain injury induces biphasic upregulation of ApoE and ApoJ protein in rats," *Journal of Neuroscience Research*, vol. 82, no. 1, pp. 103–114, 2005.

[215] H. V. De Silva, J. A. K. Harmony, W. D. Stuart, C. M. Gil, and J. Robbins, "Apolipoprotein J: structure and tissue distribution," *Biochemistry*, vol. 29, no. 22, pp. 5380–5389, 1990.

[216] R. W. Bailey, A. K. Dunker, C. J. Brown, E. C. Garner, and M. D. Griswold, "Clusterin, a binding protein with a molten globule-like region," *Biochemistry*, vol. 40, no. 39, pp. 11828–11840, 2001.

[217] G. M. Cole and M. D. Ard, "Influence of lipoproteins on microglial degradation of Alzheimer's amyloid beta-protein," *Microscopy Research and Technique*, vol. 50, no. 4, pp. 316–324, 2000.

[218] M. Shibata, S. Yamada, S. Ram Kumar et al., "Clearance of Alzheimer's amyloid-β1-40 peptide from brain by LDL receptor-related protein-1 at the blood-brain barrier," *Journal of Clinical Investigation*, vol. 106, no. 12, pp. 1489–1499, 2000.

[219] R. D. Bell, R. Deane, N. Chow et al., "SRF and myocardin regulate LRP-mediated amyloid-β clearance in brain vascular cells," *Nature Cell Biology*, vol. 11, no. 2, pp. 143–153, 2009.

[220] D. Lütjohann, S. Meichsner, and H. Pettersson, "Lipids in Alzheimer's disease and their potential for therapy," *Journal of Clinical Lipidology*, vol. 7, no. 1, pp. 65–78, 2012.

[221] J. Popp, P. Lewczuk, H. Kölsch et al., "Cholesterol metabolism is associated with soluble amyloid precursor protein production in Alzheimer's disease," *Journal of Neurochemistry*, vol. 123, no. 2, pp. 310–316, 2012.

[222] S. Ye, Y. Huang, K. Müllendorff et al., "Apolipoprotein (apo) E4 enhances amyloid β peptide production in cultured neuronal cells: ApoE structure as a potential therapeutic target," *Proceedings of the National Academy of Sciences of the United States of America*, vol. 102, no. 51, pp. 18700–18705, 2005.

[223] N. Marks and M. J. Berg, "BACE and γ-secretase characterization and their sorting as therapeutic targets to reduce amyloidogenesis," *Neurochemical Research*, vol. 35, no. 2, pp. 181–210, 2010.

[224] H. S. Hoe, D. Wessner, U. Beffert, A. G. Becker, Y. Matsuoka, and G. W. Rebeck, "F-spondin interaction with the apolipoprotein E receptor ApoEr2 affects processing of amyloid precursor protein," *Molecular and Cellular Biology*, vol. 25, no. 21, pp. 9259–9268, 2005.

[225] A. Rietveld and K. Simons, "The differential miscibility of lipids as the basis for the formation of functional membrane rafts," *Biochimica et Biophysica Acta*, vol. 1376, no. 3, pp. 467–479, 1998.

[226] M. Koistinaho, S. Lin, X. Wu et al., "Apolipoprotein E promotes astrocyte colocalization and degradation of deposited amyloid-β peptides," *Nature Medicine*, vol. 10, no. 7, pp. 719–726, 2004.

[227] J. El Khoury and A. D. Luster, "Mechanisms of microglia accumulation in Alzheimer's disease: therapeutic implications," *Trends in Pharmacological Sciences*, vol. 29, no. 12, pp. 626–632, 2008.

[228] L. M. Billings, S. Oddo, K. N. Green, J. L. McGaugh, and F. M. LaFerla, "Intraneuronal Aβ causes the onset of early Alzheimer's disease-related cognitive deficits in transgenic mice," *Neuron*, vol. 45, no. 5, pp. 675–688, 2005.

[229] K. R. Bales, T. Verina, R. C. Dodel et al., "Lack of apolipoprotein E dramatically reduces amyloid beta-peptide deposition," *Nature genetics*, vol. 17, no. 3, pp. 263–264, 1997.

[230] J. Abad-Rodriguez, M. D. Ledesma, K. Craessaerts et al., "Neuronal membrane cholesterol loss enhances amyloid peptide generation," *Journal of Cell Biology*, vol. 167, no. 5, pp. 953–960, 2004.

[231] C. Kaether and C. Haass, "A lipid boundary separates APP and secretases and limits amyloid β-peptide generation," *Journal of Cell Biology*, vol. 167, no. 5, pp. 809–812, 2004.

[232] M. Simons, P. Keller, B. De Strooper, K. Beyreuther, C. G. Dotti, and K. Simons, "Cholesterol depletion inhibits the generation of β-amyloid in hippocampal neurons," *Proceedings of the National Academy of Sciences of the United States of America*, vol. 95, no. 11, pp. 6460–6464, 1998.

[233] R. Ehehalt, P. Keller, C. Haass, C. Thiele, and K. Simons, "Amyloidogenic processing of the Alzheimer β-amyloid precursor protein depends on lipid rafts," *Journal of Cell Biology*, vol. 160, no. 1, pp. 113–123, 2003.

4

Current Views on Genetics and Epigenetics of Cholesterol Gallstone Disease

Agostino Di Ciaula,[1] David Q.-H. Wang,[2] Leonilde Bonfrate,[3] and Piero Portincasa[3,4]

[1] *Division of Internal Medicine Hospital of Bisceglie, 76011 Bisceglie, Italy*
[2] *Saint Louis University School of Medicine, Division of Gastroenterology and Hepatology, Department of Internal Medicine, Edward Doisy Research Center, St. Louis, MO 63104, USA*
[3] *Clinica Medica "A. Murri", Department of Biomedical Sciences & Human Oncology, University "Aldo Moro" of Bari Medical School, 70124 Bari, Italy*
[4] *European Society for Clinical Investigation (ESCI), 3584 CJ Utrecht, The Netherlands*

Correspondence should be addressed to Piero Portincasa; piero.portincasa@uniba.it

Academic Editor: Gloria L. Vega

Cholesterol gallstone disease, one of the commonest digestive diseases in western countries, is induced by an imbalance in cholesterol metabolism, which involves intestinal absorption, hepatic biosynthesis, and biliary output of cholesterol, and its conversion to bile acids. Several components of the metabolic syndrome (e.g., obesity, type 2 diabetes, dyslipidemia, and hyperinsulinemia) are also well-known risk factors for gallstones, suggesting the existence of interplay between common pathophysiological pathways influenced by insulin resistance, genetic, epigenetic, and environmental factors. Cholesterol gallstones may be enhanced, at least in part, by the abnormal expression of a set of the genes that affect cholesterol homeostasis and lead to insulin resistance. Additionally, epigenetic mechanisms (mainly DNA methylation, histone acetylation/deacetylation, and noncoding microRNAs) may modify gene expression in the absence of an altered DNA sequence, in response to different lithogenic environmental stimuli, such as diet, lifestyle, pollutants, also occurring *in utero* before birth. In this review, we will comment on various steps of the pathogenesis of cholesterol gallstones and interaction between environmental and genetic factors. The epigenomic approach may offer new options for therapy of gallstones and better possibilities for primary prevention in subjects at risk.

1. Introduction

Cholesterol gallstone disease is one of the most prevalent and most costly digestive diseases requiring hospital admission, since its prevalence ranges from 10% to 15% in adults. Medical expenses for gallstone treatment exceeded $4 billion in facility charges in 2004 in the United States [1] and rise to $6.5 billion when surgical complications occur [2]. The formation and growth of cholesterol gallstones, which accounts for 75% of the gallstones in westernized countries [3–5], are secondary to abnormal cholesterol homeostasis [6]. Of note, the main risk factors for cholesterol gallstone disease (e.g., obesity, type 2 diabetes, dyslipidemia, and hyperinsulinemia) are also well-known components of the metabolic syndrome [7–11], supporting the hypothesis that gallstone disease is just another component of the metabolic syndrome [12–14] (Table 1). Due to the high prevalence of the metabolic syndrome, it has been suggested that the phenotype of cholesterol gallstones may result from the interaction between insulin resistance, genetic factors, and a number of environmental factors [15]. A series of gallstone (*LITH*) genes have been identified, which affect cholesterol homeostasis and promote cholesterol gallstone formation and growth [15]. Also, a strong interest has developed to investigate the epigenetic mechanisms that are able to influence gene expression in the absence of an altered DNA sequence [16], in response to several environmental stimuli [15].

A comprehensive analysis of these latter aspects as key factors in linking cholesterol homeostasis to gene expression and to the environment might provide a clue for both the

Table 1: Major risk factors for cholesterol gallstones.

Independent
(i) Increasing age
(ii) Female gender
(iii) Race
(iv) Family history
Dietary
(i) High calorie
(ii) High cholesterol
(iii) High fat
(iv) High *trans*-fatty acids
(v) Low fiber
(vi) Low *cis*-unsaturated fats
(vii) High refined carbohydrates
Life style
(i) Low grade physical activity
(ii) Prolonged fasting
(iii) Rapid weight loss
(iv) Pregnancy and parity
(v) Oral contraceptives
(vi) Estrogen replacement therapy
Associated conditions
(i) The metabolic syndrome
(ii) Obesity
(iii) Insulin resistance
(iv) Diabetes type 2
(v) Nonalcoholic fatty liver disease
(vi) Gallbladder and/or intestinal stasis

Adapted and modified from Portincasa et al. The Lancet, 2006 [17].

prevention of gallstone formation in subjects at risk and future therapeutic approaches via manipulation of cholesterol homeostasis.

2. Cholesterol Homeostasis and the Formation of Cholesterol Gallstones

2.1. Multifactorial Contributions to the Pathogenesis of Gallstones. Precipitation of excess cholesterol in bile as solid plate-like monohydrate crystals is a prerequisite for the formation of cholesterol gallstones [18, 19]. It is evident that all factors contributing to cholesterol homeostasis (i.e., intestinal cholesterol absorption, hepatic cholesterol biosynthesis, biliary output, and cholesterol conversion to bile acids) play a vital role in the pathogenesis of cholesterol gallstones. In fact, specific pathogenic factors concurring to the formation of cholesterol gallstones in humans must include hepatic hypersecretion of cholesterol into bile leading to a supersaturated bile, accelerated cholesterol nucleation/crystallization, defective gallbladder motility (a form of cholesterol-induced leiomyopathy leading to gallbladder stasis [6, 20, 21]), increased absorption of intestinal cholesterol, and *LITH* gene expression [17, 22–28] (Figure 1).

2.2. Liver, Bile, Intestine, Gene Expression, and Cholesterol Homeostasis. The liver plays a central role in cholesterol homeostasis and lipoprotein metabolism since it is mainly involved in synthesis and catabolism of cholesterol and lipoproteins and is the exclusive excretory route for cholesterol from the body [21].

In normal subjects with an extremely low dietary cholesterol intake (~30 mg/day, pure vegetarians), biliary cholesterol mainly derives from *de novo* synthesis [33]. In the physiological steady state, hepatic secretion of biliary cholesterol principally derives from newly synthesized cholesterol, plasma lipoproteins (the main source of biliary cholesterol is HDL cholesterol, as mainly suggested by animal models [34–37]), and intestinal absorption of cholesterol. Dietary and reabsorbed biliary cholesterol is delivered by the enterolymphatic circulation to the liver for resecretion into bile. As demonstrated by both human and animal studies, reabsorption of biliary cholesterol by the enterocytes has different absorption efficiency [38, 39] and depends on sterol transport proteins compared to dietary cholesterol [40–42]. Intestinal absorption of cholesterol is a multistep process regulated by multiple genes [41], which is determined by the balance between influx and efflux of intraluminal cholesterol molecules crossing the brush border membrane of the enterocyte [41].

The rate of whole-body cholesterol synthesis by the liver is approximately 8–10 mg/day/kg body weight in humans [43], and, under normal physiological conditions, *de novo* synthesis contributes to biliary cholesterol secretion approximately by 15% [44–47]. Interestingly, cholesterol synthesis by the liver is suppressed by a negative feedback regulatory mechanism through the sterol regulatory elementary binding protein-1 (SREBP-1) pathway when dietary cholesterol intake is increased, which also induces an enhanced secretion of cholesterol into bile, the conversion of cholesterol into bile acids (subsequently for secretion into bile), an increased cholesterol esterification and storage, and an enhanced lipoprotein secretion into the circulation [21]. In humans, the fibroblast growth factor receptor 4 (FGFR4) may have an effect on maintaining bile acid homeostasis by regulating the expression of cholesterol 7alpha-hydroxylase (CYP7A1), the rate-limiting enzyme for the classic pathway of bile acid biosynthesis [48]. Additionally, the liver X receptor (LXR) plays a main role in cholesterol homeostasis because it can activate the transcription of the genes, such as ABCG5/8, ABCA1, and ABCG1, involved in the response to excess cholesterol intake [49–51]. In mice, it has been reported that there is an increased propensity to cholesterol crystallization and gallstone formation in bile following the activation of hepatic LXR and direct upregulation of the major cholesterol efflux transporters ABCG5 and ABCG8 on the canalicular membrane of hepatocyte [52].

2.3. Altered Cholesterol Homeostasis: The Lithogenic State. Pathologic conditions linked to cholesterol gallstone formation in humans are characterized by a "lithogenic state," in which the *de novo* synthesis could provide the liver with more cholesterol for secretion into bile. The current view on the physical chemistry of cholesterol carriers in bile is

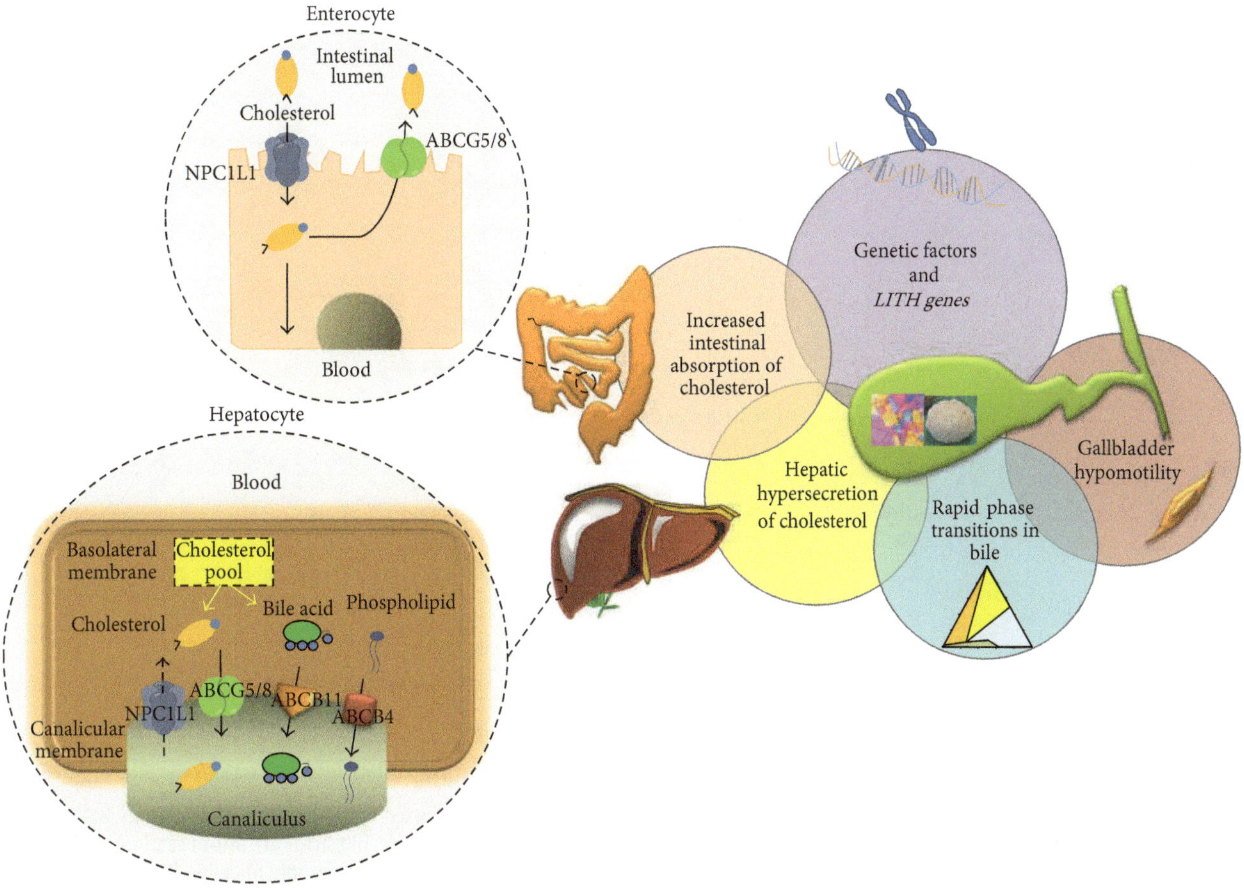

FIGURE 1: Current view on the complex interplay of pathogenic factors in cholesterol gallstone formation. The combination of multiple disturbances affecting cholesterol homeostasis in bile is essential for cholesterol gallstone formation. *LITH* genes and genetic defects play a crucial role in the formation of cholesterol gallstones. A large number of *LITH* genes have been identified in mouse models of cholesterol gallstones, and based on mouse studies, several human *LITH* genes have been identified, and their contributions to the formation of cholesterol gallstones are now being investigated. Hepatic hypersecretion of biliary cholesterol leads to unphysiological supersaturation of gallbladder bile with cholesterol. At the enterocyte (small intestine) level, absorption of cholesterol is enhanced via the Niemann-Pick C1-like 1 (NPC1L1) pathway. In bile, as a consequence, accelerated phase transitions of cholesterol occur, which are facilitated by prolonged gallbladder stasis due to impaired gallbladder motility and immune-mediated gallbladder inflammation, as well as hypersecretion of mucins and accumulation of mucin gel in the gallbladder lumen [6, 17]. In bile, growth of solid plate-like cholesterol monohydrate crystals to form gallstones is a consequence of persistent hepatic hypersecretion of biliary cholesterol together with enhanced gallbladder mucin secretion and incomplete evacuation by the gallbladder due to its impaired motility function [6, 29]. The two inlets on the left depict the major pathways of cholesterol absorption and secretion at the enterocyte level and at the hepatocyte level, respectively, as mediated by specific transporter proteins. Also, relative cholesterol hypersecretion into hepatic bile may or may not be accompanied by normal, high, or low secretion rates of biliary bile acids or phospholipids. Although NPC1L1 is expressed in the liver, its mRNA expression and protein concentrations are very low compared to those in the small intestine, thereby suggesting that hepatic NPC1L1 could have a minor role in regulating biliary cholesterol secretion.

summarized in Figure 2. Bile contains the three classes of biliary lipids (i.e., bile acids, phospholipids, and cholesterol), and specific cholesterol carriers in health include simple and mixed micelle and small and large vesicles. Sustained cholesterol supersaturation in bile will lead to a cascade of events in which excess cholesterol will lead to nucleation and crystallization and finally precipitate as solid plate-like monohydrate crystals, the first key step in cholesterol gallstone formation.

Bile becomes desaturated with cholesterol after long-term administration of statins, the competitive inhibitors of HMG-CoA reductase, and the rate-limiting enzyme in cholesterol biosynthesis [53–60].

Compared to gallstone-resistant AKR mice, susceptible C57L mice on the lithogenic diet still display higher HMG-CoA reductase activities together with lower activities of both bile acid synthetic enzymes cholesterol 7α-hydroxylase and sterol 27-hydroxylase [61]. Furthermore, higher HMG-CoA reductase activities have been found in gallstone patients compared with control subjects [62–65]. This evidence underscores the role of *de novo* cholesterol synthesis in the formation of lithogenic bile in humans at risk for gallstones.

The small intestine also plays a key role in the absorption of both dietary and biliary cholesterol, which is present in bile solely in the unesterified form (at least 97% of total sterols in bile) [15].

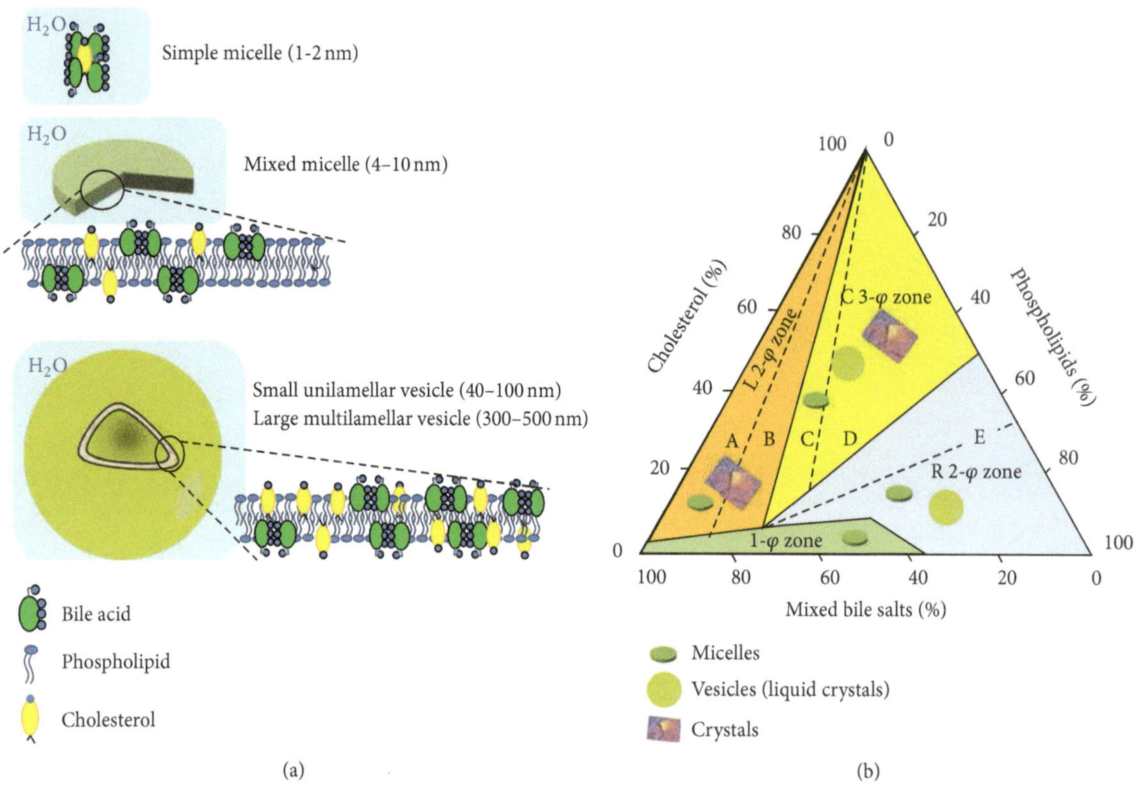

FIGURE 2: (a) The figure shows the physical states of lipids in human bile [21]. Bile is composed mainly of water (more than 90%) [30]. Bile acids are highly soluble, while cholesterol and phospholipids are highly insoluble in water. In bile, bile acids are found as monomers up to the critical micellar concentration (≈1–3 mM), a cut-off value after which bile acids can self-aggregate as simple micelles, binding a molecule of cholesterol. This step leads to increased aqueous solubility of cholesterol. Phospholipids in an aqueous environment can self-aggregate to form stable bilayer vesicles containing also a trace amount of bile acids, if any. A large amount of the cholesterol molecules is inserted into these bilayers of vesicles between the hydrophobic acyl chains of phospholipids. With typical gallbladder lipid concentrations and compositions, simple bile acid and mixed bile acid-lecithin micelles coexist in a ratio of 1 : 5. Unilamellar vesicles are larger spherical carriers in which even more cholesterol is solubilized into the bilayers of phospholipids. The ratio of unilamellar vesicles to micelles depends on the bile acid and phospholipid concentrations of bile, which is the greatest in bile with low bile acid and high phospholipid concentrations. Furthermore, at low bile acid concentrations and high phospholipid concentrations, these biliary phospholipids often form large multilamellar layers of vesicles. High concentrations of bile acids can dissolve these vesicles to form mixed micelles. (b) The picture depicts the ternary bile salt-cholesterol-phospholipid phase diagram in which the different pathways of cholesterol solubilization and/or precipitation in bile are shown [17]. The concentrations of three biliary lipids (bile acids, cholesterol, and phospholipids) are shown as percentages on the three axes of the triangle with a total lipid concentration of 7.2 g/dL, pH 7, and a temperature of 37°C [31, 32]. Different zones occupying areas within the triangle are shown, with each one containing different cholesterol carriers. The one-phase (φ) zone under the saturation curve contains only micelles and represents the bile being unsaturated with cholesterol. Above, three other zones exist with cholesterol supersaturation: a right two-phase (R 2-φ) zone containing saturated micelles and vesicles; a central three-phase (C 3-φ) zone containing saturated micelles, vesicles, and solid cholesterol crystals; and a left two-phase (L 2-φ) zone containing saturated micelles and solid cholesterol crystals. Whereas cholesterol precipitation is rapid in case of excess bile acids, at increasing amounts of phospholipids, cholesterol may reside in vesicles with phospholipids. At this moment, solid cholesterol crystal formation is slower or absent. Cholesterol crystallization, the first key step in cholesterol gallstone disease, is increasing at increasing concentrations of cholesterol, in the central and left zones, above the "safe" and physiological micellar zone.

The importance of the gallbladder on the regulation of reabsorption of biliary cholesterol has been underlined by an animal model showing that the gallbladder can modulate the physical states of cholesterol, which may in turn influence the intestinal absorption of biliary cholesterol. In this model, crystallized bile markedly reduced cholesterol uptake and absorption by the enterocyte [42].

The average intake of cholesterol in the western diet is approximately 300–500 mg per day (predominantly animal origin). The small intestine contains both unesterified and esterified cholesterol, with the latter usually in small proportion [66]. Any cholesteryl ester entering the intestine must be hydrolyzed by pancreatic cholesterol esterase in order to be absorbed. Bile delivers 500–2400 mg of cholesterol per day to the intestine [67], and this amount is approximately two to three times the dietary cholesterol. An additional source of intraluminal cholesterol (about 300 mg of cholesterol per day) comes from the turnover of intestinal mucosal epithelium [41]. It has been demonstrated that intestinal factors have a major role in the pathogenesis of mouse gallstone formation

[68], since the deficiency of cholesterol esterification in the intestine of ACAT2 knockout mice leads to a marked reduction in intestinal cholesterol absorption and complete resistance to diet-induced cholesterol gallstones.

Additionally, the lack of expression of intestinal Apo-B48 (but not Apo-B100) leads to a significant reduction in biliary cholesterol secretion and gallstone formation, possibly by decreasing intestinal absorption and hepatic bioavailability of cholesterol [69]. Apo-E knockout mice on the lithogenic diet show reduced biliary cholesterol secretion and gallstone prevalence, possibly due to a decreased availability of chylomicron-derived cholesterol in the liver for biliary cholesterol secretion [70]. Although results from animal studies underscore the role of cholesterol derived from the intestine on biliary cholesterol secretion and provide clear evidence that high dietary cholesterol through this pathway enhances cholelithogenesis, human studies concerning this topic gave conflicting results. It has been demonstrated that biliary cholesterol saturation increases with increasing cholesterol intake, inducing the formation of lithogenic bile and solid cholesterol crystals in some subjects [71]. Conversely, a group of 9 healthy women showed no increase in biliary cholesterol saturation after a high-cholesterol diet [72], and 6 normolipidemic women and 6 hyperlipidemic patients without gallstones showed no change in biliary cholesterol saturation when dietary cholesterol was increased from 300 mg to 1,500 mg daily [73]. An increase in biliary cholesterol saturation with modest increments in dietary cholesterol has been noticed in a group of 12 patients with asymptomatic gallstones (six men and six women), as compared with 7 healthy women (the diets containing 500, 750, and 1,000 mg of cholesterol daily for 3-week periods in random sequence). Interestingly, the biliary cholesterol saturation increased in this study group independently from the presence of gallstones [74]. Results from this study showed that women with gallstones had higher biliary cholesterol saturation than normal women at corresponding levels of cholesterol consumption, and six of the seven normal women formed lithogenic bile when ingesting a diet containing 1,000 mg of cholesterol. The discrepancies in human studies might be explained, at least in part, by differences in population sampling, by dissimilar diets, and by variations in the absorption efficiency of intestinal cholesterol.

3. Genetic, Epigenetic, and Environmental Factors

The analysis of the mechanisms linking environmental factors to the genes in the determination of human health is of importance in the field of life sciences and biomedical research. Several studies have demonstrated that family history, genetics, dietary, and cultural habits have a main role in the onset of gallstones [75–77]. Furthermore, a number of observations have found that a complex genetic basis could play a key role in determining individual predisposition to develop cholesterol gallstones in response to environmental factors [22, 23, 26, 28], and a wide spectrum of environmental and genetic risk factors may influence the onset of gallstone disease in humans [78, 79]. The analysis of twin pairs from The Swedish Twin Registry showed that genetic factors are estimated to account for about 25% of gallstone risk [80] and that twins carrying a heterozygous or homozygous ABCG8 D19H genotype have a significantly increased risk of gallstone disease [81]. The *ABCG8* p.D19H may lead to lower intestinal cholesterol absorption, lower serum cholesterol levels, and higher hepatic cholesterol synthesis, and polymorphisms in the ABCG5/ABCG8 genes are certainly related to the variations in plasma lipid levels, cholesterol saturation of bile [82], and insulin resistance [83]. An inventory of human cholesterol gallstone (*LITH*) genes has been depicted [15], and this list is rapidly growing. It has been recently suggested that susceptibility to gallstone disease may be influenced in humans by mucin gene polymorphisms [84] or FGFR4 polymorphism [48] and that the mucin-like protocadherin gene (MUPCDH) polymorphism rs3758650 has been considered a genetic marker to predict symptomatic gallstone disease [85]. Furthermore, carriers of CG genotype of ABCG8 rs11887534 showed higher risk of gallstones, as well as gallbladder and bile duct cancer compared with carriers of the GG genotype [86].

On the other hand, besides genes, the role of epigenetics has been highlighted by a number of human studies as the key factor in the onset of several chronic metabolic [87–92] and nonmetabolic diseases, such as cancer [93–95] cardiovascular diseases [96], neurodegenerative diseases [97], and birth defects [98], as a consequence of exposure to "toxic" agents occurring *in utero* before birth [16, 99]. They occur when the function of a gene is altered by various mechanisms, although its DNA sequence remains stable [16]. Transgenerational effects and fetal programming result from a mother's exposure and are inherited through successive generations in the absence of direct exposure of the offspring. Fetal programming, in turn, results in the onset of diseases in adult age, underlying the importance of developmental factors in influencing the risk of later-life disease [100]. Diet [101, 102] or environmental exposition to a number of chemical agents like heavy metals (e.g., cadmium, arsenic, nickel, chromium, and methylmercury) [103–107], air pollutants (e.g., particulate matter, black carbon, and benzene), and endocrine-disrupting/reproductive toxicants (e.g., diethylstilbestrol, bisphenol A, persistent organic pollutants, dioxin, and pesticides [108–112]) are able to induce epigenetic changes (mainly DNA methylation, histone acetylation/deacetylation [113], and noncoding microRNAs) [114, 115], which are involved in a wide range of metabolic diseases including obesity [90, 116], abnormal hepatic triglyceride accumulation [91], and the metabolic syndrome [92, 117], type 2 diabetes [87–89], all well-known risk factors for gallstone disease and mainly attributable to insulin resistance. Interestingly, it has been recently reported by a cluster of analyses a significant association of gallbladder diseases with environmental pollutants (heavy metals) in drinking water [118].

The interaction of histone acetyltransferases (HATs) and histone deacetylases (HDACs) and histones strongly affects gene transcription, and, in particular, it has been suggested that HDACs are important in the regulation of lipid homeostasis [113]. Of note, microRNAs (miR-122, miR-370, and miR-33) have a major influence on cholesterol homeostasis. They are important posttranscriptional regulators of gene expression [119–121] and strongly affect cholesterol metabolism [122]. It has been recently reported by an animal model that maternal low-protein diet during gestation and lactation significantly alters cholesterol homeostasis in weaning piglets through altered epigenetic regulation (promoter hypomethylation, decreased histone H3, H3 lysine 9 monomethylation, H3 lysine 27 trimethylation, and increased H3 acetylation) of the *HMGCR* (the rate-limiting enzyme in cholesterol biosynthesis) and *CYP7A1* (the rate-limiting enzyme for conversion of cholesterol to bile acids) genes, with possible long-term consequences in cholesterol homeostasis later in adult life [101]. In the rat, maternal undernutrition leads to long-term dysregulation of cholesterol metabolism in the offspring through epigenetic mechanisms [102].

In humans, it has been reported that placental insufficiency-induced intrauterine growth restriction secondary to adverse events *in utero* may be responsible for metabolic events leading to the metabolic syndrome [102, 123, 124].

The bile acid receptor farnesoid X receptor (FXR) is currently considered to be the intracellular "sensor" of bile acids [125, 126]. Cells synthesize oxysterols under conditions of cholesterol overload, and oxysterols in turn bind and activate LXR, which acts to reduce systemic cholesterol burden [125–127]. FXR is highly expressed in the enterohepatic system and regulates the expression of the genes involved in the maintenance of cholesterol, bile acid, and triglyceride homeostasis [128]. Of note, it has been recently suggested by a comparison of genomic FXR-binding sites in healthy control and obese mice that FXR transcriptional signaling is altered in diet-induced obese mice, which may underlie aberrant metabolism and liver function in obesity [129].

In conclusion, frequent metabolic abnormalities such as atherosclerosis, obesity, metabolic syndrome, and gallstone disease are related to impaired cholesterol homeostasis. The current view that such abnormalities gain clinical relevance only during adulthood and elderly age is dramatically changing. Both genetic and epigenetic studies suggest a very early onset of chronic disease already *in utero*. Epigenetic mechanisms underlying such developmental events are still under investigation, in particular in the case of cholesterol homeostasis and gallstone disease. Starting from these particular metabolic conditions, a better understanding of mechanisms resulting in chromatin remodeling in response to environmental stimuli acting on the epigenome may offer new options for therapy of cholesterol cholelithiasis and better possibilities for primary prevention in subjects at risk.

Abbreviations

ABC: ATP-binding cassette (transporter)
NPC1L1: Niemann-Pick C1-like 1 protein. Adapted from de Bari et al. [130], Wang et al. [21], and Portincasa and Wang [6].

References

[1] J. E. Everhart and C. E. Ruhl, "Burden of digestive diseases in the united states part I: overall and upper gastrointestinal diseases," *Gastroenterology*, vol. 136, no. 2, pp. 376–386, 2009.

[2] E. A. Shaffer, "Epidemiology and risk factors for gallstone disease: has the paradigm changed in the 21st century?" *Current Gastroenterology Reports*, vol. 7, no. 2, pp. 132–140, 2005.

[3] A. F. Attili, R. Capocaccia, N. Carulli et al., "Factors associated with gallstone disease in the MICOL experience," *Hepatology*, vol. 26, no. 4, pp. 809–818, 1997.

[4] A. F. Attili, N. Carulli, E. Roda et al., "Epidemiology of gallstone disease in Italy: prevalence data of the multicenter Italian study on cholelithiasis (M.I.COL.)," *The American Journal of Epidemiology*, vol. 141, no. 2, pp. 158–165, 1995.

[5] A. K. Diehl, "Epidemiology and natural history of gallstone disease," *Gastroenterology Clinics of North America*, vol. 20, no. 1, pp. 1–19, 1991.

[6] P. Portincasa and D. Q. Wang, "Intestinal absorption, hepatic synthesis, and biliary secretion of cholesterol: where are we for cholesterol gallstone formation?" *Hepatology*, vol. 55, no. 5, pp. 1313–1316, 2012.

[7] R. H. Eckel, S. M. Grundy, and P. Z. Zimmet, "The metabolic syndrome," *The Lancet*, vol. 365, no. 9468, pp. 1415–1428, 2005.

[8] S. M. Grundy, "Metabolic syndrome scientific statement by the American heart association and the national heart, lung, and blood institute," *Arteriosclerosis, Thrombosis, and Vascular Biology*, vol. 25, no. 11, pp. 2243–2244, 2005.

[9] S. M. Grundy and J. P. Barnett, "Metabolic and health complications of obesity," *Disease-a-Month*, vol. 36, no. 12, pp. 641–731, 1990.

[10] S. M. Grundy, J. I. Cleeman, S. R. Daniels et al., "Diagnosis and management of the metabolic syndrome: an American heart association/national heart, lung, and blood institute scientific statement," *Circulation*, vol. 112, no. 17, pp. 2735–2752, 2005.

[11] C. J. Tsai, M. F. Leitzmann, W. C. Willett, and E. L. Giovannucci, "Prospective study of abdominal adiposity and gallstone disease in US men," *The American Journal of Clinical Nutrition*, vol. 80, no. 1, pp. 38–44, 2004.

[12] N. Méndez-Sánchez, N. C. Chavez-Tapia, D. Motola-Kuba et al., "Metabolic syndrome as a risk factor for gallstone disease," *World Journal of Gastroenterology*, vol. 11, no. 11, pp. 1653–1657, 2005.

[13] F. Nervi, J. F. Miquel, M. Alvarez et al., "Gallbladder disease is associated with insulin resistance in a high risk Hispanic population," *Journal of Hepatology*, vol. 45, no. 2, pp. 299–305, 2006.

[14] N. Ata, M. Kucukazman, B. Yavuz et al., "The metabolic syndrome is associated with complicated gallstone disease," *Canadian Journal of Gastroenterology*, vol. 25, no. 5, pp. 274–276, 2011.

[15] D. Q. Wang, D. E. Cohen, and M. C. Carey, "Biliary lipids and cholesterol gallstone disease," *Journal of Lipid Research*, vol. 50, supplement, pp. S406–S411, 2009.

[16] E. A. Mazzio and K. F. Soliman, "Basic concepts of epigenetics: impact of environmental signals on gene expression," *Epigenetics*, vol. 7, no. 2, pp. 119–130, 2012.

[17] P. Portincasa, A. Moschetta, and G. Palasciano, "Cholesterol gallstone disease," *The Lancet*, vol. 368, no. 9531, pp. 230–239, 2006.

[18] A. F. Hofmann, A. Amelsberg, and E. Vansonnenberg, "Pathogenesis and treatment of gallstones," *The New England Journal of Medicine*, vol. 328, 25, pp. 1854–1855, 1993.

[19] J. T. Lamont and M. C. Carey, "Cholesterol gallstone formation. 2. Pathobiology and pathomechanics," *Progress in liver diseases*, vol. 10, pp. 165–191, 1992.

[20] P. Portincasa, A. Di Ciaula, G. Baldassarre et al., "Gallbladder motel function in gallstone patients: sonographic and in vitro studies on the role of gallstones; smooth muscle function and gallbladder wall inflammation," *Journal of Hepatology*, vol. 21, no. 3, pp. 430–440, 1994.

[21] D. Q. Wang, B. A. Neuschwander-Tetri, and P. Portincasa, *The Biliary System*, Morgan & Claypool Life Sciences, Princeton, NJ, USA, 2012.

[22] F. Lammert and J. F. Miquel, "Gallstone disease: from genes to evidence-based therapy," *Journal of Hepatology*, vol. 48, supplement 1, pp. S124–S135, 2008.

[23] F. Lammert and T. Sauerbruch, "Mechanisms of disease: the genetic epidemiology of gallbladder stones," *Nature Clinical Practice Gastroenterology and Hepatology*, vol. 2, no. 9, pp. 423–433, 2005.

[24] P. Portincasa, A. Di Ciaula, H. H. Wang et al., "Coordinate regulation of gallbladder motor function in the gut-liver axis," *Hepatology*, vol. 47, no. 6, pp. 2112–2126, 2008.

[25] P. Portincasa, A. Moschetta, F. Puglisi, and D. Q. H. Wang, "Medical treatment of gallstone disease," in *Biliary Lithiasis: Basic Science, Current Diagnosis and Management*, G. Borzellino and C. Cordiano, Eds., pp. 149–157, Springer Italia S.r.l., Milan, Italy, 2008.

[26] D. Q. H. Wang, L. Zhang, and H. H. Wang, "High cholesterol absorption efficiency and rapid biliary secretion of chylomicron remnant cholesterol enhance cholelithogenesis in gallstone-susceptible mice," *Biochimica et Biophysica Acta*, vol. 1733, no. 1, pp. 90–99, 2005.

[27] H. H. Wang, P. Portincasa, and D. Q. H. Wang, "Molecular pathophysiology and physical chemistry of cholesterol gallstones," *Frontiers in Bioscience*, vol. 13, no. 2, pp. 401–423, 2008.

[28] H. Wittenburg and F. Lammert, "Genetic predisposition to gallbladder stones," *Seminars in Liver Disease*, vol. 27, no. 1, pp. 109–121, 2007.

[29] D. Q. H. Wang and N. H. Afdhal, "Gallstone disease," in *Sleisenger and Fordtran's Gastrointestinal and Liver Disease*, M. Feldman, L. S. Friedman, and L. J. Brand, Eds., vol. 9, pp. 1089–1120, Elsevier, Philadelphia, Pa, USA, 2010.

[30] P. Portincasa and G. Calamita, "Water channel proteins in bile formation and flow in health and disease: when immiscible becomes miscible," *Molecular Aspects of Medicine*, vol. 33, no. 5-6, pp. 651–664, 2012.

[31] W. H. Admirand and D. M. Small, "The physicochemical basis of cholesterol gallstone formation in man," *Journal of Clinical Investigation*, vol. 47, no. 5, pp. 1043–1052, 1968.

[32] D. Q. H. Wang and M. C. Carey, "Characterization of crystallization pathways during cholesterol precipitation from human gallbladder biles: identical pathways to corresponding model biles with three predominating sequences," *Journal of Lipid Research*, vol. 37, no. 12, pp. 2539–2549, 1996.

[33] J. J. Clarenbach, M. Reber, D. Lütjohann, K. von Bergmann, and T. Sudhop, "The lipid-lowering effect of ezetimibe in pure vegetarians," *Journal of Lipid Research*, vol. 47, no. 12, pp. 2820–2824, 2006.

[34] K. F. Kozarsky, M. H. Donahee, A. Rigotti, S. N. Iqbal, E. R. Edelman, and M. Krieger, "Overexpression of the HDL receptor SR-BI alters plasma HDL and bile cholesterol levels," *Nature*, vol. 387, no. 6631, pp. 414–417, 1997.

[35] S. J. Robins and J. M. Fasulo, "High density lipoproteins, but not other lipoproteins, provide a vehicle for sterol transport to bile," *Journal of Clinical Investigation*, vol. 99, no. 3, pp. 380–384, 1997.

[36] E. Sehayek, J. G. Ono, S. Shefer et al., "Biliary cholesterol excretion: a novel mechanism that regulates dietary cholesterol absorption," *Proceedings of the National Academy of Sciences of the United States of America*, vol. 95, no. 17, pp. 10194–10199, 1998.

[37] J. F. Oram and J. W. Heinecke, "ATP-binding cassette transporter A1: a cell cholesterol exporter that protects against cardiovascular disease," *Physiological Reviews*, vol. 85, no. 4, pp. 1343–1372, 2005.

[38] Y. A. Kesaniemi and T. A. Miettinen, "Cholesterol absorption efficiency regulates plasma cholesterol level in the Finnish population," *European Journal of Clinical Investigation*, vol. 17, no. 5, pp. 391–395, 1987.

[39] M. S. Bosner, L. G. Lange, W. F. Stenson, and R. E. Ostlund Jr., "Percent cholesterol absorption in normal women and men quantified with dual stable isotopic tracers and negative ion mass spectrometry," *Journal of Lipid Research*, vol. 40, no. 2, pp. 302–308, 1999.

[40] S. W. Altmann, H. R. Davis Jr., L. J. Zhu et al., "Niemann-pick C1 like 1 protein is critical for intestinal cholesterol absorption," *Science*, vol. 303, no. 5661, pp. 1201–1204, 2004.

[41] D. Q. H. Wang, "Regulation of intestinal cholesterol absorption," *Annual Review of Physiology*, vol. 69, pp. 221–248, 2007.

[42] D. Q. H. Wang and S. P. Lee, "Physical chemistry of intestinal absorption of biliary cholesterol in mice," *Hepatology*, vol. 48, no. 1, pp. 177–185, 2008.

[43] S. D. Turley and J. M. Dietschy, "The metabolism and excretion of cholesterol by the liver," in *The Liver: Biology and Pathobiology*, I. M. Arias, W. B. Iakoby, H. Popper, D. Schachter, and D. A. Shafritz, Eds., pp. 617–641, Raven Press, New York, NY, USA, 1988.

[44] M. A. Long, E. W. Kaler, and S. P. Lee, "Structural characterization of the micelle-vesicle transition in lecithin-bile salt solutions," *Biophysical Journal*, vol. 67, no. 4, pp. 1733–1742, 1994.

[45] S. H. Quarfordt, B. Oswald, B. Landis, H. S. Xu, S. H. Zhang, and N. Maeda, "In vivo cholesterol kinetics in apolipoprotein E-deficient and control mice," *Journal of Lipid Research*, vol. 36, no. 6, pp. 1227–1235, 1995.

[46] S. J. Robins and H. Brunengraber, "Origin of biliary cholesterol and lecithin in the rat: contribution of new synthesis and preformed hepatic stores," *Journal of Lipid Research*, vol. 23, no. 4, pp. 604–608, 1982.

[47] C. C. Schwartz, M. Berman, and Z. R. Vlahcevic, "Multicompartmental analysis of cholesterol metabolism in man. Characterization of the hepatic bile acid and biliary cholesterol precursor sites," *Journal of Clinical Investigation*, vol. 61, no. 2, pp. 408–423, 1978.

[48] Q. Chen, W. J. Li, Y. Y. Wan, C. D. Yu, and W. G. Li, "Fibroblast growth factor receptor 4 Gly388Arg polymorphism associated with severity of gallstone disease in a Chinese population," *Genetics and Molecular Research*, vol. 11, no. 1, pp. 548–555, 2012.

[49] S. W. Beaven and P. Tontonoz, "Nuclear receptors in lipid metabolism: targeting the heart of dyslipidemia," *Annual Review of Medicine*, vol. 57, pp. 313–329, 2006.

[50] D. J. Peet, B. A. Janowski, and D. J. Mangelsdorf, "The LXRs: a new class of oxysterol receptors," *Current Opinion in Genetics and Development*, vol. 8, no. 5, pp. 571–575, 1998.

[51] P. Tontonoz and D. J. Mangelsdorf, "Liver X receptor signaling pathways in cardiovascular disease," *Molecular Endocrinology*, vol. 17, no. 6, pp. 985–993, 2003.

[52] H. Uppal, Y. Zhai, A. Gangopadhyay et al., "Activation of liver X receptor sensitizes mice to gallbladder cholesterol crystallization," *Hepatology*, vol. 47, no. 4, pp. 1331–1342, 2008.

[53] C. J. Tsai, M. F. Leitzmann, W. C. Willett, and E. L. Giovannucci, "Statin use and the risk of cholecystectomy in women," *Gastroenterology*, vol. 136, no. 5, pp. 1593–1600, 2009.

[54] R. Erichsen, T. Frøslev, T. L. Lash, L. Pedersen, and H. T. Sørensen, "Long-term statin use and the risk of gallstone disease: a population-based case-control study," *The American Journal of Epidemiology*, vol. 173, no. 2, pp. 162–170, 2011.

[55] B. A. Chapman, M. J. Burt, R. J. Chisholm, R. B. Allan, K. H. J. Yeo, and A. G. Ross, "Dissolution of gallstones with simvastatin, an HMG CoA reductase inhibitor," *Digestive Diseases and Sciences*, vol. 43, no. 2, pp. 349–353, 1998.

[56] D. S. Hanson and W. C. Duane, "Effects of lovastatin and chenodiol on bile acid synthesis, bile lipid composition, and biliary lipid secretion in healthy human subjects," *Journal of Lipid Research*, vol. 35, no. 8, pp. 1462–1468, 1994.

[57] J. W. A. Smit, K. J. van Erpecum, P. Portincasa, W. Renooij, D. W. Erkelens, and G. P. van Berge-Henegouwen, "Effects of simvastatin and cholestyramine on bile lipid composition and gall bladder motility in patients with hypercholesterolaemia," *Gut*, vol. 37, no. 5, pp. 654–659, 1995.

[58] J. C. Mitchell, G. M. Logan, B. G. Stone, and W. C. Duane, "Effects of lovastatin on biliary lipid secretion and bile acid metabolism in humans," *Journal of Lipid Research*, vol. 32, no. 1, pp. 71–78, 1991.

[59] J. L. Smith, P. D. Roach, L. N. Wittenberg et al., "Effects of simvastatin on hepatic cholesterol metabolism, bile lithogenicity and bile acid hydrophobicity in patients with gallstones," *Journal of Gastroenterology and Hepatology*, vol. 15, no. 8, pp. 871–879, 2000.

[60] H. Vanhanen, Y. A. Kesaniemi, and T. A. Miettinen, "Pravastatin lowers serum cholesterol, cholesterol-precursor sterols, fecal steroids, and cholesterol absorption in man," *Metabolism: Clinical and Experimental*, vol. 41, no. 6, pp. 588–595, 1992.

[61] F. Lammert, D. Q. H. Wang, B. Paigen, and M. C. Carey, "Phenotypic characterization of Lith genes that determine susceptibility to cholesterol cholelithiasis in inbred mice: integrated activities of hepatic lipid regulatory enzymes," *Journal of Lipid Research*, vol. 40, no. 11, pp. 2080–2090, 1999.

[62] S. M. Grundy, A. L. Metzger, and R. D. Adler, "Mechanisms of lithogenic bile formation in American Indian women with cholesterol gallstones," *Journal of Clinical Investigation*, vol. 51, no. 12, pp. 3026–3043, 1972.

[63] P. H. Key, G. G. Bonorris, and J. W. Marks, "Biliary lipid synthesis and secretion in gallstone patients before and during treatment with chenodeoxycholic acid," *Journal of Laboratory and Clinical Medicine*, vol. 95, no. 6, pp. 816–826, 1980.

[64] F. O. Nervi, C. F. Covarrubias, V. D. Valdivieso, B. O. Ronco, A. Solari, and J. Tocornal, "Hepatic cholesterogenesis in Chileans with cholesterol gallstone disease. Evidence for sex differences in the regulation of hepatic cholesterol metabolism," *Gastroenterology*, vol. 80, no. 3, pp. 539–545, 1981.

[65] G. Salen, G. Nicolau, S. Shefer, and E. H. Mosbach, "Hepatic cholesterol metabolism in patients with gallstones," *Gastroenterology*, vol. 69, no. 3, pp. 676–684, 1975.

[66] E. F. Stange and J. M. Dietschy, "Cholesterol absorption and metabolism by the intestinal epithelium," in *Sterols and Bile Acids*, H. Danielsson and J. Sjovall, Eds., pp. 121–149, Elsevier, Amsterdam, The Netherlands, 1985.

[67] H. Y. I. Mok, K. von Bergmann, and S. M. Grundy, "Effects of continuous and intermittent feeding on biliary lipid outputs in man: application for measurements of intestinal absorption of cholesterol and bile acids," *Journal of Lipid Research*, vol. 20, no. 3, pp. 389–398, 1979.

[68] K. K. Buhman, M. Accad, S. Novak et al., "Resistance to diet-induced hypercholesterolemia and gallstone formation in ACAT2-deficient mice," *Nature Medicine*, vol. 6, no. 12, pp. 1341–1347, 2000.

[69] H. H. Wang and D. Q. H. Wang, "Reduced susceptibility to cholesterol gallstone formation in mice that do not produce apolipoprotein B48 in the intestine," *Hepatology*, vol. 42, no. 4, pp. 894–904, 2005.

[70] L. Amigo, V. Quiones, P. Mardones et al., "Impaired biliary cholesterol secretion and decreased gallstone formation in apolipoprotein E-deficient mice fed a high-cholesterol diet," *Gastroenterology*, vol. 118, no. 4, pp. 772–779, 2000.

[71] L. DenBesten, W. E. Connor, and S. Bell, "The effect of dietary cholesterol on the composition of human bile," *Surgery*, vol. 73, no. 2, pp. 266–273, 1973.

[72] H. Dam, I. Prange, M. K. Jensen, H. E. Kallehauge, and H. J. Fenger, "Studies on human bile—IV. Influence of ingestion of cholesterol in the form of eggs on the composition of bile in healthy subjects," *Zeitschrift für Ernährungswissenschaft*, vol. 10, no. 3, pp. 178–187, 1971.

[73] E. Andersen and K. Hellstrom, "The effect of cholesterol feeding on bile acid kinetics and biliary lipids in normolipidemic and hypertriglyceridemic subjects," *Journal of Lipid Research*, vol. 20, no. 8, pp. 1020–1027, 1979.

[74] D. W. T. Lee, C. J. Gilmore, G. Bonorris et al., "Effect of dietary cholesterol on biliary lipids in patients with gallstones and normal subjects," *The American Journal of Clinical Nutrition*, vol. 42, no. 3, pp. 414–420, 1985.

[75] T. Gilat, C. Feldman, and Z. Halpern, "An increased familial frequency of gallstones," *Gastroenterology*, vol. 84, no. 2, pp. 242–246, 1983.

[76] R. E. Sampliner, P. H. Bennett, L. J. Comess, F. A. Rose, and T. A. Burch, "Gallbladder disease in pima indians. Demonstration of high prevalence and early onset by cholecystography," *The New England Journal of Medicine*, vol. 283, no. 25, pp. 1358–1364, 1970.

[77] S. K. Sarin, V. S. Negi, R. Dewan, S. Sasan, and A. Saraya, "High familial prevalence of gallstones in the first-degree relatives of gallstone patients," *Hepatology*, vol. 22, no. 1, pp. 138–141, 1995.

[78] C. S. Stokes, M. Krawczyk, and F. Lammert, "Gallstones: environment, lifestyle and genes," *Digestive Diseases*, vol. 29, no. 2, pp. 191–201, 2011.

[79] H. Wittenburg, "Hereditary liver disease: gallstones," *Best Practice and Research: Clinical Gastroenterology*, vol. 24, no. 5, pp. 747–756, 2010.

[80] D. Katsika, A. Grjibovski, C. Einarsson, F. Lammert, P. Lichtenstein, and H. U. Marschall, "Genetic and environmental influences on symptomatic gallstone disease: a Swedish study of 43,141 twin pairs," *Hepatology*, vol. 41, no. 5, pp. 1138–1143, 2005.

[81] D. Katsika, P. Magnusson, M. Krawczyk et al., "Gallstone disease in Swedish twins: risk is associated with ABCG8 D19H genotype," *Journal of Internal Medicine*, vol. 268, no. 3, pp. 279–285, 2010.

[82] M. Acalovschi, A. Ciocan, O. Mostean et al., "Are plasma lipid levels related to ABCG5/ABCG8 polymorphisms? A preliminary study in siblings with gallstones," *European Journal of Internal Medicine*, vol. 17, no. 7, pp. 490–494, 2006.

[83] H. Gylling, M. Hallikainen, J. Pihlajamäki et al., "Polymorphisms in the ABCG5 and ABCG8 genes associate with cholesterol absorption and insulin sensitivity," *Journal of Lipid Research*, vol. 45, no. 9, pp. 1660–1665, 2004.

[84] S. C. Chuang, E. Hsi, and K. T. Lee, "Mucin genes in gallstone disease," *Clinica Chimica Acta*, vol. 413, no. 19-20, pp. 1466–1471, 2012.

[85] S. C. Chuang, E. Hsi, S. N. Wang, M. L. Yu, K. T. Lee, and S. H. Juo, "Polymorphism at the mucin-like protocadherin gene influences susceptibility to gallstone disease," *Clinica Chimica Acta*, vol. 412, no. 23-24, pp. 2089–2093, 2011.

[86] H. L. Xu, J. R. Cheng, G. Andreotti et al., "Cholesterol metabolism gene polymorphisms and the risk of biliary tract cancers and stones: a population-based case-control study in Shanghai, China," *Carcinogenesis*, vol. 32, no. 1, pp. 58–62, 2011.

[87] L. M. Berends and S. E. Ozanne, "Early determinants of type-2 diabetes," *Best Practice and Research Clinical Endocrinology and Metabolism*, vol. 26, no. 5, pp. 569–580, 2012.

[88] E. R. Gilbert and D. Liu, "Epigenetics: the missing link to understanding beta-cell dysfunction in the pathogenesis of type 2 diabetes," *Epigenetics*, vol. 7, no. 8, pp. 841–852, 2012.

[89] M. S. Martin-Gronert and S. E. Ozanne, "Metabolic programming of insulin action and secretion," *Diabetes, Obesity and Metabolism*, vol. 14, supplement 3, pp. 29–39, 2012.

[90] F. I. Milagro, M. L. Mansego, M. C. De, and J. A. Martinez, "Dietary factors, epigenetic modifications and obesity outcomes: progresses and perspectives," *Molecular Aspects of Medicine*, 2012.

[91] S. Sookoian and C. J. Pirola, "DNA methylation and hepatic insulin resistance and steatosis," *Current Opinion in Clinical Nutrition and Metabolic Care*, vol. 15, no. 4, pp. 350–356, 2012.

[92] J. Wang, Z. Wu, D. Li et al., "Nutrition, epigenetics, and metabolic syndrome," *Antioxidants and Redox Signaling*, vol. 17, no. 2, pp. 282–301, 2012.

[93] M. A. Dawson and T. Kouzarides, "Cancer epigenetics: from mechanism to therapy," *Cell*, vol. 150, no. 1, pp. 12–27, 2012.

[94] M. A. Dawson, T. Kouzarides, and B. J. Huntly, "Targeting epigenetic readers in cancer," *The New England Journal of Medicine*, vol. 367, no. 7, pp. 647–657, 2012.

[95] C. Marsit and B. Christensen, "Blood-derived DNA methylation markers of cancer risk," *Advances in Experimental Medicine and Biology*, vol. 754, pp. 233–252, 2013.

[96] S. Udali, P. Guarini, S. Moruzzi, S. W. Choi, and S. Friso, "Cardiovascular epigenetics: from DNA methylation to microRNAs," *Molecular Aspects of Medicine*, 2012.

[97] J. B. Kwok, "Role of epigenetics in Alzheimers and Parkinsons disease," *Epigenomics*, vol. 2, no. 5, pp. 671–682, 2010.

[98] J. A. Piedrahita, "The role of imprinted genes in fetal growth abnormalities," *Birth Defects Research A*, vol. 91, no. 8, pp. 682–692, 2011.

[99] Y. J. Loke, B. Novakovic, M. Ollikainen et al., "The peri/postnatal epigenetic twins study (PETS)," *Twin Research and Human Genetics*, vol. 16, no. 1, pp. 13–20, 2013.

[100] F. M. Low, P. D. Gluckman, and M. A. Hanson, "Developmental plasticity and epigenetic mechanisms underpinning metabolic and cardiovascular diseases," *Epigenomics*, vol. 3, no. 3, pp. 279–294, 2011.

[101] R. Cong, Y. Jia, R. Li et al., "Maternal low-protein diet causes epigenetic deregulation of HMGCR and CYP7alpha1 in the liver of weaning piglets," *The Journal of Nutritional Biochemistry*, vol. 23, no. 12, pp. 1647–1654, 2012.

[102] G. Sohi, K. Marchand, A. Revesz, E. Arany, and D. B. Hardy, "Maternal protein restriction elevates cholesterol in adult rat offspring due to repressive changes in histone modifications at the cholesterol 7α-hydroxylase promoter," *Molecular Endocrinology*, vol. 25, no. 5, pp. 785–798, 2011.

[103] T. F. Cheng, S. Choudhuri, and K. Muldoon-Jacobs, "Epigenetic targets of some toxicologically relevant metals: a review of the literature," *Journal of Applied Toxicology*, vol. 32, no. 9, pp. 643–653, 2012.

[104] R. Martinez-Zamudio and H. C. Ha, "Environmental epigenetics in metal exposure," *Epigenetics*, vol. 6, no. 7, pp. 820–827, 2011.

[105] J. F. Reichard and A. Puga, "Effects of arsenic exposure on DNA methylation and epigenetic gene regulation," *Epigenomics*, vol. 2, no. 1, pp. 87–104, 2010.

[106] N. Sadli, M. L. Ackland, M. D. De, A. J. Sinclair, and C. Suphioglu, "Effects of zinc and DHA on the epigenetic regulation of human neuronal cells," *Cellular Physiology and Biochemistry*, vol. 29, no. 1-2, pp. 87–98, 2012.

[107] B. Wang, Y. Li, C. Shao, Y. Tan, and L. Cai, "Cadmium and its epigenetic effects," *Current Medicinal Chemistry*, vol. 19, no. 16, pp. 2611–2620, 2012.

[108] T. Ding, M. McConaha, K. L. Boyd, K. G. Osteen, and K. L. Bruner-Tran, "Developmental dioxin exposure of either parent is associated with an increased risk of preterm birth in adult mice," *Reproductive Toxicology*, vol. 31, no. 3, pp. 351–358, 2011.

[109] R. McKinlay, J. A. Plant, J. N. B. Bell, and N. Voulvoulis, "Calculating human exposure to endocrine disrupting pesticides via agricultural and non-agricultural exposure routes," *Science of the Total Environment*, vol. 398, no. 1–3, pp. 1–12, 2008.

[110] E. Nilsson, G. Larsen, M. Manikkam, C. Guerrero-Bosagna, M. I. Savenkova, and M. K. Skinner, "Environmentally induced epigenetic transgenerational inheritance of ovarian disease," *PloS ONE*, vol. 7, no. 5, Article ID e36129, 2012.

[111] T. Takeda, M. Fujii, J. Taura, Y. Ishii, and H. Yamada, "Dioxin silences gonadotropin expression in perinatal pups by inducing histone deacetylases: a new insight into the mechanism for the imprinting of sexual immaturity by dioxin," *The Journal of Biological Chemistry*, vol. 287, pp. 18440–18450, 2012.

[112] B. Weinhold, "More chemicals show epigenetic effects across generations," *Environmental Health Perspectives*, vol. 120, article A228, 2012.

[113] A. Ferrari, E. Fiorino, M. Giudici et al., "Linking epigenetics to lipid metabolism: focus on histone deacetylases," *Molecular Membrane Biology*, vol. 29, no. 7, pp. 257–266, 2012.

[114] J. C. Chuang and P. A. Jones, "Epigenetics and microRNAs," *Pediatric Research*, vol. 61, no. 5, pp. 24R–29R, 2007.

[115] W. Y. Tang and S. M. Ho, "Epigenetic reprogramming and imprinting in origins of disease," *Reviews in Endocrine and Metabolic Disorders*, vol. 8, no. 2, pp. 173–182, 2007.

[116] J. A. Martinez, P. Cordero, J. Campion, and F. I. Milagro, "Interplay of early-life nutritional programming on obesity, inflammation and epigenetic outcomes," *The Proceedings of the Nutrition Society*, vol. 71, no. 2, pp. 276–283, 2012.

[117] S. Y. Rhee, Y. C. Hwang, J. T. Woo et al., "Blood lead is significantly associated with metabolic syndrome in Korean adults: an analysis based on the Korea national health and nutrition examination survey (KNHANES), 2008," *Cardiovascular Diabetology*, vol. 12, no. 1, article 9, 2013.

[118] S. Unisa, P. Jagannath, V. Dhir, C. Khandelwal, L. Sarangi, and T. K. Roy, "Population-based study to estimate prevalence and determine risk factors of gallbladder diseases in the rural Gangetic basin of North India," *HPB*, vol. 13, no. 2, pp. 117–125, 2011.

[119] V. Ambros, "The functions of animal microRNAs," *Nature*, vol. 431, no. 7006, pp. 350–355, 2004.

[120] D. P. Bartel, "MicroRNAs: genomics, biogenesis, mechanism, and function," *Cell*, vol. 116, no. 2, pp. 281–297, 2004.

[121] D. P. Bartel, "MicroRNAs: target recognition and regulatory functions," *Cell*, vol. 136, no. 2, pp. 215–233, 2009.

[122] K. J. Moore, K. J. Rayner, Y. Suárez, and C. Fernández-Hernando, "MicroRNAs and cholesterol metabolism," *Trends in Endocrinology and Metabolism*, vol. 21, no. 12, pp. 699–706, 2010.

[123] M. G. Ross and M. H. Beall, "Adult sequelae of intrauterine growth restriction," *Seminars in Perinatology*, vol. 32, no. 3, pp. 213–218, 2008.

[124] B. Lamarche, S. Lemieux, G. R. Dagenais, and J. P. Després, "Visceral obesity and the risk of ischaemic heart disease: insights from the Québec cardiovascular study," *Growth Hormone and IGF Research*, vol. 8, pp. 1–8, 1998.

[125] M. Makishima, A. Y. Okamoto, J. J. Repa et al., "Identification of a nuclear receptor for bite acids," *Science*, vol. 284, no. 5418, pp. 1362–1365, 1999.

[126] D. J. Parks, S. G. Blanchard, R. K. Bledsoe et al., "Bile acids: natural ligands for an orphan nuclear receptor," *Science*, vol. 284, no. 5418, pp. 1365–1368, 1999.

[127] J. J. Repa and D. J. Mangelsdorf, "The liver X receptor gene team: potential new players in atherosclerosis," *Nature Medicine*, vol. 8, no. 11, pp. 1243–1248, 2002.

[128] N. Y. Kalaany and D. J. Mangelsdorf, "LXRs and FXR: the Yin and Yang of cholesterol and fat metabolism," *Annual Review of Physiology*, vol. 68, pp. 159–191, 2006.

[129] J. Lee, S. Seok, P. Yu et al., "Genomic analysis of hepatic farnesoid X receptor binding sites reveals altered binding in obesity and direct gene repression by farnesoid X receptor in mice," *Hepatology*, vol. 56, no. 1, pp. 108–117, 2012.

[130] O. de Bari, B. A. Neuschwander-Tetri, M. Liu, P. Portincasa, and D. Q. Wang, "Ezetimibe: its novel effects on the prevention and the treatment of cholesterol gallstones and nonalcoholic fatty liver disease," *Journal of Lipids*, vol. 2012, Article ID 302847, 16 pages, 2012.

Traditional Dietary Recommendations for the Prevention of Cardiovascular Disease: Do They Meet the Needs of Our Patients?

Johannes Scholl

Prevention First, 65385 Ruedesheim, Germany

Correspondence should be addressed to Johannes Scholl, scholl@preventionfirst.de

Academic Editor: Jeffrey Cohn

The characteristics of patients with CVD have changed: whereas smoking prevalence declines, obesity and metabolic syndrome are on the rise. Unfortunately, the traditional *low-fat diet* for the prevention of cardiovascular disease (CVD) still seems to be the "mainstream knowledge" despite contradicting evidence. But lowering LDL-cholesterol by the wrong diet even may be counterproductive, if sd-LDL is raised and HDL is lowered. New insights into the pathophysiology of insulin resistance and its influence on the effects of dietary changes have led to a better approach: (1) the higher a patient's insulin resistance, the more important is the glycemic load of the diet. (2) Fat quality is much more important than fat quantity. (3) The best principle for a reduced calorie intake is not fat counting, but a high volume diet with low energy density, which means fibre rich vegetables and fruits. (4) And finally, satiation and palatability of a diet is very important: there is no success without the patient's compliance. Thus, the best approach to the dietary prevention of CVD is a Mediterranean style low-carb diet represented in the LOGI pyramid. Dietary guidelines for the prevention of CVD should to be revised accordingly.

1. Introduction

In nutritional medicine evidence is more difficult to obtain than in cardiovascular drug studies, where RCTs with hard end-points are the gold standard. Conclusions in nutritional medicine are frequently drawn from epidemiological studies, which are subject to many possible confounders. There are very few randomised studies with coronary heart disease (CHD) or total mortality as the endpoint, and those studies (like some trials in mental hospitals in the 1970s) do not meet our current ethical and scientific standards. Unlike laboratory animals, human beings cannot be fed over a long time; thus most nutritional intervention studies are short to medium term and focus on surrogate parameters.

Controlled dietary intervention studies nevertheless can give important insights into the possibilities of dietary changes. If there are known pathophysiological mechanisms, a dose-response relation in the intervention, biological plausibility, and consistency with epidemiological studies, then effects of dietary changes can be considered as plausible.

One big misconception should be avoided: hardly any food is "bad" or "good" for health *per se*. When people eat less of one kind of food, they will likely exchange it for a different one, because they usually eat "ad libitum", meaning until they are satisfied. So it is always about exchanging one food item for another one—and the main question is, which changes are best for our patient's health.

The intention of this paper is to stimulate discussions about whether the current guidelines should be adapted to the latest evidence and to give an insight into the ongoing debate, which diets are best for the prevention of cardiovascular disease.

2. Diet and Heart Disease

Traditionally, low-cholesterol (LC) and low-fat-high-carb (LFHC) diets have been recommended with the intention to reduce cardiovascular disease (CVD) and obesity risk. The evidence behind this dietary strategy is questionable.

Recent data from NHANES show trends in dietary macronutrient composition, total energy intake, and the prevalence of overweight and obesity from 1971 to 2006. While relative percentage of fat in the diet decreased significantly from 36,6% to 33,7% and the percentage of carbohydrates increased from 44,0 to 48,7%, which complied with the official LFHC recommendations, total energy intake increased, too, and US people became fatter and fatter [2]. This casts doubt on whether the recommendation to "eat less fat" has had any beneficial effect on a population level.

A recent "systematic review of the evidence supporting a causal link between dietary factors and coronary heart disease" came to the conclusion that strong evidence supported a protective associations between vegetables, nuts, monounsaturated fatty acids and a "mediterranean" style, high-quality diet and coronary heart disease (CHD), and harmful associations with the intake of transfatty acids and foods with a high glycemic index or load. Neither for saturated fat nor for eggs, there was sufficient evidence for any harm [3].

For more than ten years, leading experts in the field have been advocating a paradigm shift in dietary recommendations for the prevention of heart disease [1, 4, 5]. They are opposed by strong lobbyism of the food industry, who is against any regulations, for example, of sugar-sweetened beverages or labelling of processed food with high energy density.

In routine, daily patient care, doctors still take remarkably little notice of this controversy and of the new, high-quality evidence about the effects of dietary changes, which has been accumulated within the last decade.

3. Changing Patients, Changing Recommendations?

The "typical patient" with CHD may have changed in the last decades. Smoking prevalence has declined whereas overweight and obesity, Metabolic Syndrome (MetS), and Type 2 diabetes mellitus (T2DM) are on the rise.

About two-thirds of patients with coronary heart disease have either T2DM or an impaired glucose tolerance (IGT) [6]. The increasing prevalence of the MetS and the increasing incidence of T2DM in industrialized countries may lead in a long-term perspective to a greater lifetime burden of cardiovascular disease.

Recommendations must meet the needs of the target population and must thus be adapted to their metabolic profile. Within the last 10–15 years, high-quality evidence has been accumulated through dietary intervention studies in dyslipidemic, prediabetic, and/or diabetic subjects, in lean and in obese subjects with and without insulin resistance, which have clarified the influence of dietary changes on lipids and apolipoproteins, weight reduction, glycaemia, and insulinemia. It is important to incorporate this new evidence into dietary guidelines for cardiovascular prevention.

4. Who Is the Target Population?

The *target population* is individuals with

(a) the metabolic syndrome (MS) and insulin resistance,

(b) hypertension,

(c) hypercholesterolemia,

(d) overweight and obesity,

and very often combinations of the four.

Patients with MS have a twofold increased risk for CVD already before the manifestation of T2DM and are typically characterized by the (pre)diabetic dyslipoproteinemia (small-dense LDL, high ApoB, low HDL, low Apo-A1, high triglycerides) and fasting as well as postprandial hyperinsulinemia, in many cases by arterial hypertension and signs of premature atherosclerosis (raised IMT), too.

5. What Are the Objectives of Dietary Changes in Target Population?

The main objective is to lower the individuals' overall cardiovascular disease (CVD) risk. Dietary recommendations for this target population should therefore

(i) improve dyslipoproteinemia (lower TG, increase HDL, lower TC : HDL ratio, lower small dense LDL, and ApoB),

(ii) lower blood pressure,

(iii) lower postprandial glycaemia and insulinemia,

(iv) facilitate weight control,

(v) ensure adequate intake of essential nutrients,

(vi) ensure eating pleasure and thus compliance,

(vii) finally reduce the risk for CVD morbidity and mortality.

6. Dietary Changes to Improve Dyslipoproteinemia

Traditionally, low-cholesterol (LC) and low-fat-high-carb (LFHC) diets have been recommended to improve dyslipoproteinemia. Yet the value of reducing dietary cholesterol has never been established according to EBM criteria.

The individual response to dietary cholesterol has been extensively studied [7]: whereas about 25% experience a makeable increase of both circulating LDL and HDL cholesterol (hyperresponders), about 75% of the population experiences only a mild increase or no alterations in plasma cholesterol concentrations when challenged with high amounts of dietary cholesterol (normal responders and hyporesponders). Egg intake promotes the formation of large LDL and HDL subclasses, which are less atherogenic [8]. It may even be triggered by the question, whether an individual was breast-fed as an infant, which seems to downregulate cholesterol synthesis.

Although it had been shown very early in the 1950s that dietary cholesterol and eggs are not relevant for serum cholesterol levels [9–11], it took many years to exculpate eggs from being a cause of myocardial infarction (MI) and stroke of CVD [12, 13].

Most cohort studies, among them a recent analysis of NHANES, did not find an association between egg consumption and CVD [14]. Contrasting to that, an analysis from the Physicians' Health Study found an association between egg consumption and total mortality (but not MI and stroke), which was pronounced in diabetic physicians, the reason for which is unclear [15]. Cohort studies are subject to possible

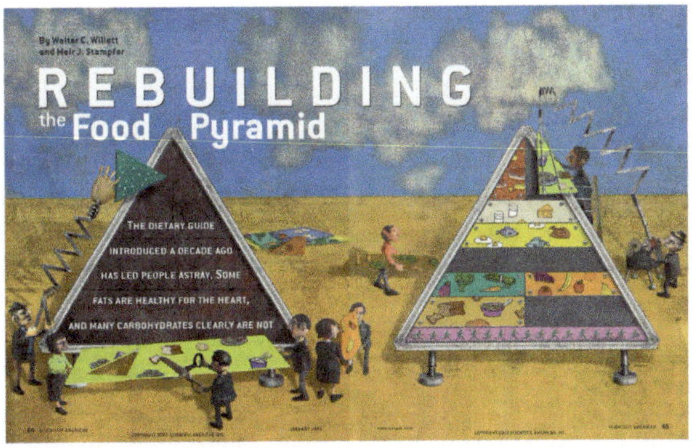

Figure 1: Cover of Willet's 2003 review article [1], with kind permission of Nature Publishing Group.

confounders. It is not known if there were lifestyle differences between physicians eating less than one egg per week and those eating more than six eggs per week. Interestingly, in the context of a carbohydrate-restricted diet, consumption of three eggs per day compared with no eggs favourably influenced the lipoprotein profile in overweight/obese male subjects [16, 17]. So the effect of egg consumption in individuals with the metabolic syndrome and/or diabetes may be modified by the carbohydrate content of the diet. In conclusion, there is no sufficient evidence to recommend a general restriction of egg consumption, which is still part of many dietary guidelines [12].

Further, the much advocated LFHC diets never had been proven to reduce CVD risk, although this still is the assumption of many physicians and nutritionists [18]. As Walter Willett put it in his remarkable 2003 review (Figure 1) in the Scientific American, "*The dietary guide we introduced a decade ago has lead people astray. Some fats are healthy for the heart, and many carbohydrates clearly are not.*" [1].

Besides, the last statement considering carbohydrates made lobbyists of the food industry to accuse Willett of a "political statement". This finally led to his exclusion from the 2005 committee, which revised the "Dietary Guidelines for Americans". Food politics always had a great influence on dietary recommendations.

It is noteworthy that before LFHC diets became popular, carbohydrates had been blamed for decades as the main culprit for diabetes, obesity, and coronary heart disease (CHD) [19].

High-quality evidence from meta-analyses of controlled nutrition intervention studies [20, 21] has now contradicted the traditional assumption that LFHC diets are the best recommendation to improve blood lipids. It has been clearly demonstrated that *fat quality* is the most important determinant of changes in blood lipids, not *total fat content* nor the *relative percentage of fat* in a diet [20].

(i) Exchanging saturated fats (less) for carbohydrates (more) will moderately lower LDL cholesterol but shift LDL subclasses to an unfavourable pattern B (small-dense LDL and higher ApoB). It will lower HDL stronger than LDL and raise triglycerides (TG), thus possibly deteriorating CVD risk, instead of improving it [22–24]. Exchanging carbohydrates (less) for saturated fats (more) induces only a small rise in TC : HDL ratio but will raise LDL size to a more favourable pattern [20, 25]. Of the four major sources of saturated fat (Lauric, myristic, palmitic, and stearic acid) only palmitic acid raises TC : HDL ratio, myristic acid is neutral, and lauric acid and stearic acid lower TC : HDL ratio and may even be beneficial [20, 26].

(ii) Exchanging carbohydrates (less) for mono- or polyunsaturated fats (more) will strongly reduce TC : HDL ratio, lower TG, and favourably influence CVD risk [27].

(iii) Exchanging saturated fats for mono- or polyunsaturated fats will improve TC : HDL ratio, too.

(iv) Only transfatty acids significantly deteriorate TC : HDL ratio if they substitute carbohydrates [20].

Low-fat-high-carb (LFHC) diets are apparently contraproductive and induce unfavourable lipid changes in overweight and obese individuals, who are insulin resistant. The metabolic profile is important for the patient's response to dietary changes: the more insulin resistant, the worse they do with a low-fat-high-carb diet. To the contrary, diets high in monounsaturated fatty acids and lower in carbohydrate content perform much better in T2DM according to a meta-analysis [27–30].

A randomised, controlled, high-quality nutrition intervention study by the group of Ronald Krauss from San Francisco clearly demonstrated the benefit of a low-carb-high-fat diet (LCHF) on blood lipids in overweight men: it compared a "prudent" LFHC diet (54% Carb, 16% Protein, 30% Fat) with a low-fat-high-protein-moderate-carb diet (39% Carb, 29% Protein, 31% Fat), an LCHF diet with predominantly monounsaturated fatty acids (26% Carb, 29% Protein, 46% Fat), and an LCHF diet higher in saturated fat (26% Carb, 29% Protein, 45% Fat). After a 1-week-run-in-phase, where all men ate a control-diet with 54% Carbs, it randomised the participants on the respective four diets for 3 weeks with stable weight (isocaloric). After this period the most favourable changes were seen in the LCHF diet with predominantly monounsaturated fatty acids: TC : HDL ratio was reduced by 13% in the LCHF group, whereas the LFHC group did not show an improvement. Lowering of ApoB was much better in the LCHF groups than in the LFHC group [31].

In the following weight-loss period all participants lost weight by calorie restriction on their respective diets. After 9 more weeks, there were improvements in all groups, which clearly separated the effects of diet alone and diet in combination with weight-loss.

This is an important aspect in the discussion, because long-term weight loss, as desirable as it may be, will remain an illusion for many individuals with weight problems. Therefore the more important is the fact that favourable changes in blood lipids are achievable *without weight loss*, if insulin resistant individuals follow an LCHF diet [32].

Thus, isocaloric exchanges of mono/polyunsaturated fatty acids (more) for carbohydrates (less) and/or protein (more) for carbohydrates (less) both improve TC : HDL ratio and LDL : HDL ratio and lower TG levels [20, 31]. The effect of LCHF diets is especially strong in overweight, obese, and/or insulin-resistant individuals.

7. Sidestep: Transfatty Acids

A widely neglected, but still very important aspect, is the problem of transfatty acids (TFAs) in fast food, bakery fats, and especially in snack foods [33, 34]. Transfatty acids in human nutrition mainly stem from partially hydrogenated vegetable oils. They raise LDL cholesterol, lower HDL-cholesterol, promote systemic inflammation, and deteriorate insulin sensitivity [35–37]. Unlike Denmark (since 2002), New York (2007), Switzerland (2008), and recently California, there is no ban on the use of TFA nor any obligation to declare its content in foods in Germany or in the European Union. Considering the importance of TFA with strong evidence for a causal link with CVD, there is an urgent need for political action towards a Europeanwide ban.

8. Effects of Different Diets on Hypertension

Reducing the dietary sodium content [38, 39] and raising the intake of potassium- and calcium-rich foods [40, 41] (e.g., fruits, vegetables, or dairy products) have been shown to lower blood pressure. The exchange of carbohydrates for either more protein or more unsaturated fatty acids lowered blood pressure and improved lipid profiles in the OmniHEART-Trial [42].

The DASH Diet is in fact a Mediterranean-style diet with 10 portions of fruits and vegetables per day, more dairy products, low sodium content, and less sugar and starch. Its glycemic load (GL) is reduced in comparison to the average American diet by preferring whole grain products instead of refined carbohydrates.

9. Effects of Different Diets on the Risk for T2DM

For quite a while now, the same low-fat-high-carb (LFHC) diet that was proposed for CVD prevention has been recommended in official guidelines to individuals with overweight, MetS, and T2DM. The main focus was lowering of TC and LDL-C, irrespective of the also known effects of such a high glycaemic load on HDL-C and glucose metabolism. A rise in glucose was lowered by medication (oral antidiabetics or insulin). Lately, the negative effects of such an approach, which favours hyperinsulinemia and ß-cell-exhaustion, have been demonstrated [43–45]. In the EPIC study and in a recently published meta-analysis of prospective studies, carbohydrate quantity and quality (GI/GL) were associated with a higher risk for T2DM [43, 46, 47].

Gerald Reaven, the "father" of the concept of insulin resistance and the Metabolic Syndrome, concluded in his 2005 review on dietary approaches in insulin resistance: *"There is considerable evidence that isocaloric diets, low in fat and enriched in CHO, will accentuate the manifestations of the IRS. The more insulin resistant an individual, the greater is the amount of insulin that must be secreted in response to a CHO-enriched diet in order to maintain glucose homeostasis. Thus, the inevitable, and consistently replicated, effect of replacing SF with CHO in insulin-resistant individuals is to increase daylong concentration of glucose or insulin, or both. In addition, this dietary approach has consistently been shown to stimulate hepatic VLDL-TG synthesis and secretion, leading to an increase in concentration of TG-rich lipoproteins, both in the fasting and postprandial states. The increase in the ambient TG-rich lipoproteins seen following low-fat/high-CHO diets has previously been shown to be associated with a decrease in HDL-C concentration, and it appears that such diets will change the LDL subclass pattern to B in 36 of 87 individuals (41%) who had either pattern A or an intermediate pattern at the outset."* [48].

Interestingly, in the preinsulin era, the dietary approach to treat T2DM was quite different and is experiencing its renaissance in the last years [19].

A recent meta-analysis of 37 prospective observational studies concluded that diets with a high GI or GL independently increased the risk of type 2 diabetes, heart disease, gallbladder disease, breast cancer, and all diseases combined [49].

The pathophysiological basis for the detrimental effects of carbohydrates in susceptible individuals has been clarified by the landmark studies of Petersen et al. from Yale University [50–52]. They discovered that an impaired mitochondrial function with a lower rate of conversion of diacyl-glycerol (DAG) to triglycerides (TGs) due to a genetic predisposition will lead to intracellular DAG accumulation, which impairs insulin signalling pathways [53] (Figure 2).

In combination with physical inactivity especially this causes muscular insulin resistance with reduced glucose uptake. After a high carbohydrate meal under these conditions, glucose will be redirected to the liver, where it induces de novo lipogenesis, fat storage in the liver, and finally hepatic insulin resistance with visceral obesity and all its known consequences. From the same amount of ingested carbohydrates, lean, but insulin resistant students will have a more than doubled de novo lipogenesis in liver as their insulin-sensitive controls. One short bout of physical activity can reverse this effect, underlining the importance of a lifestyle approach

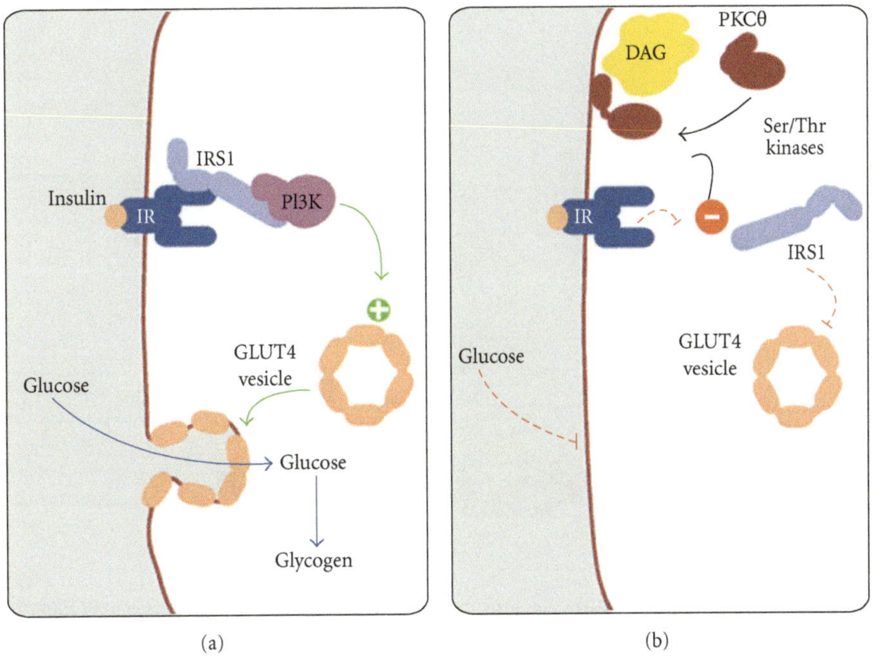

Figure 2: Pathophysiology of muscular insulin resistance: normal (a) and impaired (b) insulin signalling pathway (from [53], reprint with kind permission of Elsevier Limited).

combining dietary with physical activity recommendations in insulin resistant subjects [54].

Also, genetic deficits in insulin secretion may play a role in the development of T2DM [55]. The higher the glycaemic load of the diet, the more difficult it is for individuals with this frequent genetic mutation, to achieve glucose homeostasis. Besides, muscular activity can reverse the negative effects of this genetic deficiency, too, as has been shown in the American Diabetes Prevention Study [55].

On the other hand, controlled nutrition intervention studies have validated the influence of glycaemic load on postprandial glycaemia and have shown a benefit of carbohydrate-restricted diets with a higher content of protein and fat in prediabetic subjects as well as in diabetics [56–65].

Considering this, it is not a surprise that the latest publication from the Kuopio study published in February 2011 showed the GI/GL to be associated with a significant increase in the risk for acute myocardial infarction in overweight and/or physically inactive men [66].

10. Dietary Changes and Weight Loss

Controlled dietary intervention studies have demonstrated that low-carb-high-fat (LCHF) diets or low-glycaemic-index (LOGI) diets in comparison to low-fat-high-carb (LFHC) diets double the weight loss achieved over 6 months [67–73]. Also Low-Glycemic Load Diets (LOGI) have shown superior weight loss [74–76]. In insulin-resistant subjects especially, there is a better weight loss, when carbohydrates and/or glycaemic index are reduced. The myth that fat content of a diet is the main culprit for weight gain and obesity has been contradicted by these studies.

Interestingly, most studies tested *calorie-restricted* low-fat diets against *ad libitum* low-carb diets, and still low-carb performed better. The explanation is that low-carb but high-protein and high-fat diets promote better satiety than the traditional low-fat, low-protein, high-carb diets.

And furthermore, the energy density of a diet, which is responsible for the initial satiating effect, depends more on the *water and fibre content* of a diet than on the *relative* fat content. A "high-fat" diet with a *relative* fat content of 40–50% en but with plenty of fruits and vegetables can still be "low-caloric", because of a low energy density of the combined meal. This common misunderstanding of the term "high-fat" should be clarified at this point.

As the compliance with all dietary changes tends to degrade with time, regain of weight is initiated typically after 6–12 months. But still after 12 to 24 months there is a trend for higher weight loss on LCHF diets [73].

A recent meta-analysis of weight loss diets by the Cochrane Collaboration leads the authors to the following conclusions: *"Overweight or obese people on low glycaemic index diets lost more weight than those on high glycaemic index diets or conventional energy restricted weight loss diets, with the change in body mass, total fat mass and body mass index all significantly decreasing after the low glycaemic index diet compared to the comparison diet. It may be easier to adhere to a low glycaemic index diet than a conventional weight loss diet, since there is less need to restrict the intake of food as long as low glycaemic index carbohydrates are predominantly consumed. In studies comparing ad libitum reduced glycaemic index or load diets to conventional restricted low fat diets, even though participants could eat as much as desired on the low glycaemic index or load diets, they fared as well, or better, in the outcomes than those on the comparison diet. Hence, lowering*

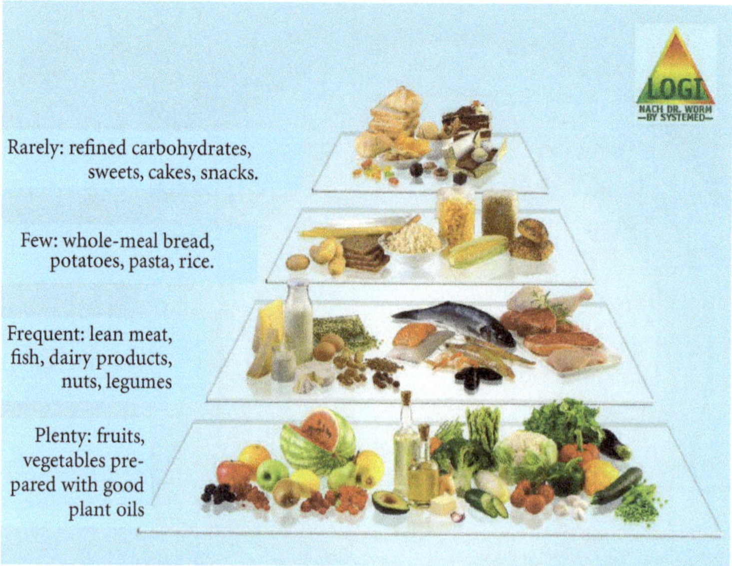
LOGI
NACH DR. WORM
—BY SYSTEMED—
Rarely: refined carbohydrates, sweets, cakes, snacks.
Few: whole-meal bread, potatoes, pasta, rice.
Frequent: lean meat, fish, dairy products, nuts, legumes
Plenty: fruits, vegetables prepared with good plant oils

FIGURE 3: The "LOGI pyramid" according to Dr. Nicolai Worm, revised version 08/2009.

the glycaemic index of foods in the diet appears to be an effective method of losing weight, particularly for the obese." [74].

11. Conclusion and Practical Approach

The aforementioned cited evidence convincingly argues for a change in dietary recommendations towards the prevention of CHD. In those patients with preponderance to overweight and diabetes especially, and in those who are most of the day physically inactive, reducing carbohydrates (low GL) is beneficial, if carbs are exchanged for good fats and/or protein.

Renowned institutions like the Joslin Diabetes Center already have revised their nutrition guidelines (Clinical nutrition guideline for overweight and obese adults with type 2 diabetes, prediabetes, or those at high risk for developing type 2 diabetes).

As any dietary strategy should be evidence-based, effective, and—in a real-life setting—practical from the patients' point of view, it has to be palatable, too.

One of most successful approaches into this direction is the LOGI concept created by David Ludwig, Harvard University, which was made popular in the German version by Dr. Nicolai Worm (Figure 3).

LOGI is "mediterranian-style low-carb" and combines practicability and palatability: it is based on an abundance of plant-based foods (fruits, low-starch vegetables, and salads), combined with "good fats" (monounsaturated and omega-3-polyunsaturated, olive oil, canola oil, nuts, seeds, fish), more protein (low-fat dairy products, legumes, fish, poultry), and only small amounts of the classical carbohydrate-rich foods like pasta, whole-meal-bread, rice, and potatoes.

Breakfast cereals, snacks, sweets, and sugar-sweetened beverages should be strictly limited. From the two basic levels (fruits/vegetables/salads/good fats, and protein sources), patients can eat ad libitum, which makes compliance very good with LOGI. There is a wealth of literature about LOGI with excellent cooking book for patients, containing easy-to-prepare recipes with calculations for energy density, carb/fat/protein content, and nutritional values (see http://www.logi-methode.de/).

12. Proposed Practical Dietary Recommendations for the Prevention of CVD

(i) Change *fat quality* to improve dyslipoproteinemia:

  (1) good fats: olive oil, canola/rapeseed oil, nut oils, nuts, seeds, and fish with omega-3-fatty acids,

  (2) neutral fats: saturated fats in milk products and cheese,

  (3) bad fats: fat in processed meat, sausages, trans-fatty acids in bakery products, cookies, sweets, and so forth.

(ii) Eat plenty high-volume-low-calorie foods: vegetables, salads, and fruits.

(iii) Reduce total carb intake, prefer low-glycaemic index foods, and reduce glycaemic load to lower fasting and postprandial glucose and insulin levels (the more insulin resistant, the stronger this recommendation is to be followed!):

  (1) good carbs: nonstarchy vegetables, salads, legumes, most fruits, and whole and minimally processed grains,

  (2) if you eat carbs, eat few and prefer whole grain bread, brown rice, and pasta,

  (3) carbs to avoid: low-fibre cereals, sugars, HFCS (high-fructose-corn-sirup) sweetened softdrinks, snacks, pizza, fries, baked potatoes, sweets,

white and brown bread, and all foods containing refined starch.

(iv) Eat more protein for better and longer lasting satiety:

(1) good protein sources: fish, poultry, low-fat dairy products, and lean-cut meat.

(2) protein sources to avoid: processed red meat and sausages.

(v) Moderate alcohol consumption:

(1) regular small amounts of alcohol (preferably wine) can be part of a healthy diet (10–20 g per day),

(2) if individuals prefer to drink small amounts of wine on a regular basis, it is OK,

(3) excessive drinking is detrimental to health,

(4) nobody should start drinking alcohol for preventive reasons,

(5) alcohol consumption should always be part of a culture of healthy good cooking (Mediterranean style).

(vi) Physical activity recommendations: 30 min daily of moderate physical activity is the minimum amount necessary for health (and should be part of the nutrition guideline, too).

Conflict of Interests

The author declares that he has no conflict of interests.

References

[1] W. C. Willett and M. J. Stampfer, "Rebuilding the food pyramid," *Scientific American*, vol. 288, no. 1, pp. 64–71, 2003.

[2] G. L. Austin, L. G. Ogden, and J. O. Hill, "Trends in carbohydrate, fat, and protein intakes and association with energy intake in normal-weight, overweight, and obese individuals: 1971–2006," *American Journal of Clinical Nutrition*, vol. 93, no. 4, pp. 836–843, 2011.

[3] A. Mente, L. De Koning, H. S. Shannon, and S. S. Anand, "A systematic review of the evidence supporting a causal link between dietary factors and coronary heart disease," *Archives of Internal Medicine*, vol. 169, no. 7, pp. 659–669, 2009.

[4] W. C. Willett, "Dietary fat and obesity: an unconvincing relation," *American Journal of Clinical Nutrition*, vol. 68, no. 6, pp. 1149–1150, 1998.

[5] F. B. Hu, "Diet and cardiovascular disease prevention. The need for a paradigm shift," *Journal of the American College of Cardiology*, vol. 50, no. 1, pp. 22–24, 2007.

[6] M. Bartnik, L. Rydén, R. Ferrari et al., "The prevalence of abnormal glucose regulation in patients with coronary artery disease across Europe: the Euro Heart Survey on diabetes and the heart," *European Heart Journal*, vol. 25, no. 21, pp. 1880–1890, 2004.

[7] P. J. Jones, "Dietary cholesterol and the risk of cardiovascular disease in patients: a review of the Harvard Egg Study and other data," *International Journal of Clinical Practice. Supplement*, no. 163, pp. 1–8, 2009.

[8] M. L. Fernandez, "Effects of eggs on plasma lipoproteins in healthy populations," *Food and Function*, vol. 1, no. 2, pp. 156–160, 2010.

[9] A. Keys, J. T. Anderson, O. Mickelsen, S. F. Adelson, and F. Fidanza, "Diet and serum cholesterol in man; lack of effect of dietary cholesterol," *Journal of Nutrition*, vol. 59, no. 1, pp. 39–56, 1956.

[10] M. W. Porter, W. Yamanaka, S. D. Carlson, and M. A. Flynn, "Effect of dietary egg on serum cholesterol and triglyceride of human males," *American Journal of Clinical Nutrition*, vol. 30, no. 4, pp. 490–495, 1977.

[11] M. A. Flynn, G. B. Nolph, and T. C. Flynn, "Effect of dietary egg on human serum cholesterol and triglycerides," *American Journal of Clinical Nutrition*, vol. 32, no. 5, pp. 1051–1057, 1979.

[12] F. B. Hu, M. J. Stampfer, E. B. Rimm et al., "A prospective study of egg consumption and risk of cardiovascular disease in men and women," *Journal of the American Medical Association*, vol. 281, no. 15, pp. 1387–1394, 1999.

[13] R. M. Weggemans, P. L. Zock, and M. B. Katan, "Dietary cholesterol from eggs increases the ratio of total cholesterol to high-density lipoprotein cholesterol in humans: a meta-analysis," *American Journal of Clinical Nutrition*, vol. 73, no. 5, pp. 885–891, 2001.

[14] C. G. Scrafford, N. L. Tran, L. M. Barraj, and P. J. Mink, "Egg consumption and CHD and stroke mortality: a prospective study of US adults," *Public Health Nutrition*, vol. 14, no. 2, pp. 261–270, 2011.

[15] L. Djoussé and J. M. Gaziano, "Egg consumption in relation to cardiovascular disease and mortality: the Physicians' Health Study," *American Journal of Clinical Nutrition*, vol. 87, no. 4, pp. 964–969, 2008.

[16] G. Mutungi, D. Waters, J. Ratliff et al., "Eggs distinctly modulate plasma carotenoid and lipoprotein subclasses in adult men following a carbohydrate-restricted diet," *Journal of Nutritional Biochemistry*, vol. 21, no. 4, pp. 261–267, 2010.

[17] G. Mutungi, J. Ratliff, M. Puglisi et al., "Dietary cholesterol from eggs increases plasma HDL cholesterol in overweight men consuming a carbohydrate-restricted diet," *Journal of Nutrition*, vol. 138, no. 2, pp. 272–276, 2008.

[18] F. M. Sacks and M. Katan, "Randomized clinical trials on the effects of dietary fat and carbohydrate on plasma lipoproteins and cardiovascular disease," *American Journal of Medicine*, vol. 113, no. 9, pp. 13S–24S, 2002.

[19] E. C. Westman, W. S. Yancy Jr., and M. Humphreys, "Dietary treatment of diabetes mellitus in the pre-insulin era (1914–1922)," *Perspectives in Biology and Medicine*, vol. 49, no. 1, pp. 77–83, 2006.

[20] R. P. Mensink, P. L. Zock, A. D. M. Kester, and M. B. Katan, "Effects of dietary fatty acids and carbohydrates on the ratio of serum total to HDL cholesterol and on serum lipids and apolipoproteins: a meta-analysis of 60 controlled trials," *American Journal of Clinical Nutrition*, vol. 77, no. 5, pp. 1146–1155, 2003.

[21] M. B. Katan, P. L. Zock, and R. P. Mensink, "Effects of fats and fatty acids on blood lipids in humans: an overview," *American Journal of Clinical Nutrition*, vol. 60, no. 6, pp. 1017S–1022S, 1994.

[22] R. M. Krauss, "Dietary and genetic effects on low-density lipoprotein heterogeneity," *Annual Review of Nutrition*, vol. 21, pp. 283–295, 2001.

[23] S. Ip, A. H. Lichtenstein, M. Chung, J. Lau, and E. M. Balk, "Systematic review: association of low-density lipoprotein subtractions with cardiovascular outcomes," *Annals of Internal Medicine*, vol. 150, no. 7, pp. 474–484, 2009.

[24] K. Musunuru, "Atherogenic dyslipidemia: cardiovascular risk and dietary intervention," *Lipids*, vol. 45, no. 10, pp. 907–914, 2010.

[25] V. Guay, B. Lamarche, A. Charest, A. J. Tremblay, and P. Couture, "Effect of short-term low- and high-fat diets on low-density lipoprotein particle size in normolipidemic subjects," *Metabolism*, vol. 61, no. 1, pp. 76–83, 2012.

[26] R. P. Mensink, "Effects of the individual saturated fatty acids on serum lipids and lipoprotein concentrations," *American Journal of Clinical Nutrition*, vol. 57, no. 5, pp. 711S–714S, 1993.

[27] Y. Cao, D. T. Mauger, C. L. Pelkman, G. Zhao, S. M. Townsend, and P. M. Kris-Etherton, "Effects of moderate (MF) versus lower fat (LF) diets on lipids and lipoproteins: a meta-analysis of clinical trials in subjects with and without diabetes," *Journal of Clinical Lipidology*, vol. 3, no. 1, pp. 19–32, 2009.

[28] M. Lefevre, C. M. Champagne, R. T. Tulley, J. C. Rood, and M. M. Most, "Individual variability in cardiovascular disease risk factor responses to low-fat and low-saturated-fat diets in men: body mass index, adiposity, and insulin resistance predict changes in LDL cholesterol," *American Journal of Clinical Nutrition*, vol. 82, no. 5, pp. 957–963, 2005.

[29] A. Garg, "High-monounsaturated-fat diets for patients with diabetes mellitus: a meta-analysis," *American Journal of Clinical Nutrition*, vol. 67, no. 3, pp. 577S–582S, 1998.

[30] S. Kodama, K. Saito, S. Tanaka et al., "Influence of fat and carbohydrate proportions on the metabolic profile in patients with type 2 diabetes: a meta-analysis," *Diabetes Care*, vol. 32, no. 5, pp. 959–965, 2009.

[31] R. M. Krauss, P. J. Blanche, R. S. Rawlings, H. S. Fernstrom, and P. T. Williams, "Separate effects of reduced carbohydrate intake and weight loss on atherogenic dyslipidemia," *American Journal of Clinical Nutrition*, vol. 83, no. 5, pp. 1025–1031, 2006.

[32] R. D. Feinman and J. S. Volek, "Low carbohydrate diets improve atherogenic dyslipidemia even in the absence of weight loss," *Nutrition and Metabolism*, vol. 3, article no. 24, 2006.

[33] D. Mozaffarian, M. B. Katan, A. Ascherio, M. J. Stampfer, and W. C. Willett, "Trans fatty acids and cardiovascular disease," *New England Journal of Medicine*, vol. 354, no. 15, pp. 1601–1613, 2006.

[34] S. Stender, J. Dyerberg, and A. Astrup, "High levels of industrially produced trans fat in popular fast foods," *New England Journal of Medicine*, vol. 354, no. 15, pp. 1650–1651, 2006.

[35] R. Micha and D. Mozaffarian, "Trans fatty acids: effects on cardiometabolic health and implications for policy," *Prostaglandins Leukotrienes and Essential Fatty Acids*, vol. 79, no. 3–5, pp. 147–152, 2008.

[36] R. Micha, I. B. King, R. N. Lemaitre et al., "Food sources of individual plasma phospholipid trans fatty acid isomers: the cardiovascular health study," *American Journal of Clinical Nutrition*, vol. 91, no. 4, pp. 883–893, 2010.

[37] R. Micha and D. Mozaffarian, "Trans fatty acids: effects on metabolic syndrome, heart disease and diabetes," *Nature Reviews Endocrinology*, vol. 5, no. 6, pp. 335–344, 2009.

[38] N. R. Cook, J. A. Cutler, E. Obarzanek et al., "Long term effects of dietary sodium reduction on cardiovascular disease outcomes: observational follow-up of the trials of hypertension prevention (TOHP)," *British Medical Journal*, vol. 334, no. 7599, pp. 885–888, 2007.

[39] V. J. Stevens, E. Obarzanek, N. R. Cook et al., "Long-term weight loss and changes in blood pressure: results of the trials of hypertension prevention, phase II," *Annals of Internal Medicine*, vol. 134, no. 1, pp. 1–11, 2001.

[40] L. J. Appel, T. J. Moore, E. Obarzanek et al., "A clinical trial of the effects of dietary patterns on blood pressure," *New England Journal of Medicine*, vol. 336, no. 16, pp. 1117–1124, 1997.

[41] F. M. Sacks, L. P. Svetkey, W. M. Vollmer et al., "Effects on blood pressure of reduced dietary sodium and the dietary approaches to stop hypertension (dash) diet," *New England Journal of Medicine*, vol. 344, no. 1, pp. 3–10, 2001.

[42] L. J. Appel, F. M. Sacks, V. J. Carey et al., "Effects of protein, monounsaturated fat, and carbohydrate intake on blood pressure and serum lipids: results of the OmniHeart randomized trial," *Journal of the American Medical Association*, vol. 294, no. 19, pp. 2455–2464, 2005.

[43] I. Sluijs, Y. T. van der Schouw, D. L. van der A et al., "Carbohydrate quantity and quality and risk of type 2 diabetes in the European Prospective Investigation into Cancer and Nutrition-Netherlands (EPIC-NL) study," *The American Journal of Clinical Nutrition*, vol. 92, no. 4, pp. 905–911, 2010.

[44] J. N. Davis, E. E. Ventura, M. J. Weigensberg et al., "The relation of sugar intake to β cell function in overweight Latino children," *American Journal of Clinical Nutrition*, vol. 82, no. 5, pp. 1004–1010, 2005.

[45] K. Kærch, A. Vaag, J. J. Holst, T. Hansen, T. Jøhnsen, and K. Borch-Johnsen, "Natural history of insulin sensitivity and insulin secretion in the progression from normal glucose tolerance to impaired fasting glycemia and impaired glucose tolerance: The inter99 study," *Diabetes Care*, vol. 32, no. 3, pp. 439–444, 2009.

[46] J.-Y. Dong, L. Zhang, Y.-H. Zhang, and L.-Q. Qin, "Dietary glycaemic index and glycaemic load in relation to the risk of type 2 diabetes: a meta-analysis of prospective cohort studies," *British Journal of Nutrition*, vol. 106, no. 11, pp. 1649–1654, 2011.

[47] K. Færch, A. Vaag, D. R. Witte, T. Jørgensen, O. Pedersen, and K. Borch-Johnsen, "Predictors of future fasting and 2-h post-OGTT plasma glucose levels in middle-aged men and women—the Inter99 study," *Diabetic Medicine*, vol. 26, no. 4, pp. 377–383, 2009.

[48] G. M. Reaven, "The insulin resistance syndrome: definition and dietary approaches to treatment," *Annual Review of Nutrition*, vol. 25, pp. 391–406, 2005.

[49] A. W. Barclay, P. Petocz, J. McMillan-Price et al., "Glycemic index, glycemic load, and chronic disease risk—a metaanalysis of observational studies," *American Journal of Clinical Nutrition*, vol. 87, no. 3, pp. 627–637, 2008.

[50] K. F. Petersen, S. Dufour, D. Befroy, R. Garcia, and G. I. Shulman, "Impaired mitochondrial activity in the insulin-resistant offspring of patients with type 2 diabetes," *New England Journal of Medicine*, vol. 350, no. 7, pp. 664–671, 2004.

[51] K. F. Petersen and G. I. Shulman, "New insights into the pathogenesis of insulin resistance in humans using magnetic resonance spectroscopy," *Obesity*, vol. 14, pp. 34S–40S, 2006.

[52] K. F. Petersen, S. Dufour, D. B. Savage et al., "The role of skeletal muscle insulin resistance in the pathogenesis of the metabolic syndrome," *Proceedings of the National Academy of Sciences of the United States of America*, vol. 104, no. 31, pp. 12587–12594, 2007.

[53] V. T. Samuel, K. F. Petersen, and G. I. Shulman, "Lipid-induced insulin resistance: unravelling the mechanism," *The Lancet*, vol. 375, no. 9733, pp. 2267–2277, 2010.

[54] R. Rabøl, K. F. Petersen, S. Dufour, C. Flannery, and G. I. Shulman, "Reversal of muscle insulin resistance with exercise reduces postprandial hepatic de novo lipogenesis in insulin resistant individuals," *Proceedings of the National Academy of*

Sciences of the United States of America, vol. 108, no. 33, pp. 13705–13709, 2011.

[55] J. C. Florez, K. A. Jablonski, N. Bayley et al., "TCF7L2 polymorphisms and progression to diabetes in the Diabetes Prevention Program," *New England Journal of Medicine*, vol. 355, no. 3, pp. 241–250, 2006.

[56] E. C. Westman, R. D. Feinman, J. C. Mavropoulos et al., "Low-carbohydrate nutrition and metabolism," *American Journal of Clinical Nutrition*, vol. 86, no. 2, pp. 276–284, 2007.

[57] M. C. Gannon and F. Q. Nuttall, "Effect of a high-protein, low-carbohydrate diet on blood glucose control in people with type 2 diabetes," *Diabetes*, vol. 53, no. 9, pp. 2375–2382, 2004.

[58] F. Q. Nuttall and M. C. Gannon, "The metabolic response to a high-protein, low-carbohydrate diet in men with type 2 diabetes mellitus," *Metabolism: Clinical and Experimental*, vol. 55, no. 2, pp. 243–251, 2006.

[59] M. C. Gannon and F. Q. Nuttall, "Control of blood glucose in type 2 diabetes without weight loss by modification of diet composition," *Nutrition and Metabolism*, vol. 3, article no. 16, 2006.

[60] F. Q. Nuttall and M. C. Gannon, "Dietary management of type 2 diabetes: a personal odyssey," *Journal of the American College of Nutrition*, vol. 26, no. 2, pp. 83–94, 2007.

[61] J. Galgani, C. Aguirre, and E. Díaz, "Acute effect of meal glycemic index and glycemic load on blood glucose and insulin responses in humans," *Nutrition Journal*, vol. 5, article no. 22, 2006.

[62] J. C. Brand-Miller, "Postprandial glycemia, glycemic index, and the prevention of type 2 diabetes," *American Journal of Clinical Nutrition*, vol. 80, no. 2, pp. 243–244, 2004.

[63] J. C. Brand-Miller, M. Thomas, V. Swan, Z. I. Ahmad, P. Petocz, and S. Colagiuri, "Physiological validation of the concept of glycemic load in lean young adults," *Journal of Nutrition*, vol. 133, no. 9, pp. 2728–2732, 2003.

[64] J. Brand-Miller, S. Hayne, P. Petocz, and S. Colagiuri, "Low-glycemic index diets in the management of diabetes: a meta-analysis of randomized controlled trials," *Diabetes Care*, vol. 26, no. 8, pp. 2261–2267, 2003.

[65] F. Q. Nuttall, K. Schweim, H. Hoover, and M. C. Gannon, "Effect of the LoBAG30 diet on blood glucose control in people with type 2 diabetes," *British Journal of Nutrition*, vol. 99, no. 3, pp. 511–519, 2008.

[66] J. Mursu, J. K. Virtanen, T. H. Rissanen et al., "Glycemic index, glycemic load, and the risk of acute myocardial infarction in Finnish men: the Kuopio Ischaemic Heart Disease Risk Factor Study," *Nutrition, Metabolism and Cardiovascular Diseases*, vol. 21, no. 2, pp. 144–149, 2011.

[67] F. F. Samaha, N. Iqbal, P. Seshadri et al., "A low-carbohydrate as compared with a low-fat diet in severe obesity," *New England Journal of Medicine*, vol. 348, no. 21, pp. 2074–2081, 2003.

[68] L. Stern, N. Iqbal, P. Seshadri et al., "The effects of low-carbohydrate versus conventional weight loss diets in severely obese adults: one-year follow-up of a randomized trial," *Annals of Internal Medicine*, vol. 140, no. 10, pp. 778–785, 2004.

[69] P. Seshadri, N. Iqbal, L. Stern et al., "A randomized study comparing the effects of a low-carbohydrate diet and a conventional diet on lipoprotein subfractions and C-reactive protein levels in patients with severe obesity," *American Journal of Medicine*, vol. 117, no. 6, pp. 398–405, 2004.

[70] F. F. Samaha, "Effect of very high-fat diets on body weight, lipoproteins, and glycemic status in the obese," *Current Atherosclerosis Reports*, vol. 7, no. 6, pp. 412–420, 2005.

[71] C. D. Gardner, A. Kiazand, S. Alhassan et al., "Comparison of the Atkins, Zone, Ornish, and LEARN diets for change in weight and related risk factors among overweight premenopausal women: the A to Z weight loss study: A randomized trial," *Journal of the American Medical Association*, vol. 297, no. 9, pp. 969–977, 2007.

[72] I. Shai, D. Schwarzfuchs, Y. Henkin et al., "Weight loss with a low-carbohydrate, Mediterranean, or low-fat diet," *New England Journal of Medicine*, vol. 359, no. 3, pp. 229–241, 2008.

[73] M. Hession, C. Rolland, U. Kulkarni, A. Wise, and J. Broom, "Systematic review of randomized controlled trials of low-carbohydrate vs. low-fat/low-calorie diets in the management of obesity and its comorbidities," *Obesity Reviews*, vol. 10, no. 1, pp. 36–50, 2009.

[74] D. E. Thomas, E. J. Elliott, and L. Baur, "Low glycaemic index or low glycaemic load diets for overweight and obesity," *Cochrane Database of Systematic Reviews*, no. 3, Article ID CD005105, 2007.

[75] A. Esfahani, J. M. W. Wong, A. Mirrahimi, C. R. Villa, and C. W. C. Kendall, "The application of the glycemic index and glycemic load in weight loss: a review of the clinical evidence," *IUBMB Life*, vol. 63, no. 1, pp. 7–13, 2011.

[76] J. M. Shikany, R. Desmond, R. Mccubrey, and D. B. Allison, "Meta-analysis of studies of a specific delivery mode for a modified-carbohydrate diet," *Journal of Human Nutrition and Dietetics*, vol. 24, no. 6, pp. 525–535, 2011.

6

Discordance of Non-HDL and Directly Measured LDL Cholesterol: Which Lipid Measure is Preferred When Calculated LDL Is Inaccurate?

Lawrence Baruch,[1,2] Valerie J. Chiong,[1] Sanjay Agarwal,[3] and Bhanu Gupta[4]

[1] *James J. Peters VA Medical Center, Bronx, NY 10468, USA*
[2] *Mt. Sinai School of Medicine, NY, USA*
[3] *Confluence Health, Moses Lake, WA 98837, USA*
[4] *St. Luke's Hospital, University of Missouri, Kansas City, MO 64111, USA*

Correspondence should be addressed to Lawrence Baruch; lawrence.baruch@va.gov

Academic Editor: Gerhard M. Kostner

Objective. To determine if non-HDL cholesterol (N-HDL) and directly measured LDL cholesterol (D-LDL) are clinically equivalent measurements. *Patients and Methods.* Eighty-one subjects recruited for 2 cholesterol treatment studies had at least 1 complete fasting lipid panel and D-LDL performed simultaneously; 64 had a second assessment after 4 to 6 weeks, resulting in 145 triads of C-LDL, D-LDL, and N-HDL. To directly compare N-HDL to D-LDL and C-LDL, we normalized the N-HDL by subtracting 30 from the N-HDL (N-HDL_A). *Results.* There was significant correlation between N-HDL_A, D-LDL, and C-LDL. Correlation was significantly greater between N-HDL_A and C-LDL than between N-HDL_A and D-LDL. A greater than 20 mg/dL difference between measures was observed more commonly between N-HDL_A and D-LDL, 29%, than between C-LDL and N-HDL_A, 11% ($P < 0.001$), and C-LDL and D-LDL, 17% ($P = 0.028$). Clinical discordance was most common, and concordance was least common between N-HDL and D-LDL. *Conclusions.* Our findings suggest that N-HDL cholesterol and D-LDL cholesterol are not clinically equivalent and frequently discordant. As N-HDL may be superior to even C-LDL for predicting events in statin-treated patients, utilizing N-HDL to guide therapy would appear to be preferable to D-LDL when C-LDL is inaccurate.

1. Introduction

Calculated low density lipoprotein cholesterol (LDL) is the cornerstone of lipid lowering therapy [1–3]. In certain clinical situations, namely, the fed state or when triglycerides are greater than 400 mg/dL, calculated LDL is inaccurate and the guidelines recommend the use of directly measured LDL cholesterol [1].

We previously reported that calculated and directly measured LDL are not clinically equivalent when targeting ATP III goals with lipid lowering therapy in a significant number of patients [4]. Based on this finding, we recommended that non-HDL cholesterol (N-HDL), an accepted, inexpensive, and guideline-based measure of atherogenic particles, available from the routine lipid panel, replace directly measured LDL (D-LDL) when the calculated LDL (C-LDL) is inaccurate [4]. However, few studies are available comparing the clinical equivalence of calculated LDL, directly measured LDL, and non-HDL cholesterol measurements. Therefore, we evaluated the clinical equivalence of N-HDL and D-LDL which would allow us to determine which lipid measure is more appropriate when C-LDL is inaccurate.

2. Methods

Our population consisted of 81 subjects from the Bronx Veterans Affairs Medical Center recruited for 2 research studies from January 2007 through March 2009. The studies incorporated simultaneous measurement of direct LDL with a Siemens Advia Chemistry System and a complete fasting lipid panel at 2 time intervals, baseline, and after 4 to 6 weeks of therapy. C-LDL was calculated using the Friedwald formula: total cholesterol—HDL − triglycerides/5. Non-HDL cholesterol was calculated as total cholesterol—HDL cholesterol. The studies were approved by the institutional review board of the Bronx VA Medical Center and registered at http://clinicaltrials.gov/ (NCT00762164 and NCT00762229). All subjects signed an informed consent document.

The NCEP ATP III guidelines, which established that N-HDL goals are 30 mg/dL above those for LDL (e.g., an individual with an LDL goal <100 has an N-HDL goal of <130), formed the basis for our comparisons between the measures of LDL (direct and calculated) and N-HDL [1, 3]. Thus, for assessment of placement in the same lipid goal cut points, LDL goals of <160, <130, <100, and <70 mg/dL corresponded to N-HDL goals of <190, <160, <130, and <100 mg/dL, respectively [1, 3]. To "normalize" N-HDL to LDL values for direct numerical comparisons, 30 was subtracted from N-HDL (e.g., an N-HDL of 155 was "normalized" to a value of 125, 155 − 30 = 125) to create the "adjusted" N-HDL (N-HDL_A).

Correlation between the lipid parameters was determined using Pearson's correlation coefficient.

The relationship between C-LDL, D-LDL, and N-HDL was also evaluated from a clinical perspective based on the following rationale. In clinical practice, adjustment of lipid lowering therapy is primarily based on the LDL numerical value (e.g., 112 mg/dL) and the ATP III goal (e.g., LDL < 100 mg/dL, N-HDL < 130 mg/dL in a patient with diabetes) [1, 3]. Furthermore, doubling the dose of any statin results in an additional 6% reduction in LDL [5]. Finally, minor changes in LDL are not generally considered to be clinically meaningful. As such, when comparing any 2 of the lipid values (e.g., N-HDL to D-LDL, N-HDL to C-LDL) they were considered *"clinically concordant"* when fulfilling the following criteria: (1) placement in the same ATP III goal cut point range (e.g., 100–129 when comparing C-LDL and D-LDL, an N-HDL of 100–129 and a C-LDL 70–99) [1, 3], (2) <6% difference between the values (e.g., C-LDL versus N-HDL_A, and C-LDL versus D-LDL) which represents the incremental LDL lowering provided by a single titration of statin dose (e.g., from simvastatin 20 to 40 mg [5]), and (3) <10 mg/dL difference between the 2 values (a difference that clinicians may consider meaningful, thus not concordant, even when the values being compared are in the same ATP III cut point and differ by <6%, e.g., when D-LDL is 181 mg/dL and N-HDL_A is 171 mg/dL).

We considered the numerical values *"clinically discordant"* when they fulfilled the following criteria: (1) placement in different ATP III goal cut point ranges [1, 3], (2) ≥12% difference between the 2 values (representing the incremental LDL lowering provided by two statin titration steps, e.g., from atorvastatin 20 to 80 mg [5]), and (3) ≥10 mg/dL difference between the values (as clinicians may *not* consider the values discordant, even when they are in different ATP III cut points and differ by ≥12% when the values being compared differ by <10 mg/dL, e.g., when N-HDL_A is 66 mg/dL and D-LDL is 75 mg/dL).

Categorical data were compared using descriptive statistics from Minitab 15th Edition (State College, PA). One sample t-test and analysis of variance (ANOVA) were used to assess within-group and between-group differences in lipid values. A P value < 0.05 was considered statistically significant for these analyses. Differences in correlation coefficients were evaluated by Fisher's z-transformation. A z-value ≥ 2.0 was considered significant for these analyses. Microsoft Excel 2007 and SPSS, version 19.0 (SPSS Inc., an IBM company), were used to analyze study data.

Our sample size was limited by the number of subjects who enrolled in each of the respective protocols.

TABLE 1: Baseline characteristics.

Variable	Initiation (n = 81)
Age (years)	60
Weight (kg)*	92
Height (cm)*	176
Male	38 (100%)
Hypertension	25 (66%)
Diabetes mellitus	9 (24%)
Low density lipoprotein (mg/dL)—calculated*	141
Low density lipoprotein (mg/dL)—direct*	149
Total cholesterol (mg/dL)	216
HDL (mg/dL)	49
Non-HDL (mg/dL)	160
"Adjusted" non-HDL (mg/dL)	130
Triglycerides (mg/dL)	130

*One patient had nonfasting lipids; his baseline LDL measurements, triglycerides, HDL, and "adjusted" non-HDL were therefore not included. Two patients did not have an assessment of height and weight.

3. Results

A total of 81 subjects had at least one lipid triad of C-LDL, D-LDL, and N-HDL performed simultaneously. Of these 81 subjects, 64 successfully completed their respective studies and had lipids assessed at baseline and followup. Sixteen subjects had lipids assessed only at baseline, and 1 patient only had a followup, as his baseline lipid assessment was nonfasting. This resulted in a total of 145 total triads of C-LDL, D-LDL, and N-HDL that were included in the analysis.

Baseline characteristics are shown in Table 1. Subjects tended to be elderly, overweight, hypertensive, and predominantly male. At baseline, N-HDL_A was less than direct and calculated LDL in 81% and 68% of subjects, respectively; D-LDL was greater than C-LDL in 66% of patients.

There was significant correlation between N-HDL_A, D-LDL, and C-LDL. For the entire cohort, which included all 145 baseline and follow-up values, the correlations for N-HDL_A with C-LDL, r^2 of 0.89 (Figure 1(a)), N-HDL_A with D-LDL, r^2 of 0.80 (Figure 1(b)), and C-LDL with D-LDL, r^2 of 0.86 (Figure 1(c)) were strong. The strength of the correlation between N-HDL_A and C-LDL was statistically significantly greater than between N-HDL_A and D-LDL for both the baseline (z = 2.02) and entire cohorts (z = 2.66).

At baseline, *clinical concordance* (as defined in Section 2) between D-LDL and N-HDL was present in only 20%

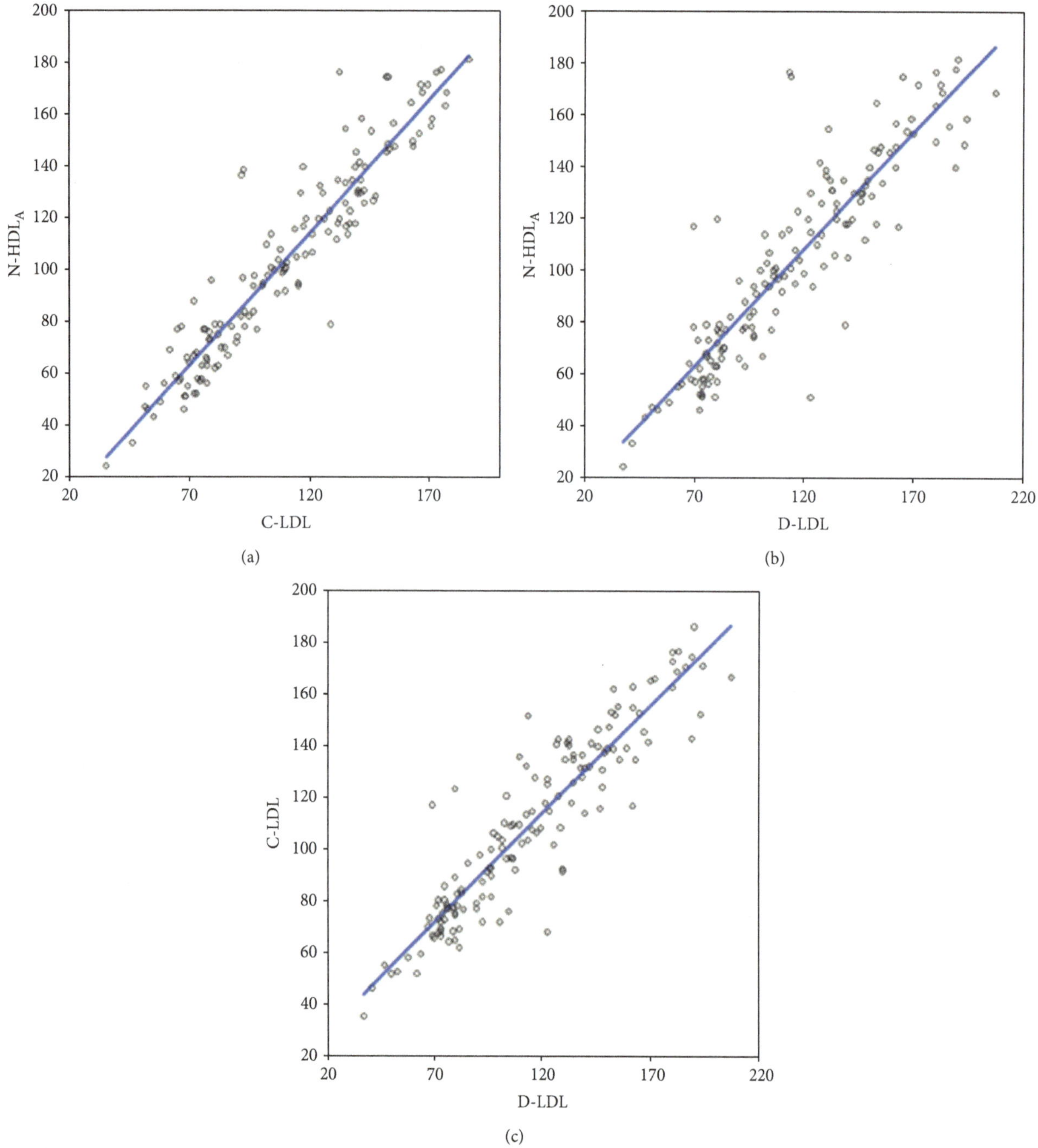

Figure 1: Regression plots for D-LDL-C, C-LDL, and N-HDL$_A$ for all values (n = 145). (a) N-HDL$_A$ with C-LDL (r^2 = 0.89). (b) N-HDL$_A$ with D-LDL (r^2 = 0.80). (c) D-LDL with C-LDL (r^2 = 0.86).

of patients, as compared to 36% between C-LDL and N-HDL and 34% between C-LDL and D-LDL. This difference approached statistical significance when comparing D-LDL and N-HDL to C-LDL (P = 0.064). Furthermore, when analyzed from a numerical perspective of clinical equivalence, values within 5 or 10 mg/dL of each other, this was least commonly observed with N-HDL$_A$ and D-LDL in the baseline and entire cohort (Figure 2). A statistically significant difference was observed between N-HDL$_A$ versus D-LDL and C-LDL versus D-LDL for both 5 and 10 mg/dL for the entire cohort (Figure 2(b)).

Clinical discordance (as defined in Section 2) between non-HDL and the 2 measures of LDL was noted on at least 1 occasion in 47% of patients with respect to D-LDL and in 37% with respect to C-LDL, while C-LDL and D-LDL were discordant in only 30% of patients (P = 0.075). A similar pattern emerged when looking at only the baseline lipid values, with discordance noted between N-HDL and

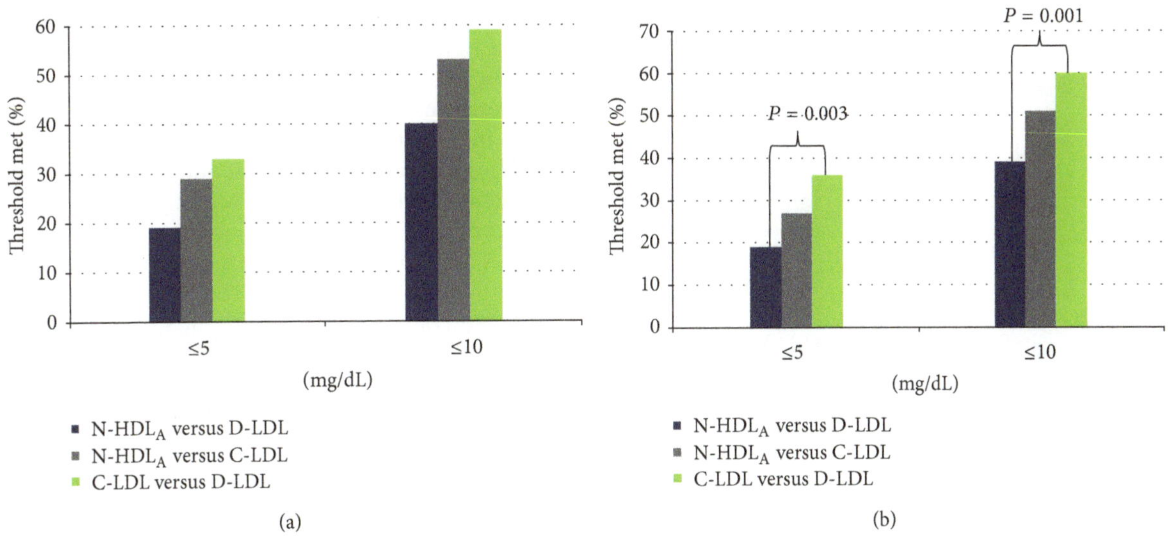

FIGURE 2: Percentage of patients whose values are near each other from a numerical perspective, <5 and <10 mg/dL. (a) Baseline values ($n = 80$), approached statistical significance for the between group differences ($P = 0.054$). (b) All values in the study ($n = 145$).

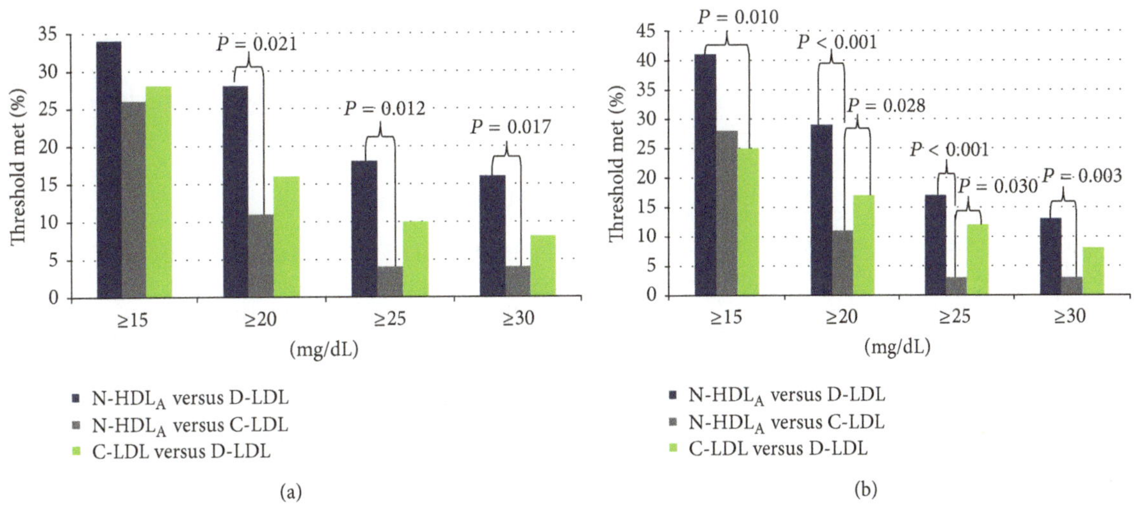

FIGURE 3: Percentage of patients with a difference between N-HDL$_A$, D-LDL and C-LDL of 15, 20, 25, and 30 mg/dL. (a) Baseline values ($n = 80$). (b) All values in the study ($n = 145$).

D-LDL in 31% of patients, as compared to 23% between N-HDL and C-LDL and 15% between direct and calculated LDL ($P = 0.039$ versus N-HDL and D-LDL).

Moreover, a clinically meaningful percentage of patients had a greater than 20 mg/dL difference between the various measures across the dataset, for both baseline and all values (Figure 3). This was statistically significantly more common when analyzing all values, between N-HDL$_A$ and D-LDL, 29%, when compared to C-LDL and N-HDL$_A$, 11% ($P < 0.001$) or C-LDL and D-LDL, 17% ($P = 0.028$) (Figure 3(b)). Similar statistically significant and clinically meaningful findings were observed when analyzing only the baseline values (Figure 3(a)). A number of patients manifested even larger differences between the lipid measures, differences that clinicians would consider highly meaningful. This was observed most frequently when comparing N-HDL$_A$ and D-LDL, and was statistically significant for a number of values and lipid comparisons (Figure 3).

Similarly, the mean absolute difference between the various lipid measures was the greatest between D-LDL and N-HDL$_A$, approximately 16 mg/dL, as compared to approximately 11 mg/dL for N-HDL$_A$ to C-LDL and D-LDL to C-LDL (Figure 4).

4. Discussion

Our analysis demonstrates a linear correlation between "adjusted" N-HDL and measures of LDL used in clinical practice, calculated and direct LDL. Despite this correlation, clinical discordance was observed in more than one in

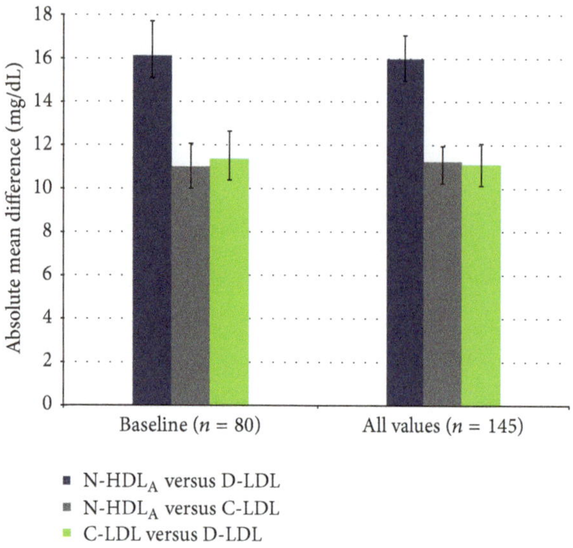

Figure 4: Mean absolute difference with standard deviation between N-HDL$_A$, D-LDL, and C-LDL for baseline values (n = 80) and all values (n = 145) in the study. The difference and standard deviation are the largest between N-HDL$_A$ and D-LDL in both cohorts. Between-group differences were statistically significant, with N-HDL$_A$ and D-LDL significantly different from both of the other lipid measurements for the baseline and entire cohorts, P = 0.010 and <0.001, respectively.

three patients, and it was more common for N-HDL to be discordant than concordant with either C-LDL or D-LDL. It is evident that N-HDL does not consistently provide similar clinical information to either measures of LDL in individual patients, a finding parallel to what we had seen previously when comparing C-LDL to D-LDL. This dissociation between clinical concordance and correlation results from the correlation coefficient being a summary statistic, rather than a statistic that defines relationships in individual patients.

Moreover, N-HDL and D-LDL, the recommended alternative lipid measures when C-LDL is inaccurate [1, 3] appear to be the most divergent of the three lipid "pairs," with N-HDL$_A$ generally lowest, D-LDL highest, and C-LDL intermediate. Similarly, the average difference between lipid "pairs" was the greatest between N-HDL$_A$ and D-LDL. N-HDL$_A$ and D-LDL had the fewest number of patients whose values were very close to each other, within 5 mg/dL, and the greatest number with highly discrepant values (e.g., >20 mg/dL). Furthermore, N-HDL$_A$ and D-LDL had the fewest concordant and most discordant values. Consistent with these findings, the weakest correlation was between N-HDL and D-LDL.

Consequently, when C-LDL is inaccurate, recommending measurement of either N-HDL or D-LDL appears questionable, as these 2 lipid measures may not reliably provide the same clinical information in individual patients. Adopting such an approach will result in different treatment decisions, resulting in less intensive therapy when the primary target is N-HDL, and more intensive therapy, even with respect to C-LDL, when D-LDL is the primary target. As there are fewer extreme differences from a numerical perspective between N-HDL and C-LDL, and N-HDL affords the additional advantages of the absence of additional cost and potential superiority to even C-LDL in predicting cardiovascular risk [6–11], the use of N-HDL seems preferable in situations where C-LDL is inaccurate. The use of non-HDL in this setting is consistent with the growing body of support for non-HDL as a target of therapy [6–11], with some even advocating that it replaces *calculated* LDL as the primary target of therapy [12].

4.1. Study Limitations. Our study is limited by the use of a single commercial assay, in a modest number of a select, male, veteran population from a single center. Criteria for clinical concordance and discordance were based on our understanding of what clinicians would consider clinically meaningful. In addition, our patients are not representative of those in whom assessment of D-LDL is recommended, as all were fasting and had triglyceride levels of less than 400 mg/dL. Despite these limitations, our study remains relevant for a number of reasons. Clinicians routinely use commercially available D-LDL assays, while our criteria for clinical concordance and discordance consisted of 3 criteria, any 1 of which clinicians may consider clinically meaningful. Moreover, N-HDL becomes more valuable as a predictor of risk as the triglycerides increase and non-HDL-C represents a secondary target of therapy when triglycerides are greater than 200 mg/dL [1].

5. Conclusion

N-HDL and D-LDL are the most divergent of the various lipid "pairs", on opposite "poles" of C-LDL, and thus do not appear to be clinically equivalent. The current findings strengthen our previous recommendation that N-HDL, and not D-LDL, be used in clinical situations where C-LDL is inaccurate, as N-HDL is a validated target of therapy, free of additional cost, and incorporated into existing guidelines. The clinical discordance between all 3 lipid measures, N-HDL, D-LDL, and C-LDL, raises the issue of whether any of these lipid measures is the best predictor of cardiovascular risk and begs the question of whether alternative lipid measures, such as apoB or LDL particle number, should become the primary target of therapy [13–16]. Prospective research is needed to compare all these lipid measures to identify the best predictor of cardiovascular risk.

Conflict of Interests

There are no conflict of interests to report on the part of any of the authors.

References

[1] J. I. Cleeman, "Executive summary of the third report of the National Cholesterol Education Program (NCEP) expert panel on detection, evaluation, and treatment of high blood cholesterol in adults (adult treatment panel III)," *Journal of the American Medical Association*, vol. 285, no. 19, pp. 2486–2497, 2001.

[2] R. McPherson, J. Frohlich, G. Fodor, and J. Genest, "Canadian Cardiovascular Society position statement—recommendations for the diagnosis and treatment of dyslipidemia and prevention of cardiovascular disease," *Canadian Journal of Cardiology*, vol. 22, no. 11, pp. 913–927, 2006.

[3] S. M. Grundy, J. I. Cleeman, C. N. Merz et al., "National Heart, Lung, and Blood Institute, American College of Cardiology Foundation, American Heart Association. Implications of recent clinical trials for the National Cholesterol Education Program Adult Treatment Panel III guidelines," *Circulation*, vol. 110, pp. 227–239, 2004.

[4] L. Baruch, S. Agarwal, B. Gupta et al., "Is directly measured low-density lipoprotein clinically equivalent to calculated low-density lipoprotein?" *Journal of clinical lipidology*, vol. 4, no. 4, pp. 259–264, 2010.

[5] K. A. Foley, R. J. Simpson, J. R. Crouse, T. W. Weiss, L. E. Markson, and C. M. Alexander, "Effectiveness of statin titration on low-density lipoprotein cholesterol goal attainment in patients at high risk of atherogenic events," *American Journal of Cardiology*, vol. 92, no. 1, pp. 79–81, 2003.

[6] J. J. Kastelein, W. A. van der Steeg, I. Holme et al., "Lipids, apolipoproteins, and their ratios in relation to cardiovascular events with statin treatment," *Circulation*, vol. 117, pp. 3002–3009, 2008.

[7] P. M. Ridker, N. Rifai, N. R. Cook, G. Bradwin, and J. E. Buring, "Non-HDL cholesterol, apolipoproteins A-I and B100, standard lipid measures, lipid ratios, and CRP as risk factors for cardiovascular disease in women," *Journal of the American Medical Association*, vol. 294, no. 3, pp. 326–333, 2005.

[8] T. Pischon, C. J. Girman, F. M. Sacks, N. Rifai, M. J. Stampfer, and E. B. Rimm, "Non-high-density lipoprotein cholesterol and apolipoprotein B in the prediction of coronary heart disease in men," *Circulation*, vol. 112, no. 22, pp. 3375–3383, 2005.

[9] Y. Cui, R. S. Blumenthal, J. A. Flaws et al., "Non-high-density lipoprotein cholesterol level as a predictor of cardiovascular disease mortality," *Archives of Internal Medicine*, vol. 161, pp. 1413–1419, 2001.

[10] B. J. Arsenault, J. S. Rana, E. S. G. Stroes et al., "Beyond low-density lipoprotein cholesterol. Respective contributions of non-high-density lipoprotein cholesterol levels, triglycerides, and the total cholesterol/high-density lipoprotein cholesterol ratio to coronary heart disease risk in apparently healthy men and women," *Journal of the American College of Cardiology*, vol. 55, no. 1, pp. 35–41, 2009.

[11] J. G. Robinson, S. Wang, B. J. Smith, and T. A. Jacobson, "Meta-analysis of the relationship between non-high-density lipoprotein cholesterol reduction and coronary heart disease risk," *Journal of the American College of Cardiology*, vol. 53, no. 4, pp. 316–322, 2009.

[12] M. J. Blaha, R. S. Blumenthal, E. A. Brinton, and T. A. Jacobson, "The importance of non-HDL cholesterol reporting in lipid management," *Journal of Clinical Lipidology*, vol. 2, no. 4, pp. 267–273, 2008.

[13] J. D. Brunzell, M. Davidson, C. D. Furberg et al., "Lipoprotein management in patients with cardiometabolic risk. Consensus conference report from the american diabetes association and the american college of cardiology foundation," *Journal of the American College of Cardiology*, vol. 51, no. 15, pp. 1512–1524, 2008.

[14] J. H. Contois, J. P. McConnell, A. A. Sethi et al., "Apolipoprotein B and cardiovascular disease risk: position statement from the AACC lipoproteins and vascular diseases division working group on best practices," *Clinical Chemistry*, vol. 55, no. 3, pp. 407–419, 2009.

[15] M. H. Davidson, C. M. Ballantyne, T. A. Jacobson et al., "Clinical utility of inflammatory markers and advanced lipoprotein testing: advice from an expert panel of lipid specialists," *Journal of Clinical Lipidology*, vol. 5, pp. 338–567, 2011.

[16] S. M. Boekholdt, B. J. Arsenault, S. Mora et al., "Association of LDL cholesterol, non-HDL cholesterol, and apolipoprotein B levels with risk of cardiovascular events among patients treated with statins: a meta-analysis," *The Journal of the American Medical Association*, vol. 307, pp. 1302–1309, 2012.

7

Quality Assessment of the Genetic Test for Familial Hypercholesterolemia in The Netherlands

Iris Kindt,[1] Roeland Huijgen,[2] Marieke Boekel,[1] Kristiaan J. van der Gaag,[3] Joep C. Defesche,[2] John J. P. Kastelein,[2] and Peter de Knijff[3]

[1] *Foundation for the Identification of Persons with Inherited Hypercholesterolemia (StOEH), Amsterdam, The Netherlands*
[2] *Department of Vascular Medicine, Academic Medical Center (AMC), 1105 AZ Amsterdam, The Netherlands*
[3] *Department of Human Genetics, Forensic Laboratory for DNA Research, Leiden, The Netherlands*

Correspondence should be addressed to Roeland Huijgen; r.huijgen@amc.uva.nl

Academic Editor: Gloria L. Vega

Introduction. Familial hypercholesterolemia (FH) is an inherited disorder associated with a severely increased risk of cardiovascular disease. Although DNA test results in FH are associated with important medical and ethical consequences, data on accuracy of genetic tests is scarce. *Methods.* Therefore, we performed a prospective study to assess the overall accuracy of the DNA test used in the genetic cascade screening program for FH in The Netherlands. Individuals aged 18 years and older tested for one of the 5 most prevalent FH mutations, were included consecutively. DNA samples were analyzed by the reference and a counter-expertise laboratory following a standardized procedure. *Results.* 1003 cases were included. In the end, 317 (32%) carried an FH mutation, whereas in 686 (69%) samples no mutation was found. The overall accuracy of the reference laboratory was 99.8%, with two false positive results identified by the counter-expertise laboratory. *Conclusion.* The currently used mutation analysis is associated with a very low error rate. Therefore, we do not recommend routine use of duplicate testing.

1. Introduction

The number of hereditary disorders for which a genetic test is available has increased from less than 200 in 1993 to more than 1,800 in 2009 [1]. Molecular genetic testing for these diseases raises a plethora of concerns, including the quality of test performance and interpretation of results [2].

Familial hypercholesterolemia (FH) is a condition that meets every criterion for genetic screening. FH is an autosomal codominant disorder of lipid metabolism with a prevalence of 1 : 500 in most Western countries [3]. Patients with FH have high plasma LDL cholesterol levels and an increased risk of coronary artery disease (CAD) [3, 4]. Statin therapy, intervening in the causal pathway of the disease, lowers CAD risk to a very significant extent in these individuals [5]. Defects in genes that code for proteins involved in hepatic clearance of low-density lipoprotein (LDL) cholesterol underlie the disorder [3]. In fact, more than a 1000 different mutations in the genes coding for the LDL-receptor (*LDLR*), apolipoprotein B (*APOB*), and proprotein convertase subtilisin/kexin type 9 (*PCSK9*) are known to cause FH [6]. Such a causal mutation can be identified by DNA analysis in a varying percentage of patients with a clinical FH diagnosis, ranging from 20% to more than 90%, with highest rates of detection in children strictly selected for severe clinical FH [7–13]. Knowledge of the causal monogenetic mutation enables rapid screening of family members for the presence of the same mutation. In fact, such a genetic cascade screening programme for FH started in The Netherlands in 1994 and was scaled up in 2003 with the aid of government support [14].

On an individual level, FH tests can have important medical and social/ethical consequences. The vast majority of individuals initiate cholesterol-lowering treatment after such a diagnosis [15]. Conversely, a person's test result may affect employment or the ability to secure life insurance [16, 17]. Because the results of genetic testing can have such a profound impact on the life of screened individuals, a high standard is required for the accuracy of DNA analysis. However, the reproducibility of DNA testing for FH has not been evaluated and hitherto no gold standard exists for DNA-based diagnostic testing for this condition.

Therefore, we decided to assess the quality of the DNA test results in our screening programme. To arrive at this, we conducted a prospective study in which two independent laboratories tested samples in duplicate using a systematic procedure. Here, we present our results.

2. Methods and Materials

2.1. Selection and Recruitment of Patients. In a prospective study, we aimed to include 1000 consecutive subjects that were tested for genetic FH. These subjects were recruited from the participants of the cascade screening program for FH in The Netherlands from November 2007 until December 2009. We only selected individuals aged 18 and older and those that were to be tested for one of the five most prevalent FH mutations. In general, the carriers of these five mutations represent approximately 50% of the molecularly diagnosed FH patients [18, 19].

The selected subjects were asked for consent for the genetic screening for FH and, in addition, for this study, that is, assessment of the reproducibility of the FH mutation analysis. The genetic cascade screening for FH and this sub study was approved and financed by the Dutch Government (RIVM).

After written informed consent was obtained, trained nurses from the StOEH drew blood from each participant. From heparinized blood the lipid profiles were measured with the LDX analyser [20]. The LDL cholesterol was estimated based on the Friedewald formula [21]. Age and sex specific percentiles of LDL cholesterol were calculated using the reference values of the Caucasian population [22].

Four vacutainers (DB Vacultainer, 5.0 mL) containing EDTA as anticoagulant were drawn for DNA extraction for mutation analysis.

2.2. Mutation Analysis. Two samples were sent to and processed by the laboratory for Experimental Vascular Medicine of the Academic Medical Center at the University of Amsterdam (referred to as the reference laboratory). The other two vacutainers were sent to and processed by the counter-expertise laboratory of the National Forensic Institute laboratory in Leiden (referred to as the counter-expertise laboratory). The counter-expertise laboratory performed its tests after the reference laboratory and was blinded for the findings of the reference laboratory.

Four mutations in *LDLR* and one in *APOB* were tested in this study (See Supplemental Table 1 (main characteristics of mutations) in Supplementary Material available online at http://dx.doi.org/10.1155/2013/531658). Mutations were described according to the nomenclature as proposed by den Dunnen and Antonarakis [23].

2.3. DNA Analysis in the Reference Laboratory. Genomic DNA was isolated from the tubes with 5 mL whole blood on an AutopureLS apparatus according to a protocol provided by the manufacturer (Gentra Systems, Minneapolis, USA). The remainder of the blood was stored at −20°C. Mutations were detected by amplification of the exon harbouring the mutation in question by polymerase chain reaction (PCR), followed by digestion of the PCR products with an appropriate restriction endonuclease and gel electrophoresis on agarose gels to separate the digestion products. The primer sequences and conditions for PCR are available upon request. The presence or absence of a mutation was determined by the difference in digestion pattern, as described previously [24, 25].

2.4. DNA Analysis in the Counter-Expertise Laboratory. From each tube 200 μL blood was used for DNA extraction using the Qiacube DNA isolation robot (Qiagen Germany) using standard protocols provided by the manufacturer. The remainder of the blood was stored at −20°C. DNA typing was performed using a multiplex SNaPshot assay designed to detect the specific mutations studied in this study. Reference sequences for each mutation of the *LDLR* and *APOB* were obtained from the literature [6, 26, 27]. The primers that were designed are available upon request. Specifics of DNA typing reactions are described in Supplemental File 1. Data was analyzed using GeneMapper ID v3.2.1 (Applied). After background subtraction and colour separation, peaks were sorted into bins according to sizes by comparison to the internal size standard. An Excel-sheet was used to transfer exported allele tables and automatically call mutations.

The overall costs of setting up the logistics for the DNA typing of the 5 different mutations, including personnel and materials, were €150 per individual tested.

2.5. Combining the DNA Test Results of Both Laboratories. The test results of the two laboratories were reported to the StOEH, and two individuals (MB RH) independently reviewed the test results for discrepancies. Samples with discrepant results between the two laboratories were analysed according to the subsequent steps until the cause of the discrepancy was discovered. If required, we used the following steps.

(i) Step 2: re-analysis of the same DNA sample as in the first analysis (performed at both labs);

(ii) Step 3: new DNA extraction and analysis from the second tube of the sample (both labs);

(iii) Step 4: re-analysis of the second DNA sample (both labs);

(iv) Step 5: exchange of DNA sample from the first DNA extraction between the reference and counter-expertise lab and re-analysis of this DNA sample;

(v) Step 6: new sampling of blood from the subject in question and initiation of Step 1 and subsequent steps in both labs.

2.6. Outcomes. In case of discrepant results between the laboratories, the end conclusion of subsequent steps was that the

Table 1: Baseline characteristics of the participants.

	All
N	1003
Age (±SD) years	49 ± 16
Male gender (%)	523 (52%)
Body mass index (±SD) kg/m^2	25.6 ± 3.9
Medication use at diagnosis (%)	250 (25%)
Tested for mutation (% of total)	
LDLR-c.313+1/2	140 (14%)
LDLR-p.S306L	80 (8%)
LDLR-c.1359–1G>A	110 (11%)
LDLR-p.N564H/2393del9bp	317 (32%)
APOB-p.R3527 L/Q/W	348 (35%)
LDLR-c.313+1/2+c.191–2	8 (1%)

Based on the per protocol study population: subjects tested when aged under 18 years were excluded.

initial conclusion of the reference laboratory was erroneous or not, and, if an error was discovered, whether the initial mutation analysis result was false positive or negative. The main study outcome was to answer whether the current DNA analysis for genetic FH by the reference laboratory provided test results that were compatible in at least 99.5% of cases with the gold standard. The gold standard was the presence or absence of the mutation based on the overall conclusion of stepwise analysis of the counter-expertise laboratory and the reference laboratory.

Secondary outcomes were (i) the stage at which an error had been made during meta-analysis and (ii) the costs made by the counter-expertise laboratory to identify one erroneous result made by the reference laboratory and the added value of routinely typing of all 5 mutations in duplicate.

2.7. Statistical Analysis

2.7.1. Sample Size Calculation. Assuming a discrepancy percentage of 0.5% between the results of the two laboratories with a confidence interval of 2% and using a 2-sided alpha level of 0.05 at 80% power, 1000 patients would be needed.

We compared differences in lipid levels between carriers and noncarriers with an independent t-test. All data were analyzed using SPSS software (version 16.0.2, SPSS, Chicago, MI, USA). A P value of less than 0.05 was considered to be statistically significant.

3. Results

In total, 1003 participants were included. Table 1 summarizes the main characteristics of the participants and the mutations tested. The participants had a mean age of 49 years, and 520 (52%) were males. The two mutations that were analyzed most often were those that resulted in changes of the arginine at position 3527 in *APOB* ($N = 348$) and the p.N564H/2393del9 bp in *LDLR* ($N = 317$), as could be expected based on the prevalence of these mutations. The other three mutations were tested in 330 individuals. In addition, eight individuals had been tested for a special mutation, which consisted of the c.191–2 and the c.313+1 mutations residing on the same allele of the *LDLR*.

Mutation analysis of the 1003 DNA samples in the reference laboratory revealed the presence of a mutation in 317 (32%) samples, whereas in the other 686 (69%) samples the mutation proved absent. Figure 1 illustrates the diagnostic procedure followed for the participants. Table 2 summarizes the overall test results and clinical characteristics of specific persons of interest. In case of subject A (Figure 1 and Table 2), the trained nurse suspected that the conclusion by the reference laboratory was incorrect, even before the counter-expertise laboratory had initiated the analysis. This case involved a 43-year-old male who, according to the initial findings of the reference laboratory, did not carry the p.N564H/2393del9 bp mutation. He had experienced a myocardial infarction at the age of 41 years. Because his medical history and his lipid profile were indicative of FH (Table 2), the cascade screening organization requested that the reference laboratory reanalyzed this individual. When retrieving the different steps of the analytical procedure it became clear that the blood sample of individual A was exchanged for that of individual B, who was analyzed for the same mutation (Table 2). Re-analysis of the DNA extracted from the spare tube of A and B revealed the presence of p.N564H/2393del9 bp variant in individual A and the absence of it in individual B. These findings were confirmed by the counter-expertise laboratory (Figure 1).

Mutation analysis of the other 1001 samples resulted in 10 discrepant results between the counter-expertise and reference laboratories. Supplemental Table 2 illustrates the end conclusion on the test results which initially gave discrepant results between both laboratories. In three cases, the counter-expertise laboratory identified a mutation, whereas the reference laboratory did not (cases C, D, and E, Figure 1). In these cases the LDL-cholesterol levels were below the 40th percentile for age and gender, which made the presence of FH less credible (Table 2). Based on the subsequent re-analyses by both laboratories, we concluded that those three individuals did indeed not carry a mutation. An error had occurred in the counter-expertise laboratory, where the samples of these subjects were exchanged for three others that carried a mutation (Supplemental Table 2). Thus, the initial findings of the reference laboratory were correct.

The counter-expertise laboratory identified absence of the mutation in seven samples in their first test, where the reference laboratory initially had found a mutation (Figure 1). In individuals F and G, subsequent analyses in both labs revealed that the first test result from the reference laboratory was indeed false positive (Figure 1). Both individuals had not experienced cardiovascular disease and had normal cholesterol levels, with LDL-cholesterol levels below the 40th percentile for age and gender (Table 2). Individual F was repeatedly tested homozygous positive for the 313+1G>C mutation in the first analysis in the reference laboratory, while in tests on the spare sample the mutation was absent. Ultimately, sequence analysis of the first and the spare sample confirmed the absence of this mutation. The reason for a repeated homozygous but false positive test result in PCR

TABLE 2: Clinical characteristics of participants of interest.

ID	Sex	Age	Medication use	TC (perc.)	HDL (perc.)	LDL (perc.)	TG (perc.)	Mutation tested	Initial finding[#]	End conclusion[*]
A	Male	43	Simva 40	6.33 (86)	0.59 (<5)	3.87 (67)	4.09 (>95)	p.N564H/2393del9bp	Absent > present	Carrier
B	Female	65	Simva 40	4.26 (<5)	0.80 (<5)	2.80 (<5)	3.02 (>95)	p.N564H/2393del9bp	Present > absent	Noncarrier
C	Male	54	No	5.92 (68)	1.55 (93)	3.36 (36)	2.20 (83)	p.N564H/2393del9bp	Absent	Noncarrier
D	Male	55	No	4.86 (24)	1.50 (82)	2.64 (10)	1.56 (62)	p.S306L	Absent	Noncarrier
E	Female	56	No	4.05 (<5)	2.22 (91)	1.61 (<5)	0.50 (<5)	p.N564H/2393del9bp	Absent	Noncarrier
F	Male	54	No	5.17 (37)	1.14 (51)	3.42 (39)	1.32 (41)	c.313+1G>C	Present	Noncarrier
G	Male	38	No	3.20 (<5)	1.33 (82)	1.22 (<5)	1.41 (57)	p.R3527W	Present	Noncarrier
H	Female	65	Rosuva 40 + Ezetimibe 10	3.09 (<5)	0.84 (<5)	1.49 (<5)	1.66 (69)	p.R3527W	Present	Carrier
I	Female	58	Simva 40	6.15 (61)	1.81 (70)	3.76 (51)	1.27 (50)	c.313+1G>C	Present	Carrier
J	Male	26	No	7.00 (>95)	1.71 (>95)	4.88 (>95)	0.89 (39)	p.S306L	Present	Carrier
K	Female	35	No	n.p.	n.p.	n.p.	n.p.	p.R3527Q	Present	Carrier
L	Male	18	No	n.p.	n.p.	n.p.	n.p.	p.R3527Q	Present	Carrier
M	Male	32	Rosuva 40	5.34 (69)	0.90 (16)	4.15 (88)	0.61 (9)	c.1359–1G>A	Absent	Noncarrier c.1359-1, carrier c.313+1G>A
N	Male	68	Atorva 80 + Ezetimibe 10	5.37 (44)	1.09 (33)	3.68 (45)	1.30 (53)	c.313+1G>A	Present	Carrier of both c.313+11G>A and p.R3527Q mutations

[#]Initial finding indicates the conclusion after the initial test by the reference laboratory only. [*]End conclusion on mutation carriership was defined by the end result of the gold standard test in this study, which was the conclusion based on results from analyses in the reference laboratory and the counter-expertise laboratory. Abbreviations: TC: total cholesterol, HDL: high-density lipoprotein cholesterol, LDL: low-density lipoprotein cholesterol, TG: triglycerides, Perc.: percentile for age and sex. Simva: simvastatin, Rosuva: rosuvastatin, n.p.: not performed (lipid profile not measured because subject was not in fasted state).

Table 3: Frequencies of mutation detection in the per-protocol study population.

Test result	Gold standard test#		Total
	Mutation present	Mutation absent	
Reference lab: mutation present	314	2	**316**
Reference lab: mutation absent	0	685	**685**
Total*	**314**	**687**	**1001**

*Excluded the 2 individuals in whom switch of DNA samples was discovered before counter-expertise test had been performed (subjects A and B from Figure 1 and Table 2).

#Gold standard test is defined as the overall conclusion after following the steps for mutation analysis in both the reference laboratory and the counter-expertise laboratory.

Overall accuracy = 999/1001 = 0.998, 95%. Confidence interval: 0.998 − (1.96 ∗ sqr(0.998 ∗ (1.0–0.998))) to 0.998 + (1.96 ∗ sqr(0.998 ∗ (1–0.998))) = 0.911 to 1.00.

Sensitivity = 314/314 = 1.0, 95%. Confidence interval: 1.0 − (1.96 ∗ sqr(1.0 ∗ (1.0–1.0))) to 1.0 + (1.96 ∗ sqr(1.0 ∗ (1–1.0))) = 1.00.

Specificity = 685/687 = 0.997, 95%. Confidence interval: 0.997 − (1.96 ∗ sqr(0.997 ∗ (1–0.997))) to 0.997 + (1.96 ∗ sqr(0.997 ∗ (1–0.997))) = 0.891 to 1.00.

Likelihood ratio for a positive test = sensitivity/(1 − specificity) = 344, indicating that a positive result is 344 times more likely to occur in someone with the mutation according to the gold standard than in one without it.

analysis remains unknown, but maybe related to the quality of the DNA sample (Supplemental Table 2). Sample switch during DNA extraction was excluded because re-analysis of the spare samples, which were processed in the same batch, did not yield conflicting results with the contra-expertise laboratory. The false positive result in individual G was shown to be caused by a sample switch between the consecutive sample of an individual that was analyzed for the same mutation (Supplemental Table 2).

The five other discrepancies involved individuals H, I, J, K, and L, in whom the initial test of the counter-expertise laboratory had identified absence of the mutation. The clinical characteristics of individuals H, I, and J were indicative of presence of an FH mutation, while clinical data of K and L were incomplete (Table 2). Indeed, the end conclusion after stepwise analyses was that the FH mutation was present in these five individuals, and the findings of the reference laboratory were correct. In cases H and I the counter-expertise laboratory failed to identify the mutation during the first test, because the diagnostics were initially only designed to detect the common nucleotide changes at that position. Cases H and I, should have been tested for the mutations c.10579C>T (or p.R3527W) in *APOB* and 313+1G>C in *LDLR*, respectively. However, the counter-expertise laboratory was initially only equipped to detect these common variants at those positions, which were c.10580G>A for p.R3527Q in *APOB* and c.313+1G>A in *LDLR*, respectively (Supplemental Table 1). The mismatch was solved after counter check laboratory expanded the diagnostic procedure to also detect those rare variants. The mismatches in cases J, K, and L were due to the exchange of the samples with those of noncarriers C, D, and E by the counter-expertise laboratory, as described before (Supplemental Table 2).

Supplemental Table 3 shows the mean lipid levels and proportion of medication use for carriers and noncarriers categorized for the different mutations. This table illustrates the extent of dyslipidemia observed in the carriers of one of those specific mutations.

Overall, two false positive test results were discovered by the counter-expertise laboratory (subjects F+G). As a consequence, the sensitivity of the first DNA test by the reference laboratory was 1.0, and the specificity (95% CI) was 0.997 (0.891 to 1.00) (Table 3). Conversely, eight incorrect conclusions of the first tests of the counter-expertise laboratory were discovered during this study. Two of those were caused by a mistake in setting up the replication of the mutations, where the rare variants were initially "not covered." The other errors were due to three erroneous exchanges of samples in the pre-analytic phase.

4. Additional Findings by the Counter-Expertise Laboratory

The counter-expertise laboratory used a mutation analysis test where all 5 different mutations were tested simultaneously. As a consequence of this procedure, the counter-expertise laboratory identified an unexpected mutation—so another mutation than the one requested to analyse in duplicate—in two subjects.

In one 32-year-old male (Individual M, Table 2), the requested mutation was the *LDLR*-c.1359−1, which was absent according to the analyses of both labs. However, the counter-expertise laboratory did identify the *LDLR*-c.313+1G>A mutation. The patient had been identified with elevated total cholesterol by the general physician before the study visit and used rosuvastatin 40 mg. Despite this treatment, the patient still had a rather unfavourable lipid profile. Thus, the presence of the *LDLR*-c.313+1G>A mutation fully accounts for the clinical FH phenotype (Table 2), whereas the first test result of the reference laboratory, that is, absence of the initial FH mutation *LDLR*-c.1359−1, would have left the phenotype with hypercholesterolemia unexplained.

Similarly, both labs excluded the presence of the *LDLR*-c.313+1G>A mutation in a 62-year-old man from another family (no complete lipid profile determined because of high triglycerides), but the counter-expertise laboratory identified an *APOB*-p.R3527Q mutation. Subsequently, his direct relatives were tested for the presence of this *APOB* mutation as well, and this led to the identification of a relative that carried both *LDLR*-c.313+1G>A and the *APOB*-p.R3527Q mutation (Individual N, Table 2). This involved a 68-year-old male,

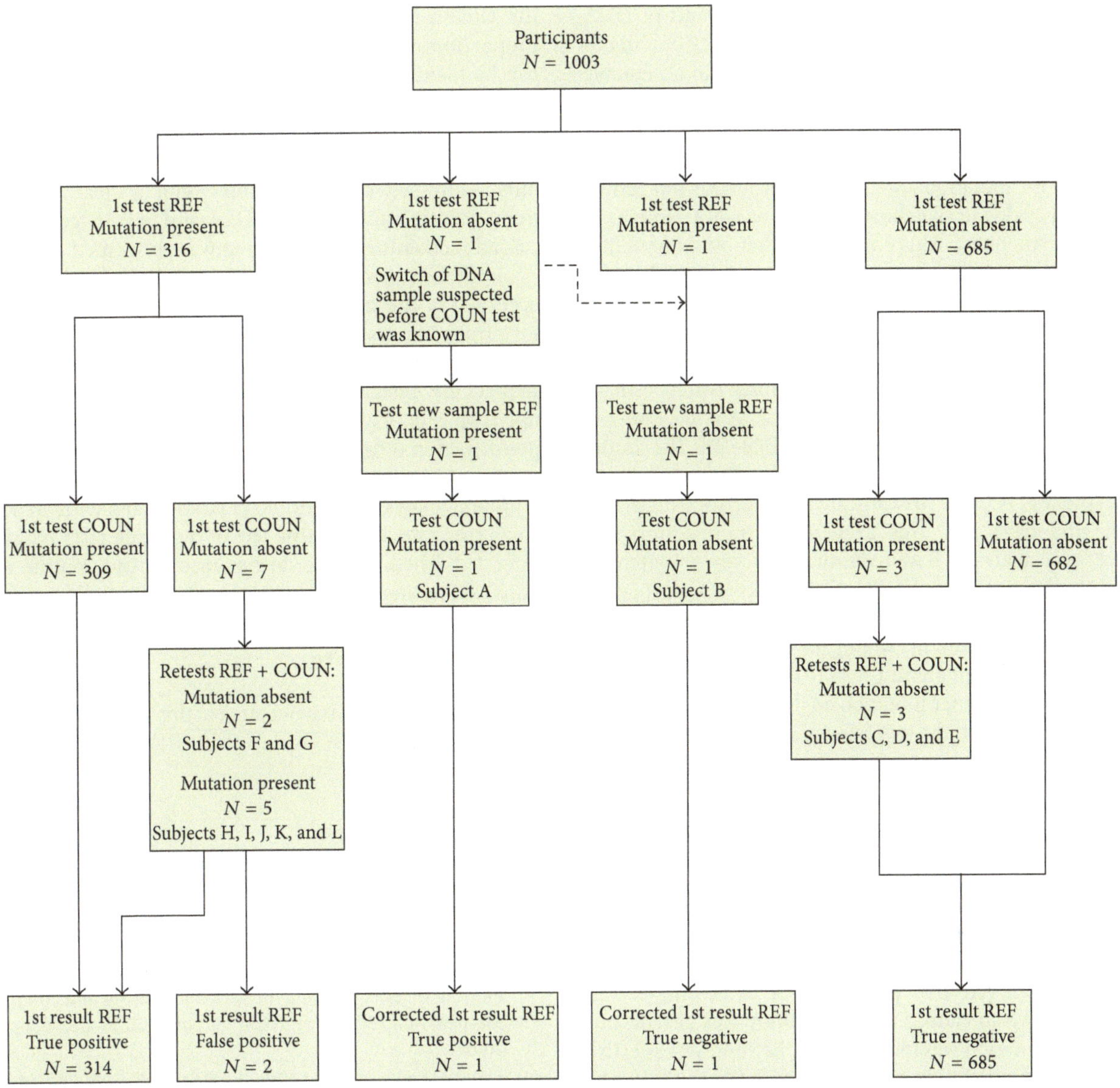

FIGURE 1: Patient enrolment and flow diagram based on mutation analysis. Diagnostic steps used for the participants. "True positive", "False positive," and "True negative" were based on end conclusion on mutation carriership after stepwise analyses in both laboratories, which indicate whether the laboratory result from the reference laboratory proved correct (True positive or True negative), or incorrect (False positive). Abbreviation: COUN = counter-expertise laboratory, REF = reference laboratory.

whose total cholesterol level was 17.5 mmol/L before he had initiated treatment.

5. Discussion

In our study, a duplicate DNA analysis for the molecular diagnosis of FH was performed in 1003 relatives of patients with an established DNA diagnosis of FH. The findings suggest that the DNA mutation analysis, currently being used by the cascade screening for FH (including a second analysis in case of conflicting clinical and mutation results), is associated with a low error rate. In fact, the counter-expertise laboratory discovered no more than two false positive cases (0.2%) from the national reference laboratory.

Implementing a duplicate test for the 1003 individuals came at a cost of approximately €150,000. This would constitute an increase of 37%, compared to the original cost per visited family member, including DNA analysis. Thus, the price tag was €150,000 for the discovery of two erroneous test results from the reference laboratory. In particular, this price was based on the costs associated with setting up an assay and duplicate testing of the five most prevalent mutations in The Netherlands. The cost efficiency of implementing a duplicate DNA test will likely be much lower if specific duplicate tests would have to be set up for all the mutations that were found to cause FH in The Netherlands. Of note, more than 400 pathogenic FH mutations have now been identified in The Netherlands, and most of these are rare [18, 28]. In general, it is highly desirable to eliminate erroneous results of DNA tests. We argue, however, that the overall accuracy of 1001 out of 1003 (99.8%) of the initial DNA test is within acceptable limits. The efficiency of the duplicate DNA test is too little, in our opinion, to routinely implement such a procedure.

Even so, the study findings can assist us in improving the logistics for mutation analysis. The erroneous test results were primarily due to switching of blood or DNA samples in the pre-analytic phase. This emphasizes that blood handling during DNA extraction and preparation of the DNA for mutation analysis should always be performed at utmost accuracy and guarded by standard operating procedures.

Furthermore, our findings show that good clinical judgement and critical evaluation of mutation test results remain essential to conclude on genetic FH status. A good example of this is individual A (Figure 1 and Table 2). The initial genetic test did not reveal presence of the mutation, which was surprising, because his clinical characteristics suggested that he did have FH. This triggered a trained nurse to request a re-analysis. Based on that process a switch of blood samples was discovered before the counter-expertise laboratory confirmed the mistake.

If systematic follow up would have been performed in those cases where genetic test results did not fit the clinical phenotype, several other mutation analysis errors could have been detected. In fact, the two false positive test results from the reference laboratory were not supported by a clinical FH phenotype.

Additional findings were (1) most of the false negative and false positive tests from the counter-expertise laboratory could have been discovered based on a mismatch between mutation analysis result and the clinical phenotype (Table 2 and Supplemental Table 3) (2) the discovery of 2 mutations which were not found in the initial analysis. In our study cohort we observed this phenomenon twice: the initial mutation known to cause FH in the family was absent, but another FH mutation was picked up by the counter-expertise laboratory (see Individuals M and N from Table 2). (3) Lastly, in case a person with a genetic diagnosis of heterozygous FH has exceptionally severe dyslipidemia, homozygous FH or compound heterozygosity should be considered [29]. This is what we observed for individual N, who had pre-treatment total cholesterol level of 17.5 mmol/L and who was shown to carry pathogenic mutationsin both *LDLR* and *APOB* genes.

Our study design had several limitations. First, a proper gold reference for DNA testing does not exist. In absence of a gold standard, we used a composite measure where, if applicable, several steps of the standard DNA-test and a comparator DNA test would lead to a best estimate.

Second, errors in the pre-analytic phase might have remained unnoticed, for example, if blood samples were accidentally switched between family members visited simultaneously before these were send to the two labs. Therefore, our results should primarily be used to get a sound impression on the processes of extraction of DNA, typing and interpretation of the results.

Third, our study results are only applicable to a subset of families with FH with clear monogenetic FH. An elegant analysis performed in large clinical FH population in the United Kingdom and Belgium showed that in a large proportion of patients no causal monogenic FH mutation can be identified [30]. In the mutation negative clinical FH patients more than half had a high allele count of common LDL cholesterol-raising variants, suggesting a polygenic cause of their hypercholesterolemia. By design, our analysis only addressed the FH families with a clear large effect monogenetic mutation in *LDLR* and *APOB* genes, where cascade screening of that variant was performed.

Last, our analysis was solely designed to assess the accuracy of the methodology used in the reference laboratory from the cascade screening programme. Because other professional laboratories might use SNP assays or direct sequencing instead, the results of the current study can not always be extrapolated for genetic testing programmes performed in other countries.

In conclusion, we would argue that the currently used mutation analysis methodology is associated with an acceptable error rate and routine use of duplicate tests has a high price tag. Therefore, we do not recommend routine use of duplicate testing.

Acknowledgments

The authors thank all participants of this study. This study was financed by the Dutch Government (RIVM).

References

[1] A. L. Beaudet, "Which way for genetic-test regulation? Leave test interpretation to specialists," *Nature*, vol. 466, no. 7308, pp. 816–817, 2010.

[2] B. Chen, M. Gagnon, S. Shahangian, N. L. Anderson, D. A. Howerton, and D. Joe Boone, "Good laboratory practices for molecular genetic testing for heritable diseases and conditions," *Morbidity and Mortality Weekly Report*, vol. 58, no. -6, pp. 1–29, 2009.

[3] J. L. Goldstein, H. H. Hobbs, and M. S. Brown, *The Metabolic and Molecular Bases of Inherited Disease*, McGraw-Hill, New York, NY, USA, 2001.

[4] R. Huijgen, M. N. Vissers, J. C. Defesche, P. J. Lansberg, J. J. P. Kastelein, and B. A. Hutten, "Familial hypercholesterolemia: current treatment and advances in management," *Expert Review of Cardiovascular Therapy*, vol. 6, no. 4, pp. 567–581, 2008.

[5] J. Versmissen, D. M. Oosterveer, M. Yazdanpanah et al., "Efficacy of statins in familial hypercholesterolaemia: a long term cohort study," *BMJ*, vol. 337, p. a2423, 2008.

[6] S. E. A. Leigh, A. H. Foster, R. A. Whittall, C. S. Hubbart, and S. E. Humphries, "Update and analysis of the university college London low density lipoprotein receptor familial hypercholesterolemia database," *Annals of Human Genetics*, vol. 72, no. 4, pp. 485–498, 2008.

[7] A. van der Graaf, H. J. Avis, D. M. Kusters et al., "Molecular basis of autosomal dominant hypercholesterolemia: assessment in a large cohort of hypercholesterolemic children," *Circulation*, vol. 123, no. 11, pp. 1167–1173, 2011.

[8] D. Damgaard, M. L. Larsen, P. H. Nissen et al., "The relationship of molecular genetic to clinical diagnosis of familial hypercholesterolemia in a Danish population," *Atherosclerosis*, vol. 180, no. 1, pp. 155–160, 2005.

[9] E. S. van Aalst-Cohen, A. C. M. Jansen, M. W. T. Tanck et al., "Diagnosing familial hypercholesterolaemia: the relevance of genetic testing," *European Heart Journal*, vol. 27, no. 18, pp. 2240–2246, 2006.

[10] L. Assouline, E. Levy, J. C. Feoli-Fonseca, C. Godbout, and M. Lambert, "Familial hypercholesterolemia: molecular, biochemical, and clinical characterization of a French-Canadian pediatric population," *Pediatrics*, vol. 96, no. 2, pp. 239–246, 1995.

[11] F. Campagna, F. Martino, M. Bifolco et al., "Detection of familial hypercholesterolemia in a cohort of children with hypercholesterolemia: results of a family and DNA-based screening," *Atherosclerosis*, vol. 196, no. 1, pp. 356–364, 2008.

[12] C. A. Graham, B. P. McIlhatton, C. W. Kirk et al., "Genetic screening protocol for familial hypercholesterolemia which includes splicing defects gives an improved mutation detection rate," *Atherosclerosis*, vol. 182, no. 2, pp. 331–340, 2005.

[13] F. E. R. Punzalan, R. G. Sy, R. S. Santos et al., "Low density lipoprotein-receptor (LDL-R) gene mutations among Filipinos with familial hypercholesterolemia," *Journal of Atherosclerosis and Thrombosis*, vol. 12, no. 5, pp. 276–283, 2005.

[14] M. A. W. Umans-Eckenhausen, J. C. Defesche, E. J. G. Sijbrands, R. L. J. M. Scheerder, and J. J. P. Kastelein, "Review of first 5 years of screening for familial hypercholesterolaemia in the Netherlands," *The Lancet*, vol. 357, no. 9251, pp. 165–168, 2001.

[15] R. Huijgen, I. Kindt, S. B. J. Verhoeven et al., "Two years after molecular diagnosis of familial hypercholesterolemia: majority on cholesterol-lowering treatment but a minority reaches treatment goal," *PLoS ONE*, vol. 5, no. 2, Article ID e9220, 2010.

[16] R. Huijgen, S. J. Homsma, B. A. Hutten et al., "Improved access to life insurance after genetic diagnosis of familial hypercholesterolaemia: cross-sectional postal questionnaire study," *European Journal of Human Genetics*, vol. 20, no. 7, pp. 722–728, 2012.

[17] S. J. M. Homsma, R. Huijgen, S. Middeldorp, E. J. G. Sijbrands, and J. J. P. Kastelein, "Molecular screening for familial hypercholesterolaemia: consequences for life and disability insurance," *European Journal of Human Genetics*, vol. 16, no. 1, pp. 14–17, 2008.

[18] R. Huijgen, I. Kindt, S. W. Fouchier et al., "Functionality of sequence variants in the genes coding for the low-density lipoprotein receptor and apolipoprotein B in individuals with inherited hypercholesterolemia," *Human Mutation*, vol. 31, no. 6, pp. 752–760, 2010.

[19] R. Huijgen, I. Kindt, J. C. Defesche, and J. J. Kastelein, "Cardiovascular risk in relation to functionality of sequence variants in the gene coding for the low-density lipoprotein receptor: a study among 29 365 individuals tested for 64 specific low-density lipoprotein-receptor sequence variants," *European Heart Journal*, vol. 33, no. 18, pp. 2325–2330, 2012.

[20] C. Cobbaert, G. J. M. Boerma, and J. Lindemans, "Evaluation of the Cholestech L.D.X. desktop analyser for cholesterol, HDL-cholesterol, and triacylglycerols in heparinized venous blood," *European Journal of Clinical Chemistry and Clinical Biochemistry*, vol. 32, no. 5, pp. 391–394, 1994.

[21] W. T. Friedewald, R. I. Levy, and D. S. Fredrickson, "Estimation of the concentration of low-density lipoprotein cholesterol in plasma, without use of the preparative ultracentrifuge," *Clinical Chemistry*, vol. 18, no. 6, pp. 499–502, 1972.

[22] A. M. Gotto Jr., E. L. Bierman, and W. E. Connor, "Recommendations for treatment of hyperlipidemia in adults. A joint statement of the nutritism committee and the Council on arteriosclerosis," *Circulation*, vol. 69, no. 5, 1984.

[23] J. T. den Dunnen and S. E. Antonarakis, "Mutation nomenclature extensions and suggestions to describe complex mutations: a discussion," *Human Mutation*, vol. 15, no. 1, pp. 7–12, 2000.

[24] M. P. Lombardi, E. J. W. Redeker, J. C. Defesche et al., "Molecular genetic testing for familial hypercholesterolemia : spectrum of LDL receptor gene mutations in the Netherlands," *Clinical Genetics*, vol. 57, no. 2, pp. 116–124, 2000.

[25] S. W. Fouchier, J. J. P. Kastelein, and J. C. Defesche, "Update of the molecular basis of familial hypercholesterolemia in The Netherlands," *Human Mutation*, vol. 26, no. 6, pp. 550–556, 2005.

[26] S. Castillo, D. Tejedor, P. Mozas et al., "The apolipoprotein B R3500Q gene mutation in Spanish subjects with a clinical diagnosis of familial hypercholesterolemia," *Atherosclerosis*, vol. 165, no. 1, pp. 127–135, 2002.

[27] I. F. A. C. Fokkema, J. T. Den Dunnen, and P. E. M. Taschner, "LOVD: easy creation of a locus-specific sequence variation database using an "LSDB-in-a-Box" approach," *Human Mutation*, vol. 26, no. 2, pp. 63–68, 2005.

[28] D. M. Kusters, R. Huijgen, J. C. Defesche et al., "Founder mutations in the Netherlands: geographical distribution of the most prevalent mutations in the low-density lipoprotein receptor and apolipoprotein b genes," *Netherlands Heart Journal*, vol. 19, no. 4, pp. 175–182, 2011.

[29] R. Huijgen, A. D. M. Stork, J. C. Defesche et al., "Extreme xanthomatosis in patients with both familial hypercholesterolemia and cerebrotendinous xanthomatosis," *Clinical Genetics*, vol. 81, no. 1, pp. 24–28, 2012.

[30] P. J. Talmud, S. Shah, R. Whittall et al., "Use of low-density lipoprotein cholesterol gene score to distinguish patients with polygenic and monogenic familial hypercholesterolaemia: a case-control study," *The Lancet*, vol. 381, no. 9874, pp. 1293–1301, 2013.

8

Modulation of Lipoprotein Cholesterol Levels in *Plasmodium berghei* Malarial Infection by Crude Aqueous Extract of *Ganoderma lucidum*

Olarewaju M. Oluba,[1] Augustine O. Olusola,[2] George O. Eidangbe,[3] Leye J. Babatola,[1] and E. Chukwu Onyeneke[4]

[1] *Department of Biochemistry, College of Natural Science, Joseph Ayo Babalola University, Ikeji-Arakeji, Osun, Nigeria*
[2] *Department of Biochemistry, Faculty of Science, Adekunle Ajasin University, Akungba Akoko, Ondo, Nigeria*
[3] *Department of Medical Biochemistry, College of Medicine, Ambrose Alli University, Ekpoma, Nigeria*
[4] *Department of Biochemistry, Faculty of Life Sciences, University of Benin, Benin, Nigeria*

Correspondence should be addressed to Olarewaju M. Oluba, olubamike2000@yahoo.co.uk

Academic Editor: Gerhard M. Kostner

In this study, attempt is made to establish changes in serum and liver lipoprotein cholesterols accompanying *Plasmodium berghei* malarial infection in mice treated with aqueous extract of *Ganoderma lucidum* at 100, 250, and 500 mg/kg body weight in comparison with 15 mg/kg chloroquine (CQ). Significant increases in all the lipoprotein fractions were observed in infected untreated mice compared with normal control mice. Treatment with 100 and 250 mg/kg *G. lucidum* extract produced significant reduction in serum total cholesterol (TC) and low-density cholesterol (LDL-C) contents compared with 500 mg/kg *G. lucidum* and CQ. Treatment with CQ, however, produced significant reduction in hepatic TC and LDL-C compared with the extract. A dose-dependent significant increase in serum high-density lipoprotein cholesterol (HDL-C) was observed in the *G. lucidum* treated mice compared with normal control but significantly lower compared with CQ-treated mice. Liver HDL-C level was significantly higher in CQ-treated mice compared with normal control and significantly lower compared with *G. lucidum*-treated and infected untreated mice. A dose-dependent effect of the extract was observed in both serum and liver very-low density lipoprotein cholesterol (VLDL-C). The implication of these results is discussed with respect to the parasite survival and proliferation in the serum and liver.

1. Introduction

The malarial parasite has been observed to have a tremendous requirement for lipids during the replicative stages that take place in the mammalian host. Biochemical studies on blood-stage *Plasmodium* malarial parasites have demonstrated the parasite's proficiency at scavenging and modifying lipids obtained from the host [1]. Studies have also shown that the parasites could obtain free fatty acids (FFAs) directly from the serum or from sources such as high-density lipoprotein (HDL) [2–4]. Within the parasite, scavenged phospholipids can be incorporated without modification [3, 5]. In addition, *Plasmodium* parasites have the capacity to modify fatty acids as needed by elongation or desaturation and incorporate them into phospholipids, diacylglycerols (DAGs), and triacylglycerols (TAGs) [6, 7].

Indeed, such biochemical revelations have not been possible for liver-stage parasites because of the difficulty in isolating the parasite from the host hepatocytes and the low rate of infection during this stage. However, early studies of malaria in genetically obese Zucker rats (fa/fa) gave indication that host cell lipids are important for *Plasmodium* liver-stage development [8]. These studies demonstrated that obese Zucker rats, which have hepatocytes with increased fatty acid synthesis, triglyceridemia and triglyceride content, supported growth of four times the number of liver-stage schizonts than their lean counterparts. Additionally, 45 hours after infection, schizonts in the obese rats were observed to be twice the size of those in control rats.

While most scavenged and synthesized lipids are likely incorporated into the membranes of the rapidly growing parasite, additional roles for fatty acids remain to be elucidated. For example, studies have yet to identify the source of fatty acids that are incorporated into GPI, which anchors numerous proteins, including MSP-1, to the merozoite plasma membrane. The low expression of MSP-1 in *fab* knockout parasites suggests that the FAS-II pathway may act together with elongases and desaturases to generate the lipid anchor for some surface proteins, including merozoite surface protein-1 (MSP-1) [9]. Alternatively, the fatty acid synthesis type II (FAS-II) pathway activity may provide a signal for progression to the merozoite formation phase of intrahepatic development. The specific upregulation of the FAS-II pathway during the liver stage may allow the parasite to synthesize its own lipids to supplement those provided by the host hepatocytes during a particularly explosive period of growth in the *Plasmodium* life cycle.

Elucidating stage-specific requirements for import, synthesis, and utilization of fatty acids and lipids in malarial parasite infection is both of considerable promise for developing novel antimalarial intervention strategies and of fundamental interest in understanding how these parasites are so successful in establishing infection in the human host. Thus, monitoring of serum and liver lipid concentrations during malarial infection could be of immense contribution in establishing the parasite source of lipids for its propagation.

Mushrooms have been known to have medicinal properties since 1200AD in Chinese folk medicine [10]. In recent years there has been renewed interest in cholesterol lowering properties of mushrooms, including *Ganoderma lucidum* (Reishi mushroom) [11, 12], *Pleurotus ostreatus* (Oyster mushroom) [13], and *Agaricus bisporus* (champignon) [14]. In this study, our focus is *G. lucidum*, an important medicinal fungus belonging to the Ganodermataceae family that has been studied for its many interesting health promoting properties, including antitumour, anti-inflammatory, antiplatelet aggregation, antidiabetic, and hypocholesterolemic properties [15–19]. The cholesterol lowering property of *G. lucidum* is explored in this study for its possible effects in preventing the proliferation of malarial parasites in mice.

2. Materials and Methods

2.1. Fungal Materials. Fruiting bodies of *G. lucidum* were obtained locally from open forest at Ipele in Ose Local Government Area of Ondo State, Nigeria. The fungal material was identified by Dr. S. Fakoya of the Department of Biological Sciences, Joseph Ayo Babalola University, Ikeji-Arakeji, Osun State, Nigeria, where voucher specimen number 1103 has been deposited.

2.2. Extract Preparation. Fruiting bodies of *G. lucidum* were sorted, washed to remove debris and dust particles, and then dried under shade for two weeks. The dried materials were cut into pieces and ground into powder using mechanical grinder. The powdered sample was kept in airtight container and stored at 4°C until required for further analysis. One hundred gram (100 g) of the powdered fungal material was soaked in 1000 mL distilled water and placed in an orbital shaker at room temperature for 48 hr. The aqueous extract was filtered with a muslin cloth. The resulting filtrate was evaporated to dryness at 37°C by the help of a Speed Vac (Model 7811001, Labconco, USA). The recovered extract was weighed and formulated in distilled water to give the required dose.

2.3. Animals and Treatment. A total of forty-eight (48) male Swiss albino mice (15–22 g body weight) obtained from the animal laboratory of the Department of Medical Biochemistry, University of Ibadan, Nigeria were used for the study. The animals were housed in stainless steel cages with raised wired floor at 30°C under standard conditions of humidity and 12 h light/dark cycle. They were fed standard feed (Guinea Feeds Ltd) and water *ad libitum*. The animals were kept for an initial period of two feed to acclimatize with their new environment. Before the commencement of the experiment animals were fasted overnight (but allowed access to water *ad libitum*) and weighed. All experimental protocols complied with NIH guidelines [20].

2.4. Malarial Parasite. Chloroquine sensitive *Plasmodium berghei* berghei (NK-65) obtained from the Institute for Advanced Medical Research and Training (IMRAT), University College Hospital, University of Ibadan, Nigeria, and kept at the Department of Biochemistry, Joseph Ayo Babalola University, Ikeji-Arakeji, was used for the study. The parasite was subsequently maintained in our laboratory by serial blood passage from mouse to mouse [21] every four days.

2.5. Inoculums. One milliliter parasitized erythrocytes were obtained from a donor-infected mouse by cardiac puncture in heparin and made up to 5 mL with normal saline. Mice were inoculated intraperitoneally with 0.2 mL blood suspension containing 10^6–10^7 parasitized erythrocytes on day zero. Infected mice with parasitemia of 10–12% were allocated to five groups. The fungal extract and the standard drug (CQ) administration were carried out for four days postinfection.

2.6. Treatment Regimen. Forty-eight mice (consisting of 40 infected divided into five groups of eight animals each; a sixth group of eight normal mice, as positive control) were used for this study. The four day postinfection treatment commenced at the establishment of parasitemia in the mice. The treatment administered to each group is as follows:

(i) negative control—infected mice treated with 0.2 mL normal saline;

(ii) extract test group I (AQ_{100})—infected mice treated with 100 mg/kg *G. lucidum* aqueous extract;

(iii) extract test group II (AQ_{250})—infected mice treated with 250 mg/kg *G. lucidum* aqueous extract;

(iv) extract test group III (AQ_{500})—infected mice treated with 500 mg/kg *G. lucidum* aqueous extract;

(v) reference test group (CQ)—Infected mice treated with 15 mg/kg chloroquine phosphate;

(vi) positive control—normal mice treated with 0.2 mL distilled water.

Treatments were given once daily by gavage using intubator for four consecutive days according to the method of Builders et al. [22]. On the fifth day (postinfection) thick smears of blood films were obtained from the peripheral blood on the tail from each mouse and used in the determination of the suppressive effect of the extract on the parasitemia level. Thereafter, extract and drug treatment were stopped while mice in each group were placed under surveillance until signs of death were noticed in the infected untreated group (negative control) after which mice in each group were sacrificed.

2.7. Blood Collection and Serum Preparation. As soon as signs of death were noticed in the infected untreated mice group (negative control) mice in each group were weighed anesthetized (in chloroform saturated chamber) and sacrificed by jugular puncture. Blood was obtained through their jugular vein into plain sterile bottles and allowed to clot for 2 h and then centrifuged at 3,000 ×g for ten minutes at room temperature to obtain the sera. The sera samples were collected by aspiration using a pasture pipette into sterile bijou bottles and stored frozen until required for analysis, which was done within 72 h.

2.8. Tissue Preparation. Upon sacrifice, liver and kidneys of each mouse were quickly excised, rinsed in normal saline, blotted dry on tissue paper, and weighed. Each tissue was placed in separate plastic vial containing ice-cold normal saline and stored at −8°C until required for further analysis.

2.9. Preparation of Tissue Homogenate. A weighed portion of liver and kidneys of each mouse was cut out, chopped into small pieces and homogenized using precooled pestle and mortar in a bowl of ice cubes. A 5% homogenate of each tissue was obtained in buffer solution (50 mM Tris-HCl) using normal saline solution, and stored at −8°C until further analysis was carried out.

2.10. Assays. Total cholesterol (TC), low-density lipoprotein (LDL) cholesterol, and high-density lipoprotein (HDL) cholesterol were determined using commercial kits (Randox Laboratory Ltd., UK) following the manufacturer's instruction while very low-density lipoprotein (VLDL) cholesterol concentration was determined by difference.

2.11. Statistical Analysis. Results presented are means ± SEM of eight independent determinations. Results obtained from this study were statistically analyzed using one way analysis of variance (ANOVA) and Duncan's Multiple Range Test (DMRT) using SPSS 17.0. Significant differences between the treatment means were determined at 95% confidence level.

3. Results

The effects of the extracts treatment compared with CQ and SP as reference drugs on percentage suppression and mean survival time are presented in Table 1. There was no significant difference in % suppression observed in mice treated with 100 mg/kg and those treated with 250 mg/kg aqueous extract and aqueous 200 and aqueous 500 groups, though a significant decrease was noticed in % suppression on comparing aqueous 100 and aqueous 500 treated groups.

From Table 2, serum cholesterol fractions (TC, LDL, HDL, and VLDL) were observed to be significantly elevated ($P < 0.01$) above normal control level in the infected control mice and infected mice treated with CQ (Table 1). However, significant decreases ($P < 0.05$) were observed in serum TC, LDL, HDL, and VLDL levels in infected mice treated with aqueous extract of *Ganoderma lucidum* (at 100, 250 and 500 mg/kg body weight) compared to infected untreated mice though these values were significantly higher compared to normal control level. Serum TC and LDL-C concentrations were not significantly ($P > 0.05$) changed in mice treated with 100 mg/kg and 250 mg/kg body weight of the extract. The extract at 100 mg/kg and 250 mg/kg body weight produced significantly lower reductions in serum TC and LDL-C compared to 500 mg/kg extract concentration.

As shown in Table 3, liver TC, LDL-C, HDL-C, and VLDL-C concentrations were significantly ($P < 0.01$) higher in infected control mice compared with normal control. The liver concentration of these cholesterol fractions were significantly ($P < 0.05$) reduced in *P. berghei* infection as a result of treatment with aqueous extract of *G. lucidum*. Liver TC, LDL, HDL and VLDL cholesterol were significantly ($P < 0.05$) higher in infected mice treated with 100, 250, and 500 mg/kg body weight *G. lucidum* aqueous extract compared to those administered CQ.

4. Discussion

Lipids have been observed to play important roles in pathological changes observed in disease conditions and are implicated in the production of immunity against diseases [23]. Serum lipids primarily bound to lipoproteins can be elevated by an increase in biosynthesis and/or by a decrease in their removal. Both of these processes appear to contribute to the hyperlipidemia that is often produced by some pathological changes. Although the source of increase in erythrocyte lipid component in malaria infection is not from lipid of the parasite there is no indication that the increase in the serum lipid is due to the lipid content of the parasite [24].

The results obtained from the suppressive, curative, and prophylactic tests indicate that the aqueous, chloroform and ethanol extracts of *G. lucidum* possessed significant antiplasmodial activity as evident from the chemosuppression obtained during the four day early infection test. However, on established infection the plant extracts also exhibited significant activity as evident from the curative effect of the extracts. Agents with suppressive activity against *Plasmodium berghei* were known for antimalarial activity

Table 1: Suppressive effect of aqueous extract of *Ganoderma lucidum* on parasitemia in mice infected with *Plasmodium berghei*.

Treatment groups		Parasite count	% suppression
Controls	Normal (P-CTR)	—	—
	Infected (N-CTR)	31.10 ± 1.20	—
Aqueous extract	AQ_{100}	14.20 ± 0.60	54.20 ± 3.70^{a}
	AQ_{250}	17.40 ± 1.20	$43.82 \pm 6.03^{a,b}$
	AQ_{500}	19.40 ± 0.90	$37.42 \pm 5.31^{b,c}$
Reference drug	CQ	2.25 ± 0.85	93.65 ± 0.47^{c}

Results are means ± SEM of eight independent determinations. Values in the same row carrying different superscripts are significant ($P < 0.05$) from each other.
Note. AQ_{100}: infected mice treated with 100 mg/kg aqueous extract; AQ_{250}: infected mice treated with 250 mg/kg aqueous extract; AQ_{500}: infected mice treated with 500 mg/kg aqueous extract; CQ: infected mice treated with chloroquine.

Table 2: Serum TC, LDL-, HDL-, and VLDL-cholesterol levels in mice *Plasmodium berghei* infected mice treated with aqueous extract of *Ganoderma lucidum*.

Treatment groups		TC	LDL	HDL	VLDL
Controls	Normal	8.75 ± 0.86^{a}	5.29 ± 0.57^{a}	1.46 ± 0.01^{a}	2.01 ± 0.01^{a}
	Infected	68.43 ± 5.33^{b}	36.56 ± 5.64^{b}	16.14 ± 0.01^{b}	15.74 ± 0.01^{b}
Aqueous extract	AQ_{100}	33.76 ± 2.27^{c}	21.77 ± 1.47^{c}	3.88 ± 0.01^{c}	8.10 ± 0.17^{c}
	AQ_{250}	39.97 ± 1.29^{c}	25.58 ± 0.83^{c}	4.40 ± 0.01^{d}	9.99 ± 0.06^{d}
	AQ_{500}	63.87 ± 5.03^{b}	40.87 ± 3.22^{b}	8.33 ± 0.01^{e}	14.69 ± 0.01^{e}
Reference drug	CQ	66.17 ± 4.50^{b}	39.86 ± 2.40^{b}	10.43 ± 0.01^{f}	15.88 ± 0.02^{b}

Results are means ± SEM of eight independent determinations. Values in the same row carrying different superscripts are significant ($P < 0.05$) from each other.
Note. P-CTR: positive control mice; N-CTR: negative control mice; AQ_{100}: infected group treated with 100 mg/kg *G. lucidum*; AQ_{250}: infected group treated with 250 mg/kg *G. lucidum*; AQ_{500}: infected mice treated with 500 mg/kg *G. lucidum*; CQ: infected mice treated with chloroquine.

Table 3: Liver TC, LDL-, HDL-, and VLDL-cholesterol levels in *Plasmodium berghei*-infected mice treated with aqueous extract of *Ganoderma lucidum*.

Treatment groups		TC	LDL	HDL	VLDL
Controls	Normal	66.03 ± 6.97^{a}	37.51 ± 3.82^{a}	12.67 ± 0.01^{a}	15.85 ± 0.06^{a}
	Infected	171.78 ± 8.70^{b}	99.25 ± 8.46^{b}	31.31 ± 0.01^{b}	41.22 ± 0.02^{b}
Aqueous extract	AQ_{100}	146.42 ± 4.34^{c}	93.70 ± 2.78^{b}	19.29 ± 0.25^{c}	33.68 ± 0.02^{c}
	AQ_{250}	$150.94 \pm 9.54^{b,c}$	96.60 ± 6.10^{b}	16.60 ± 0.11^{d}	37.74 ± 0.02^{d}
	AQ_{500}	172.00 ± 8.35^{b}	110.08 ± 5.34^{b}	22.36 ± 0.01^{e}	39.56 ± 0.06^{e}
Reference drug	CQ	111.56 ± 4.99^{d}	71.40 ± 3.19^{c}	13.39 ± 0.01^{f}	26.78 ± 0.02^{f}

Results are means ± SEM of eight independent determinations. Values in the same row carrying different superscripts are significant ($P < 0.05$) from each other.
Note. P-CTR: positive control mice; N-CTR: negative control mice; AQ_{100}: infected group treated with 100 mg/kg *G. lucidum*; AQ_{250}: infected group treated with 250 mg/kg *G. lucidum*; AQ_{500}: infected mice treated with 500 mg/kg *G. lucidum*; CQ: infected mice treated with chloroquine.

[21]. It is noteworthy that the antiplasmodial activity of the extract at all doses during early and established infections was comparable to that of the standard drug, CQ. There was a dose-dependent chemosuppression of parasitemia seen with the extract. In infected untreated mice, the parasite count increased daily until the death of the animals which was also observed in other studies [25, 26].

It is evident based on the findings from this study that aqueous extract of the fruiting bodies of *G. lucidum* represent potential antiplsmodial agent. The activity (antiplasmodial) may be attributed to terpenes, sterols, and flavonoids present in the extract as confirmed in this study. Antiplasmodial screening of plant substances has implicated terpenes, flavonoids and alkaloids [27–29]. These compounds could be acting singly or in synergy with one another to exert the antiplasmodial activity observed in this study.

Results obtained in the present study show significant increases in serum and liver total, LDL, VLDL, and HDL cholesterol in mice infected with *Plasmodium berghei*. This observation is consistent with reports from earlier studies by Onyeneke et al. [30] and Onongbu and Onyeneke [31] which showed increased serum lipoprotein fractions in malarial patients compared with apparently healthy control subjects. The observed increases in hepatic lipoproteins content are also in agreement with the report of Lombard et al. [8]. According to Lombard et al. [8] increase in hepatic lipid in malarial subjects is consistent with the degree of parasitemia. Again, observations from the present study support this assertion as the level of parasitemia correlates with hepatic lipoprotein composition.

As observed from this study, administration of aqueous extract of *G. lucidum* downregulates serum and liver lipoprotein content. The observed effect of the extract was to be negatively correlated with parasitemia level. The hypocholesterolemic property of *G. lucidum* has been established in our earlier study [19].

Malaria disturbs liver function though there is no evidence of hepatic insufficiency. In malarial infection, the liver is commonly enlarged and congested with parasitized red cells in sinusoids and centrilobular veins and swollen parenchymatous and kupffer cells [32]. Lipid metabolism is therefore deranged and the resulting lipoprotein particles synthesized by the liver undergo drastic changes in composition. Maurois et al. [33] have demonstrated that increased lipolysis induced by threshold of parasitemia promotes VLDL synthesis and their metabolism into LDL. Thus, with increase in parasitemia there was a progressive increase in LDL fraction and with the resulting incorporation of cholesterol particles, the overall LDL cholesterol was found to be increased. There is also the possibility of a reduction in the breakdown of LDL by the infective liver tissue thereby leading to an increase in these particles. It is also likely that the elevation in LDL cholesterol may be due to decrease uptake by the infected erythrocytes as a result of increased levels of parasitemia.

In conclusion, results obtained from this study show that aqueous extract of *G. lucidum* reduces serum and liver lipoprotein cholesterol with a corresponding decrease in parasitemia levels in both tissues. Therefore, it could thus be inferred that the antimalarial property of the extract could possibly be mediated by mechanisms involving reduction in liver lipids.

Conflict of Interests

The authors do not have a direct financial relationship with the commercial identity mentioned in this paper.

Acknowledgments

The authors wish to acknowledge the Director of institute for Advance Medical Research and Training (IAMRAT), University College Hospital, Ibadan, for the gift of the malaria parasite. The technical assistance of Mr. Famuyiwa Olajide also of IAMRAT in microscopic determination of parasite count is also acknowledged.

References

[1] H. J. Vial, M. J. Thuet, and J. R. Philippot, "Phospholipid biosynthesis in synchronous *Plasmodium falciparum* cultures," *Journal of Protozoology*, vol. 29, no. 2, pp. 258–263, 1982.

[2] P. Grellier, D. Rigomier, V. Clavey, J. C. Fruchart, and J. Schrevel, "Lipid traffic between high density lipoproteins and *Plasmodium falciparum*-infected red blood cells," *Journal of Cell Biology*, vol. 112, no. 2, pp. 267–277, 1991.

[3] G. Krishnegowda and D. C. Gowda, "Intraerythrocytic *Plasmodium falciparum* incorporates extraneous fatty acids to its lipids without any structural modification," *Molecular and Biochemical Parasitology*, vol. 132, no. 1, pp. 55–58, 2003.

[4] A. V. O. Ofulla, V. C. N. Okoye, B. Khan et al., "Cultivation of *Plasmodium falciparum* parasites in a serum-free medium," *American Journal of Tropical Medicine and Hygiene*, vol. 49, no. 3, pp. 335–340, 1993.

[5] G. N. Moll, H. J. Vial, M. L. Ancelin, J. A. F. Op den Kamp, B. Roelofsen, and L. L. M. Van Deenen, "Phospholipid uptake by *Plasmodium knowlesi* infected erythrocytes," *FEBS Letters*, vol. 232, no. 2, pp. 341–346, 1988.

[6] F. Mi-Ichi, K. Kita, and T. Mitamura, "Intraerythrocytic *Plasmodium falciparum* utilize a broad range of serum-derived fatty acids with limited modification for their growth," *Parasitology*, vol. 133, no. 4, pp. 399–410, 2006.

[7] N. M. Q. Palacpac, Y. Hiramine, F. Mi-Ichi et al., "Developmental-stage-specific triacylglycerol biosynthesis, degradation and trafficking as lipid bodies in *Plasmodium falciparum*-infected erythrocytes," *Journal of Cell Science*, vol. 117, no. 8, pp. 1469–1480, 2004.

[8] M. N. Lombard, R. Bazin, G. Durand et al., "Rodent *Plasmodium* development in livers of genetically obese Zucker rats (fa/fa)," *European Journal of Protistology*, vol. 34, no. 1, pp. 78–81, 1998.

[9] P. Gratraud, E. Huws, B. Falkard et al., "Oleic acid biosynthesis in *Plasmodium falciparum*: characterization of the stearoyl-CoA desaturase and investigation as a potential therapeutic target," *PloS ONE*, vol. 4, no. 9, article e6889, 2008.

[10] A. T. Borchers, J. S. Stern, R. M. Hackman, C. L. Keen, and M. E. Gershwin, "Mushrooms, tumors, and immunity," *Proceedings of the Society for Experimental Biology and Medicine*, vol. 221, no. 4, pp. 281–293, 1999.

[11] Y. Kabir, S. Kimura, and T. Tamura, "Dietary effect of *Ganoderma lucidum* mushroom on blood pressure and lipid levels in spontaneously hypertensive rats (SHR)," *Journal of Nutritional Science and Vitaminology*, vol. 34, no. 4, pp. 433–438, 1988.

[12] R. Li Khva, A. V. Vasil'ev, A. N. Orekhov, V. V. Tertov, and V. A. Tutel'ian, "Anti-atherosclerotic properties of higher mushrooms (a clinico-experimental investigation)," *Voprosy Pitaniia*, vol. 1, pp. 16–19, 1989.

[13] P. C. K. Cheung and M. Y. Lee, "Fractionation and characterization of mushroom dietary fiber (nonstarch polysaccharides) as potential nutraceuticals from sclerotia of *Pleurotus tuber-regium* (fries) singer," *Journal of Agricultural and Food Chemistry*, vol. 48, no. 8, pp. 3148–3151, 2000.

[14] M. Fukushima, M. Nakano, Y. Morii, T. Ohashi, Y. Fujiwara, and K. Sonoyama, "Hepatic LDL receptor mRNA in rats is increased by dietary mushroom (*Agaricus bisporus*) fiber and sugar beet fiber," *Journal of Nutrition*, vol. 130, no. 9, pp. 2151–2156, 2000.

[15] J. Tao and K. Feng, "Experimental and clinical studies on inhibitory effect of *Ganoderma lucidum* on platelet aggregation," *Journal of Tongji Medical University*, vol. 10, no. 4, pp. 240–243, 1990.

[16] S. T. Chang, "Ganoderma-the leader in production and technology of mushroom neutraceuticals," in *Recent Advances in Ganoderma lucidum Research*, B. K. Kim and Y. S. Kim, Eds., pp. 43–52, The Pharmaceutical Society of Korea, Seoul, Korea, 1995.

[17] A. W. Chen and P. G. Miles, "Biomedical research and the application of the mushroom nutriceuticals from *Ganoderma lucidum*," in *Mushroom Biology and Mushroom Products*, D. J. Royse, Ed., pp. 161–175, The Pennsylvania State University, University Park, Pa, USA, 1996.

[18] S. T. Chang and J. A. Buswell, "Medicinal Mushrooms—a prominent source of nutriceuticals for the 21st century," *Current Topics in Nutraceutical Research*, vol. 1, pp. 257–280, 2003.
[19] O. M. Oluba, E. C. Onyeneke, G. C. Ojieh, B. O. Idonije, and T. I. Ojiezeh, "Hepatoprotective potential of aqueous extract of *Ganoderma lucidum* against carbon tetrachloride intoxication in rats," *Der Pharmacia Lettre*, vol. 2, no. 4, pp. 432–439, 2010.
[20] National Research Council, *Guides For the Care and Use of Laboratory Animals*, National Institutes of Health, Bethesda, Md, USA, 1985.
[21] L. H. Carvalho, M. G. L. Brandao, D. Santos-Filho, J. L. C. Lopes, and A. U. Krettli, "Antimalarial activity of crude extracts from Brazilian plants studied *in vivo* in *Plasmodium berghei*-infected mice and *in vitro* against *Plasmodium falciparum* in culture," *Brazilian Journal of Medical and Biological Research*, vol. 24, no. 11, pp. 1113–1123, 1991.
[22] M. I. Builders, N. N. Wannang, G. A. Ajoku, P. F. Builders, A. Onsadipe, and J. C. Aguiyi, "Evaluation of the antimalarial potential of *Vernonia ambigua* kotschy and peyr (Asteraceae)," *International Journal of Pharmacology*, vol. 7, no. 2, pp. 238–247, 2011.
[23] R. Beckwith, R. H. Schenkel, and P. H. Silverman, "Qualitative analysis of phospholipids isolated from nonviable *Plasmodium* antigen," *Experimental Parasitology*, vol. 37, no. 2, pp. 164–172, 1975.
[24] D. H. Beach, I. W. Sherman, and G. G. Holz, "Lipids of *Plasmodium lophurae*, and of erythrocytes and plasmas of normal and P. lophurae infected Pekin ducklings," *Journal of Parasitology*, vol. 63, no. 1, pp. 62–75, 1977.
[25] G. C. Akuodor, M. Idris-Usman, T. C. Ugwu, J. L. Akpan, S. I. Ghasi, and U. A. Osunkwo, "*In vivo* schizonticidal activity of ethanolic leaf extract of *Ganoderma latifolium* on *Plasmodium berghei berghei* in mice," *African Journal of Biotechnology*, vol. 9, no. 5, pp. 2316–2321, 2010.
[26] S. Dewanjee, A. Maiti, M. Kundu, and S. G. Mandal, "Evaluation of anthelmintic activity of crude extracts of *Diospyros peregrina, Coccinia grandis* and *Schima wallichii*," *Dhaka University Journal of Pharmaceutical Sciences*, vol. 6, no. 2, pp. 121–123, 2007.
[27] J. D. Philipson and C. W. Wright, "Antiprotozoal compounds from plants source," *Planta Medica*, vol. 57, pp. 553–559, 1990.
[28] W. Milliken, "Malaria and antimalarial plants in Roraima, Brazil," *Tropical Doctor*, vol. 27, no. 1, pp. 20–25, 1997.
[29] S. B. Christensen and A. Kharazmi, "Antimalarial natural products: isolation, characterization and biological properties," in *Bioactive Compounds From Natural Sources*, Tringali, Ed., pp. 379–432, Taylor & Francis, London, UK, 2001.
[30] E. C. Onyeneke, E. O. Alumanah, and F. E. Mba, "Serum lipoprotein cholesterol of malarial patients: possible effects of chloroquine administration," *Journal of Environmental Toxicology*, vol. 1, pp. 15–21, 1997.
[31] I. C. Onongbu and E. C. Onyeneke, "Plasma lipid changes in human malaria," *Tropenmedizin und Parasitologie*, vol. 34, no. 3, pp. 193–196, 1983.
[32] C. Seshadri, B. R. Shetty, N. Gowri et al., "Biochemical changes at different levels of parasitaemia in *Plasmodium vivax* malaria," *Indian Journal of Medical Research*, vol. 77, no. 4, pp. 437–442, 1983.
[33] P. Maurois, P. Charet, A. Nouvelot, J. C. Fruchart, A. Vernes, and J. Biguet, "Kinetic study of serum lipoproteins, total cholesterol and triacylglycerides in various models of experimental rodent malaria," *Annals of Tropical Medicine and Parasitology*, vol. 74, no. 1, pp. 17–28, 1980.

9

Ezetimibe and Simvastatin Reduce Cholesterol Levels in Zebrafish Larvae Fed a High-Cholesterol Diet

Ji Sun Baek, Longhou Fang, Andrew C. Li, and Yury I. Miller

Department of Medicine, University of California, San Diego, La Jolla, CA 92093, USA

Correspondence should be addressed to Yury I. Miller, yumiller@ucsd.edu

Academic Editor: Jeffrey Cohn

Cholesterol-fed zebrafish is an emerging animal model to study metabolic, oxidative, and inflammatory vascular processes relevant to pathogenesis of human atherosclerosis. Zebrafish fed a high-cholesterol diet (HCD) develop hypercholesterolemia and are characterized by profound lipoprotein oxidation and vascular lipid accumulation. Using optically translucent zebrafish larvae has the advantage of monitoring vascular pathology and assessing the efficacy of drug candidates in live animals. Thus, we investigated whether simvastatin and ezetimibe, the principal drugs used in management of hypercholesterolemia in humans, would also reduce cholesterol levels in HCD-fed zebrafish larvae. We found that ezetimibe was well tolerated by zebrafish and effectively reduced cholesterol levels in HCD-fed larvae. In contrast, simvastatin added to water was poorly tolerated by zebrafish larvae and, when added to food, had little effect on cholesterol levels in HCD-fed larvae. Combination of low doses of ezetimibe and simvastatin had an additive effect in reducing cholesterol levels in zebrafish. These results suggest that ezetimibe exerts in zebrafish a therapeutic effect similar to that in humans and that the hypercholesterolemic zebrafish can be used as a low-cost and informative model for testing new drug candidates and for investigating mechanisms of action for existing drugs targeting dyslipidemia.

1. Introduction

In 2009, we suggested, for the first time, to use zebrafish as a model organism to study specific vascular events relevant to development of human atherosclerosis [1]. Feeding adult zebrafish a high-cholesterol diet (HCD) results in hypercholesterolemia, with total plasma cholesterol reaching 800 mg/dL, profound lipoprotein oxidation, and formation of vascular lesions, resembling human fatty streaks. HCD-fed adult zebrafish have been used by Cho and coworkers to study effects of food supplements and sweeteners on plasma cholesterol levels and CETP activity [2–4]. The optical transparency of zebrafish larvae within first 30 days post fertilization (dpf) enables microscopic monitoring in live animals of vascular lipid accumulation, recruitment of myeloid cells, formation of macrophage foam cells, disorganization of the endothelial cell layer, and increases in vascular PLA_2 activity and vascular permeability—all induced by a short (5–14 days) HCD feeding [1, 5]. Furthermore, our recent report demonstrates applications of a transgenic *hsp70:IK17-EGFP* zebrafish, with conditional expression of the EGFP-conjugated antibody IK17 specific to oxidized LDL, in studying *in vivo* lipoprotein oxidation and in testing therapeutic effects of antioxidants [5].

Because feeding zebrafish a HCD leads to extensive lipoprotein oxidation, we further characterized the oxidized lipid milieu in HCD-fed larvae [6]. A 2-week HCD feeding resulted in up to 70-fold increases in the levels of oxidized cholesterol esters, oxidized phospholipids, and lysophospholipids in zebrafish homogenates. Remarkably, specific oxidized lipid molecules detected in HCD-fed zebrafish larvae using liquid chromatography-mass spectrometry were identical to those found in human and mouse atherosclerotic lesions [6]. Lipoproteins isolated from HCD-fed larvae activated mouse macrophages *in vitro*, with the pattern of ERK1/2, JNK, and Akt phosphorylation and cell spreading similar to that induced by minimally oxidized human LDL [6].

Thus, our work and the work of others suggest that hypercholesterolemia and lipoprotein oxidation achieved in zebrafish and characteristics of vascular lipid accumulation and inflammatory processes, relevant to human atherogenesis, make the zebrafish model an attractive *in vivo* system for testing novel therapeutic approaches and studying the mechanisms of existing drugs. The goal of the present study was to investigate whether simvastatin and ezetimibe, the principal drugs used for management of hypercholesterolemia in humans, would also reduce cholesterol levels in HCD-fed zebrafish larvae.

2. Materials and Methods

2.1. Zebrafish Maintenance and Feeding. Wild-type (AB) zebrafish embryos were obtained by *in vitro* fertilization and natural spawning of adults maintained at 28°C on a 14/10 hour light/dark cycle and staged as described [7]. Zebrafish larvae were fed twice a day, starting at the 5th day post fertilization (dpf), with either control diet (Golden Pearls, 100–200 mm size from Brine Shrimp Direct) or HCD (4% cholesterol dissolved in diethyl ether added to Golden Pearls) for 14 days, as described in our previous work [1]. All animal studies were approved by the Animal Care and Use Committee of the University of California, San Diego.

2.2. Treatment with Ezetimibe and Simvastatin. Ezetimibe (Santa Cruz Biotechnology, cat. no. sc-205690) was added directly to the fish tank water at concentrations of 0.1–50 μM. This concentration range was chosen based on previous reports that 50 μM ezetimibe prevented approximately 75% of intestinal cholesterol absorption in zebrafish [8] and our preliminary studies showing a high efficiency of ezetimibe at lower doses. Simvastatin (Cayman Chemicals, cat. no. 10010344) was initially added to the fish tank water, in the same manner as it was done with ezetimibe. We observed that even at low doses of simvastatin, added directly to water, it was toxic to zebrafish larvae. Thus, we changed the protocol and mixed simvastatin into the fish food using the same procedure as described above for making a HCD. Simvastatin was added at 0.1–50 μg per gram food. We estimated that 20 larvae in a fish tank consumed approximately one half of 1.5 mg food administered 2 times a day. Given that larvae at this age weigh 0.8–1.0 mg, we calculated that the dose was between 9 and 3,750 ng simvastatin per mg body weight. This translates into an equivalent of 0.6–260 mg simvastatin per 70 kg body weight given to humans. Since clinical doses of simvastatin range from 5–80 mg, we consider doses of simvastatin administered to zebrafish larvae being roughly within a therapeutic range used to treat patients. The ezetimibe and/or simvastatin treatments described above did not affect zebrafish feeding behavior, swimming pattern, nor their growth (apparent body size).

2.3. Lipid Extraction from Zebrafish Homogenates and Cholesterol Measurements. At the end of the feeding/treatment period, 20 zebrafish larvae in each experimental group were euthanized by exposure to 0.05% tricaine (Sigma). Abdomens containing undigested food were removed, and the remaining bodies were pooled and gently homogenized in 200 μL of ice-cold PBS in an eppendorf tube using a plastic pestle. After spinning down tissue debris, the supernatant representing body fluids was used for further analysis. Protein content in the homogenates was determined using the Bradford assay with a BCA Protein Assay kit (Pierce). Total lipid was extracted from zebrafish homogenates as we previously described [6]. In brief, the tissue homogenates were supplemented with 50 μg stigmasterol, an internal standard to control for recovery of extracted sterols. Total lipid extraction was performed with 1 : 2 methanol/dichloromethane. Cholesterol esters were saponified and total free cholesterol and stigmasterol were measured with a Shimadzu GC-2014 gas chromatograph using a 30 m × 0.25 mm (i.d.) ZB-5HT inferno capillary column, film thickness 0.2 μm (Phenomenex). Cholesterol and stigmasterol standards were analyzed in parallel with experimental samples.

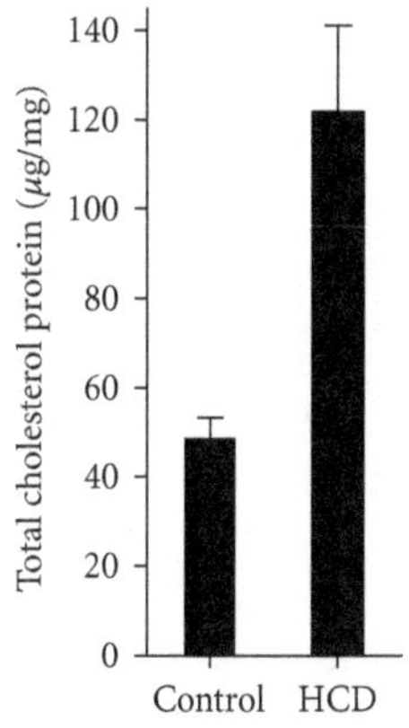

FIGURE 1: Total cholesterol levels in HCD-fed zebrafish larvae. Zebrafish larvae were fed control or high-cholesterol diets starting at the 5th dpf and continued for 14 days. Total cholesterol levels are expressed in μg cholesterol per mg protein of larvae lysate. Mean ± SEM from 6 independent experiments; 15–20 larvae were pooled for each experimental data point in each individual experiment. $P < 0.005$.

2.4. Statistics. Student's t-test was used to analyze differences between means of 2 groups. $P < 0.05$ was used as the significance threshold.

3. Results and Discussion

We have previously reported that plasma cholesterol levels in adult zebrafish rise from 200 to 800 mg/dL following 12 weeks of HCD feeding. Zebrafish larvae are too small to draw blood. Thus, we measured cholesterol levels in body fluids isolated from the larvae from which abdomens were removed and remaining bodies were gently homogenized. The homogenates were centrifuged to pellet tissue debris, and supernatants were used to extract total lipid and measure cholesterol using a gas chromatography method. A 2-week HCD feeding resulted in a 2.5-fold increase in cholesterol levels in zebrafish larvae (Figure 1). These results suggest that the experimental conditions used in experiments with zebrafish larvae reported in our earlier work [1, 5, 6] lead to significant elevations in cholesterol levels in larvae body

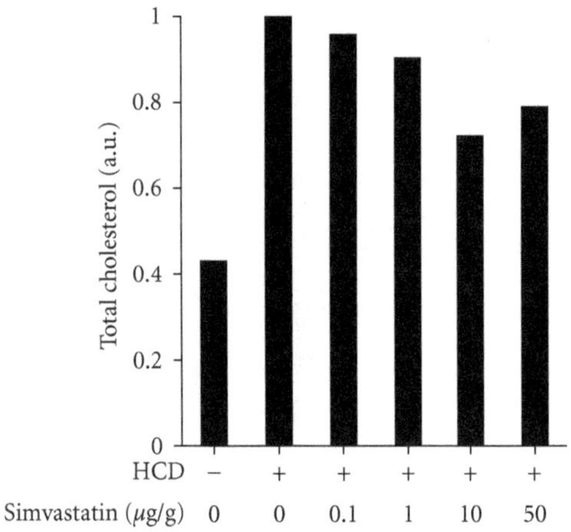

FIGURE 2: Effect of simvastatin on cholesterol levels in HCD-fed zebrafish larvae. Zebrafish larvae were fed a HCD with simvastatin mixed into zebrafish food at indicated quantities (μg simvastatin per gram food) for 14 days. Total cholesterol was measured in lipid extracts from larvae homogenates. Values of total cholesterol per larva were normalized to the values in the group that received HCD only (second column). Homogenates of 20 animals were pooled together for each data point in each individual experiment. Experiments with 0, 10, and 50 μg/g simvastatin were repeated twice, and average values from these two experiments are presented in the graph.

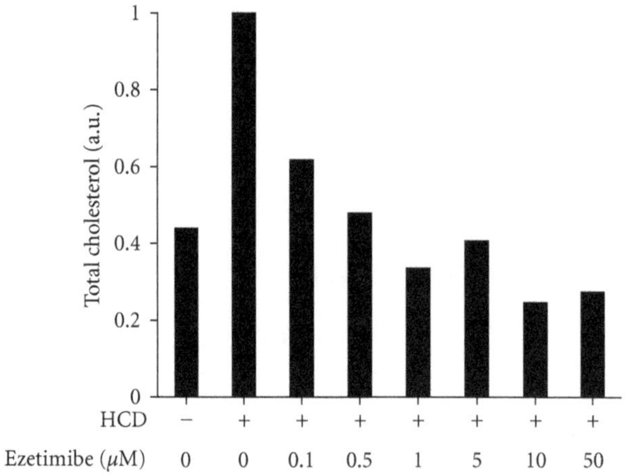

FIGURE 3: Effect of ezetimibe on cholesterol levels in HCD-fed zebrafish larvae. Zebrafish larvae were fed a HCD for 14 days. Ezetimibe was added at indicated concentrations directly to fish tank water, and the water was changed every day. Total cholesterol was measured in lipid extracts from larvae homogenates. Values of total cholesterol per larva were normalized to the values in the group that received HCD only (second column). Homogenates of 20 animals were pooled together for each data point in each individual experiment. Experiments with 0, 1, and 5 μM ezetimibe were repeated three times, and average values from these three experiments are presented in the graph.

fluids, comparable with hypercholesterolemia reported for adult zebrafish fed a HCD [1].

To study the effect of simvastatin, we initially added it directly to water, as it has been reported in short-term studies [9]. However, we found that a prolonged exposure to simvastatin in water was toxic to zebrafish larvae. Varying the doses of simvastatin and the larval age at the beginning of treatment did not help improve zebrafish survival. Next, we mixed simvastatin into fish food at doses ranging from 0.1 to 50 μg per gram of food (μg/g). As estimated in Methods, a dose of, for example, 10 μg/g simvastatin administered with zebrafish food is roughly an equivalent of a 50 mg simvastatin dose administered to human patients. As shown in Figure 2, these doses of simvastatin were less effective than expected from short-term studies, with no significant difference between the group that received HCD alone and the group that received HCD with higher doses of simvastatin ($P = 0.11$, $n = 4$ for the combined 10 and 50 μg/g simvastatin group). As pharmacokinetics of simvastatin administered with food to zebrafish larvae has not been explored, these negative results could be due to a low effective dose of simvastatin. However, a higher dose is problematic given the toxicity of simvastatin added to water.

In contrast to simvastatin, adding ezetimibe to water did not affect survival of larvae, their swimming pattern nor apparent food intake. Based on the range of doses of ezetimibe that has been reported to inhibit intestinal cholesterol absorption in zebrafish larvae [8], we tested 0.1–50 μM ezetimibe added to water. We found that ezetimibe was very effective in reducing cholesterol levels in HCD-fed larvae (Figure 3). Already at the concentration of 1 μM, ezetimibe reduced cholesterol to the levels observed in larvae fed control diet ($P = 0.39$ for the hypothesis that means of "control" and "HCD + ezetimibe" are different, $n = 3$).

In humans, ezetimibe targets intestinal Niemann-Pick C1-like protein 1 (NPC1L1). The ezetimibe-binding domain in zebrafish Npc1l1 is highly homologues to the corresponding domain in human NPC1L1, with preserved phenylalanine and methionine required for high-affinity binding of ezetimibe [8]. Larvae treated with 6.25–50 μM ezetimibe shows 25–75% reductions in gallbladder formation and in intestinal fluorescence derived from nitrobenzoxadiazole (NBD)-cholesterol [8]. These data suggest that the mechanism of inhibition of intestinal cholesterol absorption by ezetimibe in zebrafish is similar to that in humans, but direct evidence of the involvement of Npc1l1 in zebrafish cholesterol metabolism targeted by ezetimibe has not yet been reported.

Next, we tested whether a combined treatment with ezetimibe (in water) and simvastatin (in food) would result in greater reductions in cholesterol levels in HCD-fed larvae. Concentrations of ezetimibe of 1 and 5 μM, combined with 10 or 50 μg/g simvastatin, reduced cholesterol to lower levels than individual treatments with ezetimibe or simvastatin (Figures 4(a), 4(b), and 4(c)), while combinations of higher concentrations of ezetimibe with simvastatin did not have any additive effect (Figures 4(d), 4(e), and 4(f)). Thus, even though simvastatin, under our experimental conditions, had little effect on cholesterol levels in zebrafish larvae, selected combinations of simvastatin with ezetimibe produced a

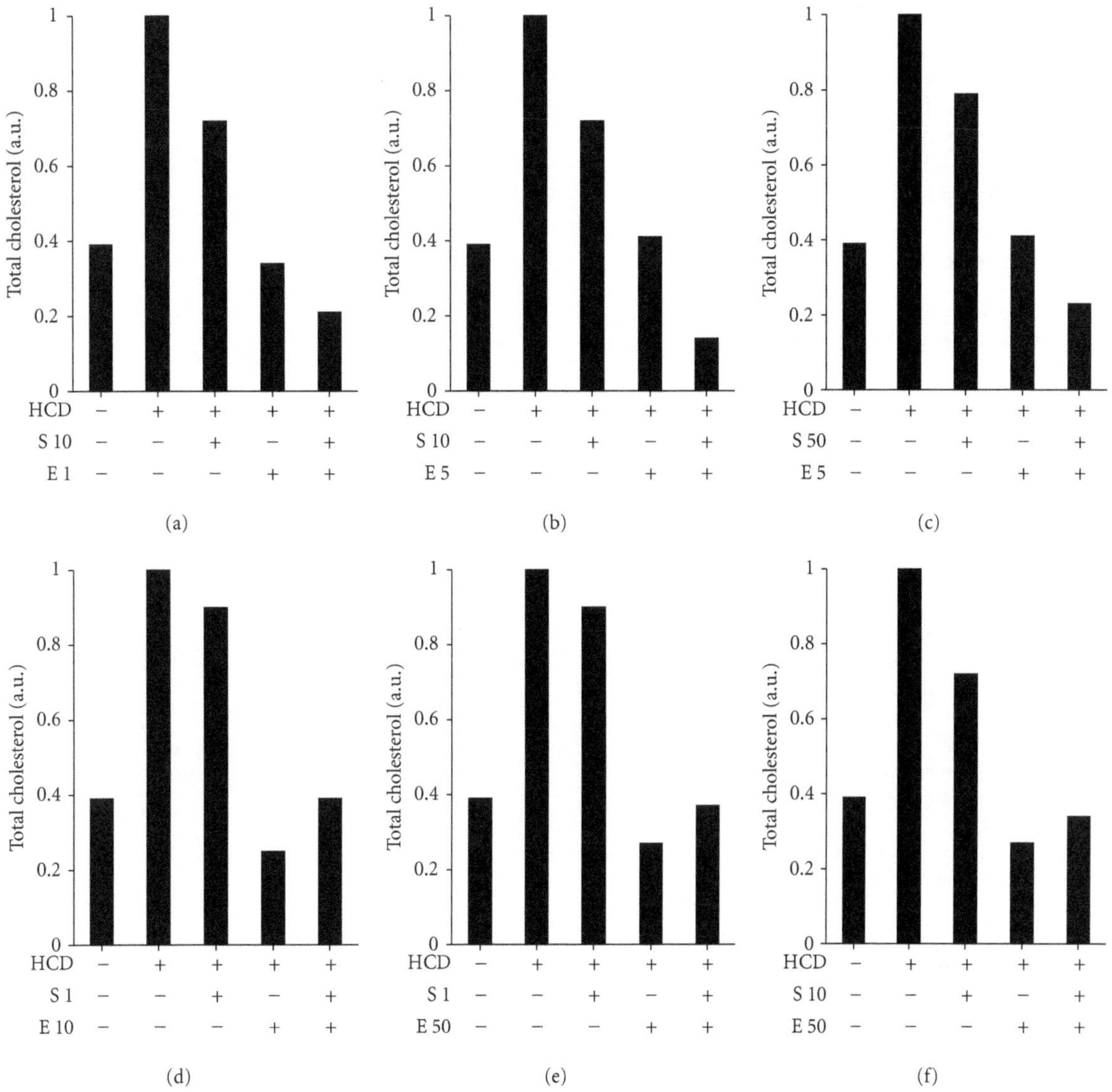

FIGURE 4: Effect of combined simvastatin and ezetimibe treatments on cholesterol levels in HCD-fed zebrafish larvae. Zebrafish larvae were fed a HCD for 14 days. Simvastatin and ezetimibe were administered as described in legends to Figures 1 and 2. Total cholesterol was measured in lipid extracts from larvae homogenates. Values of total cholesterol per larva were normalized to the values in the group that received HCD only (second column). Homogenates of 20–40 animals were pooled together for each data point in each individual experiment.

greater effect in reducing cholesterol levels than each drug alone.

Note, that in several experiments, treatments of HCD-fed zebrafish with ezetimibe or with a ezetimibe/simvastatin combination reduced cholesterol levels as much as 4-fold lower than in zebrafish that received control diet and no other treatment (Figures 3 and 4). Fish preferentially use lipids rather than carbohydrates as an energy source and would be classified, using standards applied to mammals, as hyperlipidemic and hypercholesterolemic, even when consuming their normal diet [10]. Treatments with ezetimibe and ezetimibe/simvastatin were able to reduce "normal" zebrafish hypercholesterolemia, without any apparent detrimental effects on larvae survival, swimming pattern, or feeding behavior.

4. Conclusions

Cholesterol feeding of zebrafish larvae resulted in 2.5-fold increases in cholesterol levels in body fluids isolated from larvae homogenates. These results agree well with our earlier findings of elevated cholesterol levels in plasma of adult zebrafish fed a similar HCD and suggest that HCD-feeding likely induces hypercholesterolemia in larvae as well. We found that ezetimibe is well tolerated by zebrafish larvae and effectively reduces cholesterol levels in HCD-fed larvae to or even below the levels observed in control animals. In contrast, simvastatin added to water is poorly tolerated by zebrafish larvae and, when added to food at the doses tested, has little effect on cholesterol levels in HCD-fed larvae. Combination of low doses of ezetimibe and simvastatin may have an additive effect in reducing cholesterol levels in zebrafish. These results suggest that, similar to its therapeutic effect in humans, ezetimibe effectively reduces cholesterol levels in HCD fed zebrafish larvae and can be used in the hypercholesterolemic zebrafish model to study its effects on vascular lipid accumulation and inflammation, processes relevant to the pathogenesis of human atherosclerosis.

Acknowledgments

The study was supported by the Investigator-Initiated Study Program (IISP 38001) from Merck, Inc. and the NIH Grant HL093767.

References

[1] K. Stoletov, L. Fang, S. H. Choi et al., "Vascular lipid accumulation, lipoprotein oxidation, and macrophage lipid uptake in hypercholesterolemic zebrafish," *Circulation Research*, vol. 104, no. 8, pp. 952–960, 2009.

[2] S. Jin, J. H. Hong, S. H. Jung, and K. H. Cho, "Turmeric and laurel aqueous extracts exhibit *in vitro* anti-atherosclerotic activity and *in vivo* hypolipidemic effects in a zebrafish model," *Journal of Medicinal Food*, vol. 14, no. 3, pp. 247–256, 2011.

[3] S. Jin and K. H. Cho, "Water extracts of cinnamon and clove exhibits potent inhibition of protein glycation and anti-atherosclerotic activity *in vitro* and *in vivo* hypolipidemic activity in zebrafish," *Food and Chemical Toxicology*, vol. 49, no. 7, pp. 1521–1529, 2011.

[4] J. Y. Kim, J. Seo, and K. H. Cho, "Aspartame-fed zebrafish exhibit acute deaths with swimming defects and saccharin-fed zebrafish have elevation of cholesteryl ester transfer protein activity in hypercholesterolemia," *Food and Chemical Toxicology*, vol. 49, pp. 2899–2905, 2011.

[5] L. Fang, S. R. Green, J. S. Baek et al., "*In vivo* visualization and attenuation of oxidized lipid accumulation in hypercholesterolemic zebrafish," *Journal of Clinical Investigation*, vol. 121, pp. 4861–4869, 2011.

[6] L. Fang, R. Harkewicz, K. Hartvigsen et al., "Oxidized cholesteryl esters and phospholipids in zebrafish larvae fed a high cholesterol diet: macrophage binding and activation," *Journal of Biological Chemistry*, vol. 285, no. 42, pp. 32343–32351, 2010.

[7] C. B. Kimmel, W. W. Ballard, S. R. Kimmel, B. Ullmann, and T. F. Schilling, "Stages of embryonic development of the zebrafish," *Developmental Dynamics*, vol. 203, no. 3, pp. 253–310, 1995.

[8] J. D. Clifton, E. Lucumi, M. C. Myers et al., "Identification of novel inhibitors of dietary lipid absorption using zebrafish," *PLoS One*, vol. 5, no. 8, Article ID e12386, 2010.

[9] L. S. Wen, K. Eng, J. Lee, and P. McGrath, "Use of a monoclonal antibody specific for activated endothelial cells to quantitate angiogenesis *in vivo* in zebrafish after drug treatment," *Angiogenesis*, vol. 7, no. 3, pp. 243–253, 2004.

[10] P. J. Babin and J. M. Vernier, "Plasma lipoproteins in fish," *Journal of Lipid Research*, vol. 30, no. 4, pp. 467–489, 1989.

10

Immune Response to Lipoproteins in Atherosclerosis

Sonia Samson,[1] Lakshmi Mundkur,[1] and Vijay V. Kakkar[1,2]

[1] *Department of Molecular Immunology, Thrombosis Research Institute, Narayana Hrudayalaya Hospital, 258/A, Bommasandra Industrial Area, Bangalore 560099, India*
[2] *Scientific Chairman, Thrombosis Research Institute, London, UK*

Correspondence should be addressed to Lakshmi Mundkur, lakshmi.mundkar@triindia.org.in

Academic Editor: Michael Ibrahim

Atherosclerosis, the underlying cause of cardiovascular disease, is characterized by chronic inflammation and altered immune response. Cholesterol is a well-known risk factor associated with the development of cardiovascular diseases. Elevated serum cholesterol is unique because it can lead to development of atherosclerosis in animals and humans even in the absence of other risk factors. Modifications of low-density lipoproteins mediated by oxidation, enzymatic degradation, and aggregation result in changes in their function and activate both innate and adaptive immune system. Oxidized low-density lipoprotein (LDL) has been identified as one of the most important autoantigens in atherosclerosis. This escape from self-tolerance is dependent on the formation of oxidized phospholipids. The emerging understanding of the importance of immune responses against oxidized LDL in atherosclerosis has focused attention on the possibility of development of novel therapy for atherosclerosis. This review provides an overview of immune response to lipoproteins and the fascinating possibility of developing an immunomodulatory therapy for atherosclerosis.

1. Introduction

Cardiovascular diseases remain the leading cause of global morbidity and mortality. As per the WHO estimates 17.3 million people died of CVD in 2008 representing almost 30% of global mortality. It is estimated that this number will rise to 23.6 million by 2030 with almost 80% of the death occurring in low and middle income countries. The most important risk factors of heart disease and stroke are unhealthy diet, physical inactivity, tobacco use, and harmful use of alcohol. These result in raised blood pressure, raised levels of glucose and lipids in blood, overweight, and obesity which constitute the metabolic syndrome [1].

Higher level of cholesterol in blood has traditionally been considered as established risk factors for CVD. However, increased total cholesterol concentrations in plasma do not accurately predict the risk of coronary heart disease as it includes the sum of all cholesterol carried not only by atherogenic lipoproteins, that is, very low-density lipoprotein [VLDL], low-density lipoprotein [LDL], and intermediate-density lipoprotein [IDL], but also by antiatherogenic lipoproteins, that is, high-density lipoprotein, [HDL]. It is also known that the small, dense LDL cholesterol is more atherogenic than large, buoyant particles, and oxidation of LDL increases its atherogenicity. The relationship between LDL cholesterol and risk for CVD is well established, and measurement of LDL is routinely used for risk assessment, as well as risk management [2]. Over the last four decades, significant progress has been made towards the prevention of CVD, primarily by the use of statins which result in lowering the cholesterol levels. However, the increasing epidemic of metabolic syndrome and Type 2 diabetes mellitus (T2DM) has slown down this progress. Although the use of statins has accounted for the significant reduction in the morbidity and mortality associated with CVD, the risk is not completely eliminated despite effective lipid-lowering treatment [3]. It is estimated that the current therapies prevent only 30% of clinical events, suggesting an urgent need for newer therapeutic strategies [3].

For many years atherosclerosis was believed to be a disease of lipid accumulation in the vessel wall. Extensive research on the pathophysiology of the disease has brought about a paradigm shift in our understanding of CVD, and atherosclerosis is now accepted as a multifactorial, multiphase chronic inflammatory disease with immunological activity at every stage, from initiation to progression and plaque rupture [4–6]. This review will concentrate on immune response to lipoproteins, its role in the development of atherosclerosis, and modulation of immune response to lipoprotein as therapeutic strategy.

2. Immune Response and Atherosclerosis

Atherosclerosis, which manifests itself as acute coronary syndrome, stroke, and peripheral arterial diseases, is a chronic inflammatory disease of the arterial wall [7]. Immune system plays an important role in the development, progression, and the complications associated with atherosclerosis [5]. Both innate and adaptive immune responses are associated with the progression of the disease (Figure 1). The retention of cholesterol in the subendothelial region of the vessel is the central pathogenic event that starts the atherosclerotic lesion formation [8]. Lipids, such as cholesterol and triglycerides, are insoluble in plasma and are carried by lipoproteins that transport them to various tissues, and LDL is normally associated with the apolipoprotein (Apo) B-100. An increase in plasma LDL levels leads to an increased rate of its entry into the intima, and consequently a higher level of LDL is observed in the intimal region [9]. The interaction of positively charged ApoB to negatively charged proteoglycans leads to the retention of ApoB-linked lipoproteins in the vessel wall [10]. These sequestered lipoproteins are susceptible to modification by oxidation, enzymatic cleavage, and aggregation [11]. Immune response to these modified lipoproteins drives the pathogenic evolution of the plaque by releasing proinflammatory mediators leading to a chronic inflammatory reaction. Oxidized LDL induces the formation of foam cells and fatty streaks in the vessel wall which is the hallmark of initiation of atherosclerosis [12]. Macrophages from the host immune system try to clean up cholesterol deposits in arteries, but once they are loaded with the unhealthy form of cholesterol, they get stuck in the arteries, triggering the body's inflammatory response. These cholesterol-loaded macrophages line the artery wall and become major components of the growing plaque. As the atherosclerotic lesion evolves, other immune inflammatory cells such as T cells, dendritic cells, and mast cells accumulate in the region. Macrophages and dendritic cells are known to contribute to the innate immune response by generating free oxygen radicals, proteases, complement factors and cytokines. Macrophages also produce chemokines including the T-cell attractant CCL5 (RANTES) to attract other immune cells into the growing plaque [13, 14]. A fibrous cap of variable thickness, composed mainly of collagen, covers the lesion, while the shoulder region consists of activated T cells, macrophages, and mast cells [7]. The early fatty streaks develop into a complex lesion consisting of apoptotic and necrotic cells, cell debris, and cholesterol crystals which form the necrotic core over a long period of time [15]. Adaptive immunity recognizes specific epitopes on antigens that are processed and presented by the antigen-presenting cells to the T cells, leading to lymphocyte activation and secretion of cytokines and antigen-specific antibodies. T cells reacting to disease-related antigens such as Ox-LDL, HSP60, bacterial, and viral antigens have been found in the human lesions [16–18] (Figure 1).

3. ProAtherogenic and Atheroprotective Immune Response

Four major subsets of T helper cells are involved in the adaptive immune response: helper T-cell subsets Th1 and Th2, regulatory T cells, and the Th17 cells. The $CD8^{+}$ T cells promote atherogenesis when activated by foreign antigens, but their precise role in atherogenesis remains unclear as their depletion is not associated with any change in the lesion formation [19]. Th1 cells the induce activation of macrophages, neutrophils, and cytotoxic T lymphocytes and secrete proinflammatory cytokines such as interferon γ and IL12. They are more prevalent in the lesions of both human and $ApoE^{-/-}$ mice suggesting that atherosclerosis is a Th1-dominant disease [20, 21]. Th2 cells are involved in allergic diseases such as atopic allergy and asthma [22]. Their role in atherosclerosis seems to depend on the stage and site of the disease. Increased concentrations of Th2 cytokines in lymphoid organs and atheroprotective anti-oxLDL IgM antibodies in the serum resulted in a significant reduction in atherosclerotic plaque development [23]. However in mice deficient in IL4, the archetypical Th2 cytokine, atherosclerosis was less severe than in IL4-sufficient mice [24]. Th17 cells produce the proinflammatory cytokine IL17 and promote autoimmune diseases [25, 26]. Significant increase in peripheral Th17 cells, cytokines IL17, IL6 and IL23, and transcription factor RORγ levels was reported in patients with acute coronary syndrome (ACS) when compared to control [27]. A functional imbalance between the Th17/Treg was also reported in patients with acute coronary syndrome (ACS), suggesting a potential role for these cells in plaque destabilization and the onset of ACS.

Treg cells are a subpopulation of T cells specialized in maintaining immune homeostasis and self-tolerance by suppressing pathogenic immune responses. Treg cells are heterogeneous and can be subdivided schematically into two major subsets: natural (n Treg) and induced (i Treg). These cells are characterized by expression of CD25 (a subunit of the IL2 receptor) and CD4, on the surface and intracellular expression of the transcription factor fork head box protein P3 (FoxP3) [28]. Treg cells can inhibit effector T cells by contact-dependent suppression of cell proliferation and downregulate the availability of growth factors to effector T cells by enhanced consumption of IL2, and by inhibiting the effector cell functions through secretion of the anti-inflammatory cytokines TGF-β, IL10, and IL35 [29]. The clinical manifestation of atherosclerosis can be linked to inflammation mediated by the Th1 cells, while Treg cells may be involved in the stabilization of disease. Several review articles have discussed the role of immune response in atherosclerosis in detail [5, 7, 27, 30–41].

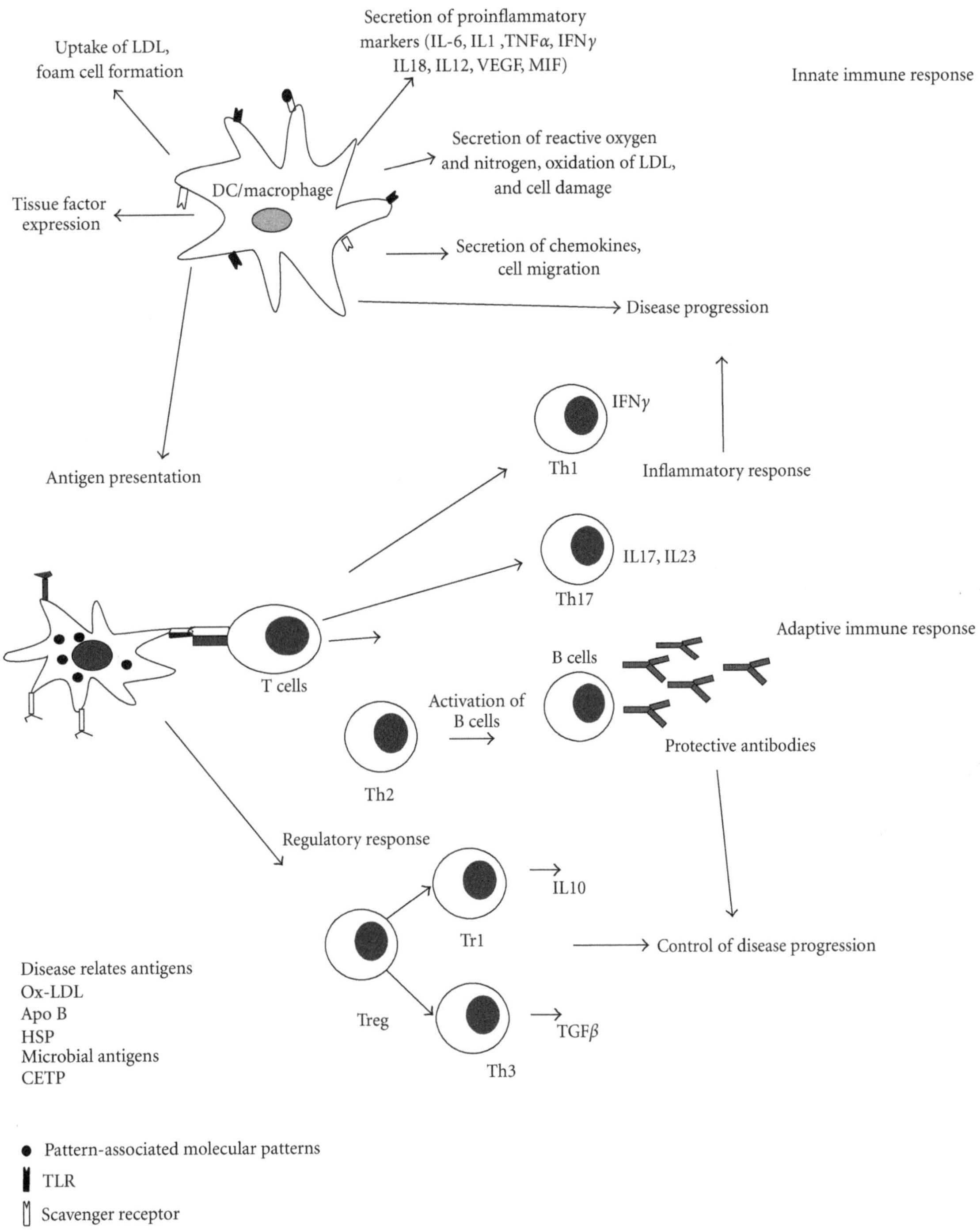

Figure 1: Immune response in atherosclerosis. Macrophages and dendritic cells are the important components of innate immune response in atherosclerosis. Uptake of modified LDL particles such as oxLDL through scavenger receptors leads to the intracellular accumulation of cholesterol leading to activation and expression of a series of genes encoding proinflammatory molecules, including cytokines, chemokines, eicosanoids, proteases, oxidases, and costimulatory molecules. Adaptive immune response is activated when self-antigens, oxidized LDL, and other disease-related antigens are presented to T cells by the macrophages/dendritic cells. The concomitant release of cytokines determines the maturation of the T cell recognizing the antigen. Differentiation into Th1 cells results in inflammatory response, while Th2 leads to activation of antigen-specific B cells. These B cells produce antibodies to the disease-specific antigens. Regulatory T cells induce a tolerogenic response mediated by Tr1 cells and Th3 cells which secrete IL10 and TGF-β respectively, which inhibit the progression of the disease. Th, T helper cells; Treg, regulatory T cell; IL, interleukin; VEGF, vascular endothelial growth factor; TNF, tumor necrosis factor; MIF, migration inhibition factor; Ox-LDL, oxidized low-density lipoprotein; HSP, heat shock protein, CETP, cholesteryl ester transfer protein.

4. Immune Response to Lipoproteins in Atherosclerosis

The positive role of lipoproteins in the development of cardiovascular diseases has been reported by several epidemiological studies so much so that atherosclerosis was considered a lipid-mediated disease. A key early step in atherogenesis is the formation of the fatty streak, consisting of a subendothelial collection of foam cells, which are cholesterol-laden macrophages or smooth muscle cells [42]. LDL does not trigger an immune response in its native state. Formation of oxidized phospholipids and aldehyde-modified breakdown fragments of apolipoprotein B-100 (apoB-100) exposes neoantigens which cause a breakdown in self-tolerance and induces inflammatory reactions [43, 44]. Oxidation of LDL generates reactive aldehydes and truncated lipids by cleaving the fatty acid double bonds in phospholipids, triglycerides, and cholesteryl esters [45]. Modified phospholipids such as lysophosphatidyl choline and trimethylamine N-oxide can trigger potent immune response by activating NKT cells, macrophages, and endothelial cells [15, 46, 47]. Oxidative modification of ApoB 100 also causes degradation of ApoB and release of small peptides which increase vascular permeability [48, 49]. Accumulation of monocytes/macrophages, smooth muscle cells, and T cells within the arterial wall in response to proinflammatory molecules constitutes a hallmark of developing plaque [5]. Oxidized LDL (OxLDL) has been identified as one of the most important autoantigens in atherosclerosis. The Activation of both innate and adaptive immune responses against OxLDL is the major cause of inflammation and its pathological consequences [31, 36, 50, 51]. Modified LDL interact with scavenger receptors while OX LDL binds to CD36 receptor on monocytes and macrophages and form foam cells [44]. Foam cells are highly immunogenic and attract the adhesion, migration, and activation of the cells of the immune system thus contributing to the development of the disease.

Antigen-presenting cells take up modified LDL and initiate an adaptive immune response by presenting these antigens to T cells, which proliferate to amplify the immune response [52]. Upon renewed exposure to the specific antigen, these T cells produce cytokines and trigger inflammation.

OxLDL is frequently present in sera of patients with coronary syndrome [53, 54] and also accumulates in atherosclerotic plaques [55]. Apart from the formation of foam cells, OxLDL exhibits a range of proatherogenic properties. It acts as a chemoattractant for circulating monocytes and can stimulate secretion of monocyte chemoattractant protein-1 by endothelial cells [56]. It is cytotoxic for endothelial cells cultured in serum-free medium, induces expression of macrophage colony stimulating factor, promotes the differentiation of monocytes to macrophages, attracts T cells into the growing atherosclerotic plaque, induces a wide variety of proinflammatory cytokines in macrophages, increases expression of vascular cell adhesion molecule-1 and is also immunogenic [57, 58]. The existence of a preexisting, natural immune response against oxidized LDL phospholipids mediated by IgM produced by B-1-cells has also been identified [43]. Immune complexes formed by modified LDL and corresponding antibodies are potent macrophage activators and direct overexpression of MHC-II, costimulatory molecules, and proinflammatory markers, thus creating an ideal conditions for Th1 activation [56–58]. Activated macrophages also release reactive oxygen radicals, enhancing the opportunity for LDL modification [5] which increases the immunogenic load, induce a more vigorous antibody response, and increase the formation of LDL immune complexes (Figure 2).

5. Natural Antibodies to Lipoproteins

Natural antibodies are defined as antibodies that are found in normal individuals in the complete absence of any exogenous antigenic stimulation and provide first line of defense against invading pathogens [59]. These antibodies bind to a number of self-antigens such as cell membrane components (phosphtidyl choline, glycolipids, etc.) [59, 60] single-stranded DNA [61] and cell surface molecules on T-cells such as Thy1 [62]. Many of these self-epitopes are also present on pathogens [63–65]. These natural antibodies are also termed as poly reactive to explain their cross reactivity with multiple self-and- non-self-antigens and are required for the immediate recognition and protection against invading pathogens [59, 66]. Natural antibodies are also involved in the removal of aging and dead cells, their debris, and self-antigens and thus protect from autoimmunity [32]. This role of protection from autoimmunity is very relevant especially under certain pathological conditions that involve increased accumulation of self-antigens such as oxidation specific epitopes during atherosclerosis [31].

Natural IgM antibodies are predominantly produced by a small subset of long-lived, self-replenishing B cells, termed B-1 cells which exhibit a conserved repertoire [65]. These antibodies are encoded in the germline genome and are not dependent on immunoglobulin gene rearrangement. They have broad specificities, but display low affinities and do not require T-cell stimulation of the B lymphocytes to produce antibodies. Presence of autoantibodies to epitopes of copper-oxidized LDL (Cu-OxLDL) and malondialdehyde-modified LDL (MDA-LDL) has been reported in human and animal models of atherosclerosis [67–69]. Cholesterol-fed ApoE$^{-/-}$ mice were found to have very high autoantibody titers, particularly IgM, to a wide variety of Ox LDL epitopes [70]. B-cell hybridomas generated from these mice revealed that most of these autoantibodies were of IgM isotype, recognized the lipid and ApoB moieties of OxLDL, but not of native LDL, and had a specific recognition for phosphorylcholine group [71, 72]. The prototypic and best-characterized antibody against OxLDL, EO6, is identical to T15, a natural antibody known to recognize phosphorylcholine (PC) expressed as a capsular epitopes on *Streptococcus pneumonia* [43] and could also block OxLDL uptake by macrophages. Binder et al. identified the functional role of antiphospholipid antibodies in atherosclerosis by immunizing LDLr$^{-/-}$ mice with heat-inactivated PC containing pneumococci [73]. The pneumococcal immunization was found to induce high titers

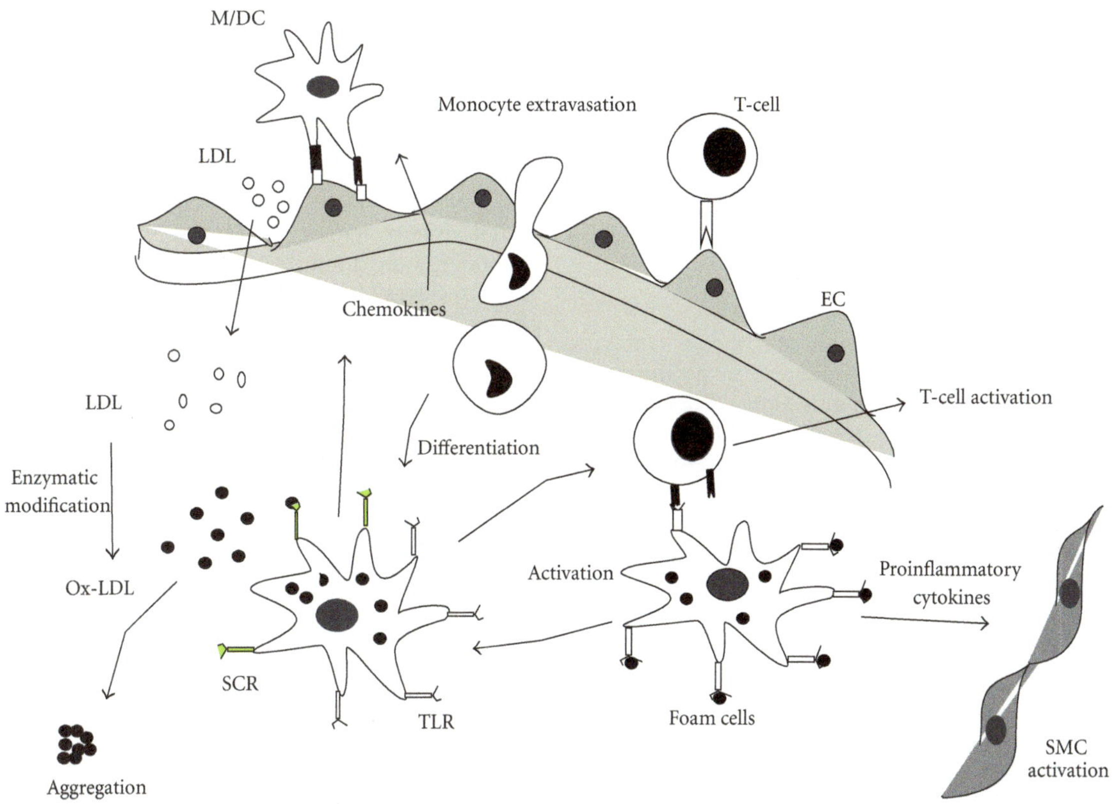

Figure 2: Immune response to LDL in atherosclerosis. The low-density lipoprotein (LDL) in the blood diffuses into the intima of the-vessel wall, where it gets oxidized by enzymes or reactive oxygen to form OxLDL. Modified LDL particles are taken up by macrophages that accumulate cholesterol and become foam cells. Ox-LDL causes overexpression of VCAM-1 and ICAM-1 by the endothelial cells, which attracts the monocytes, and T cells move into the vessel wall. Activated macrophages secrete proinflammatory mediators, such as TNFα, IL-1, MCP-1, and proteolytic enzymes (MMPs). Foam cells can process and present ApoB100 peptides to CD4+ T helper cells via MHC class II molecules. Antigen presentation to CD4+ TH1 cells triggers their activation, with ensuing release of IFN- and TNF known to have proatherogenic properties. VCAM, vascular cell adhesion molecule; ICAM, intercellular cell adhesion molecule; TNF, tumour necrosis factor; IL, interleukin; MCP, macrophage chemoattractant protein; MMP, matrix metalloproteinase, Th, T helper cells; ApoB, apolipoprotein B.

of anti-OxLDL IgM (predominantly of the T15 clonotype) and significantly reduce atherosclerotic lesion in the aortic sinus. The uptake of OxLDL by macrophages was found to be inhibited by the plasma of immunized mice. In a similar attempt to use PC as a vaccine for atherosclerosis, Caligiuri et al. immunized mice with PC covalently linked to a carrier protein, keyhole limpet hemocyanin (KLH). Immunized mice showed a 40% reduction in lesions compared to control and sera from PC-KLH-immunized mice decreased, the uptake of OxLDL compared to sera of PBS-immunized mice [74]. Further studies in human revealed that patients recovering from pneumococcal infections contain IgM antibodies to the bacterial polysaccharide that significantly correlated with levels of anti-OxLDL IgM antibodies in the same serum sample. These findings suggest that PC-specific cross-reacting IgMs are also present in humans. Human IgG1 against a specific OxLDL epitope was reported to induce rapid and substantial regression of atherosclerotic lesions, possibly by stimulating lipid efflux and inhibiting macrophage recruitment [75]. These recombinant human atheroprotective antibodies could, thus, represent a novel strategy for rapid regression/stabilization of atherosclerotic lesions.

The mechanism of protection afforded by these antibodies has not been studied in detail so far [76, 77]. Binding of OxLDL by IgM antibodies could potentially neutralize most of their proinflammatory properties, which promote atherogenesis. The formation of circulating immune complexes of these IgMs with OxLDL may have protective properties by preventing LDL from entering vulnerable sites of the artery wall. A number of in vitro studies have suggested that these IgM antibodies block the uptake of OxLDL by macrophages and thus could prevent foam cell formation in vivo [73]. They could prevent the activation of endothelial cells and monocyte binding by apoptotic cells containing oxidized lipids [67]. It is still not clear whether passive therapy with these antibodies alone would be protective. Passive transfer of antiphosphorylcholine monoclonal antibodies reduced atherosclerosis supporting the protective role of natural antibodies [78]. Thus, a number of protective mechanisms have been suggested for natural antibodies; however, the relevance of these mechanisms in vivo is still not very clear.

On the other hand existence of proatherogenic natural antibodies is also a possibility which has not been studied in detail so far, as some B-1 cell-derived IgMs have been shown to play a pathogenic role in intestinal ischemia/reperfusion injury [79]. Understanding the role of natural antibodies in health disease and autoimmunity is likely to open up novel therapeutic approaches for the control of atherosclerosis.

6. Antilipoprotein Antibodies: Friend or Foe?

Antibodies to lipoproteins are exemplary in having both proatherogenic as well as protective function against atherosclerosis (Figure 3).

6.1. Pathogenic Effects of Anti-OxLDL Antibodies. OxLDL frequently presents in the sera of patients with coronary artery disease, and the serum concentrations of circulating oxLDL may correlate with the severity of CAD and acute coronary syndrome [53, 54, 80, 81]. Analysis of several studies suggests that, in humans, the humoral immune response to modified LDL is pathogenic. Adaptive response is known to generate IgG antibodies, and the predominance of IgG over IgM antibodies favors the formation of IgG-containing immune complexes with proinflammatory properties. Immune complexes formed with modified LDL and IgG antibodies have been shown to have significantly stronger proatherogenic and proinflammatory properties than modified LDL itself [82–85]. Atherosclerotic lesions also contain immunoglobulins that specifically recognize OxLDL [86], and these antibodies are believed to be the most effective parameters for predicting the extent of coronary atherosclerosis [82]. Their presence is also associated with a higher risk for coronary restenosis after coronary angioplasty [83].

Elevated levels of anti-Ox-LDL antibody are related to hypertension, systemic vacuities, peripheral arterial disease, endothelial dysfunction, atherosclerosis, and cardiovascular disease [69, 84, 85, 87–90]. Anti-OxLDL antibodies can also induce other effects, such as complement activation, and induction of adaptive immune response leading to inflammation. Different subclasses of anti-Ox LDL antibodies with a range of pathogenic effects are reported in humans [91]. IgG1 and IgG3 antibodies have been defined as proinflammatory, based on their ability to activate the complement system by the classical pathway and to interact with Fcγ receptors in phagocytic cells [68]. The involvement of IgG1 and IgG3 antibodies in immune complex disease is also well recognized [92]. However, there are reports showing negative or no correlation between anti-LDL antibodies and atherosclerosis [93, 94]. The measurement of free circulating autoantibodies depends on the magnitude of the antibody response, antibody avidity, and on the amount of antigen present in circulation. Soluble immune complexes are formed by the high-avidity antibodies and circulating Ox-LDL leading to inaccurate estimation of anti-Ox-LDL antibodies in the serum [52, 95].

6.2. Protective Effects of Ox-LDL Antibodies. Anti-Ox-LDL antibodies are present in healthy individuals as well as in patients with atherosclerosis [69, 96]. Several experimental studies in animals using Ox-LDL immunization have shown a positive correlation between high titers of anti-Ox-LDL antibodies and the degree of protection against atherosclerosis [97–100]. Transfer of B cells from atherosclerotic apolipoprotein (Apo) E- knockout mice (ApoE−/−) to young, ApoE−/− mice protected the latter from developing advanced disease [96]. Passive administration of recombinant human antibodies against aldehyde-modified apolipoprotein B-100 peptide sequences was observed to inhibit atherosclerosis in ApoE−/− mice [101]. These antibodies were found to modulate the development of fatty streaks as well as their progression to atherosclerotic plaque [102]. Anti-Ox-LDL antibodies are present in healthy individuals as well as in patients with atherosclerosis [69, 96]. Antibodies to Ox LDL seem to play an important role in regulating the level of OX LDL in human. Circulating antibodies recognizing ox-LDL have been found in children with no risk of CVD, and an inverse correlation was observed between plasma Ox-LDL concentrations with the levels of anti-Ox-LDL antibodies in healthy subjects [103, 104]. In another study anti-Ox-LDL antibody levels were inversely related to the intima-media thickness of the carotid arteries in a healthy population with no clinical signs of atherosclerosis [105]. These studies support the protective function of anti LDL antibodies in atherosclerosis which seem to be native antibodies that neutralize Ox-LDL [104, 105].

These observations raise several pertinent questions; is it possible that different epitopes on Ox-LDL determine its protection or pathogenicity? "Can we use anti-Ox-LDL antibodies for atheroprotection? Can OX-LDL be used as an immunogen for modulation of immune response without having any serious adverse effects? Careful consideration of these aspects will be most essential before they can be taken as candidates for therapeutic intervention.

7. Vaccine against Atherosclerosis

Over the last few years, considerable efforts have been made to develop a vaccine using epitopes from lipoproteins and heat shock proteins [106–110]. Considering atherosclerosis as an autoimmune disease wherein an immune response is triggered against the autoantigens, a vaccine which can restore the tolerance to these antigens would be effective in reducing the inflammatory response. Antigen-specific immune modulation is an attractive approach to prevent chronic inflammatory diseases without affecting the normal immune function of the host. Two self-antigens which have emerged as most important ones are related to LDL and heat shock protein (HSP) [60]. Normally T cells reacting to these antigens should be eliminated by negative selection, in the thymus leading to central tolerance. If oxidation of LDL generates neoantigens, all the T cell clones reactive to these would not be removed during thymic education [15]. Similarly in the case of HSP60, molecular mimicry between HSPs of pathogens and human could trigger autoimmune response leading to chronic inflammation. Peripheral tolerance plays a role in maintaining an immune homeostasis to these self-antigens under normal circumstances. Vaccines against atherosclerosis that are being currently developed are different from traditional vaccines for infectious diseases.

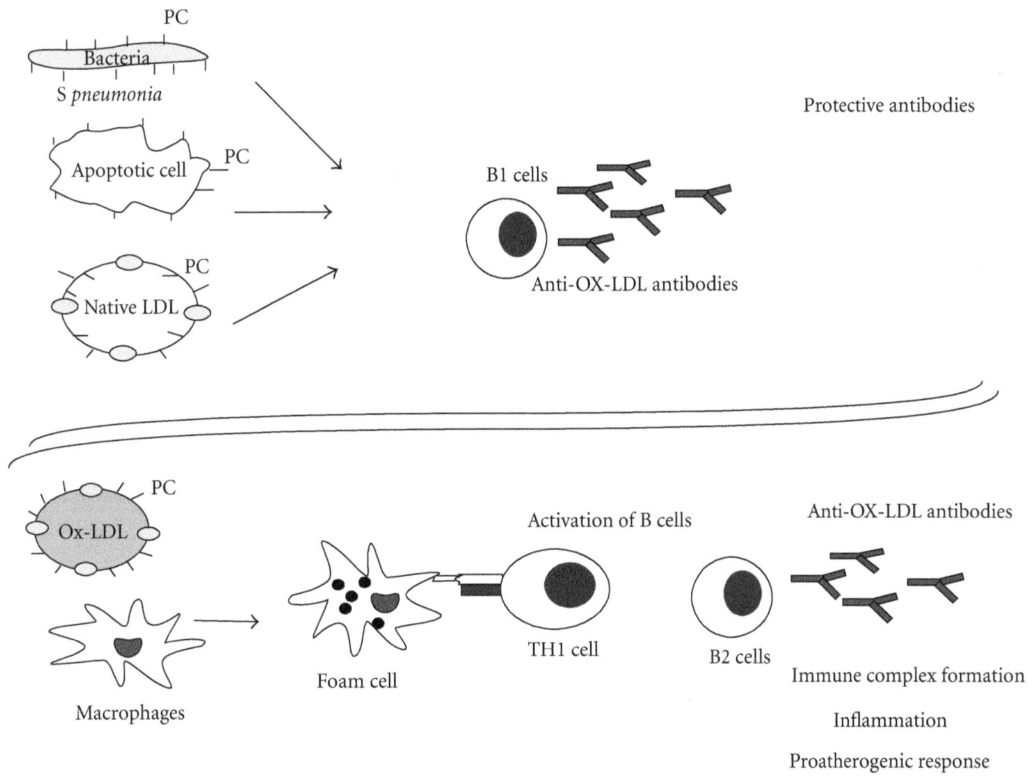

Figure 3: Protective and pathogenic antilipoprotein antibodies. Molecular mimicry occurs when LDL or a viable cell undergoes limited oxidative modification to present phosphocholine (PC) antigens like those expressed on bacteria (*Streptococcus pneumonia)*.These antigens stimulate B1 lymphocytes to produce the protective EO6/T15 autoantibodies. These antibodies are likely to block the uptake of Ox-LDL through scavenger receptors, promote the clearance of apoptotic cells, or neutralize the infecting bacteria resulting in a protective response. Extensive oxidation of LDL results in its conversion to Ox-LDL is taken up by macrophages and stimulate the T-cell-dependent immune response to produce IgG antibodies. These antibodies, along with other proinflammatory cytokines produced by foam cells, in turn accelerate lesion progression.

An ideal vaccine is aimed at restoring the self-tolerance to autoantigens like LDL and heat shock proteins, reducing the inflammation, and balancing the pro- and anti-atherogenic immune response [111].

8. Modulation of Immune Response to Lipoproteins

Lipoprotein oxidation and subsequent formation of several new antigenic epitopes renders this molecule highly immunogenic, leading to both humoral and cellular immune response. Moreover LDL is a complex particle composed of a high-molecular-weight protein, apolipoprotein B-100 (ApoB100), neutral and polar lipids, and lipophilic antioxidants. Since the different epitopes of ox-LDL induce atherogenic immune responses, it is an attractive candidate to explore immune modulation. Immunization against Ox-LDL has been shown to reduce atherosclerosis by a number of studies [73, 75, 97, 101, 109, 112–115].

Immunization of hypercholesterolemic rabbits and $LDLr^{-/-}$ mice with both MDA-LDL and Cu-Ox-LDL were found to generate high titers of antibodies and inhibit atherosclerosis development by 40–70%, suggesting an induction of atheroprotective immune response [68, 97, 100, 108]. The mechanism of protection afforded by this immunization is thought to be through IgM antibodies generated against Ox-LDL that are shown to block the uptake of Ox-LDL by CD36 receptors on macrophages, thus reducing foam cell formation [116]. Induction of oral tolerance to Cu-Ox-LDL and MDA-LDL mediated by Treg cells and TGF-β was also reported to attenuate the initiation and progression of atherosclerosis in $LDLr^{-/-}$ mice [109]. Similar effects were also observed on tolerance induction to HSP60 [110].

The protein sequence of ApoB-100 was studied by Fredrikson et al. to identify potential antigenic epitopes that could have atheroprotective effects [112]. Out of the 302 overlapping 20 amino acid peptides synthesized, few were found to provoke an atheroprotective immune response in hypercholesterolemic mice [117]. Peptide 45, corresponding to the amino acid sequence 661–680 of ApoB100 was found to be one of the most effective atheroprotective peptides [113]. The presence of autoantibodies against this peptide sequence was also shown to be associated with reduced risk for development of myocardial infarction (MI) in humans [118]. Adoptive transfer of splenocytes from immunized mice as well as monoclonal antibody against this peptide was found to passively transfer protection [101]. Treatment with human recombinant IgG1 antibodies against the same epitope ameliorated the existing atherosclerotic lesions in $ApoB^{-/-}$ and $LDLr^{-/-}$ mice. The study also demonstrated reduction in macrophage MCP1 release leading to reduced inflammatory plaques and increased reverse cholesterol transport as a possible mechanism of protection [75]. Recently intranasal immunization with ApoB100 peptides was found to induce protective immune response mediated by antigen-specific Treg and could confer protection against the disease in animal models. Our study showed a synergistic effect of immunization with a combination of ApoB and HSP60 peptides in preventing early atherosclerosis [106]. Molecular mimicry between PC of Ox-LDL and apoptotic cells and that of pneumococcus leading to generation of cross-reactive antibodies which can block uptake of LDL by macrophages has been reported [73]. Thus, immunizations with both ApoB peptides as well as oxidized phospholipids have atheroprotective effects in animal models of diet-induced atherosclerosis.

9. Conclusion

The search for alternative and more specific ways to reduce the modification of LDL, which would consequently reduce the immune response to modified lipoproteins, has received continued attention from the atherosclerosis research community. Different epitopes on Ox-LDL is shown to determine its protection or pathogenicity by various studies. The possibility of using Ox-LDL as an immunogen for modulation of response without having any serious adverse effects has to be elucidated. Anti-Ox-LDL antibodies with neutralizing activity against modified LDL may be an effective therapeutic molecule and needs to be deliberated carefully. Another important criterion for a vaccine is to elucidate its potential in preventing the progression of an established plaque. Atherosclerosis is a slow progressing disease in human. Traces of fatty streaks are also observed in children though the disease manifests itself at a much later age. Development of a proper clinical protocol, establishment of surrogate markers, and identification of right patient population to study the vaccine efficacy are some of the important criteria to be explored in the development of a therapeutic vaccine. Careful consideration of these aspects will be most essential before they can be taken as candidates for therapeutic intervention.

Acknowledgments

The authors gratefully acknowledge the support of the trustees of Thrombosis Research Institute, London and Bangalore, the Tata Social Welfare Trust, India (TSWT/IG/SNB/JP/Sdm), and the Department of Biotechnology, Ministry of Science and Technology, Government of India (BT/01/CDE/08/07).

References

[1] P. Greenland, M. D. Knoll, J. Stamler et al., "Major risk factors as antecedents of fatal and nonfatal coronary heart disease events," *Journal of the American Medical Association*, vol. 290, no. 7, pp. 891–897, 2003.

[2] J. I. Cleeman, "Executive summary of the third report of the National Cholesterol Education Program (NCEP) expert panel on detection, evaluation, and treatment of high blood cholesterol in adults (adult treatment panel III)," *Journal of the American Medical Association*, vol. 285, no. 19, pp. 2486–2497, 2001.

[3] C. Baigent, "Efficacy and safety of cholesterol-lowering treatment: prospective meta-analysis of data from 90 056 participants in 14 randomised trials of statins," *The Lancet*, vol. 366, no. 9493, pp. 1267–1278, 2005.

[4] R. Paoletti, A. M. Gotto, and D. P. Hajjar, "Inflammation in atherosclerosis and implications for therapy," *Circulation*, vol. 109, no. 23, supplement, pp. III20–III26, 2004.

[5] G. K. Hansson and P. Libby, "The immune response in atherosclerosis: a double-edged sword," *Nature Reviews Immunology*, vol. 6, no. 7, pp. 508–519, 2006.

[6] A. A. Cuneo and M. V. Autieri, "Expression and function of anti-inflammatory interleukins: the other side of the vascular response to injury," *Current Vascular Pharmacology*, vol. 7, no. 3, pp. 267–276, 2009.

[7] G. K. Hansson, "Mechanisms of disease: inflammation, atherosclerosis, and coronary artery disease," *New England Journal of Medicine*, vol. 352, no. 16, pp. 1685–1695, 2005.

[8] D. Steinberg, "Atherogenesis in perspective: hypercholesterolemia and inflammation as partners in crime," *Nature Medicine*, vol. 8, no. 11, pp. 1211–1217, 2002.

[9] D. C. Schwenke and T. E. Carew, "Initiation of atherosclerotic lesions in cholesterol-fed rabbits. II. Selective retention of LDL vs. selective increases in LDL permeability in susceptible sites of arteries," *Arteriosclerosis*, vol. 9, no. 6, pp. 908–918, 1989.

[10] K. Olin-Lewis, R. M. Krauss, M. La Belle et al., "ApoC-III content of apoB-containing lipoproteins is associated with binding to the vascular proteoglycan biglycan," *Journal of Lipid Research*, vol. 43, no. 11, pp. 1969–1977, 2002.

[11] T. Hevonoja, M. O. Pentikäinen, M. T. Hyvönen, P. T. Kovanen, and M. Ala-Korpela, "Structure of low density lipoprotein (LDL) particles: basis for understanding molecular changes in modified LDL," *Biochimica et Biophysica Acta*, vol. 1488, no. 3, pp. 189–210, 2000.

[12] E. Riley, V. Dasari, W. H. Frishman, and K. Sperber, "Vaccines in development to prevent and treat atherosclerotic disease," *Cardiology in Review*, vol. 16, no. 6, pp. 288–300, 2008.

[13] L. Gu, Y. Okada, S. K. Clinton et al., "Absence of monocyte chemoattractant protein-1 reduces atherosclerosis in low density lipoprotein receptor-deficient mice," *Molecular Cell*, vol. 2, no. 2, pp. 275–281, 1998.

[14] L. Boring, J. Gosling, M. Cleary, and I. F. Charo, "Decreased lesion formation in $CCR2^{-/-}$ mice reveals a role for chemokines in the initiation of atherosclerosis," *Nature*, vol. 394, no. 6696, pp. 894–897, 1998.

[15] G. K. Hansson and A. Hermansson, "The immune system in atherosclerosis," *Nature Immunology*, vol. 12, no. 3, pp. 204–212, 2011.

[16] Q. Xu, "Role of heat shock proteins in atherosclerosis," *Arteriosclerosis, Thrombosis, and Vascular Biology*, vol. 22, no. 10, pp. 1547–1559, 2002.

[17] S. Stemme and G. K. Hansson, "Immune mechanisms in atherosclerosis," *Coronary Artery Disease*, vol. 5, no. 3, pp. 216–222, 1994.

[18] O. J. De Boer, A. C. Van der Wal, M. A. Houtkamp, J. M. Ossewaarde, P. Teeling, and A. E. Becker, "Unstable

atherosclerotic plaques contain T-cells that respond to *Chlamydia pneumoniae*," *Cardiovascular Research*, vol. 48, no. 3, pp. 402–408, 2000.
[19] A. K. L. Robertson and G. K. Hansson, "T cells in atherogenesis: for better or for worse?" *Arteriosclerosis, Thrombosis, and Vascular Biology*, vol. 26, no. 11, pp. 2421–2432, 2006.
[20] J. Frostegård, A. K. Ulfgren, P. Nyberg et al., "Cytokine expression in advanced human atherosclerotic plaques: dominance of pro-inflammatory (Th1) and macrophage-stimulating cytokines," *Atherosclerosis*, vol. 145, no. 1, pp. 33–43, 1999.
[21] H. Methe, S. Brunner, D. Wiegand, M. Nabauer, J. Koglin, and E. R. Edelman, "Enhanced T-helper-1 lymphocyte activation patterns in acute coronary syndromes," *Journal of the American College of Cardiology*, vol. 45, no. 12, pp. 1939–1945, 2005.
[22] D. K. Agrawal and Z. Shao, "Pathogenesis of allergic airway inflammation," *Current Allergy and Asthma Reports*, vol. 10, no. 1, pp. 39–48, 2010.
[23] S. A. Huber, P. Sakkinen, C. David, M. K. Newell, and R. P. Tracy, "T helper-cell phenotype regulates atherosclerosis in mice under conditions of mild hypercholesterolemia," *Circulation*, vol. 103, no. 21, pp. 2610–2616, 2001.
[24] V. L. King, S. J. Szilvassy, and A. Daugherty, "Interleukin-4 deficiency decreases atherosclerotic lesion formation in a site-specific manner in female LDL receptor$^{-/-}$ mice," *Arteriosclerosis, Thrombosis, and Vascular Biology*, vol. 22, no. 3, pp. 456–461, 2002.
[25] L. E. Harrington, R. D. Hatton, P. R. Mangan et al., "Interleukin 17-producing CD4$^+$ effector T cells develop via a lineage distinct from the T helper type 1 and 2 lineages," *Nature Immunology*, vol. 6, no. 11, pp. 1123–1132, 2005.
[26] H. Park, Z. Li, X. O. Yang et al., "A distinct lineage of CD4 T cells regulates tissue inflammation by producing interleukin 17," *Nature Immunology*, vol. 6, no. 11, pp. 1133–1141, 2005.
[27] X. Cheng, X. Yu, Y.-j. Ding et al., "The Th17/Treg imbalance in patients with acute coronary syndrome," *Clinical Immunology*, vol. 127, no. 1, pp. 89–97, 2008.
[28] G. L. Stephens and E. M. Shevach, "Foxp3$^+$ regulatory T cells: selfishness under scrutiny," *Immunity*, vol. 27, no. 3, pp. 417–419, 2007.
[29] E. M. Shevach, "Mechanisms of Foxp3$^+$ T regulatory cell-mediated suppression," *Immunity*, vol. 30, no. 5, pp. 636–645, 2009.
[30] J. Andersson, P. Libby, and G. K. Hansson, "Adaptive immunity and atherosclerosis," *Clinical Immunology*, vol. 134, no. 1, pp. 33–46, 2010.
[31] C. J. Binder, M. K. Chang, P. X. Shaw et al., "Innate and acquired immunity in atherogenesis," *Nature Medicine*, vol. 8, no. 11, pp. 1218–1226, 2002.
[32] C. J. Binder, P. X. Shaw, M.-K. Chang et al., "The role of natural antibodies in atherogenesis," *Journal of Lipid Research*, vol. 46, no. 7, pp. 1353–1363, 2005.
[33] G. S. Getz, "Bridging the innate and adaptive immune systems," *Journal of Lipid Research*, vol. 46, no. 4, pp. 619–622, 2005.
[34] G. S. Getz, "Thematic review series: the immune system and atherogenesis. Immune function in atherogenesis," *Journal of Lipid Research*, vol. 46, no. 1, pp. 1–10, 2005.
[35] G. K. Hansson, "Immune and inflammatory mechanisms in the pathogenesis of atherosclerosis," *Journal of Atherosclerosis and Thrombosis*, vol. 1, supplement, pp. S6–S9, 1994.
[36] G. K. Hansson, "Immune mechanisms in atherosclerosis," *Arteriosclerosis, Thrombosis, and Vascular Biology*, vol. 21, no. 12, pp. 1876–1890, 2001.
[37] G. K. Hansson, "Regulation of immune mechanisms in atherosclerosis," *Annals of the New York Academy of Sciences*, vol. 947, pp. 157–166, 2001.
[38] G. K. Hansson, "Atherosclerosis-An immune disease. The Anitschkov Lecture 2007," *Atherosclerosis*, vol. 202, no. 1, pp. 2–10, 2009.
[39] G. K. Hansson, "Inflammatory mechanisms in atherosclerosis," *Journal of Thrombosis and Haemostasis*, vol. 7, supplement 1, pp. 328–331, 2009.
[40] P. Libby, "Inflammation in atherosclerosis," *Nature*, vol. 420, no. 6917, pp. 868–874, 2002.
[41] P. Libby, P. M. Ridker, and G. K. Hansson, "Inflammation in atherosclerosis. From pathophysiology to practice," *Journal of the American College of Cardiology*, vol. 54, no. 23, pp. 2129–2138, 2009.
[42] G. K. Hansson, A.-K. L. Robertson, and C. Söderberg-Nauclér, "Inflammation and atherosclerosis," *Annual Review of Pathology*, vol. 1, pp. 297–329, 2006.
[43] P. X. Shaw, S. Hörkkö, M. K. Chang et al., "Natural antibodies with the T15 idiotype may act in atherosclerosis, apoptotic clearance, and protective immunity," *Journal of Clinical Investigation*, vol. 105, no. 12, pp. 1731–1740, 2000.
[44] W. Palinski and J. L. Witztum, "Immune responses to oxidative neoepitopes on LDL and phospholipids modulate the development of atherosclerosis," *Journal of Internal Medicine*, vol. 247, no. 3, pp. 371–380, 2000.
[45] H. Esterbauer, M. Dieber-Rotheneder, G. Waeg, G. Striegl, and G. Jurgens, "Biochemical, structural, and functional properties of oxidized low-density lipoprotein," *Chemical Research in Toxicology*, vol. 3, no. 2, pp. 77–92, 1990.
[46] S. Yia-Herttuala, W. Palinski, M. E. Rosenfeld et al., "Evidence for the presence of oxidatively modified low density lipoprotein in atherosclerotic lesions of rabbit and man," *Journal of Clinical Investigation*, vol. 84, no. 4, pp. 1086–1095, 1989.
[47] N. M. Gharavi, J. A. Alva, K. P. Mouillesseaux et al., "Role of the JAK/STAT pathway in the regulation of interleukin-8 transcription by oxidized phospholipids in vitro and in atherosclerosis in vivo," *Journal of Biological Chemistry*, vol. 282, no. 43, pp. 31460–31468, 2007.
[48] E. Svensjö, P. Boschcov, D. F. J. Ketelhuth, S. Jancar, and M. Gidlund, "Increased microvascular permeability in the hamster cheek pouch induced by oxidized low density lipoprotein (oxLDL) and some fragmented apolipoprotein B proteins," *Inflammation Research*, vol. 52, no. 5, pp. 215–220, 2003.
[49] D. F. J. Ketelhuth and G. K. Hansson, "Cellular immunity, low-density lipoprotein and atherosclerosis: break of tolerance in the artery wall," *Thrombosis and Haemostasis*, vol. 106, no. 5, pp. 779–786, 2011.
[50] D. Steinberg, S. Parthasarathy, T. E. Carew, J. C. Khoo, and J. L. Witztum, "Beyond cholesterol: modifications of low-density lipoprotein that increase its atherogenicity," *New England Journal of Medicine*, vol. 320, no. 14, pp. 915–924, 1989.
[51] G. K. Hansson, "Vaccination against atherosclerosis: acience or fiction?" *Circulation*, vol. 106, no. 13, pp. 1599–1601, 2002.
[52] S. Stemme, B. Faber, J. Holm, O. Wiklund, J. L. Witztum, and G. K. Hansson, "T lymphocytes from human atherosclerotic

plaques recognize oxidized low density lipoprotein," *Proceedings of the National Academy of Sciences of the United States of America*, vol. 92, no. 9, pp. 3893–3897, 1995.

[53] S.-I. Toshima, A. Hasegawa, M. Kurabayashi et al., "Circulating oxidized low density lipoprotein levels: a biochemical risk marker for coronary heart disease," *Arteriosclerosis, Thrombosis, and Vascular Biology*, vol. 20, no. 10, pp. 2243–2247, 2000.

[54] P. Holvoet, J. Vanhaecke, S. Janssens, F. Van De Werf, and D. Collen, "Oxidized LDL and malondialdehyde-modified LDL in patients with acute coronary syndromes and stable coronary artery disease," *Circulation*, vol. 98, no. 15, pp. 1487–1494, 1998.

[55] H. C. Boyd, A. M. Gown, G. Wolfbauer, and A. Chait, "Direct evidence for a protein recognized by a monoclonal antibody against oxidatively modified LDL in atherosclerotic lesions from a Watanabe heritable hyperlipidemic rabbit," *American Journal of Pathology*, vol. 135, no. 5, pp. 815–825, 1989.

[56] S. D. Cushing, J. A. Berliner, A. J. Valente et al., "Minimally modified low density lipoprotein induces monocyte chemotactic protein 1 in human endothelial cells and smooth muscle cells," *Proceedings of the National Academy of Sciences of the United States of America*, vol. 87, no. 13, pp. 5134–5138, 1990.

[57] D. Steinberg, "The LDL modification hypothesis of atherogenesis: an update," *Journal of Lipid Research*, vol. 50, pp. S376–S381, 2009.

[58] E. A. Dennis and J. L. Witztum, "Fifty years of research on lipids," *Journal of Lipid Research*, vol. 50, supplement, p. S1, 2009.

[59] N. Baumgarth, J. W. Tung, and L. A. Herzenberg, "Inherent specificities in natural antibodies: a key to immune defense against pathogen invasion," *Springer Seminars in Immunopathology*, vol. 26, no. 4, pp. 347–362, 2005.

[60] H. Masmoudi, T. Mota-Santos, F. Huetz, A. Coutinho, and P. A. Cazenave, "All T15 Id-positive antibodies (but not the majority of V(H)T15+ antibodies) are produced by peritoneal CD5+ B lymphocytes," *International Immunology*, vol. 2, no. 6, pp. 515–520, 1990.

[61] P. Casali, S. E. Burastero, and M. Nakamura, "Human lymphocytes making rheumatoid factor and antibody to ssDNA belong to Leu-1+ B-cell subset," *Science*, vol. 236, no. 4797, pp. 77–81, 1987.

[62] K. Hayakawa, M. Asano, S. A. Shinton et al., "Positive selection of anti-thy-1 autoreactive B-1 cells and natural serum autoantibody production independent from bone marrow B cell development," *Journal of Experimental Medicine*, vol. 197, no. 1, pp. 87–99, 2003.

[63] R. Berland and H. H. Wortis, "Origins and functions of B-1 cells with notes on the role of CD5," *Annual Review of Immunology*, vol. 20, pp. 253–300, 2002.

[64] N. A. Bos, J. J. Cebra, and F. G. M. Kroese, "B-1 cells and the intestinal microflora," *Current Topics in Microbiology and Immunology*, vol. 252, pp. 211–220, 2000.

[65] P. A. Lalor and G. Morahan, "The peritoneal Ly-1 (CD5) B cell repertoire is unique among murine B cell repertoires," *European Journal of Immunology*, vol. 20, no. 3, pp. 485–492, 1990.

[66] L. A. Herzenberg and L. A. Herzenberg, "Toward a layered immune system," *Cell*, vol. 59, no. 6, pp. 953–954, 1989.

[67] W. Palinski, S. Hörkkö, E. Miller et al., "Cloning of monoclonal autoantibodies to epitopes of oxidized lipoproteins from apolipoprotein E-deficient mice: demonstration of epitopes of oxidized low density lipoprotein in human plasma," *Journal of Clinical Investigation*, vol. 98, no. 3, pp. 800–814, 1996.

[68] W. Palinski, R. K. Tangirala, E. Miller, S. G. Young, and J. L. Witztum, "Increased autoantibody titers against epitopes of oxidized LDL in LDL receptor-deficient mice with increased atherosclerosis," *Arteriosclerosis, Thrombosis, and Vascular Biology*, vol. 15, no. 10, pp. 1569–1576, 1995.

[69] J. T. Salonen, S. Ylä-Herttuala, R. Yamamoto et al., "Autoantibody against oxidised LDL and progression of carotid atherosclerosis," *The Lancet*, vol. 339, no. 8798, pp. 883–887, 1992.

[70] W. Palinski, V. A. Ord, A. S. Plump, J. L. Breslow, D. Steinberg, and J. L. Witztum, "ApoE-deficient mice are a model of lipoprotein oxidation in atherogenesis: demonstration of oxidation-specific epitopes in lesions and high titers of autoantibodies to malondialdehyde-lysine in serum," *Arteriosclerosis and Thrombosis*, vol. 14, no. 4, pp. 605–616, 1994.

[71] P. Friedman, S. Hörkkö, D. Steinberg, J. L. Witztum, and E. A. Dennis, "Correlation of antiphospholipid antibody recognition with the structure of synthetic oxidized phospholipids. Importance of Schiff base formation and aldol condensation," *Journal of Biological Chemistry*, vol. 277, no. 9, pp. 7010–7020, 2002.

[72] S. Hörkkö, D. A. Bird, E. Miller et al., "Monoclonal autoantibodies specific for oxidized phospholipids or oxidized phospholipid-protein adducts inhibit macrophage uptake of oxidized low-density lipoproteins," *Journal of Clinical Investigation*, vol. 103, no. 1, pp. 117–128, 1999.

[73] C. J. Binder, S. Hörkkö, A. Dewan et al., "Pneumococcal vaccination decreases atherosclerotic lesion formation: molecular mimicry between *Streptococcus pneumoniae* and oxidized LDL," *Nature Medicine*, vol. 9, no. 6, pp. 736–743, 2003.

[74] G. Caligiuri, J. Khallou-Laschet, M. Vandaele et al., "Phosphorylcholine-targeting immunization reduces atherosclerosis," *Journal of the American College of Cardiology*, vol. 50, no. 6, pp. 540–546, 2007.

[75] A. Schiopu, B. Frendéus, B. Jansson et al., "Recombinant antibodies to an oxidized low-density lipoprotein epitope induce rapid regression of atherosclerosis in *Apobec-1*$^{-/-}$/low-density lipoprotein receptor$^{-/-}$ mice," *Journal of the American College of Cardiology*, vol. 50, no. 24, pp. 2313–2318, 2007.

[76] J. Hulthe, L. Bokemark, and B. Fagerberg, "Antibodies to oxidized LDL in relation to intima-media thickness in carotid and femoral arteries in 58-year-old subjectively clinically healthy men," *Arteriosclerosis, Thrombosis, and Vascular Biology*, vol. 21, no. 1, pp. 101–107, 2001.

[77] J. Karvonen, M. Päivänsalo, Y. A. Kesäniemi, and S. Hörkkö, "Immunoglobulin M type of autoantibodies to oxidized low-density lipoprotein has an inverse relation to carotid artery atherosclerosis," *Circulation*, vol. 108, no. 17, pp. 2107–2112, 2003.

[78] J. R. Faria-Neto, K. Y. Chyu, X. Li et al., "Passive immunization with monoclonal IgM antibodies against phosphorylcholine reduces accelerated vein graft atherosclerosis in apolipoprotein E-null mice," *Atherosclerosis*, vol. 189, no. 1, pp. 83–90, 2006.

[79] M. Zhang, W. G. Austen, I. Chiu et al., "Identification of a specific self-reactive IgM antibody that initiates intestinal

ischemia/reperfusion injury," *Proceedings of the National Academy of Sciences of the United States of America*, vol. 101, no. 11, pp. 3886–3891, 2004.
[80] D. Zhao, H. Ogawa, X. Wang et al., "Oxidized low-density lipoprotein and autoimmune antibodies in patients with antiphospholipid syndrome with a history of thrombosis," *American Journal of Clinical Pathology*, vol. 116, no. 5, pp. 760–767, 2001.
[81] S. Ehara, M. Ueda, T. Naruko et al., "Elevated levels of oxidized low density lipoprotein show a positive relationship with the severity of acute coronary syndromes," *Circulation*, vol. 103, no. 15, pp. 1955–1960, 2001.
[82] J. George, Y. Shoenfeld, A. Afek et al., "Enhanced fatty streak formation in C57BL/6J mice by immunization with heat shock protein-65," *Arteriosclerosis, Thrombosis, and Vascular Biology*, vol. 19, no. 3, pp. 505–510, 1999.
[83] J. George, D. Harats, B. Gilburd et al., "Immunolocalization of β2-glycoprotein I (apolipoprotein H) to human atherosclerotic plaques: potential implications for lesion progression," *Circulation*, vol. 99, no. 17, pp. 2227–2230, 1999.
[84] C. Bergmark, R. Wu, U. De Faire, A. K. Lefvert, and J. Swedenborg, "Patients with early-onset peripheral vascular disease have increased levels of autoantibodies against oxidized LDL," *Arteriosclerosis, Thrombosis, and Vascular Biology*, vol. 15, no. 4, pp. 441–445, 1995.
[85] C. Monaco, F. Crea, G. Niccoli et al., "Autoantibodies against oxidized low density lipoproteins in patients with stable angina, unstable angina or peripheral vascular disease: pathophysiological implications," *European Heart Journal*, vol. 22, no. 17, pp. 1572–1577, 2001.
[86] S. Yla-Herttuala, W. Palinski, S. W. Butler, S. Picard, D. Steinberg, and J. L. Witztum, "Rabbit and human atherosclerotic lesions contain IgG that recognizes epitopes of oxidized LDL," *Arteriosclerosis and Thrombosis*, vol. 14, no. 1, pp. 32–40, 1994.
[87] R. Wu, S. Nityanand, L. Berglund, H. Lithell, G. Holm, and A. K. Lefvert, "Antibodies against cardiolipin and oxidatively modified LDL in 50-year- old men predict myocardial infarction," *Arteriosclerosis, Thrombosis, and Vascular Biology*, vol. 17, no. 11, pp. 3159–3163, 1997.
[88] M. Puurunen, M. Mänttäri, V. Manninen et al., "Antibody against oxidized low-density lipoprotein predicting myocardial infarction," *Archives of Internal Medicine*, vol. 154, no. 22, pp. 2605–2609, 1994.
[89] J. C. Fang, S. Kinlay, D. Behrendt et al., "Circulating autoantibodies to oxidized LDL correlate with impaired coronary endothelial function after cardiac transplantation," *Arteriosclerosis, Thrombosis, and Vascular Biology*, vol. 22, no. 12, pp. 2044–2048, 2002.
[90] B. P. Swets, D. A. J. Brouwer, and J. W. Cohen Tervaert, "Patients with systemic vasculitis have increased levels of autoantibodies against oxidized LDL," *Clinical and Experimental Immunology*, vol. 124, no. 1, pp. 163–167, 2001.
[91] R. Wu, Y. Shoenfeld, Y. Sherer et al., "Anti-idiotypes to oxidized LDL antibodies in intravenous immunoglobulin preparations—possible immunomodulation of atherosclerosis," *Autoimmunity*, vol. 36, no. 2, pp. 91–97, 2003.
[92] R. Wu, E. Svenungsson, I. Gunnarsson et al., "Antibodies to adult human endothelial cells cross-react with oxidized low-density lipoprotein and β2-glycoprotein I (β2-GPI) in systemic lupus erythematosus," *Clinical and Experimental Immunology*, vol. 115, no. 3, pp. 561–566, 1999.
[93] G. N. Fredrikson, B. Hedblad, G. Berglund et al., "Association between IgM against an aldehyde-modified peptide in apolipoprotein B-100 and progression of carotid disease," *Stroke*, vol. 38, no. 5, pp. 1495–1500, 2007.
[94] J. Hulthe, J. Wikstrand, A. Lidell, I. Wendelhag, G. K. Hansson, and O. Wiklund, "Antibody titers against oxidized LDL are not elevated in patients with familial hypercholesterolemia," *Arteriosclerosis, Thrombosis, and Vascular Biology*, vol. 18, no. 8, pp. 1203–1211, 1998.
[95] U. P. Steinbrecher, S. Parthasarathy, and D. S. Leake, "Modification of low density lipoprotein by endothelial cells involves lipid peroxidation and degradation of low density lipoprotein phospholipids," *Proceedings of the National Academy of Sciences of the United States of America*, vol. 81, no. 12 I, pp. 3883–3887, 1984.
[96] G. Virella, I. Virella, R. B. Leman, M. B. Pryor, and M. F. Lopes-Virella, "Anti-oxidized low-density lipoprotein antibodies in patients with coronary heart disease and normal healthy volunteers," *International Journal of Clinical & Laboratory Research*, vol. 23, no. 1-4, pp. 95–101, 1993.
[97] S. Ameli, A. Hultgårdh-Nilsson, J. Regnström et al., "Effect of immunization with homologous LDL and oxidized LDL on early atherosclerosis in hypercholesterolemic rabbits," *Arteriosclerosis, Thrombosis, and Vascular Biology*, vol. 16, no. 8, pp. 1074–1079, 1996.
[98] W. Palinski, E. Miller, and J. L. Witztum, "Immunization of low density lipoprotein (LDL) receptor-deficient rabbits with homologous malondialdehyde-modified LDL reduces atherogenesis," *Proceedings of the National Academy of Sciences of the United States of America*, vol. 92, no. 3, pp. 821–825, 1995.
[99] G. Caligiuri, A. Nicoletti, B. Poirierand, and G. K. Hansson, "Protective immunity against atherosclerosis carried by B cells of hypercholesterolemic mice," *Journal of Clinical Investigation*, vol. 109, no. 6, pp. 745–753, 2002.
[100] X. Zhou, G. Caligiuri, A. Hamsten, A. K. Lefvert, and G. K. Hansson, "LDL immunization induces T-cell-dependent antibody formation and protection against atherosclerosis," *Arteriosclerosis, Thrombosis, and Vascular Biology*, vol. 21, no. 1, pp. 108–114, 2001.
[101] A. Schiopu, J. Bengtsson, I. Söderberg et al., "Recombinant human antibodies against aldehyde-modified apolipoprotein B-100 peptide sequences inhibit atherosclerosis," *Circulation*, vol. 110, no. 14, pp. 2047–2052, 2004.
[102] D. Nicolo, B. I. Goldman, and M. Monestier, "Reduction of atherosclerosis in low-density lipoprotein receptor-deficient mice by passive administration of antiphospholipid antibody," *Arthritis and Rheumatism*, vol. 48, no. 10, pp. 2974–2978, 2003.
[103] Y. Shoenfeld, R. Wu, L. D. Dearing, and E. Matsuura, "Are anti-oxidized low-density lipoprotein antibodies pathogenic or protective?" *Circulation*, vol. 110, no. 17, pp. 2552–2558, 2004.
[104] T. Shoji, Y. Nishizawa, M. Fukumoto et al., "Inverse relationship between circulating oxidized low density lipoprotein (oxLDL) and anti-oxLDL antibody levels in healthy subjects," *Atherosclerosis*, vol. 148, no. 1, pp. 171–177, 2000.
[105] M. Fukumoto, T. Shoji, M. Emoto, T. Kawagishi, Y. Okuno, and Y. Nishizawa, "Antibodies against oxidized LDL and carotid artery intima-media thickness in a healthy population," *Arteriosclerosis, Thrombosis, and Vascular Biology*, vol. 20, no. 3, pp. 703–707, 2000.
[106] R. Klingenberg, M. Lebens, A. Hermansson et al., "Intranasal immunization with an apolipoprotein B-100 fusion protein

induces antigen-specific regulatory T cells and reduces atherosclerosis," *Arteriosclerosis, Thrombosis, and Vascular Biology*, vol. 30, no. 5, pp. 946–952, 2010.

[107] R. Maron, G. Sukhova, A. M. Faria et al., "Mucosal administration of heat shock protein-65 decreases atherosclerosis and inflammation in aortic arch of low-density lipoprotein receptor-deficient mice," *Circulation*, vol. 106, no. 13, pp. 1708–1715, 2002.

[108] J. Nilsson, G. N. Fredrikson, H. Björkbacka, K. Y. Chyu, and P. K. Shah, "Vaccines modulating lipoprotein autoimmunity as a possible future therapy for cardiovascular disease," *Journal of Internal Medicine*, vol. 266, no. 3, pp. 221–231, 2009.

[109] G. H. M. Van Puijvelde, A. D. Hauer, P. De Vos et al., "Induction of oral tolerance to oxidized low-density lipoprotein ameliorates atherosclerosis," *Circulation*, vol. 114, no. 18, pp. 1968–1976, 2006.

[110] G. H. M. Van Puijvelde, T. Van Es, E. J. A. Van Wanrooij et al., "Induction of oral tolerance to HSP60 or an HSP60-peptide activates t cell regulation and reduces atherosclerosis," *Arteriosclerosis, Thrombosis, and Vascular Biology*, vol. 27, no. 12, pp. 2677–2683, 2007.

[111] Z. Mallat and A. Tedgui, "Immunomodulation to combat atherosclerosis: the potential role of immune regulatory cells," *Expert Opinion on Biological Therapy*, vol. 4, no. 9, pp. 1387–1393, 2004.

[112] G. N. Fredrikson, B. Hedblad, G. Berglund et al., "Identification of immune responses against aldehyde-modified peptide sequences in apoB associated with cardiovascular disease," *Arteriosclerosis, Thrombosis, and Vascular Biology*, vol. 23, no. 5, pp. 872–878, 2003.

[113] G. N. Fredrikson, M. W. Lindholm, I. Ljungcrantz, I. Söderberg, P. K. Shah, and J. Nilsson, "Autoimmune responses against the apo B-100 LDL receptor-binding site protect against arterial accumulation of lipids in LDL receptor deficient mice," *Autoimmunity*, vol. 40, no. 2, pp. 122–130, 2007.

[114] S. Hörkkö, C. J. Binder, P. X. Shaw et al., "Immunological responses to oxidized LDL," *Free Radical Biology and Medicine*, vol. 28, no. 12, pp. 1771–1779, 2000.

[115] P. X. Shaw, S. Hörkkö, S. Tsimikas et al., "Human-derived anti-oxidized LDL autoantibody blocks uptake of oxidized LDL by macrophages and localizes to atherosclerotic lesions in vivo," *Arteriosclerosis, Thrombosis, and Vascular Biology*, vol. 21, no. 8, pp. 1333–1339, 2001.

[116] G. Virella, M. F. Lopes-Virella, C. J. Binder, and J. L. Witztum, "Humoral immunity and atherosclerosis," *Nature Medicine*, vol. 9, no. 3, pp. 243–245, 2003.

[117] G. N. Fredrikson, I. Söderberg, M. Lindholm et al., "Inhibition of atherosclerosis in apoE-null mice by immunization with apoB-100 peptide sequences," *Arteriosclerosis, Thrombosis, and Vascular Biology*, vol. 23, no. 5, pp. 879–884, 2003.

[118] G. N. Fredrikson, A. Schiopu, G. Berglund, R. Alm, P. K. Shah, and J. Nilsson, "Autoantibody against the amino acid sequence 661-680 in apo B-100 is associated with decreased carotid stenosis and cardiovascular events," *Atherosclerosis*, vol. 194, no. 2, pp. e188–e192, 2007.

11

Are Dietary Cholesterol Intake and Serum Cholesterol Levels Related to Nonalcoholic Fatty Liver Disease in Obese Children?

Dimitrios Papandreou,[1,2] Zaharoula Karabouta,[1] and Israel Rousso[1]

[1] *2nd Department of Pediatrics, School of Medicine and Ahepa General Hospital, Aristotle University of Thessaloniki, Street Kiriakidi 1, 54636 Thessaloniki, Greece*
[2] *Department of Life and Health Sciences, University of Nicosia, Makedonitissas Avenue, 1700 Nicosia, Cyprus*

Correspondence should be addressed to Dimitrios Papandreou, papandreoudimitrios@yahoo.gr

Academic Editor: Roya Kelishadi

Background. Nonalcoholic fatty liver disease (NAFLD) in children has been recognized as a major health burden. Serum lipids as well as dietary cholesterol (DC) intake may positively relate to development of NAFLD. The purpose of this study was to investigate anthropometric, biochemical, and dietary intake parameters of obese Greek children with and without NAFLD. *Materials and Methods.* Eighty-five obese children aged 8–15 (45 boys/40 girls) participated in the study. NAFLD was diagnosed by ultrasonography (US) in all subjects. Liver indexes were measured in all children. A 3-day dietary was recorded for all subjects. *Results.* 38 out of 85 children (44.7%) were found to have fatty liver. Obese children with increased levels of TC (95% CI: 1.721–3.191), low density lipoprotein (LDL) (95% CI: 1.829–3.058), and increased dietary cholesterol intakes (95% CI: 1.511–2.719) were 2.541, 2.612, and 2.041 times more likely to develop NAFLD compared with the children without NAFLD. *Conclusion.* The present study showed that TC, LDL, and DC were the strongest risk factors of development of NAFLD. Reducing body weight and dietary cholesterol intakes as well as decreasing serum TC and LDL levels are urgently necessary in order to prevent NAFLD and possible other health implications later in life.

1. Introduction

Nonalcoholic fatty liver disease (NAFLD), which encompasses a broad spectrum of liver disorders ranging from simple hepatic steatosis to steatohepatitis (NASH) and cirrhosis, is currently the most common cause of chronic liver disease and abnormal liver function tests in Western countries [1]. The development of hepatic steatosis is considered to be associated with an excess intake of calories, visceral obesity, and insulin resistance, which result in an increased release of free fatty acids from adipocytes and increased rates of fatty acid synthesis in the liver [1]. Therefore, nutritional management and therapeutic exercise are fundamental steps to treat NAFLD.

The "two-hit theory" is increasingly being adopted to explain the pathogenesis of NAFLD and NASH [2]. In this theory, the first hit consists of the accumulation of fatty acids/triglycerides in the liver, while the second hit involves oxidative stress, mitochondrial dysfunction, and inflammation, which ultimately cause liver damage.

Hepatic lipid homeostasis represents a balance between lipid uptake, synthesis, catabolism, and secretion. Therefore, steatosis, a typical characteristic of NAFLD, is expected to be caused by disordered lipid metabolism, particularly inhibition of fatty acid oxidation and enhanced lipogenesis. Many factors involved in hepatic lipid metabolism pathways have been identified, even though the precise cellular networks are not fully elucidated. In humans with NAFLD, cholesterol uptake in the form of LDL is limited by the intracellular accumulation of fatty acid and cholesterol, while fatty acid and cholesterol synthesis are upregulated in the NAFLD liver suggesting that the feedback system regulating and clearing up intracellular lipids levels is disrupted in NAFLD [3].

The prevalence of NAFLD in children remains unknown because of the lack of population-based studies and reliable screening tools. The available data suggests a prevalence range from 2.6% to 9.6% among children and adolescents in the United States and Asia which may reach to 12–80% in overweight and obese children [4]. Even though there is no consensus for the treatment for NAFLD in children, a recent review shoed that many studies have been attempted to treat NAFLD using weight loss and exercise, antioxidants, and pharmacological agents [5].

Some studies have been suggesting that high-fat, high-fat plus low-protein, high-carbohydrate, and/or high-cholesterol diets are the main causes of NAFLD [6–8]. The reason for this is that cholesterol overload can upregulate gene expression and activate fatty acid synthesis by increasing oxysterol levels, metabolites of cholesterol that act as agonists for these genes indicating that excess cholesterol intake (i.e., cholesterol supply) itself can be a strong stimulant for the development of steatosis [9].

The purpose of this study was to investigate possible differences of certain parameters such as anthropometric, biochemical, and dietary of obese Greek children with and without NAFLD.

2. Materials and Methods

Eighty-five (85) obese children aged 8–15 y (45 boys/40 girls) were initially referred for obesity assessment to the outpatient 2nd Pediatric Department of Aristotle University of Thessaloniki, between January 2007 and January 2011. All children were screened for parameters of NAFLD. Written, informed consent was also obtained from each child's parents who participated in the study.

2.1. Anthropometrics and Biochemical Indexes. Anthropometrical indices such as height, weight, Tanner stage, and waist circumference were assessed in all children. Obesity was defined by International Obesity Task Force criteria for age and sex [10]. BMI was calculated by dividing weight (kg) by height squared (m^2). Biochemical indices such as liver transaminases (ALT, AST), lipid profile, total cholesterol (TC), low density lipoprotein (LDL), high density lipoprotein (HDL), and triglycerides (TG) were measured in all children. All children had normal serum levels of alanine aminotransferase (ALT) <40 U/L and aspartate aminotransferase (AST) <37 U/L. Participants were free of a history of clinical evidence of diabetes, cardiovascular, liver disease, hepatits B or C, use of alcohol, drugs, or other disease (e.g., Wilson's disease, autoimmune hepatitis). NAFLD was diagnosed by ultrasonography (US) and was classified as having no or moderate hepatic steatosis (Grade II). The examination was performed by a radiologist with a convex probe (3.5–5 MHZ) with Elegra-Siemens equipment. The echogenicity of the liver was estimated in a longitudinal US slice, showing the liver parenchyma and the neighboring right kidney [11].

Insulin resistance (IR) was calculated by means of the homeostasis model assessment (HOMA). IR was defined by HOMA >3.2 μU/mL [12].

2.2. Dietary Intake. A validated dietary intake [13] was used to collect information for a total of 3 days (2 weekdays and 1 weekend day). Study participants together with their parents were asked to describe the type and amount of food consumed after a detailed explanation and guidance provided by a registered dietician of our clinic. To improve the accuracy of food description, food models were used to describe the portion sizes. The dietary record was then analyzed using a software program (Sciencetech Diet 200A, Science Technologies, Athens, Greece, 2001) which consisted of more than 2500 Greek food items and recipes.

2.3. Statistical Analysis. Standard descriptive statistics were used for all patient characteristics. Data for continuous variables is expressed as mean values ± standard deviation. *t*-test was used to compare characteristics of obese children with and without NAFLD. Partial correlation was estimated by using Spearman's correlation coefficient. Logistic regression analysis was used to estimate the relationship between ultrasound findings (normal or pathological) with HOMA, BMI, WC, HDL, LDL, dietary cholesterol, saturated fatty acid, sugar, and fiber consumed daily. P values < 0.05 were considered statistically significant, while all confidence intervals (C.I.) represent 95% intervals.

3. Results

Based on ultrasonography, 38 out of 85 children (44.7%) were found to have fatty liver.

Anthropometric and biochemical characteristics of all subjects were presented in Table 1. Children with NAFLD were having higher BMI, WC TC, and LDL and lower HDL levels compared to children without NAFLD. In addition IR was significantly higher in obese children with NAFLD.

The dietary intakes of energy and major nutrients in the three categories are reported in Table 2. SFA, cholesterol, and sugar intakes were significantly higher in group with NAFLD compared with the group without NAFLD.

In Spearman's correlation model, BMI, WC, TC, LDL, and dietary cholesterol were found to be positively correlated with NAFLD, while HDL levels were negatively associated with NAFLD (Table 3).

In logistic regression analysis, obese children with increased levels of TC (95% CI: 1.721–3.191), low density lipoprotein (LDL) (95% CI: 1.829–3.058), and increased dietary cholesterol intakes (95% CI: 1.511–2.719) were 2.541, 2.612, and 2.041 times more likely to develop NAFLD compared with the obese children without NAFLD (Table 4).

4. Discussion

In the current study, we presented clinical data of 85 obese children with and without NAFLD proven by ultrasonography and its association with anthropometric and clinical

Table 1: Clinical characteristics of subjects based on fatty liver.

	Absent ($n = 47$)	Moderate (Grade II) ($n = 38$)	P value
Sex (M/F)	25/22	20/18	0.451
Age (y)	11 ± 2.1	11.5 ± 1.1	0.369
BMI (kg/m^2)	25 ± 3.6	31 ± 2.9	**0.001**
WC (cm)	85.2 ± 11.2	97 ± 10.9	**0.001**
ALT (U/L)	22.7 ± 6.2	26 ± 4.1	0.942
AST (U/L)	21.1 ± 7.4	25.1 ± 3.2	0.212
TC (mg/dL)	168.7 ± 27.4	179 ± 19.8	**0.006**
HDL (mg/dL)	50.3 ± 13.1	40 ± 12.1	**0.002**
LDL (mg/dL)	103.7 ± 22.1	94 ± 9.6	**0.043**
TG (mg/dL)	110.2 ± 54.3	109.1 ± 60	0.294
CRP	2.2 ± 2.8	2.4 ± 2.6	0.591
HOMA-IR	4.3 ± 1.9	6.2 ± 2.1	**0.001**

Values are presented as means ± SD. Statistical significant difference ($P < 0.05$). Abbreviations: BMI: body mass index, WC: waist circumference, ALT: alanine aminotransferase, AST: aspartate aminotransferase, TC: total cholesterol, LDL: low density lipoprotein, HDL: high density lipoprotein, TG: triglycerides, CRP: C-reactive protein, HOMA-IR: homeostasis model assessment of insulin resistance.

Table 2: Dietary intake of subjects based on fatty liver.

	Absent ($n = 47$)	Moderate (Grade II) ($n = 38$)	P value
Energy (kcal)	2444 ± 539	2605 ± 489	0.641
PRO (g)	103.1 ± 27.7	97 ± 23.3	0.323
CHO (g)	244.5 ± 67.5	276.1 ± 51.9	0.051
FAT (g)	139.7 ± 45.1	138 ± 41.9	0.079
SFA (g)	45.1 ± 12.6	61.9 ± 11.8	**0.032**
CHOL (mg)	321 ± 29.7	378 ± 28.7	**0.001**
Sugar (g)	10.8 ± 15.3	21 ± 12.9	**0.002**
Fiber (g)	20.0 ± 8.0	15 ± 9.1	0.081

Values are presented as means ± SD. Statistical significant difference ($P < 0.05$). Abbreviations: PRO: protein, CHO: carbohydrates, SFA: saturated fatty acid, CHOL: dietary cholesterol.

parameters as well as with dietary intakes. The prevalence of our sample data was 38/85 (44.7%) which is between the prevalence (12–80%) found by other authors in a review study of different regions of the world such as Europe, America, and Asia [4].

It has been reported that the degree of steatosis in NAFLD is proportional to the degree of obesity [14]. BMI and WC were found in our study positively correlated with hepatic fat content. However, none of them were of the strongest risk factors of developing NAFLD in the logistic regression model analysis, suggesting that obesity and splanchnic fat distribution might also be effects of insulin resistance, rather than being directly involved in the etiology of fatty liver.

In our study the obese children with NAFLD were presented to have increased levels of insulin resistance, dyslipidemia, and WC. NAFLD is strongly associated with obesity, insulin resistance, hypertension, and dyslipidemia and is now regarded as the liver manifestation of the metabolic syndrome (MetS) [15], a highly atherogenic condition.

Diets rich in fatty acids mainly saturated and trans-fatty acids, as well as carbohydrate-rich diets, favor an acute increase in IR independent of adiposity [16]. High SFA intake may also promote steatohepatitis directly by modulating hepatic triglyceride accumulation and oxidative activity as well as indirectly by affecting insulin sensitivity and postprandial triglyceride metabolism [17]. SFA consumption where found to be significantly higher in children with NAFLD compared with the children without NAFLD.

The consumption of sugar has been linked to risks for obesity, diabetes, metabolic syndrome, fatty liver, and heart disease, possibly by providing excess calories and large amounts of rapidly absorbable sugars [18, 19]. Our results showed that obese children with NAFLD had significantly higher intakes compared to children without NAFLD.

The most important finding of our study was that the children with NAFLD consumed significantly higher levels of dietary cholesterol compared to children without NAFLD. In addition, the total serum cholesterol levels of the same group were also found to significantly higher, compared with the group without NAFLD.

Observational studies have been conflicting with regard to our findings. Some studies did not demonstrate different dietary intakes of cholesterol between NAFLD patients and controls [20, 21]. However, Musso et al. [17] did demonstrate a higher cholesterol consumption among normal weight NASH patients versus BMI matched controls. A recent study supported the role of dietary cholesterol in NAFLD. In this study, 12 normal weight NAFLD patients were compared to 44 obese NAFLD patients. A characteristic feature was that dietary cholesterol intake was significantly higher, while the intake of polyunsaturated fatty acids (PUFAs) was significantly lower, in the nonobese group. Similar differences were noted in comparison to 15 healthy nonobese controls. Therefore, this altered cholesterol and PUFA intake may be associated with the development of NAFLD in nonobese patients [9]. In addition, studies using nonobese animal models have confirmed that a diet high in cholesterol can induce NASH [22].

Obese children with NAFLD should be informed that a healthy diet has benefits beyond weight reduction. They should be advised to reduce saturated/trans-fat and increase polyunsaturated fat with special emphasize on omega-3 fatty acids. They should reduce added sugar to its minimum, and increase fiber intake. Physical activity should be integrated into behavioral therapy in NAFLD, as even small gains in PA and fitness may have significant health benefits. A combination of educational, behavioral, and motivational strategies is required to help patients achieve lifestyle change.

5. Conclusion

The present study showed that TC, LDL, and DC were the strongest risk factors of development of NAFLD. Reducing body weight and dietary cholesterol intakes as well as

Table 3: Parameters associating with NAFLD by Spearman's correlation coefficient.

Parameters	r	P value
BMI (kg/m^2)	0.521	**0.001**
WC (cm)	0.296	**0.001**
HOMA-IR	0.175	0.501
TC (mg/dL)	0.533	**0.001**
HDL (mg/dL)	−0.281	**0.031**
LDL (mg/dL)	0.419	**0.021**
SFA (g)	0.081	0.092
CHOL (mg)	0.312	**0.009**
Sugar (g)	0.109	0.290

Statistical significant difference ($P < 0.05$). Abbreviations: BMI: body mass index, WC: waist circumference, HDL: high density lipoprotein, HOMA-IR, homeostasis model assessment of insulin resistance, TC: total cholesterol, SFA: saturated fatty acids, CHOL: dietary cholesterol.

Table 4: Parameters associating with NAFLD by logistic regression analysis*.

Parameters	Odds Ratio	95% CI	P value
BMI (kg/m^2)	1.141	(0.871–1.645)	0.349
WC (cm)	1.192	(0.941–1.779)	0.452
HOMA-IR	1.488	(1.108–1.877)	0.229
TC (mg/dL)	**2.541**	(1.721–3.191)	**0.001**
HDL (mg/dL)	1.228	(0.877–1.524)	0.612
LDL (mg/dL)	**2.612**	(1.829–3.058)	**0.001**
SFA (g)	1.211	(0.544–1.612)	0.053
CHOL (mg)	**2.041**	(1.511–2.719)	**0.009**
Sugar (g)	0.448	(0.156–0.997)	0.319

Statistical significant difference ($P < 0.05$). *Adjusted for age, gender, and energy intake. Abbreviations: BMI: body mass index, WC: waist circumference, HDL: high density lipoprotein, HOMA-IR: homeostasis model assessment of insulin resistance, CHOL: dietary cholesterol, SFA: saturated fatty acids.

decreasing serum TC and LDL levels is urgently necessary in order to prevent NAFLD and possible other health implications later in life.

6. Limitations

Limitations of our study include the small size of the participants and the lack of liver biopsy. We also did not present activity level of patients as well as socioeconomic data.

References

[1] O. Cheung and A. J. Sanyal, "Recent advances in nonalcoholic fatty liver disease," *Current Opinion in Gastroenterology*, vol. 25, no. 3, pp. 230–237, 2009.

[2] O. F. W. James and C. P. Day, "Non-alcoholic steatohepatitis (NASH): a disease of emerging identity and importance," *Journal of Hepatology*, vol. 29, no. 3, pp. 495–501, 1998.

[3] M. Nakamuta, T. Fujino, R. Yada et al., "Impact of cholesterol metabolism and the LXRα-SREBP-1c pathway on nonalcoholic fatty liver disease," *International Journal of Molecular Medicine*, vol. 23, no. 5, pp. 603–608, 2009.

[4] D. Papandreou, I. Rousso, and I. Mavromichalis, "Update on non-alcoholic fatty liver disease in children," *Clinical Nutrition*, vol. 26, no. 4, pp. 409–415, 2007.

[5] L. Peng, J. Wang, and F. Li, "Weight reduction for non-alcoholic fatty liver disease," *Cochrane Database of Systematic Reviews*, no. 6, Article ID CD003619, 2011.

[6] G. Musso, R. Gambino, F. De Michieli et al., "Dietary habits and their relations to insulin resistance and postprandial lipemia in nonalcoholic steatohepatitis," *Hepatology*, vol. 37, no. 4, pp. 909–916, 2003.

[7] S. Solga, A. R. Alkhuraishe, J. M. Clark et al., "Dietary composition and nonalcoholic fatty liver disease," *Digestive Diseases and Sciences*, vol. 49, no. 10, pp. 1578–1583, 2004.

[8] K. Toshimitsu, B. Matsuura, I. Ohkubo et al., "Dietary habits and nutrient intake in non-alcoholic steatohepatitis," *Nutrition*, vol. 23, no. 1, pp. 46–52, 2007.

[9] K. Yasutake, M. Nakamuta, Y. Shima et al., "Nutritional investigation of non-obese patients with non-alcoholic fatty liver disease: the significance of dietary cholesterol," *Scandinavian Journal of Gastroenterology*, vol. 44, no. 4, pp. 471–477, 2009.

[10] T. J. Cole, C. M. Bellizzi, M. K. Flegal, and W. H. Dietz, "Establishing a standarddefinition for child overweight and obesity worldwide: international survey," *British Medical Journal*, vol. 320, no. 7244, pp. 1240–1243, 2000.

[11] J. A. Zagzebski, in *Essentials of Ultrasound Physics*, Mosby, 1996.

[12] D. R. Matthews, J. P. Hosker, A. S. Rudenski, B. A. Naylor, D. F. Treacher, and R. C. Turner, "Homeostasis model assessment: insulinresistance and β-cell function from fasting plasma glucose and insulin concentrations in man," *Diabetologia*, vol. 28, no. 7, pp. 412–419, 1985.

[13] H. R. H. Rockett, M. Breitenbach, A. L. Frazier et al., "Validation of a youth/adolescent food frequency questionnaire," *Preventive Medicine*, vol. 26, no. 6, pp. 808–816, 1997.

[14] I. R. Wanless and J. S. Lentz, "Fatty liver hepatitis (steatohepatitis) and obesity: an autopsy study with analysis of risk factors," *Hepatology*, vol. 12, no. 5, pp. 1106–1110, 1990.

[15] A. Kotronen and H. Yki-Järvinen, "Fatty liver: a novel component of the metabolic syndrome," *Arteriosclerosis, Thrombosis, and Vascular Biology*, vol. 28, no. 1, pp. 27–38, 2008.

[16] K. McAuley and J. Mann, "Nutritional determinants of insulin resistance," *Journal of Lipid Research*, vol. 47, no. 8, pp. 1668–1676, 2006.

[17] C. M. Reynolds, F. C. McGillicuddy, K. A. Harford, O. M. Finucane, K. H. Mills, and H. M. Roche, "Dietary saturated fatty acids prime the NLRP3 inflammasome via TLR4 in dendritic cells-implications for diet-induced insulin resistance," *Molecular Nutrition & Food Research*. Epub ahead of print.

[18] A. R. Gaby, "Adverse effects of dietary fructose," *Alternative Medicine Review*, vol. 10, no. 4, pp. 294–306, 2005.

[19] L. R. Vartanian, M. B. Schwartz, and K. D. Brownell, "Effects of soft drink consumption on nutrition and health: a systematic review and meta-analysis," *American Journal of Public Health*, vol. 97, no. 4, pp. 667–675, 2007.

[20] S. Zelber-Sagi, D. Nitzan-Kaluski, R. Goldsmith et al., "Long term nutritional intake and the risk for non-alcoholic fatty

liver disease (NAFLD): a population based study," *Journal of Hepatology*, vol. 47, no. 5, pp. 711–717, 2007.

[21] H. Cortez-Pinto, L. Jesus, H. Barros, C. Lopes, M. C. Moura, and M. E. Camilo, "How different is the dietary pattern in non-alcoholic steatohepatitis patients?" *Clinical Nutrition*, vol. 25, no. 5, pp. 816–823, 2006.

[22] M. Kainuma, M. Fujimoto, N. Sekiya et al., "Cholesterol-fed rabbit as a unique model of nonalcoholic, nonobese, non-insulin-resistant fatty liver disease with characteristic fibrosis," *Journal of Gastroenterology*, vol. 41, no. 10, pp. 971–980, 2006.

12

Macronutrient Intake Influences the Effect of 25-Hydroxy-Vitamin D Status on Metabolic Syndrome Outcomes in African American Girls

Anna L. Newton,[1] Lynae J. Hanks,[1] Ambika P. Ashraf,[2] Elizabeth Williams,[1] Michelle Davis,[1] and Krista Casazza[1]

[1] *Department of Nutrition Sciences, University of Alabama at Birmingham, 1675 University Boulevard, WEBB 439 Birmingham, AL 35294-3360, USA*
[2] *Division of Pediatric Endocrinology, Department of Medicine, University of Alabama at Birmingham, Birmingham, AL 35294-3360, USA*

Correspondence should be addressed to Krista Casazza, kristac@uab.edu

Academic Editor: Roya Kelishadi

The objectives were to determine the effect of macronutrient modification on vitamin D status and if change in 25-hydroxy-vitamin D concentration influences components of metabolic syndrome in obese African American girls. *Methods.* Five-week intervention using reduced CHO (43% carbohydrate; 27% fat: SPEC) versus standard CHO (55% carbohydrate; 40% fat: STAN) eucaloric diet. Subjects were 28 obese African American females, aged 9–14 years. Dual energy X-ray absorptiometry and meal test were performed at baseline and five weeks. *Results.* Approximately 30% of girls had metabolic syndrome. Serum 25OHD increased in both groups at five weeks [STAN: 20.3 ± 1.1 to 22.4 ± 1.1 ($P < 0.05$) versus SPEC: 16.1 ± 1.0 to 16.8 ± 1.0 ($P = 0.05$)]. The STAN group, increased 25OHD concentration over five weeks ($P < 0.05$), which was positively related to triglycerides ($P < 0.001$) and inversely associated with total cholesterol ($P < 0.001$) and LDL ($P < 0.001$). The SPEC group, had increase in 25OHD ($P = 0.05$), which was positively related to fasting insulin ($P < 0.001$) and insulin sensitivity while inversely associated with fasting glucose ($P < 0.05$). The contribution of vitamin D status to metabolic syndrome parameters differs according to macronutrient intake. Improvement in 25OHD may improve fasting glucose, insulin sensitivity, and LDL; however, macronutrient intake warrants consideration.

1. Introduction

The steady rise in prevalence of pediatric obesity over the past three decades has been accompanied by accumulation of risk factors for metabolic syndrome (MetSyn) in childhood and adolescence. The occurrence of hypovitaminosis D (expressed as levels <20 ng/mL of circulating 25-hydroxy vitamin D (25OHD)) has been increasingly documented in the same population [1, 2]. Moreover, children/adolescents with hypovitaminosis D have been reported to experience greater instances of hypertension, hypertriglyceridemia, hyperglycemia, and low high-density lipoprotein cholesterol (HDL) [1, 3, 4]. Further, it has been proposed that elevated parathyroid hormone (PTH), consequential to chronic low vitamin D level, is mechanistically involved in the adverse perturbations of risk factors underlying MetSyn [5]. Given the emerging identification of vitamin D as an integral player in numerous metabolic pathways, it stands to reason that vitamin D status in the pediatric populace may play a role in the prevalence of metabolic disease risk factors [6, 7].

The relationship between 25OHD status and metabolic health is not equally distributed across groups. In particular, the relationship is more apparent among African American (AA) females, particularly those who are overweight/obese [8–11]. Although greater prevalence of hypovitaminosis D among obese AA may be in part attributed to skin pigmentation and sequestering of vitamin D in adipose tissue, differences in classical endocrine effects (e.g., PTH and insulin response) likely also play a role [11]. Further, diet may modify the relationship between vitamin D bioavailability and underlying metabolic pathways. It is known that 25OHD level is dependent on intestinal absorption of dietary vitamin D, the extent to which vitamin D may exert effects on metabolic factors is at least in part dependent upon macronutrient profile of the diet. The metabolic response to dietary composition, specifically carbohydrate quantity of a meal, influences the postprandial cascade of events (increased glucose, insulin, lipogenesis, glycogenesis, etc.). Vitamin D has been independently associated with these processes, and the fact that vitamin D insufficiency stimulates secretion of PTH cannot be ignored. Data from this group has demonstrated that the physiological response to macronutrient concentration of the diet differs among racial groups [12]; however, to our knowledge there has been no investigation regarding the contribution of macronutrient profile to vitamin D involvement with metabolic components. Accordingly, the independent and interactive contribution of diet and vitamin D status (and consequent PTH level) on metabolic risk warrants investigation, particularly among obese adolescents.

Understanding the extent to which macronutrient composition influences vitamin D bioavailability may be particularly important during growth and development. Adolescence characterizes a time when risk factors for MetSyn can be identified, and modification of the dietary profile represents a strategy in which intervention may have the greatest directive impact. Therefore, the objective of this study was to determine the effect of macronutrient modifications on vitamin D status and if change in 25OHD concentration would influence components of MetSyn in obese AA girls. Further, as AA females are a population group that are at increased metabolic risk, this study seeks to evaluate the effect of macronutrient modification on associations of vitamin D concentrations and potential influence of PTH in AA adolescent females to parameters of MetSyn (fat distribution, insulin sensitivity, glucose tolerance, lipid concentrations, and blood pressure).

2. Methods

Participants included 28 overweight/obese AA girls aged 9–14 years. Obesity was defined as greater than 95th sex- and age-specific body mass index (BMI) percentile, and exclusion criteria were medical diagnosis and/or taking medications known to affect body composition, metabolism, and cardiac function. Participants were recruited through newspaper advertisements, flyers posted at various community partnerships, and by word-of-mouth. The nature, purpose, and possible risks of the study were carefully explained to each participant and guardian(s), and informed assent and consent, respectively were obtained. The protocol was approved by the Institutional Review Board for human subjects at the University of Alabama at Birmingham (UAB). All measurements were performed at the Participant and Clinical Interactions Resources (PCIRs) and the Department of Nutrition Sciences at UAB between 2008 and 2009.

2.1. Protocol. This study was part of a 16-week intervention comparing the effectiveness of a reduced CHO (43% carbohydrate: SPEC) versus a standard CHO (55% carbohydrate: STAN) diet on weight loss and metabolic health. Included data were derived from the initial five-week eucaloric phase, during which time the goal was for participants to maintain their baseline weight while consuming respective diets. Participants were block-randomized to one of the two diets which they remained on for the duration of the study. All food was provided, with the amount determined according to calculated individual needs determined by resting energy expenditure (REE; assessed via indirect calorimetry) multiplied by a 1.2 activity factor (averaging about 2000 kcal/d).

At baseline, participants attended two visits. The first visit entailed a physical examination by the study pediatrician, questionnaires on typical diet and regular physical activity, and a full-body dual energy X-ray absorptiometry (DXA) scan. At the second visit, participants reported to the PCIR in the morning in the fasted state for metabolic testing. After 30 minutes of rest, REE was assessed, and a liquid mixed-meal test (LMMT) was performed. To ensure weight stability, participants were weighed twice per week at food pickup to evaluate the caloric prescription throughout the five-week eucaloric phase. Weight changes exceeding two kilograms from baseline resulted in caloric modification in effort to maintain weight. Participants were asked to maintain their regular level of physical activity. At the duration of five weeks, the DXA scan, indirect calorimetry, and LMMT were repeated.

2.2. Diets. The SPEC diet comprised 42% of energy from CHO and 40% of energy from fat, whereas the STAN diet comprised 55% of energy from CHO and 27% of energy from fat. Both diets contained a similar content of protein (about 18%). Baseline energy levels for all diets were 1600 kcal with the addition of 100 to 400 kcal snack increments to participants who required more than 1600 kcal per day. All diets included culturally- and age-appropriate foods with no inclusion of supplements or formulas, and noncaloric fluid intake of ≥64 fluid ounces per day was recommended. All meals were prepared and packaged in the research kitchen at the UAB PCIR. A trained registered dietitian coded and entered data from each diet into the computerized Nutrition Data System for Research (NDSR).

2.3. Anthropometrics. The same registered dietitian obtained anthropometric measurements for all participants. Participants were weighed (Scale-Tronix 6702W; Scale-Tronix, Carol Stream, IL, USA) to the nearest 0.1 kg in minimal clothing without shoes. Height was also recorded without shoes using a digital stadiometer (Heightronic 235; Measurement Concepts, Snoqualmie, WA, USA). BMI percentile and obesity status (≥95th percentile) was calculated using sex- and age-specific CDC growth charts based on these measurements (http://apps.nccd.cdc.gov/dnpabmi/).

2.4. Body Composition and Fat Mass Index. Body composition was measured by DXA using GE Lunar Prodigy densitometer (GE LUNAR Radiation Corp., Madison, WI, USA). Participants were scanned in light clothing, while lying flat on their backs with arms at their sides. Due to size limitations, participants not fitting within the scanning box were right-sided hemiscanned with the left side estimated as per instrument protocol. Fat mass index calculated as total body fat divided by height was used as a covariate [13].

2.5. Liquid Mixed Meal Test/Insulin Sensitivity. Insulin response to a standardized meal was determined from an index of insulin sensitivity and secretion through frequent blood sampling following ingestion of a LMMT (Carnation Instant Breakfast prepared with whole milk). To perform the LMMT, a flexible intravenous catheter was placed in the antecubital space of the left arm. The "dose" for the liquid meal test was obtained according to amount of lean body mass (LBM) of the participant (1.75 g CHO/kg LBM). Participants were required to consume the meal within five minutes. Blood was drawn at baseline (three samples over 15 minutes) prior to initiation of meal consumption at time "zero." Subsequent blood samples were drawn every five minutes from time zero to 30 minutes, every 10 minutes from time 40 to 180 minutes, and at 210 and 240 minutes. Using the obtained measures, the insulin sensitivity index (SI) was calculated by oral glucose model [14].

2.6. Assay of Metabolites. Glucose was measured in 12 μL sera with the glucose oxidase method using a SIRRUS analyzer (interassay CV 2.56%). Insulin was analyzed using a TOSOH 1800 Automated Immunoassay Analyzer. Assay sensitivity is 15.42 pmol/L, mean intraassay CV is 4.69%, and interassay CV is 6.0%. Triglycerides (TGs) were assessed with the glyceryl phosphate method. HDL was analyzed using a two-reagent system involving stabilization of low-density lipoprotein cholesterol (LDL), very low-density lipoprotein cholesterol (VLDL), and chylomicrons using cyclodextrin and dextrin sulfate, and subsequent enzymatic-colorimetric detection of HDL. 25OHD and PTH concentration was obtained from fasting sera drawn and assayed in the UAB Core Laboratory with liquid chromatography/tandem mass spectrometry technique and a two-site radiometric assay, respectively.

2.7. Statistical Analysis. Differences at baseline in descriptive characteristics between girls in the two diet groups were examined using *t*-tests. The differences between diet groups regarding metabolic parameters were evaluated using ANOVA to allow for inclusion of covariates (pubertal stage, fat mass index, and baseline measures). Multivariate linear regression (Model A) was used to analyze the contribution of the change in 25OHD concentration over five weeks to individual components of metabolic syndrome. Due to the intricate relationship with PTH, for each component that was observed to be associated with 25OHD, a second regression model (Model B) was analyzed with inclusion of PTH as a covariate. To conform to the assumptions of linear regression, all statistical models were evaluated for residual normality and logarithmic transformations were performed when appropriate. All data were analyzed using SAS 9.2 software. Subsequently, models were evaluated by presence or absence of MetSyn. MetSyn was defined as meeting the IDF criteria for at least three of the components and was coded as zero for absence and one for presence. In addition, interaction terms were created (diet by change in 25OHD) and included in regression models to test the moderation by diet and change in 25OHD of relationships between metabolic outcomes.

Table 1: Baseline descriptive characteristics.

	Total ($n = 28$)	STAN ($n = 15$)	SPEC ($n = 13$)
Age (yrs)	12.4 ± 0.3	12.5 ± 0.4	12.4 ± 0.5
Tanner stage	4.4 ± 0.2	4.4 ± 0.3	4.4 ± 0.3
Height (cm)	159.5 ± 1.5	159.3 ± 2.0	160.3 ± 2.3
Weight (kg)	89.6 ± 4.6	93.8 ± 7.5	85.1 ± 4.8
BMI %	98.0 ± 0.3	98.1 ± 0.3	97.9 ± 0.5
BMI z-score	2.4	2.5	2.2
Trunk fat (%)	46.1 ± 1.4	48.1 ± 1.7	43.9 ± 2.3
Total fat (kg)	38.6 ± 2.4	41.1 ± 3.6	35.2 ± 2.7
Percent fat (%)	43.9 ± 1.0	45.8* ± 1.2	41.8* ± 1.5
Total lean (kg)	46.0 ± 2.2	47.4 ± 3.4	44.2 ± 2.3
Energy intake (kcal/d)	2105	2031	1991
MetSyn (%)	8 (29%)	4	4

*Indicate significant difference between diet groups ($P < 0.05$).
STAN: standard diet (55% calories from carbohydrate).
SPEC: specialized diet (43% calories from carbohydrate).

Table 2: Circulating 25OHD levels at baseline and five weeks in the presence or absence of MetSyn.

	Baseline	SE	Five weeks	SE
MetSyn	17.6	1.59	17.7	1.49
No MetSyn	19.1*	0.93	21.3*	0.94

*Indicates significant difference between baseline and five weeks ($P < 0.05$).
Abbreviations: standard error (SE).

3. Results

Descriptive characteristics and body composition at baseline in the total sample and by diet group are presented in Table 1. There were no differences between groups across variables, with the exception of percent body fat, which was significantly higher in the STAN diet group versus the SPEC diet group. At baseline, 29% of participants met the criteria for MetSyn, and individual components are illustrated at baseline and five weeks in Figure 1. Differences between diet groups were observed at baseline for circulating 25OHD and all lipid parameters [TG, LDL, HDL, and total cholesterol (tot chol)], and at five weeks for circulating 25OHD and TG.

Diet group evaluations related to MetSyn components are illustrated in Figure 2. Among those consuming the STAN diet, significant differences were observed from baseline to five weeks for circulating 25OHD ($P < 0.05$) and all lipid parameters ($P < 0.001$), except HDL. A significant

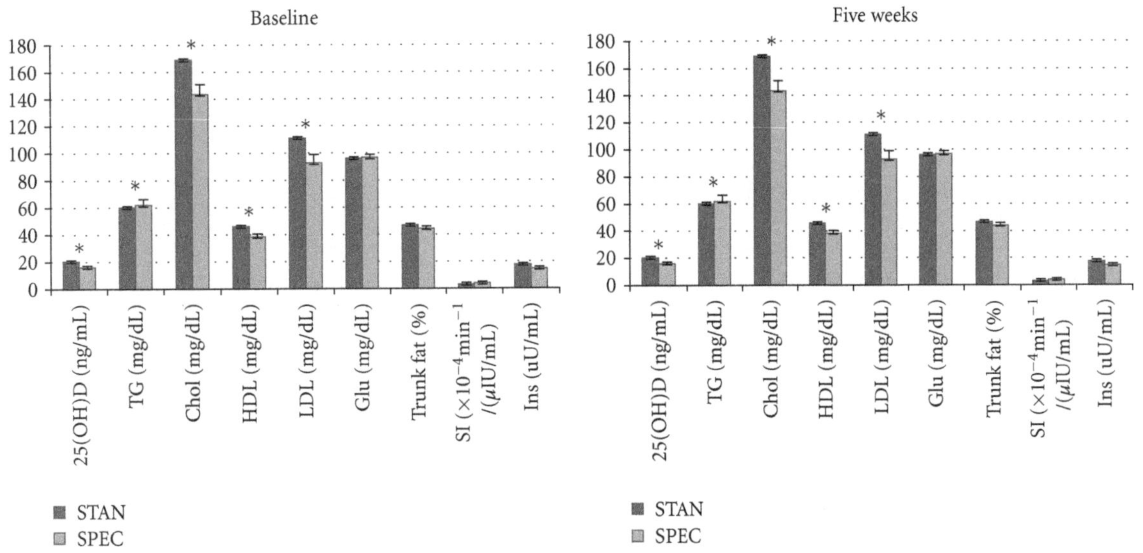

(a) (b)

Figure 1: Components of metabolic syndrome at baseline and five weeks. *Indicates significant difference between diet groups ($P < 0.5$). Abbreviations: circulating vitamin D (25OHD), triglycerides (TGs), cholesterol (Chol), high-density lipoprotein (HDL), low-density lipoprotein (LDL), fasting glucose (Glu), insulin sensitivity (SI), and insulin (Ins).

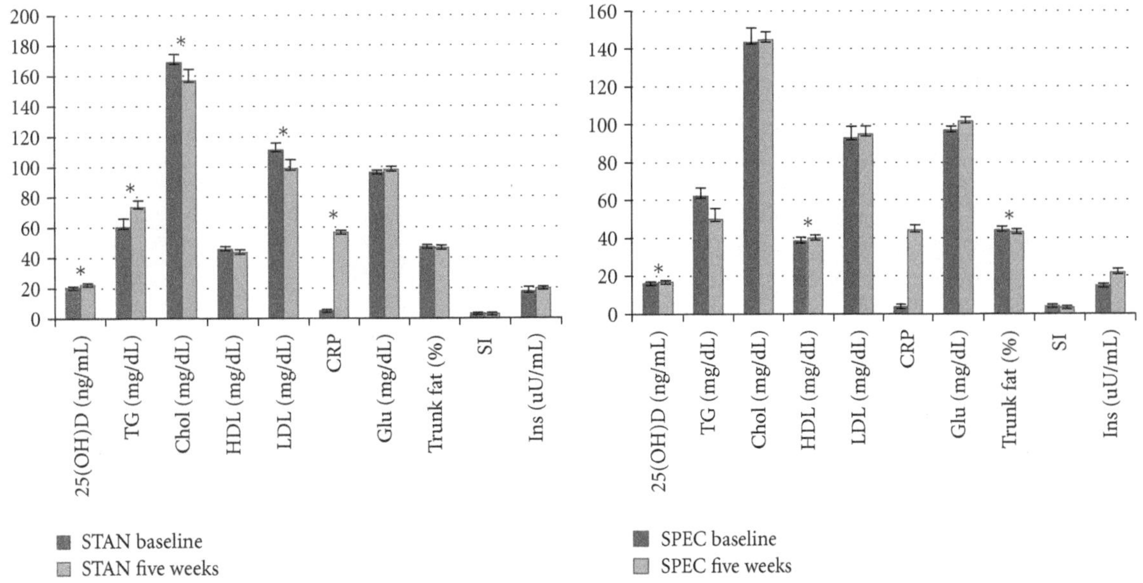

(a) (b)

Figure 2: Diet group evaluations related to MetSyn components. *Indicates significant differences between baseline and five weeks ($P < 0.05$). Abbreviations: circulating vitamin D (25OHD), triglycerides (TGs), cholesterol (Chol), high-density lipoprotein (HDL), low-density lipoprotein (LDL), fasting glucose (Glu), insulin sensitivity (SI), and insulin (Ins).

increase was revealed for circulating 25OHD and TG with a decrease in total chol and LDL across the five-week period. Among those consuming the SPEC diet, a significant increase in circulating 25OHD and insulin ($P = 0.05$ and $P < 0.001$, resp.) from baseline to five weeks was distinguished. Although an increase in circulating 25OHD was observed for both diet groups, circulating 25OHD levels were lower at baseline in participants presenting with MetSyn versus those with no MetSyn (Table 2). Similarly, greater PTH concentrations were observed in those presenting with MetSyn than those without MetSyn at both baseline and five weeks ($P < 0.001$). Further, individuals meeting criteria for MetSyn displayed no increase in circulating 25OHD across the five-week study period unlike participants without MetSyn.

The contribution of change in circulating 25OHD (ΔOHD) over the five weeks to MetSyn components is presented in Table 3. Two models were used to assess

TABLE 3: The contribution of ΔOHD over the five weeks to MetSyn components represented by two models. Model A illustrates the independent contribution of ΔOHD to metabolic parameters and Model B presents the inclusion of both ΔOHD and PTH as independent variables.

	STAN		SPEC	
REG Model A	ΔOHD[a]	P value	ΔOHD[a]	P value
Glucose (mg/dL)	−0.06 ± 0.43	0.88	−2.33 ± 1.01*	0.04
SI ($\times 10^{-4}$ min^{-1}/(μIU/mL))	−0.04 ± 0.06	0.49	0.66 ± 0.26*	0.02
LDL (mg/dL)	−1.53 ± 0.60*	0.02	0.99 ± 2.54	0.70
HDL (mg/dL)	−0.33 ± 0.38	0.39	−0.47 ± 0.89	0.60
Triglycerides (mg/dL)	0.67 ± 0.44	0.14	4.71 ± 3.46	0.19
Trunk fat (kg)	0.18 ± 0.12	0.15	0.35 ± 0.35	0.34

REG Model B	ΔOHD[a]	P value	PTH[a]	P value	ΔOHD[a]	P value	PTH[a]	P value
Glucose (mg/dL)	0.68 ± 0.36	0.07	0.29 ± 0.07*	0.0007	−2.31 ± 1.04*	0.05	−0.14 ± 0.26	0.60
SI ($\times 10^{-4}$ min^{-1}/(μIU/mL))	−0.03 ± 0.07	0.69	0.00 ± 0.01	0.73	0.66 ± 0.22*	0.01	−0.11 ± 0.05*	0.04
LDL (mg/dL)	−1.84±0.70*	0.02	−0.13 ± 0.15	0.38	1.10 ± 2.62	0.68	0.31 ± 0.55	0.58
Triglycerides (mg/dL)	0.11 ± 0.37	0.75	−0.27 ± 0.07*	0.002	4.62 ± 3.62	0.23	−0.20 ± 0.85	0.81

* Indicates significant difference ($P < 0.05$).
[a]Values represent beta coefficient and standard error.
Abbreviations: insulin sensitivity (SI), low-density lipoprotein (LDL), high-density lipoprotein (HDL), parathyroid hormone (PTH), and change in 25OHD concentration (ΔOHD).

the relationship. Model A illustrates the independent contribution of ΔOHD to metabolic parameters, and Model B presents the inclusion of both ΔOHD and PTH as independent variables. Among those consuming the STAN diet, an inverse relationship between ΔOHD and LDL ($P < 0.05$) was observed (Model A); in Model B, the association remained significant ($P < 0.05$). However, in this model a marginal association between ΔOHD and fasting glucose ($P = 0.07$) was observed as well as an independent contribution of PTH to fasting glucose concentration ($P < 0.001$). Additionally, a significant positive association between PTH and TG ($P < 0.01$) was observed. Among those consuming the SPEC diet, ΔOHD (Model A) was inversely associated with fasting glucose ($P < 0.05$) and positively associated with SI ($P < 0.05$); in Model B, these relationships remained, and an inverse relationship between PTH and SI was observed, whereas there was no relationship between PTH and fasting glucose.

At five weeks, 32% of participants met the criteria for MetSyn. There was no difference in those meeting criteria between diet groups; however, when the interaction term (ΔOHD × diet) was evaluated, those individuals who presented with MetSyn at five weeks displayed significantly positive associations between the interaction term and TG ($P < 0.001$), HDL ($P < 0.01$), LDL ($P < 0.01$), and systolic blood pressure (SysBP; $P < 0.01$). SI and insulin were inversely associated with the interaction term ($P < 0.01$) in those individuals who did not present with MetSyn at five weeks. After five weeks, there was an increase in circulating 25OHD among those without MetSyn, yet no change was observed in those with MetSyn (Figure 3). Further, 25OHD concentration among those with MetSyn was at a level that would be deemed insufficient based on currently accepted criteria [15].

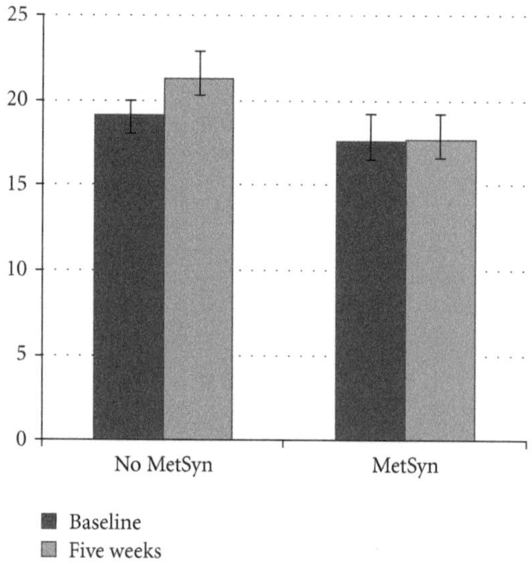

FIGURE 3: Circulating 25OHD levels at baseline and five weeks in the presence or absence of MetSyn.

4. Discussion

Vitamin D's emerging role as an integral component of metabolism is accompanied by the occurrence of risk factors for metabolic disease early in life and displays a critical conduit to which dietary intervention may facilitate improved metabolic outcomes. The objective of this study was to determine the effect of macronutrient modifications in the absence of weight loss on vitamin D status and if ΔOHD concentration would influence components of MetSyn in AA adolescent females. For those consuming a reduced carbohydrate diet, ΔOHD was inversely associated with fasting glucose and positively associated with SI. These relationships were maintained with inclusion of PTH. Clustering of metabolic parameters occurred such that glucose-related parameters in those without MetSyn, and lipid-related components in those with MetSyn were significantly associated with an interaction of diet and ΔOHD. These results provide some evidence regarding the role that vitamin D may exert on alterations in the biological response to macronutrients lending itself to further exploration.

Numerous studies in children have suggested metabolic effects of 25OHD on several markers of glucose (e.g., fasting glucose, insulin concentrations, and HOMA score) [16–19] and lipid metabolism (e.g., TG, HDL, and LDL) [18, 19]. In this sample, the interaction term (diet and ΔOHD) was positively associated with lipid profile among those meeting the criteria for MetSyn. Similarly, an independent effect of vitamin D on lipid profile was suggested by a weight-loss intervention study that found vitamin D supplementation resulted in improved lipid profile in the supplementation group despite similar weight-loss in nonsupplemented group [20]. Additionally, Al-Daghri and colleagues observed an association between total cholesterol and LDL and 25OHD which was apparent among adults with Type 2 Diabetes, but not in those without. Further, there was a reversal of MetSyn manifestations with vitamin D status correction [21]. From a physiologic standpoint, metabolic response to diet and potential relation with vitamin D status is an area in need of further exploration. The differential impact of the interaction between macronutrient composition and ΔOHD is of particular interest in light of the lack of consensus regarding optimal 25OHD concentration as it relates to vitamin D recommendations.

It has been suggested that a reduction in carbohydrate intake requires increased insulin resistance to maintain glucose homeostasis, particularly during reproductive development [22]. Among the SPEC diet group, glucose concentration increased to a greater extent in those with a lesser increase in 25OHD, respectively insulin sensitivity decreased to a greater extent in those with a lesser increase in 25OHD. It is plausible that vitamin D mediates the effect of reduced carbohydrate intake through its direct action on pancreatic β-cell function [23]. Conversely, in the STAN diet group, in which carbohydrate intake reflected that which is more typical of the adolescent population [24], manifestations of altered 25OHD concentration were apparent in lipid parameters. LDL concentration increased to a greater extent in those with a lesser increase in 25OHD. Although cross-sectional analysis has consistently identified a favorable effect of 25OHD concentration on LDL, vitamin D's function in lipid metabolism remains uncertain. The confluence of macronutrient composition adds further complexity. The relationship observed in this study is clear, and our findings suggest that effect of dietary composition on 25OHD bioavailability warrant consideration.

Establishing the role of vitamin D in relation to MetSyn is complicated by its reciprocal association with PTH; in addition, several of the proposed predictors of MetSyn are also known to be associated with PTH. Not surprisingly, in those meeting criteria, as opposed to those not meeting the criteria for MetSyn, PTH concentrations were significantly greater at both baseline and five weeks of this study. Many [25–27], but not all [28], studies report an inverse relationship between 25OHD and PTH. Moreover, AA generally present with lower 25OHD concentrations and higher PTH relative to European American counterparts [16, 26, 29, 30]. The relationship between vitamin D and PTH is influenced by various factors during growth and development, including dietary macronutrient composition, supported by findings reported herein. Independent of the positive association with vitamin D, an inverse relationship was found between PTH and SI, only apparent in those consuming the reduced carbohydrate, specialized diet. This may be translated into independent pathways of both PTH and vitamin D in linkage with MetSyn. It has been recently reported that PTH concentration, but not 25OHD, contributed to MetSyn in obese adults [5]. Support is provided for the postulation that influence by each of these factors diverges according to dietary composition.

This study had many strengths as well as evident limitations. Comprehensive phenotyping using robust measures of body composition is a major strength. The provision of food to each participant is an additional advantage because it ensured some degree of dietary control. Despite these strengths, it is important to evaluate certain shortcomings of this investigation. In noninstitutionalized subjects, dietary adherence is difficult to ascertain; beyond monitoring for weight change, the consumption of additional foods other than those provided cannot be certain. Also, the modest sample size and inclusion of only one racial group limits generalizability to other populations. Each participant was in the >99% BMI percentile, which may limit the ability to detect changes in outcome measures across body habitus. Finally, it is important to note that the short duration of the intervention may limit ability to identify the long-term effects of the diet on vitamin D.

5. Conclusions

Initiation and progression to MetSyn encompasses perturbations in glucose and lipid metabolism and is exacerbated by overweight/obesity, with AA females experiencing disproportionate incidence. Similar to what has been reported in other studies [7, 30–32], 29% of girls in this study presented with MetSyn and 25OHD was observed to be significantly lower and deemed insufficient in those presenting with MetSyn. Additionally, our results support the effect of macronutrient composition on the contribution of circulating 25OHD to parameters associated with MetSyn. Our findings also indicate that improvement in circulating 25OHD concentrations may normalize glucose parameters associated with initiation and progression to MetSyn. Additionally, though the mechanistic response of PTH to diet is unclear, its reciprocal relationship with vitamin D may mediate the effects of a reduced carbohydrate diet. This investigation builds upon previous findings which imply unique metabolic characteristics of peripubertal AA females.

In this context and considering the consistent reports of vitamin D insufficiency among this group, our findings may help inform recommendation efforts.

Declaration of interest

The authors report no conflict of interest.

Acknowledgments

This research was supported by R00DK083333 (K. Casazza); CA-47888 (L. J. Hanks); P30 DK056336 UAB Nutrition Obesity Research Center; UAB Diabetes Research Center Human Physiology Core P60DK079626, Thrasher Research Fund.

References

[1] T. D. Thacher and B. L. Clarke, "Vitamin D insufficiency," *Mayo Clinic Proceedings*, vol. 86, no. 1, pp. 50–60, 2011.

[2] A. A. Ginde, M. C. Liu, and C. A. Camargo Jr., "Demographic differences and trends of vitamin D insufficiency in the US population, 1988–2004," *Archives of Internal Medicine*, vol. 169, no. 6, pp. 626–632, 2009.

[3] S. Al-Musharaf, A. Al-Othman, N. M. Al-Daghri et al., "Vitamin D deficiency and calcium intake in reference to increased body mass index in children and adolescents," *European Journal of Pediatrics*. In press.

[4] J. P. Reis, D. von Mühlen, E. R. Miller III, E. D. Michos, and L. J. Appel, "Vitamin D status and cardiometabolic risk factors in the United States adolescent population," *Pediatrics*, vol. 124, no. 3, pp. e371–e379, 2009.

[5] J. Hjelmesæth, D. Hofsø, E. T. Aasheim et al., "Parathyroid hormone, but not vitamin D, is associated with the metabolic syndrome in morbidly obese women and men: a cross-sectional study," *Cardiovascular Diabetology*, vol. 8, article 7, 2009.

[6] L. S. Harkness and B. A. Cromer, "Vitamin D deficiency in adolescent females," *Journal of Adolescent Health*, vol. 37, no. 1, p. 75, 2005.

[7] K. Rajakumar, J. D. Fernstrom, M. F. Holick, J. E. Janosky, and S. L. Greenspan, "Vitamin D status and response to vitamin D_3 in obese vs. Non-obese African American children," *Obesity*, vol. 16, no. 1, pp. 90–95, 2008.

[8] P. Zhou, C. Schechter, Z. Cai, and M. Markowitz, "Determinants of 25(OH)D sufficiency in obese minority children: selecting outcome measures and analytic approaches," *Journal of Pediatrics*, vol. 158, no. 6, pp. 930–934.e1, 2011.

[9] C. M. Lenders, H. A. Feldman, E. Von Scheven et al., "Relation of body fat indexes to vitamin D status and deficiency among obese adolescents," *The American Journal of Clinical Nutrition*, vol. 90, no. 3, pp. 459–467, 2009.

[10] C. M. Gordon, K. C. DePeter, H. A. Feldman, E. Grace, and S. J. Emans, "Prevalence of vitamin D deficiency among healthy adolescents," *Archives of Pediatrics and Adolescent Medicine*, vol. 158, no. 6, pp. 531–537, 2004.

[11] T. Reinehr, G. de Sousa, U. Alexy, M. Kersting, and W. Andler, "Vitamin D status and parathyroid hormone in obese children before and after weight loss," *European Journal of Endocrinology*, vol. 157, no. 2, pp. 225–232, 2007.

[12] K. Casazza, M. Cardel, A. Dulin-Keita et al., "Reduced carbohydrate diet to improve metabolic outcomes and decrease adiposity in obese peripubertal African American girls," *Journal of Pediatric Gastroenterology and Nutrition*, vol. 54, no. 3, pp. 336–342, 2012.

[13] A. L. Willig, K. Casazza, A. Dulin-Keita, F. A. Franklin, M. Amaya, and J. R. Fernandez, "Adjusting adiposity and body weight measurements for height alters the relationship with blood pressure in children," *American Journal of Hypertension*, vol. 23, no. 8, pp. 904–910, 2010.

[14] E. Breda, M. K. Cavaghan, G. Toffolo, K. S. Polonsky, and C. Cobelli, "Oral glucose tolerance test minimal model indexes of β-cell function and insulin sensitivity," *Diabetes*, vol. 50, no. 1, pp. 150–158, 2001.

[15] A. C. Ross, J. E. Manson, S. A. Abrams et al., "The 2011 report on dietary reference intakes for calcium and vitamin D from the Institute of Medicine: what clinicians need to know," *Journal of Clinical Endocrinology and Metabolism*, vol. 96, no. 1, pp. 53–58, 2011.

[16] J. A. Alvarez, A. P. Ashraf, G. R. Hunter, and B. A. Gower, "Serum 25-hydroxyvitamin D and parathyroid hormone are independent determinants of whole-body insulin sensitivity in women and may contribute to lower insulin sensitivity in African Americans," *The American Journal of Clinical Nutrition*, vol. 92, no. 6, pp. 1344–1349, 2010.

[17] R. Alemzadeh, J. Kichler, G. Babar, and M. Calhoun, "Hypovitaminosis D in obese children and adolescents: relationship with adiposity, insulin sensitivity, ethnicity, and season," *Metabolism*, vol. 57, no. 2, pp. 183–191, 2008.

[18] A. J. Rovner and K. O. O'Brien, "Hypovitaminosis D among healthy children in the United States: a review of the current evidence," *Archives of Pediatrics and Adolescent Medicine*, vol. 162, no. 6, pp. 513–519, 2008.

[19] E. Rodríguez-Rodríguez, R. M. Ortega, L. G. González-Rodríguez, and A. M. López-Sobaler, "Vitamin D deficiency is an independent predictor of elevated triglycerides in Spanish school children," *European Journal of Nutrition*, vol. 50, no. 5, pp. 373–378, 2011.

[20] G. C. Major, F. Alarie, J. Doré, S. Phouttama, and A. Tremblay, "Supplementation with calcium + vitamin D enhances the beneficial effect of weight loss on plasma lipid and lipoprotein concentrations," *The American Journal of Clinical Nutrition*, vol. 85, no. 1, pp. 54–59, 2007.

[21] N. M. Al-Daghri, O. S. Al-Attas, M. S. Alokail et al., "Hypovitaminosis D associations with adverse metabolic parameters are accentuated in patients with diabetes mellitus type 2: A BMI-independent role of adiponectin?" *Journal of Endocrinological Investigation*. In press.

[22] J. C. Brand-Miller, H. J. Griffin, and S. Colagiuri, "The carnivore connection hypothesis: revisited," *Journal of Obesity*, vol. 2012, Article ID 258624, 9 pages, 2012.

[23] A. G. Pittas, J. Lau, F. B. Hu, and B. Dawson-Hughes, "Review: the role of vitamin D and calcium in type 2 diabetes. A systematic review and meta-analysis," *Journal of Clinical Endocrinology and Metabolism*, vol. 92, no. 6, pp. 2017–2029, 2007.

[24] Y. Pan and C. A. Pratt, "Metabolic syndrome and its association with diet and physical activity in US adolescents," *Journal of the American Dietetic Association*, vol. 108, no. 2, pp. 276–286, 2008.

[25] R. Kumar and J. R. Thompson, "The regulation of parathyroid hormone secretion and synthesis," *Journal of the American Society of Nephrology*, vol. 22, no. 2, pp. 216–224, 2011.

[26] S. A. Abrams, I. J. Griffin, K. M. Hawthorne, S. K. Gunn, C. M. Gundberg, and T. O. Carpenter, "Relationships among vitamin D levels, parathyroid hormone, and calcium absorption in young adolescents," *Journal of Clinical Endocrinology and Metabolism*, vol. 90, no. 10, pp. 5576–5581, 2005.

[27] R. P. Heaney, "Functional indices of vitamin D status and ramifications of vitamin D deficiency," *The The American Journal of Clinical Nutrition*, vol. 80, no. 6, supplement, pp. 1706S–1709S, 2004.

[28] K. M. Hill, G. P. McCabe, L. D. McCabe, C. M. Gordon, S. A. Abrams, and C. M. Weaver, "An inflection point of serum 25-hydroxyvitamin D for maximal suppression of parathyroid hormone is not evident from multi-site pooled data in children and adolescents," *Journal of Nutrition*, vol. 140, no. 11, pp. 1983–1988, 2010.

[29] F. Cosman, D. C. Morgan, J. W. Nieves et al., "Resistance to bone resorbing effects of PTH in black women," *Journal of Bone and Mineral Research*, vol. 12, no. 6, pp. 958–966, 1997.

[30] S. Cook, M. Weitzman, P. Auinger, M. Nguyen, and W. H. Dietz, "Prevalence of a metabolic syndrome phenotype in adolescents: findings from the Third National Health and Nutrition Examination Survey, 1988–1994," *Archives of Pediatrics and Adolescent Medicine*, vol. 157, no. 8, pp. 821–827, 2003.

[31] M. Rodríguez-Morán, B. Salazar-Vázquez, R. Violante, and F. Guerrero-Romero, "Metabolic syndrome among children and adolescents aged 10–18 years," *Diabetes Care*, vol. 27, no. 10, pp. 2516–2517, 2004.

[32] R. Weiss, J. Dziura, T. S. Burgert et al., "Obesity and the metabolic syndrome in children and adolescents," *The New England Journal of Medicine*, vol. 350, no. 23, pp. 2362–2374, 2004.

13

In Vivo Inflammation Does Not Impair ABCA1-Mediated Cholesterol Efflux Capacity of HDL

Remco Franssen,[1] Alinda W. M. Schimmel,[2] Sander I. van Leuven,[1] Simone C. S. Wolfkamp,[3] Erik S. G. Stroes,[1] and Geesje M. Dallinga-Thie[1,2]

[1] *Department of Vascular Medicine, Academic Medical Center Amsterdam, 1105 AZ Amsterdam, The Netherlands*
[2] *Department of Experimental Vascular Medicine, Academic Medical Center Amsterdam, 1105 AZ Amsterdam, The Netherlands*
[3] *Department of Gastroenterology, Tytgat Institute for Liver and Intestinal Research, Academic Medical Center Amsterdam, 1105 AZ Amsterdam, The Netherlands*

Correspondence should be addressed to Geesje M. Dallinga-Thie, g.m.dallinga@amc.nl

Academic Editor: Andrei C. Sposito

HDL provides atheroprotection by facilitating cholesterol efflex from lipid-laden macrophages in the vessel wall. In vitro studies have suggested impaired efflux capacity of HDL following inflammatory changes. We assessed the impact of acute severe sepsis and mild chronic inflammatory disease on the efflux capacity of HDL. We hypothesize that a more severe inflammatory state leads to stronger impaired cholesterol efflux capacity. Using lipid-laden THP1 cells and fibroblasts we were able to show that efflux capacity of HDL from both patients with severe sepsis or with Crohn's disease (active or in remission), either isolated using density gradient ultracentrifugation or using apoB precipitation, was not impaired. Yet plasma levels of HDL cholesterol and apoA-I were markedly lower in patients with sepsis. Based on the current observations we conclude that inflammatory disease does not interfere with the capacity of HDL to mediate cholesterol efflux. Our findings do not lend support to the biological relevance of HDL function changes *in vitro*.

1. Introduction

High-density lipoprotein (HDL) cholesterol levels exhibit strong inverse relations with cardiovascular disease risk [1–3]. In the light of this, raising HDL has been a prime target in current drug therapy. HDL exerts a variety of antiatherogenic effects [4]; it improves endothelial function, inhibits thrombosis, and has potent antioxidative properties as well as anti-inflammatory effects [5–7]. Most importantly, HDL is a key player in reverse cholesterol transport (RCT), a process that facilitates transport of cholesterol from peripheral tissues to the liver [8, 9]. In the course of this process, small HDL precursors, such as lipid-poor apoA-I and pre-β HDL, acquire free cholesterol and phospholipids through the action of ATP binding cassette transporter A1 (ABCA1) [10]. Maturation occurs through the action of lecithin cholesterol acyltransferase (LCAT), and further lipidation of these particles occurs by interaction with the ATP-binding cassette transporter G1 (ABCG1) resulting in the formation of α-HDL particles [11]. Finally, HDL lipoproteins are—as described for mice—directly taken up in the liver by scavenger-receptor-B1 (SR-B1) or HDL lipids are transferred to apo-B-containing lipoproteins via the action of cholesterol ester transfer protein (CETP) and will be subsequently cleared through hepatic low-density lipoprotein (LDL) receptors [5].

More recently, concerns have been raised that, beyond HDL quantity, HDL quality changes may also contribute to impaired cardiovascular disease (CVD) protection [12]. Inflammation is a central feature during all stages of atherosclerotic plaque formation with cytokines and chemokines orchestrating the influx of immune cells in disease vessels [12, 13]. At the same time, cellular activation status of local macrophages determines oxidation of subintimal cholesteryl esters and plaque stability [14]. Systemic inflammatory disease, such as rheumatoid arthritis, has been associated with an increased CVD risk [15]. Patients with active Crohn's disease (CD) also presented with accelerated atherogenesis [16], although a recent meta-analysis was unable to substantiate an increased CV mortality rate in CD [17].

Recent *in vitro* findings suggested that the propensity towards CVD risk in chronic inflammatory disease might in part be related to an impaired protective capacity of HDL particles. It has been shown that myeloperoxidase (MPO), a potent inflammatory mediator predominantly derived from polymorphonuclear cells, can modify apoA-I, resulting in the generation of "dysfunctional" HDL particles with attenuated capacity to mediate ABCA1-dependent cholesterol efflux [18–22]. Colocalization of MPO and apoA-I in the human plaque has fuelled the concept that MPO may also be involved in HDL modification *in vivo* [20, 23, 24].

In the present study we set out to analyse whether systemic inflammatory disease, dependent upon the severity of the disease, affects the capacity of HDL to mediate cholesterol efflux. HDL from patients in a mild chronic (Crohn's disease—CD) and acute severe inflammatory state (sepsis) was tested in *in vitro* cell-based efflux systems. A fibroblast cell line, expressing only ABCA1 was used to test the initial hypothesis that inflammation may specifically affect apoA-I-mediated cholesterol efflux. THP1 cells, a macrophage cell line expressing ABCG1, ABCA1, and SR-B1, were used to reflect total *in vivo* cholesterol efflux. These studies may imply that quantity of HDL may be more important for total cholesterol efflux than the quality of HDL.

2. Methods

2.1. Patients. Ten patients with Crohn's disease (CD) were recruited at the outpatient clinic (inflammatory bowel disease) at the AMC. During study visits, disease activity was assessed using the Harvey Bradshaw index (HBI, a research tool taking into account clinical parameters such as, general well-being, abdominal pain, number of liquid stools per day, abdominal mass and complications). Five patients with HBI > 4 were considered to have active CD and five patients with HBI < 4 were in remission. Additionally, we have selected 8 patients with severe sepsis from the ICU unit of the AMC. Sepsis was defined as the presence of a hemodynamic compromised state with temperature above 38°C and CRP levels above 50 mg/L. Additionally 5 healthy controls were recruited from the general population. The institutional review board at the AMC approved the study. All subjects gave written informed consent.

2.2. Blood Collection and Biochemical Measurements. Blood was collected after an overnight fast in EDTA-containing tubes and directly placed on ice. Blood of the patients with sepsis was collected during the admission to the hospital disregarding the fasting status of the patient. Plasma was isolated by centrifugation at 4°C, 3000 g for 15 minutes and stored at −80°C for further analyses. Cholesterol and triglycerides were analysed using a commercially available enzymatic method (Randox, Crumlin, UK) on the Cobas Mira autoanalyzer (Roche, Basel, Switzerland). HDLc and LDLc were analysed by a commercial assay (WAKO, Neuss, Germany). ApoB and apoA-I were analysed using a turbidimetric assay (WAKO, Neuss, Germany). Plasma C reactive protein (CRP) was analysed with a high-sensitivity nephelometric assay (Roche, Basel, Switzerland). Serum amyloid A (SAA) concentration was analysed with a commercial available ELISA (EL10015) from Anogen (Mississauga, Canada). HDL preparations of all patients were included in the efflux studies.

2.3. HDL Isolation. HDL (*d*: 1.063-1.21 g/mL) was isolated by gradient ultracentrifugation in a TLR 100.4 rotor (Beckman Coulter, Fullerton, USA). In short, 0.9 mL human plasma was brought to density $d = 1.31$ g/mL by addition of KBr. UC-tubes were filled with 4 ml 0.9% NaCL. 0.9 ml high density plasma was loaded underneath the NaCL using large injection needles. HDL fraction was harvested after centrifugation for 2 h, 12°C, 100,000 rpm in a Beckman Table top ultracentrifuge. HDL was subsequently dialysed against PBS (0.9% NaCL, 10.9 mmol/L $Na_2HPO_4 \cdot 2H_2O$, 1.8 mmol/L $NaH_2PO_4 \cdot 2H_2O$, pH 7.4; Fresenius Kabi), and apoA-I concentration was measured and used directly in the efflux experiments. Then, HDL was obtained by precipitation of the apoB-containing lipoprotein fraction with polyethylene glycol 8000 (Sigma P-2139) as described [25].

2.4. Preparation of MPO-Modified HDL. HDL was purchased from Calbiochem (cat. nr. 178452) and used for the MPO-modification reaction exactly as described [19]. In short, HDL (1 mg/mL apoA-I) was added to the reaction mixture containing 50 mM phosphate buffer, pH 7.0, containing 100 μM DTPA, 100 μM NaCl, 140 μM hydroperoxide, 57 nM purified human MPO (BioDesign Int; cat and A63100H). Incubations were performed at 37°C for 1 h. MPO-modified HDL was dialyzed against PBS and used as a positive control in the efflux experiments.

2.5. HDL-Mediated Cholesterol Efflux from Fibroblast and THP1 Cells. Primary human fibroblasts (NHDF-Ad- dermal fibroblasts; Cambrex, CC-2511) expressing human ABCA1 were grown in Hanks Balanced Salt Solution (HBSS) medium without Ca and Mg, containing 10% FBS (GIBCO 14170-088) and 0.1% penicillin/streptomycin at 37°C under 5% CO_2. To measure cellular cholesterol efflux, fibroblasts were plated and grown until 80% confluency; at this point cells were labelled for 24 h, with 0.5 μCi/mL ^{3}H-cholesterol in labeling medium (D-MEM : F-12 (1 : 1), Glutamax, 0.1% penicillin/streptomycin, 0.2% BSA, and 30 μg/mL cholesterol in the presence or absence of 3 μM LXR agonist T0901317 (Cayman Chemicals Comp.; art 71810) for fibroblasts. After labeling, efflux was induced by the addition of 0.5 mL of efflux medium, consisting of D-MEM : F-12 (1 : 1), Glutamax, 0.1% P/S, 0.2% BSA, and the patients HDL, or HDL from control subjects, isolated by apoB precipitation or HDL isolated by ultracentrifugation at a concentration of 10 μg/mL apoA-I, or HDL isolated from plasma obtained

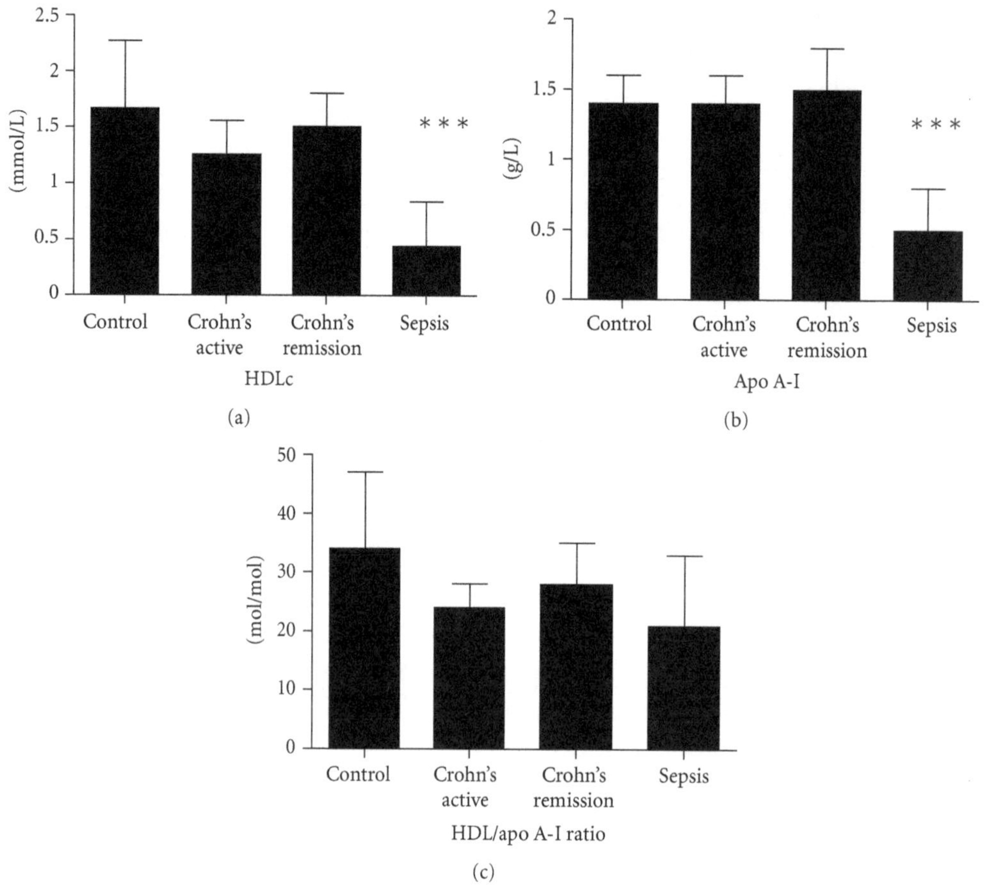

FIGURE 1: Plasma HDLc and ApoA-I levels in patients with CD, sepsis, and controls. Patients with CD exacerbation had decreased HDLc levels, whereas plasma apoA-I levels were normal. In patients with sepsis, plasma HDLc levels are strongly decreased by 73% and plasma apoA-I levels decreased by 64% as compared to controls. $^{**}P < 0.001$, $^{***}P < 0.0001$.

from controls, for a period of 4 h. Efflux medium without apoA-I was used as a negative control, and commercially available apoA-1 at a concentration of 10 μg/mL was used as a positive control. At the end of the incubation period, medium was expired. Cells were extracted with 2-propanol. Both medium and cell extracts were transferred into a vial containing scintillation fluid and counts were assessed (Packard, Tri-Carb 2900TR Liquid scintillation analyzer). Fractional cholesterol efflux was obtained by measuring the release of radio-labeled cholesterol into the medium. The percentage efflux equals the counts in medium divided by total counts in medium and cells combined, subtracted by counts to medium without HDL (control).

THP1 cells (ATCC) were grown in RPMI 1640, glutamax, 25 mM HEPES, 10% FCS, and 0.1% Penn/Strep at 37°C under 5% CO_2. One day prior to the experiment, cells were differentiated into macrophages by addition of phorbol 12-myristate 13-acetate (PMA: 50 ng/mL; Sigma p8138) to the cells. The efflux procedure was similar to that described above for fibroblasts. All experiments were performed in triplicate on the same day in different wells.

2.6. Statistical Analysis. All data are presented as mean (±SD) unless stated otherwise. Statistical analysis was performed in SPSS version 16. All differences in sepsis and controls were analyzed using unpaired Student's t-test statistics. The differences in CD-active, CD-remission, and controls were analyzed using two-way ANOVA and LSD post hoc analysis. A P value <0.05 was considered as being statistical significant.

3. Results

3.1. Baseline Characteristics. The baseline characteristics of patients with Crohn's disease are shown in Table 1. Patients with CD-active, reflecting a mild inflammatory state, had 10-fold higher plasma CRP levels than those with Crohn's disease in remission ($P < 0.05$; Table 1). In line, patients with CD-active had a tendency to lower plasma HDL levels (CD-active: 1.25 ± 1.2 mmol/L versus controls: 1.6 ± 0.6 mmol/L; $P = 0.11$; Figure 1). ApoA-I levels were similar to those in controls. As a consequence, the HDLc/apoA-I ratio in patients with active Crohn's disease was not significantly different (Figure 1).

In patients with sepsis, plasma CRP levels were very high (>200 mg/L). Subsequently, plasma HDLc levels were strongly decreased (0.44 ± 0.4 mmol/L; controls: 1.67 ± 0.6 mmol/L; $P < 0.001$; Figure 1). Plasma apoA-I levels

TABLE 1: Baseline characteristics of the subjects.

	Control	Crohn's disease active	Crohn's disease remission	Sepsis
Age, years	28 (3)	43 (10)	48 (15)	65 (12)*
Male/female	3/2	5/0	4/1	5/3
TC, mmol/L	4.7 (0.6)	4.0 (0.6)	5.12 (1.6)	1.9 (1.0)**
LDLc, mmol/L	2.57 (0.6)	2.14 (0.4)	3.06 (1.4)	1.27 (0.6)**
TG, mmol/L	1.03 (0.5)	1.25 (1.2)	1.22 (0.7)	1.70 (0.7)
CRP, mg/L	0.5 (0.2)	23.5 (27.8)	2.2 (1.8)	282 (109)**

Data are presented as mean (±SD). TC: total cholesterol; LDLc: low density lipoprotein cholesterol; HDLc: high-density lipoprotein cholesterol; TG: triglycerides; apo: apolipoprotein. $^{*}P < 0.05$; $^{**}P < 0.01$ versus controls.

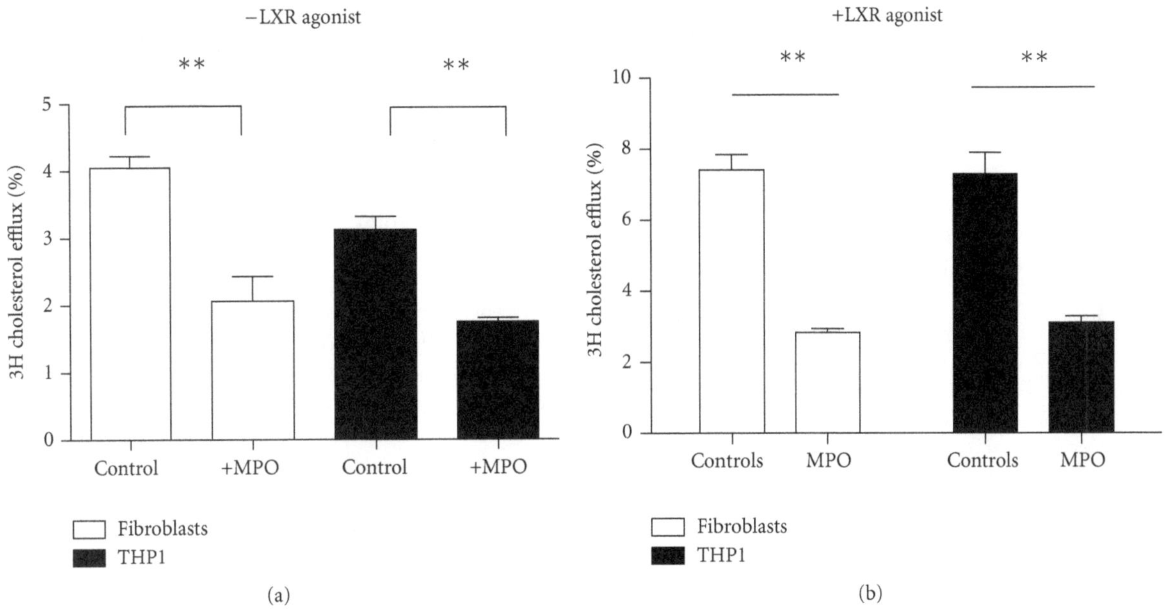

FIGURE 2: Cholesterol efflux capacity of MPO-HDL in fibroblasts and TP1 cells. HDL and MPO-HDL are used as cholesterol acceptors. Cholesterol efflux potential is measured in fibroblasts (white bars) and THP1 cells (black bars) under cholesterol-loaded conditions as described. The cells are labelled for 24 h, with ^{3}H-cholesterol in the absence (a) or presence (b) of LXR agonist. Efflux to HDL (10 μg /mL apoA-I) is measured during a 4 h time span. Efflux medium without HDL is used as a negative control. Fractional cholesterol efflux is determined by measuring the release of radio-labeled cholesterol into the medium. The percentage efflux equals the counts in medium divided by total counts in medium and cells combined, subtracted by efflux to the control. Data are presented as mean ± SD; $^{**}P < 0.01$. Experiments were performed in triplicate.

were 64% lower than in controls (0.5 g/L versus 1.4 g/L; $P < 0.0001$); (Figure 1), reflecting a strong decrease in circulating HDL particles. The HDLc/apoA-I ratio was markedly reduced as compared to controls (21 ± 12 mol/mol versus 34 ± 13 mol/mol; $P < 0.05$; Figure 1). Plasma SAA levels in patients with sepsis were significantly higher than in controls (sepsis: >400 mg/L and controls: 2.5 (range: 1.0–7.2) mg/L). Plasma SAA levels in CD-active and CD-remission were measured in a different, but comparable cohort of patients. Plasma SAA levels in CD-active was 23 mg/L (range 3–148) and in CD-remission 5.4 mg/L (range 1.2–69).

3.2. MPO-HDL Displays Impaired Cholesterol Efflux Capacity. We first tested whether *in vitro* modulation of commercially available human native HDL by MPO impaired the capacity of HDL to mediate cholesterol efflux, measured over a 4 h time span in LXR-stimulated fibroblasts to test ABCA1-mediated efflux. THP1 cells were used to test total efflux capacity mediated by ABG1, ABCA1 and SR-B1 and ABCA1-mediated efflux under LXR agonist stimulation of ABCA1. We have chosen to standardize the amount of HDL added to the incubation system based on apoA-I concentration in the HDL preparations, so that in every efflux experiment comparable amounts of apoA-I are present, reflecting an equal number of HDL particles. In line with expectations, cholesterol efflux capacity of MPO-HDL was significantly decreased by 62% ($P = 0.008$) in fibroblasts and 32% ($P = 0.01$) in THP1 cells (Figure 2) under both conditions, providing evidence that our experimental setup is viable.

3.3. Cholesterol Efflux Capacity of HDL from Patients with Crohn's Disease. HDL was isolated by ultracentrifugation as well as by precipitation to avoid bias through the presence of serum proteins in the PEG-precipitated HDL preparation, which may interfere with the cholesterol efflux measurement. Again equal amounts of apoA-I (10 μg/mL) were added to each well in the efflux experiment. Surprisingly, HDL isolated by ultracentrifugation (UC-HDL) showed similar ABCA1-mediated cholesterol efflux in fibroblasts as compared to controls; (Figure 3(a)). UC-HDL showed increased total cholesterol efflux potential in THP1 cells (CD-active: +28%, $P < 0.02$ versus controls; CD-remission: +24%; $P < 0.01$ versus controls (Figure 3(b)). PEG-HDL (10 μg/mL apoA-I), as a control, isolated from CD-active and CD-remission patient's plasma induced a similar ABCA1-mediated cholesterol efflux in fibroblasts as well as total cholesterol efflux potential in THP1 cells as compared to control PEG-HDL (Figure 3).

3.4. Cholesterol Efflux Capacity of HDL from Patients with Sepsis. UC-HDL from patients with sepsis, reflecting a severe inflammatory state, showed a similar ABCA1-mediated cholesterol efflux potential from cholesterol-laden fibroblast cells in the presence of a LXR agonist (Figure 4). Cholesterol efflux potential from THP1 cells to UC-HDL isolated from plasma of patients with sepsis was increased as compared to controls (+14%, $P < 0.05$; (Figure 4). Cholesterol efflux potential of PEG-HDL in cholesterol-laden fibroblast cells was similar to controls (Figure 4), whereas cholesterol efflux capacity of PEG-HDL in THP1 cells was significantly increased (+58%; $P < 0.005$; Figure 4).

4. Discussion

We demonstrate that the capacity of HDL (normalized for apoA-1 concentration) of patients with severe acute or mild chronic inflammatory state, to mediate cholesterol efflux from cultured cholesterol-loaded fibroblasts treated with a LXR agonist to stimulate ABCA1 expression and THP1 cells, was not decreased as compared to normolipidemic controls. Even in patients with sepsis, suffering from a severe inflammatory disease state, HDL efflux capacity is, if anything, increased compared to healthy controls. These data underline that *in vitro* findings regarding HDL "dysfunction" cannot be extrapolated to an *in vivo* situation.

In the present study we have used two different cell systems to determine HDL-mediated cholesterol efflux potential. Fibroblasts are known to express the ABCA-1 receptor abundantly which can be further increased by treating the cells with a LXR agonist, whereas THP1 cells (under lipid-laden conditions) express ABCA1, SR-B1 and ABCG-1 and thus model lipid-laden macrophages in human atherosclerotic plaques [26]. In line with previous reports, we observed that HDL when exposed to MPO in a test tube displays impaired capacity to mediate cholesterol efflux from both fibroblasts as well as THP1 cells, [20, 24] showing that ABCA1-mediated cholesterol efflux is highly impaired and thus provides validation of our efflux system. Two different disease models, one representing an acute, severe inflammatory state (sepsis) and the other representing a mild inflammatory state (Crohn's disease), have been used in the present study. Both disease states were characterized by increased plasma CRP and SAA levels, as well as decreased plasma HDLc levels, albeit not significant in CD-active, which is in line with HDL acting as an inverse acute phase reactant [5]. Our original hypothesis was based on the observation that *in vitro* inflammatory challenges modulate HDL response to induce normal cholesterol efflux from cell culture systems. We expected to see a gradual decrease in HDL efflux potential with increasing severity of inflammatory state. However, despite the inflammatory conditions of these patients we observed a modest increase in the efflux capacity of HDL, but we feel that more robust analysis are required to further investigate this.

Thus, our data clearly indicate that impaired efflux capacity of HDL in inflammatory disease states does not play a significant role *in vivo*. Obviously, these findings do not exclude a decreased total efflux capacity, since HDLc and apoA-I concentrations are profoundly lower in patients with sepsis albeit not in patients with a mild inflammatory state (active Crohn's disease) [15, 27]. The efflux data were obtained through controlling for apoA-I levels in the different HDL preparations. Plasma apoA-I levels in patients with sepsis were 45% reduced. This means in theory that, although HDL was more efficient in accepting cholesterol from cells, this cannot be compensated for by the strong decrease in number of circulating HDL particles and thus an overall decreased total efflux capacity.

Interestingly, we observed a slight increase in HDL efflux capacity in an inflammatory disease state. Van Der Westhuyzen et al. have previously shown that, besides apoA-I, SAA is also capable of promoting cholesterol efflux [28]. Since we have used similar apoA-I concentrations in all our assays and more importantly since HDL particles in the inflammatory state contain an increased number of SAA molecules, this may have been the reason for the increase in efflux capacity. However, plasma SAA levels in patients with sepsis are more than 200-fold increased as compared to controls whereas plasma SAA levels in active Crohn's disease were only increased 10-fold compared to controls. Therefore, we conclude that plasma SAA levels do not contribute to the increased cholesterol efflux observed in both CD-active and sepsis.

Previous studies have suggested that smaller lipid depleted HDL particles serve as better cholesterol acceptors via the ABCA1-mediated efflux pathway [29]. Indeed, the estimated HDL-c/apoA-I ratio between controls and patients in a severe inflammatory state was significantly reduced suggesting the presence of smaller-sized HDL particles. In line, the average number of particles was reduced in our study as reflected by the decrease in apoA-I levels. These data lend further support to the concept that HDL quantity is the main determinant of cholesterol efflux capacity under these conditions. In contrast to our findings, Mc Gillicuddy et al. reported that, following an acute endotoxin challenge, several steps in the RCT pathway were disrupted [30]. Thus, *in vitro* exposure of macrophages to LPS significantly reduced ABCA1 expression thereby attenuating cholesterol efflux capacity towards apoA-I. Cholesterol efflux acceptor capacity of HDL obtained from subjects subjected to the

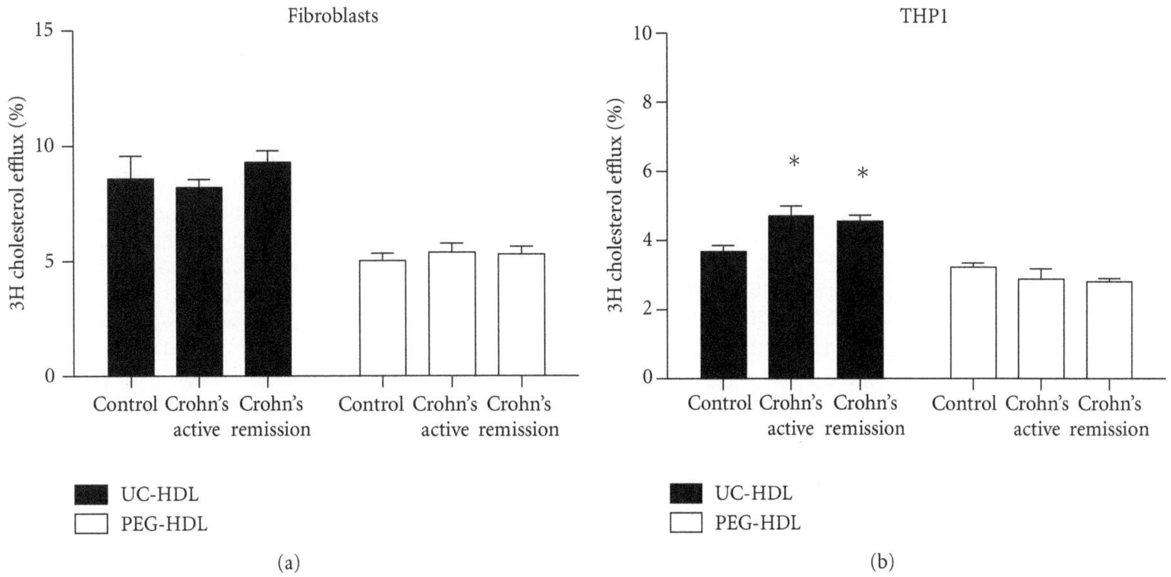

Figure 3: Efflux potential of HDL isolated from patients with Crohn's disease in fibroblasts and THP1 cells. Cholesterol acceptor capacity of UC-HDL (black bars) and PEG HDL (white bars) isolated from controls, and patients with active Crohn's disease and Crohn's disease in remission using cholesterol-laden fibroblasts and cholesterol-laden THP1 cells. Cells are labelled for 24 h with ^{3}H-cholesterol. Fibroblasts were incubated in the presence of LXR agonist TO901317. Efflux to HDL (10 μg/mL apoA-I) is measured during a 4 h time span. Efflux medium without HDL is used as a negative control. Fractional cholesterol efflux is determined by measuring the release of radio-labeled cholesterol into the medium. The percentage efflux equals the counts in medium divided by total counts in medium and cells combined and was corrected for counts to medium without acceptor HDL. Experiments were performed in triplicate. Data are presented as mean ± SD; $^*P < 0.05$.

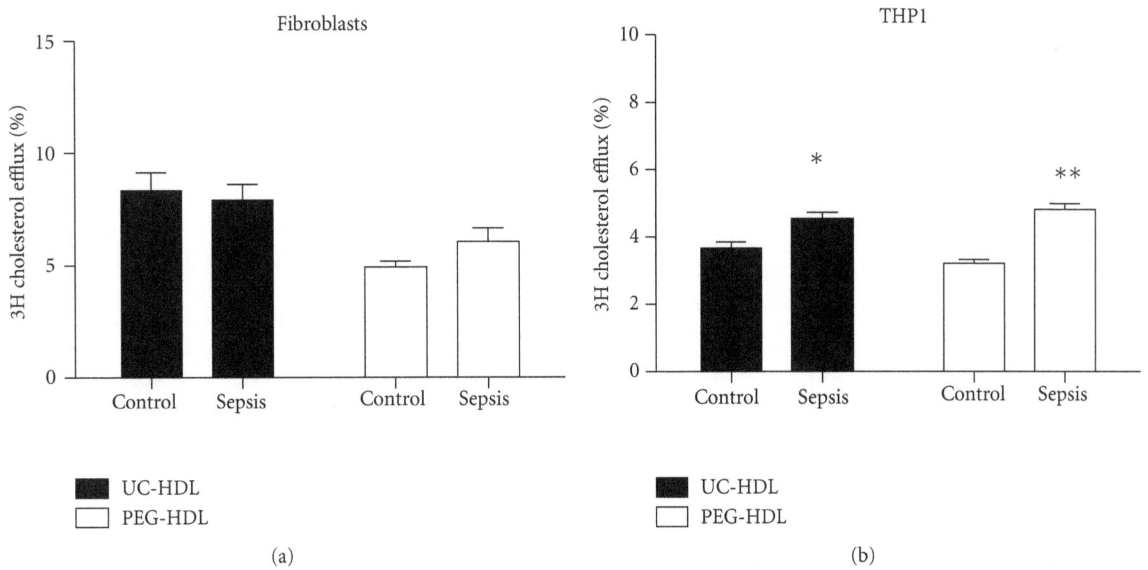

Figure 4: Efflux potential of UC-HDL and PEG-HDL isolated from patients with sepsis in fibroblasts and THP1 cells. Cholesterol acceptor capacity of UC-HDL (black bars) and PEG-HDL (white bars) from patients with sepsis using cholesterol-laden fibroblasts (and cholesterol-laden THP1 cells). Fibroblasts were incubated in the presence of LXR agonist TO901317. Cells are labelled for 24 h with ^{3}H-cholesterol. Efflux to HDL (10 μg/mL apoA-I) is measured during a 4 h time span. Efflux medium without HDL is used as a negative control. Fractional cholesterol efflux is determined by measuring the release of radio-labeled cholesterol into the medium. The percentage efflux equals the counts in medium divided by total counts in medium and cells combined and was corrected for counts to the medium without acceptor HDL. Experiments were performed in triplicate. Data are presented as mean ± SD; $^*P < 0.05$, $^{**}P < 0.01$.

LPS challenge was decreased with a concomitant decrease in plasma apoA-I level. There are several reasons that may underlie the discrepancy with the current findings. First, a single endotoxin challenge is not comparable to a more sustained inflammation, since a wide variety of adaptation mechanisms evolve over time [5, 31, 32]. Most importantly, these authors failed to normalize for the decrease in apoA-I levels after the endotoxin challenge in the cholesterol efflux assay, which invariably contributes to differences in cholesterol efflux. In fact, we demonstrated in septic patients that correction for changes in apoA-I result in a normal or even increased efflux acceptor capacity of HDL independent of the HDL preparation (PEG isolated or ultracentrifugally isolated).

4.1. Study Limitations. Our study has several limitations. First, the patients in the present study were older compared to the controls. Berrougui et al. have reported that particularly ABCA1-mediated cholesterol efflux decreased with advancing age [33]. This implies that in patients we may have observed lower values compared to the younger controls. However, since we find, if anything, higher efflux values, the age difference cannot have contributed to the present observation. Second, we included only a limited number of subjects in our study. However, since we observe an increased efflux in patients with an extreme inflammatory disease, it is unlikely that inclusion of a larger number of subjects would alter these findings.

4.2. Conclusion. Whereas exposure of HDL to MPO *ex vivo* leads to an impaired cholesterol efflux, native HDL preparations isolated from patients in mild and severe inflammatory disease states retain its ability to stimulate efflux. These findings do not lend support to the biological relevance of HDL function changes observed *in vitro*.

Acknowledgments

The authors would like to thank Mirjam van Aalderen for her assistance in the efflux studies and Joram van Miert for technical assistance. This work was supported by a Grant from the Dutch Heart Foundation 2008B070 to (R. Franssen).

References

[1] T. Gordon, W. P. Castelli, and M. C. Hjortland, "High density lipoprotein as a protective factor against coronary heart disease. The Framingham study," *American Journal of Medicine*, vol. 62, no. 5, pp. 707–714, 1977.

[2] W. B. Kannel, "High-density lipoproteins: epidemiologic profile and risks of coronary artery disease," *American Journal of Cardiology*, vol. 52, no. 4, pp. 9B–12B, 1983.

[3] P. W. F. Wilson, R. D. Abbott, and W. P. Castelli, "High density lipoprotein cholesterol and mortality. The Framingham heart study," *Arteriosclerosis*, vol. 8, no. 6, pp. 737–741, 1988.

[4] S. I. Van Leuven, E. S. Stroes, and J. J. P. Kastelein, "High-density lipoprotein: a fall from grace?" *Annals of Medicine*, vol. 40, no. 8, pp. 584–593, 2008.

[5] A. Kontush and M. J. Chapman, "Functionally defective high-density lipoprotein: a new therapeutic target at the crossroads of dyslipidemia, inflammation, and atherosclerosis," *Pharmacological Reviews*, vol. 58, no. 3, pp. 342–374, 2006.

[6] C. Mineo, H. Deguchi, J. H. Griffin, and P. W. Shaul, "Endothelial and antithrombotic actions of HDL," *Circulation Research*, vol. 98, no. 11, pp. 1352–1364, 2006.

[7] R. S. Birjmohun, S. I. Van Leuven, J. H. M. Levels et al., "High-density lipoprotein attenuates inflammation and coagulation response on endotoxin challenge in humans," *Arteriosclerosis, Thrombosis, and Vascular Biology*, vol. 27, no. 5, pp. 1153–1158, 2007.

[8] A. R. Tall, "Cholesterol efflux pathways and other potential mechanisms involved in the athero-protective effect of high density lipoproteins," *Journal of Internal Medicine*, vol. 263, no. 3, pp. 256–273, 2008.

[9] L. Yvan-Charvet, N. Wang, and A. R. Tall, "Role of HDL, ABCA1, and ABCG1 transporters in cholesterol efflux and immune responses," *Arteriosclerosis, Thrombosis, and Vascular Biology*, vol. 30, no. 2, pp. 139–143, 2010.

[10] J. F. Oram and R. M. Lawn, "ABCA1: the gatekeeper for eliminating excess tissue cholesterol," *Journal of Lipid Research*, vol. 42, no. 8, pp. 1173–1179, 2001.

[11] Y. L. Marcel, M. Ouimet, and M. D. Wang, "Regulation of cholesterol efflux from macrophages," *Current Opinion in Lipidology*, vol. 19, no. 5, pp. 455–461, 2008.

[12] P. Libby, P. M. Ridker, and A. Maseri, "Inflammation and atherosclerosis," *Circulation*, vol. 105, no. 9, pp. 1135–1143, 2002.

[13] R. Ross, "Atherosclerosis—an inflammatory disease," *New England Journal of Medicine*, vol. 340, no. 2, pp. 115–126, 1999.

[14] P. Libby, P. M. Ridker, and G. K. Hansson, "Progress and challenges in translating the biology of atherosclerosis," *Nature*, vol. 473, no. 7347, pp. 317–325, 2011.

[15] W. Khovidhunkit, M. S. Kim, R. A. Memon et al., "Effects of infection and inflammation on lipid and lipoprotein metabolism: mechanisms and consequences to the host," *Journal of Lipid Research*, vol. 45, no. 7, pp. 1169–1196, 2004.

[16] S. I. Van Leuven, R. Hezemans, J. H. Levels et al., "Enhanced atherogenesis and altered high density lipoprotein in patients with Crohn's disease," *Journal of Lipid Research*, vol. 48, no. 12, pp. 2640–2646, 2007.

[17] S. D. Dorn and R. S. Sandler, "Inflammatory bowel disease is not a risk factor for cardiovascular disease mortality: results from a systematic review and meta-analysis," *American Journal of Gastroenterology*, vol. 102, no. 3, pp. 662–667, 2007.

[18] S. L. Hazen, R. Zhang, Z. Shen et al., "Formation of nitric oxide-derived oxidants by myeloperoxidase in monocytes pathways for monocyte-mediated protein nitration and lipid peroxidation in vivo," *Circulation Research*, vol. 85, no. 10, pp. 950–958, 1999.

[19] B. Shao, C. Bergt, X. Fu et al., "Tyrosine 192 in apolipoprotein A-I is the major site of nitration and chlorination by myeloperoxidase, but only chlorination markedly impairs ABCA1-dependent cholesterol transport," *Journal of Biological Chemistry*, vol. 280, no. 7, pp. 5983–5993, 2005.

[20] L. Zheng, B. Nukuna, M. L. Brennan et al., "Apolipoprotein A-I is a selective target for myeloperoxidase-catalyzed oxidation and function impairment in subjects with cardiovascular disease," *Journal of Clinical Investigation*, vol. 114, no. 4, pp. 529–541, 2004.

[21] B. Shao and J. W. Heinecke, "Impact of HDL oxidation by the myeloperoxidase system on sterol efflux by the ABCA1

pathway," *Journal of Proteomics*, vol. 74, no. 11, pp. 2289–2299, 2011.

[22] B. Shao, S. Pennathur, and J. W. Heinecke, "Myeloperoxidase targets apolipoprotein A-I, the major HDL protein, for site-specific oxidation in human atherosclerotic lesions," *The Journal of Biological Chemistry*, vol. 287, no. 9, pp. 6375–6386, 2012.

[23] S. Pennathur, C. Bergt, B. Shao et al., "Human atherosclerotic intima and blood of patients with established coronary artery disease contain high density lipoprotein damaged by reactive nitrogen species," *Journal of Biological Chemistry*, vol. 279, no. 41, pp. 42977–42983, 2004.

[24] B. Shao, M. N. Oda, C. Bergt et al., "Myeloperoxidase impairs ABCA1-dependent cholesterol efflux through methionine oxidation and site-specific tyrosine chlorination of apolipoprotein A-I," *Journal of Biological Chemistry*, vol. 281, no. 14, pp. 9001–9004, 2006.

[25] F. Matsuura, N. Wang, W. Chen, X. C. Jiang, and A. R. Tall, "HDL from CETP-deficient subjects shows enhanced ability to promote cholesterol efflux from macrophages in an apoE- and ABCG1-dependent pathway," *Journal of Clinical Investigation*, vol. 116, no. 5, pp. 1435–1442, 2006.

[26] M. Denis, R. Bissonnette, B. Haidar, L. Krimbou, M. Bouvier, and J. Genest, "Expression, regulation, and activity of ABCA1 in human cell lines," *Molecular Genetics and Metabolism*, vol. 78, no. 4, pp. 265–274, 2003.

[27] H. J. Van Leeuwen, E. C. J. M. Heezius, G. M. Dallinga, J. A. G. Van Strijp, J. Verhoef, and K. P. M. Van Kessel, "Lipoprotein metabolism in patients with severe sepsis," *Critical Care Medicine*, vol. 31, no. 5, pp. 1359–1366, 2003.

[28] D. R. Van Der Westhuyzen, L. Cai, M. C. De Beer, and F. C. De Beer, "Serum amyloid A promotes cholesterol efflux mediated by scavenger receptor B-I," *Journal of Biological Chemistry*, vol. 280, no. 43, pp. 35890–35895, 2005.

[29] M. De La Llera-Moya, D. Drazul-Schrader, B. F. Asztalos, M. Cuchel, D. J. Rader, and G. H. Rothblat, "The ability to promote efflux via ABCA1 determines the capacity of serum specimens with similar high-density lipoprotein cholesterol to remove cholesterol from macrophages," *Arteriosclerosis, Thrombosis, and Vascular Biology*, vol. 30, no. 4, pp. 796–801, 2010.

[30] F. C. McGillicuddy, M. L. De La Moya, C. C. Hinkle et al., "Inflammation impairs reverse cholesterol transport in vivo," *Circulation*, vol. 119, no. 8, pp. 1135–1145, 2009.

[31] S. F. Lowry, "Human endotoxemia: a model for mechanistic insight and therapeutic targeting," *Shock*, vol. 24, no. 1, pp. 94–100, 2005.

[32] R. Anel and A. Kumar, "Human endotoxemia and human sepsis: limits to the model," *Critical Care*, vol. 9, no. 2, pp. 151–152, 2005.

[33] H. Berrougui, M. Isabelle, M. Cloutier, G. Grenier, and A. Khalil, "Age-related impairment of HDL-mediated cholesterol efflux," *Journal of Lipid Research*, vol. 48, no. 2, pp. 328–336, 2007.

HDL-C Response Variability to Niacin ER in US Adults

Jennifer B. Christian,[1] Eric J. Olson,[2] Jeffery K. Allen,[3] and Kimberly A. Lowe[4]

[1] *GlaxoSmithKline, Clinical Effectiveness & Safety, 5 Moore Drive, B.3116, Durham, NC 27709-3398, USA*
[2] *GlaxoSmithKline, Heart Failure DPU, Medicines Discovery and Development, King of Prussia, PA 19406, USA*
[3] *GlaxoSmithKline, Worldwide Epidemiology, Durham, NC 27709, USA*
[4] *Exponent Health Sciences, Bellevue, WA 98004, USA*

Correspondence should be addressed to Jennifer B. Christian; jennifer.b.christian@gsk.com

Academic Editor: Francisco Blanco-Vaca

Background. Niacin is the most effective treatment currently available for raising HDL-C levels. *Objective.* To evaluate if gender and baseline lipid levels have an effect on the HDL-C response of niacin ER and to identify factors that predict response to niacin ER at the 500 mg dose. *Material and Methods.* The change in HDL-C effect between baseline and follow-up levels was quantified in absolute change as well as dichotomized into high versus low response (high response was defined as an HDL-C effect of >15% increase and low response was HDL-C <5%) in a sample of 834 individuals. *Results.* Both males and females with low HDL-C levels at baseline exhibited a response to treatment in the multivariate model (males, HDL-C <40 mg/dL: OR = 5.18, 95% CI: 2.36–11.39; females, HDL-C <50 mg/dL: OR = 5.40, 95% CI: 1.84–15.79). There was also a significant difference in the mean HDL-C effect between baseline and follow-up HDL-C levels in the 500 mg niacin ER dose group for both males (mean HDL-C effect = 0.08, $P < 0.001$) and females (mean HDL-C effect = 0.10, $P = 0.019$). *Conclusion.* Baseline HDL-C levels are the biggest predictor of response to niacin ER treatment for both males and females among the factors evaluated.

1. Introduction

High-density lipoprotein cholesterol (HDL-C), also referred to as the "good cholesterol," is a known antioxidant, antithrombotic, and antiinflammatory, with properties that promote the removal of cellular cholesterol [1]. Individuals with low HDL-C levels may be at an increased risk of coronary heart disease (CHD) [2], and it has been shown in observational studies that the risk of CHD is reduced by 2%-3% for every 1 mg/dL increase in HDL-C [3]. Approximately 16% of adults in the United States have low HDL-C levels (25% of males and 7% of females) [4], while 11% of males and 4% of females of 19 years of age or younger have low HDL-C [5].

Low HDL-C is managed by three classes of dyslipidemic pharmacotherapy: niacin, statins, and fibric acid derivatives. Of these, niacin has been shown to increase HDL-C levels by as much as 35% in higher doses, which makes it the most effective pharmaceutical treatment currently available for raising HDL-C [6–9]. In addition, extended-release (ER) high-dose niacin has been shown to significantly reduce carotid atherosclerosis within 12 months among statin-treated individuals with low HDL-C who had either type II diabetes with coronary heart disease or carotid/peripheral atherosclerosis [9]. However, recently published results from the Atherothrombosis Intervention in Metabolic Syndrome with Low HDL Cholesterol/High Triglyceride and Impact on Global Health Outcomes (AIM-HIGH) study showed that high-dose niacin ER did not provide additional reduction in risk of cardiovascular-related events beyond what is observed with statin therapy alone [4]. In this modest sized trial, 3,414 subjects were randomized to niacin ER or placebo while their low-density lipoprotein cholesterol (LDL-C) levels were maintained to a median of <70 mg/dL. Importantly, the lipid community still awaits the results of a second larger niacin ER study (HSP2 THRIVE) to understand where the potential value of niacin therapy may reside in CV risk reduction, if it does at all. Therefore, due to the findings of the AIM-HIGH study and until the results of the HSP2 THRIVE results are revealed (in addition to the poor tolerability of niacin itself), administration of niacin to those who stand to achieve the most lipid benefit is important.

Therefore, our objectives were to evaluate the extent to which gender and baseline lipid levels may have an effect on the HDL-C response of niacin ER and to identify factors that predict greater response to niacin ER.

2. Materials and Methods

2.1. Data Source and Description of the Study Population. This is a retrospective cohort study using medical claims that occurred between January 1, 2000, and March 31, 2008, from the Optum Impact National Managed Care Benchmark Database (OptumInsight, Eden Prairie, MN, USA). This database includes de-identified claims for inpatient and outpatient services, laboratory results, and pharmacy fills for privately insured patients, including several hundred thousand Managed Medicare and Medicare Advantage members. It is a commonly used and reliable data source for epidemiologic research in the United States [7, 9–12]. Database administrators perform multiple cross-checks to ensure data accuracy. Such practices include tracking of historical trends to identify anomalies and outliers. Database metrics are run after each update to cross-check the data and ensure it meets known population distributions. Source-to-target validation of data quantities is also completed and prescribed rules for researching and discarding nonconforming data are followed. The patients included in the database are representative of privately insured patients in all 50 states. A large proportion of the lab results come from two major lab vendors.

The sample for the current study includes patients ≥18 years of age who met the following criteria: (1) concurrent medical and prescription coverage for the study period for at least two months while taking niacin ER, (2) a prescription of at least 28 days of niacin ER filled during the study period, (3) continuous eligibility for six months prior to the first niacin ER prescription and ≥29 days after the first prescription at the desired dose of niacin ER, (4) HDL-C measurements were available ≤6 months prior to and ≥29 days after filling the first prescription of niacin ER, and (5) gender was provided in the claims record.

2.2. Niacin ER Dose Levels. Prescription niacin ER was measured at 500 mg and 1000 mg doses. The two niacin ER dose groups were mutually exclusive, and all study participants were taking the niacin ER in combination with a statin. Individuals who qualified for the study in more than one dose group were categorized into the highest dose group for the purposes of this study.

2.3. Baseline Lipid Levels. Baseline lipid levels were taken within a six-month period prior to starting niacin ER at any dose and were dichotomized into the following groups for analysis: HDL-C levels for males and females combined (<40 mg/dL versus ≥40 mg/dL), HDL-C levels for males only (HDL-C<40 mg/dL versus ≥40 mg/dL), HDL-C levels for females only (HDL-C <50 mg/dL versus ≥50 mg/dL), LDL-C levels (<130 mg/dL versus ≥130 mg/dL), triglyceride (TG) levels <150 mg/dL versus ≥150 mg/dL), and total cholesterol (TC) levels (<200 mg/dL versus ≥200 mg/dL).

2.4. Change in HDL Effect. Follow-up HDL-C levels were included in the analysis after the first month of treatment with niacin ER (at the specific dose of interest) through 5 days after termination of niacin ER. The distribution of change in HDL-C effect was evaluated with 5% intervals by gender and also by dose of niacin ER. For the purposes of statistical analysis, the change in HDL-C effect was measured in two ways: (1) as a continuous variable and (2) dichotomized into high versus low response, in which high response was defined as an HDL-C effect of >15% and low response was HDL-C <5%. These cut points were selected based on a combination of the distribution of HDL-C response in our sample and a meaningful clinical response to niacin ER.

2.5. Statistical Analysis. Baseline demographic characteristics and lipid levels were summarized as frequencies and percentages. The change in HDL-C effect between baseline and followup was quantified by the difference and divided by the baseline value and then summarized using mean values and standard deviations. The Student's t-test was used to test the null hypothesis that there was no difference in the mean HDL-C effect by dichotomous categorical variables. The F-statistic was used to test the null hypothesis that there was no difference in the mean HDL-C effect across variables with three or more categories. Crude and adjusted multivariate logistic regression models were then developed to evaluate HDL-C response to niacin ER at the 500 mg dose level by calculating an odds ratio (OR) and 95% confidence interval (CI). As described above, our main analysis defined high responders as individuals with an HDL-C effect of >15% and low responders were defined as individuals with a <5% HDL-C effect. The outcomes in these models were high response (yes or no).

A sensitivity analysis was also conducted where high response was defined as a combination of HDL-C rise of >15% and LDL-C lowering effect of >−15%, and low response was defined as <5% HDL-C effect and LDL-C effect was >−15%. This restricted definition was used to ensure that subjects were taking their combination medications of niacin and a statin but not achieving the anticipated rise in HDL-C. Crude and adjusted multivariate logistic regression models were developed using this restricted definition to evaluate HDL-C response to niacin ER at the 500 mg dose level.

3. Results

Our sample included a total of 834 study participants (680 at the 500 mg niacin ER dose level, and 154 at the 1000 mg niacin ER dose level). Table 1 summarizes the baseline characteristics and lipid levels of the study participants by niacin ER dose level. The majority of study participants in each niacin ER dose level were 41 to 65 years of age, male, had HDL-C levels <40 mg/dL, had baseline LDL-C levels <130 mg/dL, and had baseline triglyceride levels ≥150 mg/dL. The majority of study participants in the 500 mg niacin ER dose group had baseline total cholesterol levels ≥200 mg, while the majority of the study participants in the 1000 mg niacin ER dose group had baseline total cholesterol levels <200 mg/dL. The proportion of study participants who had diabetes, stroke (within six months), hypertension (within six months), and ischemic heart disease (within six months) were similar in both dose groups. The average persistence of niacin ER was 193.6 days in the 500 mg dose group and 192.1 in the 1000 mg dose group.

Figure 1 illustrates the distribution of HDL-C effect by niacin ER dose and baseline lipid levels, and Table 2 reports the results of the inferential statistics of the overall HDL-C effect by niacin ER dose. There was a statistically significant change in the mean HDL-C effect between baseline and follow-up HDL-C levels in the 500 mg niacin ER dose group for both males (mean HDL-C effect = 0.08, $P < 0.001$) and females (mean HDL-C effect = 0.10, $P = 0.019$). Similar results were observed in the 1000 mg niacin ER dose group for males (mean HDL-C effect = 0.08, $P = 0.029$) and females (mean HDL-C effect = 0.19, $P = 0.048$). Females had statistically significantly higher levels of both baseline and follow-up HDL-C levels than males in both niacin ER dose groups. In addition, there was a statistically significant difference in the HDL-C effect observed among females across the niacin ER dose groups ($P = 0.021$). This trend was not observed among males ($P = 0.768$). There was a statistically significant change in the mean HDL-C effect between baseline and follow-up HDL-C levels in both niacin ER dose groups among individuals of 41 to 65 years of age (mean HDL-C effect in the 500 mg dose group = 0.08, $P < 0.001$; mean HDL-C effect in the 1000 mg dose group = 0.12, $P = 0.008$), but not among individuals in the 18 to 40 or ≥66 age groups. The mean HDL-C levels were statistically significantly higher in the >66-year age group than the other age groups at baseline ($P = 0.03$) and followup ($P = 0.018$) among participants in the 500 mg niacin ER dose group but not in the 1000 mg niacin ER dose group. The change in the mean HDL-C effect between baseline and follow-up HDL-C levels was statistically significant for individuals with HDL-C levels <40 mg/dL in the 500 mg niacin ER dose group (mean HDL-C effect = 0.12, $P < 0.001$) and also for individuals in the 1000 mg niacin ER dose group (mean HDL-C effect = 0.13, $P < 0.001$). There was no change in the HDL-C effect among individuals with HDL-C levels ≥40 mg/dL in either niacin ER dose group. When baseline LDL-C levels were stratified at 130 mg/dL, there was a statistically significant difference in the mean HDL-C effect between baseline and follow-up HDL-C levels among individuals who had LDL-C levels <130 mg/dL (mean HDL-C effect = 0.07, $P = 0.025$) and among those who had LDL-C ≥130 (mean HDL-C effect = 0.08, $P = 0.031$) in the 500 mg niacin ER dose. Among individuals in the 1000 mg niacin ER dose group, only individuals with LDL-C levels <130 showed a statistically significant improvement in the mean HDL-C effect (mean HDL-C effect = 0.12, $P = 0.008$). The mean HDL-C effect was statistically significantly higher among individuals with triglyceride levels ≥150 mg/dL (mean HDL-C effect = 0.08, $P < 0.001$) in the 500 mg niacin ER dose group and among individuals in that TG category in the 1000 mg niacin ER dose group (HDL-C effect = 0.12, $P = 0.005$). There were no significant changes in the HDL-C effect in either niacin ER dose group among individuals with triglyceride levels <150 mg/dL. There was a statistically significant difference in the mean HDL-C effect among individuals with total cholesterol levels <200 mg/dL (mean HDL-C effect = 0.09,

Table 1: Baseline characteristics and lipid levels[1].

Demographics and lipids	500 mg niacin ER dose (n = 680) n (%)	1000 mg niacin ER dose (n = 154) n (%)
Age (years)		
18 to 40	79 (11.6)	12 (7.8)
41 to 65	516 (75.9)	131 (85.1)
≥66	85 (12.5)	11 (7.1)
Gender		
Male	480 (70.6)	120 (77.9)
Female	200 (29.4)	34 (22.1)
HDL-C mg/dL (both genders)		
<40	419 (61.6)	87 (56.5)
40 to 59	213 (31.3)	59 (38.3)
≥60	44 (6.5)	8 (5.2)
Baseline LDL-C mg/dL		
<130	266 (39.1)	87 (56.5)
≥130	178 (26.2)	34 (22.1)
Unknown	236 (34.7)	33 (21.4)
Baseline TG mg/dL		
<150	192 (28.2)	60 (39.0)
≥150	483 (71.0)	93 (60.4)
Unknown	5 (0.7)	1 (0.7)
Baseline TC mg/dL		
<200	301 (44.3)	96 (62.3)
≥200	375 (55.2)	57 (37.0)
Unknown	4 (0.6)	1 (0.7)
Comorbidities		
Diabetes	188 (27.7)	41 (26.6)
Stroke (within 6 months)	26 (3.8)	10 (6.5)
Hypertension (within 6 months)	46 (6.8)	7 (4.6)
Ischemic heart disease (within 6 months)	130 (19.1)	32 (20.8)
Medication use		
Prestatin users	258 (37.9)	64 (41.6)
Prefibric acid users	82 (12.1)	12 (7.8)
Persistence		
Average persistence (days)	193.6	192.1
≥365 days persistence	79 (11.6)	17 (11.0)
<365 days persistence	601 (88.4)	137 (89.0)

[1]Lipid levels were measured within six months prior to any niacin ER use. Definition of lipids: HDL-C: high-density lipoprotein cholesterol; LDL-C: low-density lipoprotein cholesterol; TG: triglycerides; TC: total cholesterol.

TABLE 2: Overall HDL effect by niacin ER dose.

Demographics and lipids	500 mg niacin ER dose					1000 mg niacin ER dose					P value[b]
	n	Baseline HDL-C levels Mean (SD)	Follow-up HDL-C levels Mean (SD)	HDL-C effect Mean (SD)	P value[a]	n	Baseline HDL-C levels Mean (SD)	Follow-up HDL-C levels Mean (SD)	HDL-C effect Mean (SD)	P value[a]	
Gender											
Males	480	37.1 (0.4)	39.4 (0.4)	0.08 (0.01)	<0.001	120	39.0 (0.9)	41.6 (0.9)	0.08 (0.02)	0.029	0.768[b]
Females	200	45.5 (1.1)	49.3 (1.2)	0.10 (0.01)	0.019	34	48.5 (2.6)	57.4 (3.6)	0.19 (0.03)	0.048	0.021[b]
P value[c]		<0.001	<0.001	0.221			0.001	<0.001	0.009		0.053[d]
Age (years)											
18 to 40	79	37.9 (1.2)	40.0 (1.1)	0.10 (0.04)	0.196	12	38.9 (2.9)	40.4 (1.7)	0.07 (0.05)	0.659	0.660[b]
41 to 65	516	39.4 (0.5)	42.2 (0.6)	0.08 (0.01)	<0.001	131	41.3 (1.1)	45.8 (1.3)	0.12 (0.02)	0.008	0.057[b]
≥66	85	42.5 (1.4)	45.5 (1.4)	0.08 (0.02)	0.126	11	41.2 (2.2)	41.9 (1.8)	0.03 (0.05)	0.803	0.335[b]
P value[d]		0.032	0.018	0.842			0.799	0.343	0.242		0.613[d]
HDL-C mg/dL (both genders)											
40	423	32.8 (0.3)	36.3 (0.4)	0.12 (0.01)	<0.001	87	33.5 (0.5)	37.7 (0.8)	0.13 (0.02)	<0.001	0.437[b]
≥40	257	50.8 (0.7)	52.3 (0.8)	0.03 (0.01)	0.168	67	50.9 (1.2)	54.7 (1.9)	0.07 (0.02)	0.096	0.094[b]
P value[c]		<0.001	<0.001	<0.001			<0.001	<0.001	0.037		0[d]
LDL-C mg/dL											
<130	264	39.0 (0.7)	41.3 (0.8)	0.07 (0.01)	0.025	88	40.6 (1.1)	44.9 (1.2)	0.12 (0.02)	0.008	0.160[b]
≥130	176	41.8 (0.9)	44.6 (1.0)	0.08 (0.02)	0.031	33	44.7 (2.7)	48.9 (3.5)	0.09 (0.03)	0.344	0.802[b]
P value[c]		0.011	0.006	0.474			0.161	0.291	0.489		0.472[d]
TG mg/dL											
<150	192	44.0 (1.1)	46.5 (1.1)	0.08 (0.02)	0.102	60	46.6 (1.6)	50.4 (2.2)	0.08 (0.02)	0.166	0.899[b]
≥150	483	38.0 (0.4)	40.9 (0.5)	0.08 (0.01)	<0.001	93	37.6 (1.0)	41.8 (1.1)	0.12 (0.02)	0.005	0.060[b]
P value[c]		<0.001	<0.001	0.943			<0.001	0.001	0.111		0.362[d]
TC mg/dL											
<200	301	36.8 (0.6)	39.5 (0.6)	0.09 (0.01)	0.001	96	39.6 (1.0)	43.7 (1.2)	0.11 (0.02)	0.007	0.362[b]
≥200	375	42.2 (0.6)	44.9 (0.7)	0.08 (0.01)	0.004	57	43.7 (1.9)	47.6 (2.4)	0.10 (0.03)	0.200	0.530[b]
P value[c]		<0.001	<0.001	0.259			0.052	0.144	0.549		0.195[d]

Definition of lipids: HDL-C: high-density lipoprotein cholesterol; LDL-C: low-density lipoprotein cholesterol; TG: triglycerides; TC: total cholesterol.
[a] P value tested the null hypothesis that there is no difference in the baseline and follow-up HDL-C levels using the Student's t-test.
[b] P value tested the null hypotheses that there is no difference in the mean HDL-C effect across niacin ER dose groups using the Student's t-test.
[c] P value tested the null hypothesis that there is no difference in the mean HDL-C effect across each risk factor/lipid level category using the Student's t-test.
[d] P value tested the null hypothesis that there is no difference in the mean HDL-C effect across each risk factor/lipid level category using the F-statistic.

$P = 0.001$) and among individuals with total cholesterol levels ≥200 mg/dL (mean HDL-C effect = 0.08, $P = 0.004$) in the 500 mg niacin ER dose group, but only among individuals with total cholesterol levels <200 mg/dL in the 1000 mg niacin ER dose group (mean HDL-C effect = 0.011, $P = 0.007$).

Table 3 summarizes the results of the univariate and multivariate logistic regression models that evaluated the predictors of high response to the 500 mg dose of niacin ER. The only statistically significant predictors of response to niacin ER in the univariate models were triglyceride levels >150 mg/dL and low HDL-C levels (<40 mg/dL for males and <50 mg/dL for females). Triglyceride levels did not maintain statistical significance in the multivariate model. However, both males and females with low HDL-C levels exhibited a strong response to treatment in the multivariate model (males, HDL-C <40 mg/dL: OR = 5.18, 95% CI: 2.36–11.39; females, HDL-C <50 mg/dL: OR = 5.40, 95% CI: 1.84–15.79). Similar, but attenuated, trends were observed in the multivariate sensitivity analysis model (males, HDL-C <40 mg/dL: OR = 4.90, 95% CI: 1.56–15.46; females, HDL-C <50 mg/dL: OR = 2.34, 95% CI: 0.61–9.04) (data not shown).

4. Discussion

Approximately one-quarter of the adult population in the USA has low HDL-C [8]. The causes of low HDL-C levels are largely unknown; however, there is evidence to suggest that being overweight or obese, having limited physical activity, smoking, increased intake of carbohydrates, Type II diabetes,

Table 3: Predictors of response to niacin ER (500 mg dose).

	High responder[1] (n = 202) n (%)	Low responder[2] (n = 305) n (%)	Crude OR (95% CI)[3]	Adjusted OR (95% CI)[3,4]
Age (years, continuous)	—	—	0.10 (0.97–1.02)	1.0 (0.97–1.03)
Gender				
Female	39 (32.5%)	53 (29.1%)	1.0	1.0
Male	81 (67.5%)	129 (70.9%)	0.85 (0.52–1.40)	0.79 (0.25–2.51)
HDL-C mg/dL (males only)				
≥40	49 (40.8%)	111 (61.0%)	1.0	1.0
40	71 (59.2%)	71 (39.0%)	2.27 (1.42–3.63)	5.18 (2.36–11.39)
HDL-C mg/dL (females only)				
≥50	87 (72.5%)	155 (85.2%)	1.0	1.0
<50	33 (27.5%)	27 (14.8%)	2.18 (1.23–3.86)	5.40 (1.84–15.79)
LDL-C mg/dL				
<130	69 (57.5%)	103 (56.6%)	1.0	1.0
≥130	51 (42.5%)	79 (43.4%)	0.96 (0.61–1.54)	1.23 (0.54–2.77)
TG mg/dL				
<150	32 (26.7%)	71 (39.0%)	1.0	1.0
≥150	88 (73.3%)	111 (61.0%)	1.76 (1.06–2.91)	1.38 (0.76–2.50)
TC mg/dL				
<200	62 (51.7%)	85 (46.7%)	1.0	1.0
≥200	58 (48.3%)	97 (53.3%)	0.82 (0.52–1.30)	1.0 (0.42–2.34)
Diabetes				
No	82 (68.3%)	138 (75.8%)	1.0	1.0
Yes	38 (31.7%)	44 (24.2%)	1.45 (0.87–2.43)	1.41 (0.78–2.52)
Stroke (within 6 months)				
No	114 (95.0%)	174 (95.6%)	1.0	1.0
Yes	6 (5.0%)	8 (4.4%)	1.15 (0.39–3.39)	0.69 (0.19–2.49)
Hypertension (within 6 months)				
No	108 (90.0%)	171 (94.0%)	1.0	1.0
Yes	12 (10.0%)	11 (6.0%)	1.73 (0.74–4.05)	1.91 (0.71–5.15)
Ischemic heart disease (within 6 months)				
No	97 (80.8%)	147 (80.8%)	1.0	1.0
Yes	23 (19.2%)	35 (19.2%)	1.0 (0.56–1.79)	0.91 (0.44–1.87)
Statin use during baseline				
No	50 (41.7%)	63 (34.6%)	1.0	1.0
Yes	70 (58.3%)	119 (65.4%)	0.74 (0.46–1.19)	0.69 (0.37–1.31)
Fibric acid use during Baseline				
No	10 (8.3%)	22 (12.1%)	1.0	1.0
Yes	110 (91.7%)	160 (87.9%)	1.51 (0.69–3.32)	1.60 (0.69–3.75)

Definition of lipids: HDL-C: high-density lipoprotein cholesterol; LDL-C: low-density lipoprotein cholesterol; TG: triglycerides; TC: total cholesterol.
[1]High responder: HDL-C effect > 15%.
[2]Low responder: HDL-C effect < 5%.
[3]Outcome is high responder.
[4]Adjusted model includes all variables listed in the table.

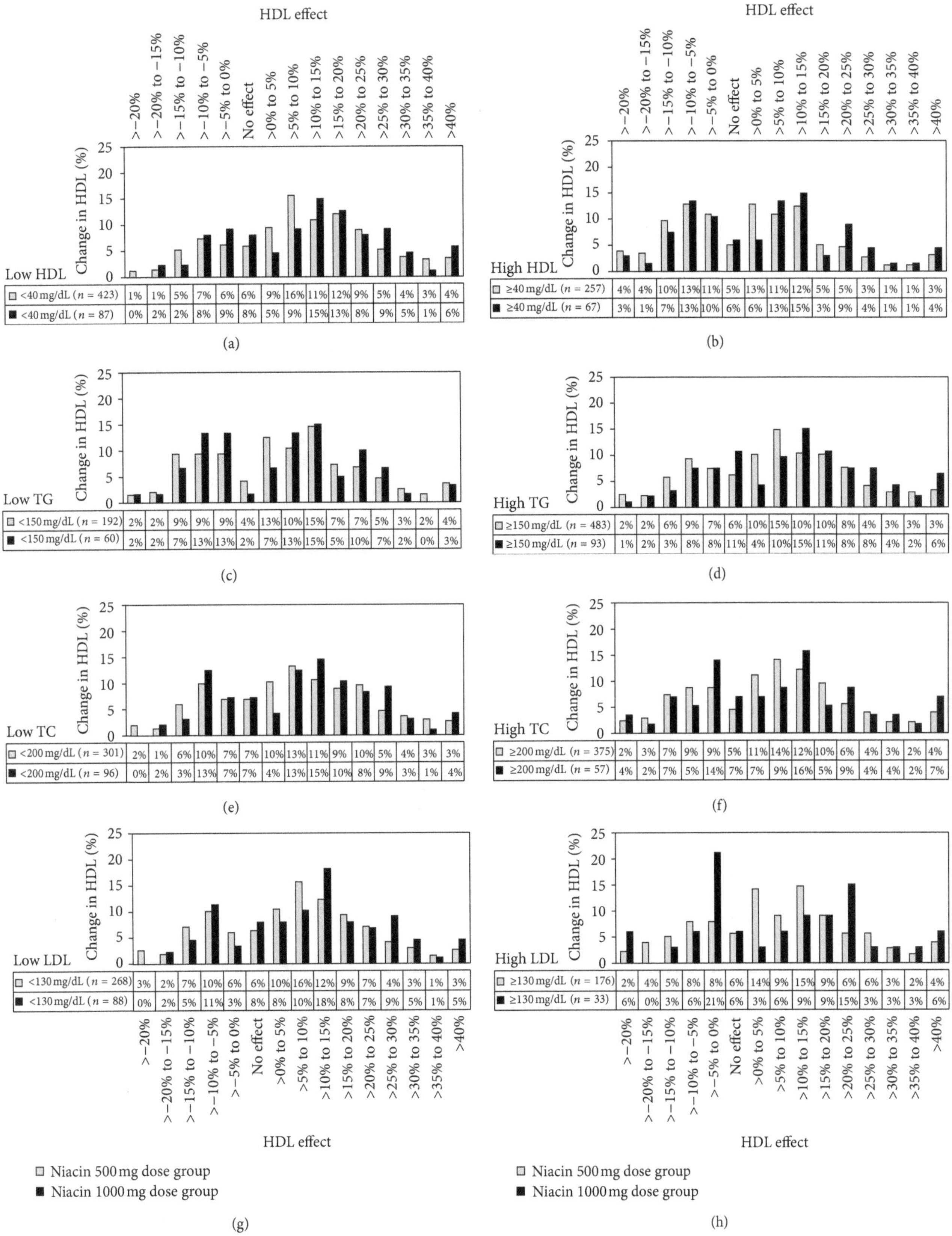

	>−20%	>−20% to −15%	>−15% to −10%	>−10% to −5%	>−5% to 0%	No effect	>0% to 5%	>5% to 10%	>10% to 15%	>15% to 20%	>20% to 25%	>25% to 30%	>30% to 35%	>35% to 40%	>40%
(a) Niacin 500 mg, <40 mg/dL (n = 423)	1%	1%	5%	7%	6%	6%	9%	16%	11%	12%	9%	5%	4%	3%	4%
(a) Niacin 1000 mg, <40 mg/dL (n = 87)	0%	2%	2%	8%	9%	8%	5%	9%	15%	13%	8%	9%	5%	1%	6%
(b) Niacin 500 mg, ≥40 mg/dL (n = 257)	4%	4%	10%	13%	11%	5%	13%	11%	12%	5%	5%	3%	1%	1%	3%
(b) Niacin 1000 mg, ≥40 mg/dL (n = 67)	3%	1%	7%	13%	10%	6%	6%	13%	15%	3%	9%	4%	1%	1%	4%
(c) Niacin 500 mg, <150 mg/dL (n = 192)	2%	2%	9%	9%	9%	4%	13%	10%	15%	7%	7%	5%	3%	2%	4%
(c) Niacin 1000 mg, <150 mg/dL (n = 60)	2%	2%	7%	13%	13%	2%	7%	13%	15%	5%	10%	7%	2%	0%	3%
(d) Niacin 500 mg, ≥150 mg/dL (n = 483)	2%	2%	6%	9%	7%	6%	10%	15%	10%	10%	8%	4%	3%	3%	3%
(d) Niacin 1000 mg, ≥150 mg/dL (n = 93)	1%	2%	3%	8%	8%	11%	4%	10%	15%	11%	8%	8%	4%	2%	6%
(e) Niacin 500 mg, <200 mg/dL (n = 301)	2%	1%	6%	10%	7%	7%	10%	13%	11%	9%	10%	5%	4%	3%	3%
(e) Niacin 1000 mg, <200 mg/dL (n = 96)	0%	2%	3%	13%	7%	7%	4%	13%	15%	10%	8%	9%	3%	1%	4%
(f) Niacin 500 mg, ≥200 mg/dL (n = 375)	2%	3%	7%	9%	9%	5%	11%	14%	12%	10%	6%	4%	3%	2%	4%
(f) Niacin 1000 mg, ≥200 mg/dL (n = 57)	4%	2%	7%	5%	14%	7%	7%	9%	16%	5%	9%	4%	4%	2%	7%
(g) Niacin 500 mg, <130 mg/dL (n = 268)	3%	2%	7%	10%	6%	6%	10%	16%	12%	9%	7%	4%	3%	1%	3%
(g) Niacin 1000 mg, <130 mg/dL (n = 88)	0%	2%	5%	11%	3%	8%	8%	10%	18%	8%	7%	9%	5%	1%	5%
(h) Niacin 500 mg, ≥130 mg/dL (n = 176)	2%	4%	5%	8%	8%	6%	14%	9%	15%	9%	6%	6%	3%	2%	4%
(h) Niacin 1000 mg, ≥130 mg/dL (n = 33)	6%	0%	3%	6%	21%	6%	3%	6%	9%	9%	15%	3%	3%	3%	6%

Figure 1: HDL effect by niacin ER dose and baseline lipid levels: (a) low HDL (<40 mg/dL), (b) high HDL (>40 mg/dL), (c) low TG (<150 mg/dL), (d) high TG (>150 mg/dL), (e) low TC (<200 mg/dL), (f) high TC (>200 mg/dL), (g) low LDL (<130 mg/dL), and (h) high LDL (≥130 mg/dL).

genetic factors, and the use of some medications (i.e., beta-blockers, anabolic steroids, and progestational agents) may increase the likelihood of having low HDL-C [13]. A recent evaluation of data from the National Health and Nutrition Examination Survey (NHANES) identified several factors that were associated with HDL-C levels among *both* men and women. Specifically, being obese, having high apolipoprotein B levels (>117 mg/dL), and having high triglyceride levels (≥200 mg/dL) were shown to be associated with low HDL-C levels, while increased age (65 years or older) and having elevated total cholesterol (>240 mg/dL) were shown to be associated with elevated HDL-C levels [4].

The clinical management of HDL-C is a somewhat vexing topic for several reasons. First, treatment with dyslipidemic pharmacotherapy, primarily niacin, has been shown to increase HDL-C levels by as much as 35% in some populations [6–9]. However, the manner in which these positive increases translate into reduced morbidity and mortality has been disappointing in recent studies. Results from the AIM-HIGH study showed a lack of efficacy in reducing cardiovascular-related events after 3.5 years, which led to the early termination of this study [4]. Second, niacin is known to cause cutaneous vasodilatation with flushing, which may include itching, tingling, warmth, and redness, which can lead to poor adherence or early discontinuation [14, 15]. A cohort study of 2,369 individuals who were newly prescribed dyslipidemic agents reported a one-year probability of discontinuation of 46% for niacin versus 15% for lovastatin [4, 16].

Overall, our results showed that treatment with niacin ER at both the 500 mg and 1000 mg dose levels significantly increased HDL-C levels in both men and women. However, the average increase we observed was much lower than the 35% increase that has been observed in some populations. In our study, females had significantly higher levels of both baseline and follow-up HDL-C levels than males in both niacin ER dose groups. Furthermore, there was a statistically significant difference in the HDL-C effect observed among females across the niacin ER dose groups. This trend was not observed among males. When the association between age and effect of treatment was evaluated, the only statistically significant change in the mean HDL-C effect between baseline and follow-up HDL-C levels in both niacin ER dose groups was among individuals of 41 to 65 years of age. The mean HDL-C levels were statistically significantly higher in the >66-year age group compared with the younger age groups at both baseline and follow-up HDL-C measurements among participants in the 500 mg niacin ER dose group but not in the 1000 mg niacin ER dose group.

It is because of these paradoxical associations that we sought to identify factors that predict response to niacin ER, with the goal of providing useful information that may lead to the most efficient and successful prescription patterns for this treatment. Unfortunately, we were not able to conduct univariate and multivariate models for those treated with niacin ER at the 1000 mg dose due to a smaller sample size. However, we did find that baseline HDL-C levels were the only factor that significantly predicted a high response to treatment with niacin ER at the 500 mg dose level in the multivariate models. These results provide some insight into the factors that are associated with the effect of niacin treatment.

Limitations of our study may include the manner in which high response to niacin ER was classified. High response was defined as an HDL-C effect of >15% and low response was defined as <5% HDL-C effect. These thresholds were selected based on the distribution of response in our sample irrespective of characteristics and determined to be clinically meaningful responses. Modifications in these thresholds may have resulted in a slight change in our findings. However, we conducted a sensitivity analysis among people who were responding to taking their medications by including only those who had an LDL-C decrease of 15% or greater and our findings were consistent. Although monitoring prescription fills and biomarker response is not identical to consuming the medication, this method was the most accurate way of estimating actual medication use in a large population. In addition, clinical variables such as body mass index, exercise, diet, and smoking were not available in this healthcare claims database. We did not include other medications that may control HDL-C levels, such as statins, in our models. However, the majority of the patients included in this study were taking simvastatin at 20 mg or 40 mg doses. There is evidence to suggest that statins (as a drug class) only modestly increase HDL-C levels, with less than a 10% increase reported in two studies [16, 17]. Finally, the quality control of laboratory measurements is assumed but cannot be verified. The laboratory values provided in the database are those that were provided by the laboratory vendor. As such, the specific laboratory methods or reference ranges that correspond with the lipid values are not available. Despite these limitations, the strengths of this study include the large sample size, which allowed us to evaluate a highly stratified matrix of response to treatment.

In summary, individuals with low HDL-C levels at baseline may have an increased risk of CHD-related events; however, the issues surrounding the pharmacological management of HDL-C are complex. We have shown that low baseline HDL-C levels are the strongest predictor of high response from the treatment of niacin ER at the 500 mg dose level, among statin-treated individuals. We have also shown that both men and women had a significant increase in the mean HDL-C effect between baseline and followup, regardless of niacin ER dose. These findings can help clinicians and researchers better understand the extent to which response to niacin ER is variable and the importance of baseline HDL-C influencing response size while further data is generated to elucidate the value of HDL-C-raising therapy.

Acknowledgments

All the authors met the criteria for authorship set forth by the International Committee for Medical Journal Editors. J. B. Christian and E. J. Olson made substantial contributions to conception, study design, and interpretation of data. J. B. Christian and J. K. Allen were responsible for the acquisition of data and analytic plan. K. A. Lowe was responsible for preparing the figures and tables, drafting a significant portion of the paper, and providing editorial support. J. B. Christian, E. J. Olson, and J. K. Allen are employees of and hold equity interest in GlaxoSmithKline. None of the authors have a financial conflict associated with paper. Editorial support in the form of development of draft outline and first draft of paper, editorial suggestions to draft versions of this paper, assembling tables and figures, collating author comments, copyediting, fact checking, and referencing were provided by Exponent Health Sciences and was funded by GlaxoSmithKline.

References

[1] B. J. Ansell, K. E. Watson, A. M. Fogelman, M. Navab, and G. C. Fonarow, "High-density lipoprotein function: recent advances," *Journal of the American College of Cardiology*, vol. 46, no. 10, pp. 1792–1798, 2005.

[2] A. Morrison and J. E. Hokanson, "The independent relationship between triglycerides and coronary heart disease," *Vascular Health and Risk Management*, vol. 5, pp. 89–95, 2009.

[3] E. J. Schaefer, S. Lamon-Fava, J. M. Ordovas et al., "Factors associated with low and elevated plasma high density lipoprotein cholesterol and apolipoprotein A-I levels in the Framingham Offspring Study," *Journal of Lipid Research*, vol. 35, no. 5, pp. 871–882, 1994.

[4] W. E. Boden, J. L. Probstfield, T. Anderson et al., "Niacin in patients with low HDL cholesterol levels receiving intensive statin therapy," *The New England Journal of Medicine*, vol. 365, no. 24, pp. 2255–2267, 2011.

[5] "Prevalence of abnormal lipid levels among youths—United States, 1999-2006," *MMWR. Morbidity and Mortality Weekly Report*, vol. 59, no. 2, pp. 29–33, 2010.

[6] R. S. Birjmohun, J. J. P. Kastelein, D. Poldermans, E. S. G. Stroes, U. Hostalek, and G. Assmann, "Safety and tolerability of prolonged-release nicotinic acid in statin-treated patients," *Current Medical Research and Opinion*, vol. 23, no. 7, pp. 1707–1713, 2007.

[7] P. P. Toth, V. Zarotsky, J. M. Sullivan, and D. Laitinen, "Niacin and fibrate use among patients with high triglycerides and low high-density lipoprotein cholesterol," *Current Medical Research and Opinion*, vol. 25, no. 6, pp. 1355–1363, 2009.

[8] J. B. Christian, N. E. Bourgeois, and K. A. Lowe, "Prevalence, clinical characteristics and treatment patterns of low high-density lipoprotein cholesterol in the US population: National Health and Nutrition Examination Survey 2005-2008," *Journal of Cardiovascular Medicine*, vol. 12, no. 10, pp. 714–722, 2011.

[9] P. P. Toth, V. Zarotsky, J. M. Sullivan, and D. Laitinen, "Dyslipidemia treatment of patients with diabetes mellitus in a US managed care plan: a retrospective database analysis," *Cardiovascular Diabetology*, vol. 8, article 26, 2009.

[10] B. Alemayehu, E. Buysman, D. Parry, L. Becker, and F. Nathan, "Economic burden and healthcare utilization associated with castration-resistant prostate cancer in a commercial and Medicare Advantage US patient population," *Journal of Medical Economics*, vol. 13, no. 2, pp. 351–361, 2010.

[11] J. B. Christian, B. Arondekar, E. K. Buysman et al., "Clinical and economic benefits observed when follow-up triglyceride levels are less than 500 mg/dL in patients with severe hypertriglyceridemia," *Journal of Clinical Lipidology*, vol. 6, no. 5, pp. 450–461, 2012.

[12] S. A. Williams, E. K. Buysman, E. M. Hulbert et al., "Hemoglobin A1c outcomes and health care resource use in type 2 diabetes mellitus patients treated with combination oral antidiabetic drugs through step therapy and loose-dose and fixed-dose combinations," *Managed Care*, vol. 21, pp. 40–48, 2012.

[13] "Third Report of the National Cholesterol Education Program (NCEP) Expert Panel on Detection, Evaluation, and Treatment of High Blood Cholesterol in Adults (Adult Treatment Panel III) final report," *Circulation*, vol. 106, no. 25, pp. 3143–3421, 2002.

[14] T. A. Jacobson, "A "hot" topic in dyslipidemia management—"how to beat a flush": optimizing Niacin tolerability to promote long-term treatment adherence and coronary disease prevention," *Mayo Clinic Proceedings*, vol. 85, no. 4, pp. 365–379, 2010.

[15] S. Kamal-Bahl, D. J. Watson, and B. M. Ambegaonkar, "Patients' experiences of niacin-induced flushing in clinical practice: a structured telephone interview," *Clinical Therapeutics*, vol. 31, no. 1, pp. 130–140, 2009.

[16] C. L. Shear, F. A. Franklin, S. Stinnett et al., "Expanded Clinical Evaluation of Lovastatin (EXCEL) Study results: effect of patient characteristics on lovastatin-induced changes in plasma concentrations of lipids and lipoproteins," *Circulation*, vol. 85, no. 4, pp. 1293–1303, 1992.

[17] A. S. Wierzbicki and D. P. Mikhailidis, "Dose-response effects of atorvastatin and simvastatin on high-density lipoprotein cholesterol in hypercholesterolaemic patients: a review of five comparative studies," *International Journal of Cardiology*, vol. 84, no. 1, pp. 53–57, 2002.

Leishmania major Self-Limited Infection Increases Blood Cholesterol and Promotes Atherosclerosis Development

Luciana R. Fernandes,[1] Ana Cecília C. Ribeiro,[1] Marcela Segatto,[1] Luís Felipe F. F. Santos,[1] Joana Amaral,[2] Luciane R. Portugal,[1] and Jacqueline I. A. Leite[1]

[1] *Departamento de Bioquímica e Imunologia, Universidade Federal Minas Gerais, 31270-901 Belo Horizonte, MG, Brazil*
[2] *Centro Universitário, Av. Prof. Mário Werneck, 1685-Estoril, 30455-610 Belo Horizonte, MG, Brazil*

Correspondence should be addressed to Jacqueline I. A. Leite; jalvarezleite@gmail.com

Academic Editor: Gloria L. Vega

Leishmania major infection of resistant mice causes a self-limited lesion characterized by macrophage activation and a Th1 proinflammatory response. Atherosclerosis is an inflammatory disease involving hypercholesterolemia and macrophage activation. In this study, we evaluated the influence of *L. major* infection on the development of atherosclerosis using atherosclerosis-susceptible apolipoprotein E-deficient (apoE KO) mice. After 6 weeks of infection, apoE KO mice exhibited reduced footpad swelling and parasitemia similar to C57BL/6 controls, confirming that both strains are resistant to infection with *L. major*. *L. major*-infected mice had increased plasma cholesterol levels and reduced triacylglycerols. With regard to atherosclerosis, noninfected mice developed only fatty streak lesions, while the infected mice presented with advanced lesions containing a necrotic core and an abundant inflammatory infiltrate. CD36 expression was increased in the aortic valve of the infected mice, indicating increased macrophage activation. In conclusion, *L. major* infection, although localized and self-limited in resistant apoE KO mice, has a detrimental effect on the blood lipid profile, increases the inflammatory cell migration to atherosclerotic lesions, and promotes atherogenesis. These effects are consequences of the stimulation of the immune system by *L. major*, which promotes the inflammatory components of atherosclerosis, which are primarily the parasite-activated macrophages.

1. Introduction

Leishmania major is a protozoan parasite transmitted by sandflies of the genus *Lutzomyia* that inject the promastigote form into the dermis of the host. Once injected, the parasite is rapidly enclosed by phagocytic cells and transforms into the replicative intracellular amastigote form [1]. In immunocompetent hosts, such as C57BL/6 mice, *L. major* infection is a self-contained cutaneous lesion that elicits a Th1 immune response. In infected mice, the immune cells (macrophages, dendritic cells, natural killer cells, and T cells) produce cytokines and bioactive molecules, such as IFN-γ, IL-12, and nitric oxide (NO), which act against the protozoan [1].

Atherosclerosis is a chronic inflammatory disease associated with a high level of total cholesterol and proatherogenic lipoproteins (VLDL, IDL, and LDL), a prothrombotic status, and a Th1-polarized immune response [2, 3]. Macrophage and endothelial cell activation by atypical lipoproteins and proinflammatory cytokines induces the production of adhesion molecules, cytokines and chemokines, and causes oxidative stress [4]. Among atherosclerosis risk factors, infection plays an important role in the perpetuation of chronic inflammation at the atherosclerotic site [5, 6]. Several studies suggest that pathogens, such as bacteria, viruses, and protozoa, contribute to the atherogenesis process [7–11]. The increased inflammation caused by these pathogens promotes macrophage activation and migration to the atheroprone site. Alternatively, proatherogenic status may be attributed to the systemic oxidative stress induced by infection, which enhances lipoprotein or endothelium oxidation. Pathogens involved in atherosclerosis development usually induce a systemic infection instead of a localized infection such as an *L. major* infection. However, even localized infections, such as odontologic ones, may be associated with the development of atherosclerosis [12].

Apolipoprotein (apo) E is a component of chylomicron and very low-density lipoproteins (VLDL) and mediates the uptake of these lipoproteins and possesses anti-inflammatory and antioxidant effects [13]. ApoE KO mice have impaired clearance of VLDL and chylomicrons from the blood, which results in hypercholesterolemia and favors the development of atherosclerotic lesions [11]. ApoE also has anti-inflammatory and antioxidative properties, and its absence is partially responsible for the higher inflammatory profile of apoE-deficient animals compared to the wild-type control, C57BL/6 mice [14]. ApoE KO mice spontaneously develop atherosclerosis even when fed a normolipidemic diet [15]. The atherosclerotic lesions of apoE KO mice exhibit a similar distribution, microscopic appearance, and cellular composition to those found in humans. The atherosclerotic lesions are characterized by endothelial dysfunction, macrophage, and T cell infiltration and production of proinflammatory cytokines, such as TNF-α, INF-γ, and IL-6, which indicates a typical Th1 polarized immune response [2].

This work aimed to determine if a self-limited *L. major* infection would be sufficient to modify the lipid metabolism and promote the development of atherosclerosis similar to what occurs with systemic infections.

2. Material and Methods

This protocol was approved by the Animal Care Committee of Universidade Federal de Minas Gerais (CETEA #147/05).

2.1. Mice and Diet. Twenty-eight 11-week-old female apoE KO mice were separated into control (noninfected) and *Leishmania major* (*L. major*) infected groups. For the background control, twenty wild-type C57BL/6 mice were divided into control (noninfected) or *L. major* infected groups. Animals of both strains were equally distributed according to weight and blood cholesterol and were fed on AIN-93G standard diet [15].

2.2. Leishmania major Infection. The mice were infected with *L. major* (clone WHO MHOM/IL/80/Friedlin). The inoculum was prepared under sterile conditions from five-day *L. major* cultures, which corresponds to the stationary growth phase rich in the promastigote metacyclic infectious forms. The medium containing *L. major* was centrifuged, and the pellet was resuspended in 1 mL of PBS. Approximately 1×10^6 parasites were inoculated into the left footpad, and the right footpad was used as a control after inoculation with PBS as previously described [16]. The footpad was measured weekly with a caliper, and the amount of swelling was calculated as the difference between the measures of the infected (left) and control (right) footpads.

The animals' body weight and food intake were measured weekly for 6 weeks after infection. All groups received the same amount of food to avoid confounding the experiment with different amounts of nutrients. After 6 weeks and an overnight fast, the mice were euthanized under anesthesia. Plasma, footpads, and tissues were collected for subsequent analyses. The infected footpad was weighed without the skin and used for parasite quantification as previously described [16].

2.3. Lipids Assay. The total cholesterol, cholesterol in high density lipoprotein (HDLc) form, and triacylglycerols in the plasma were measured using commercial kits (Doles, Brazil) as previously described [17]. The amount of non-HDLc (that represents the atherogenic fractions VLDLc and IDLc) in the plasma was determined by calculating the difference between the total cholesterol and the HDLc.

The liver was washed in PBS and dried on filter paper. The contents of the cecum were separated from the lumen. The hepatic and cecal lipid extractions were performed as previously described by Folch et al. [18].

2.4. Histological Analysis. For the analysis of atherosclerosis, the aortic valves were washed with PBS, gently perfused with 10% neutral buffered formalin, and embedded in paraffin. The analysis was performed on 10 samples per group. The specimens were fixed in 3.7% paraformaldehyde and processed in paraffin. Briefly, every consecutive section (10 μm thick) through the aortic valve (300 μm) was taken and stained with hematoxylin and eosin [19]. The sections used for immunofluorescence were deparaffinized by 2 xylene washes (30 min) and then transferred to 3 washes (15 minutes each) of ethanol at concentrations of 100%, 85%, and 70%. The atherosclerotic lesion area was quantified using the Image Pro Plus software (Media Cybernetics, USA) from the sum of the atherosclerotic lesion areas obtained from the selected 10 sections, spaced 20 μm apart, as previously described [11]. The inflammatory cells per field were counted automatically by the Image Pro Plus software ($n = 5$ mice, 3 nonconsecutive sections per animal) [11].

2.5. L. major Parasitism. The DNA in liver and spleen was extracted with proteinase K (Qiagen USA) according to the manufacturer's instructions. A PCR analysis was conducted [20]. Briefly, 2 μL of DNA sample was added to 1.2 μL of Taq polymerase buffer, 1.0 μL of dNTPs (2.5 mM), 1.0 μL of primers, 0.05 μL of Taq polymerase, and 5.75 μL of Milli-Q sterile H_2O. The samples were placed in a thermocycler and the amplification conditions were as follows (35 cycles): denaturation at 94°C for 1 min, annealing at 54°C for 1 min, elongation at 72°C for 1.5 min, and extension at 72°C for 10 min. The PCR products were then subjected to gel electrophoresis polyacrylamide and visualized by silver staining. The sequences of the primers used, which correspond to the minicircle kDNA [20], are Uni 21-5′GGGGTTGGTGTAAAATAGGCC 3′ and LmJ4-5′CTA.

2.6. Immunofluorescence Staining. Cross-sections of the aortic roots were blocked with 4% (wt/vol) BSA in PBS. Next, sections were incubated for 1 h at 22°C with FITC-goat antibody to mouse CD11b (0.2 mg/mL, 1 : 200 dilution; Santa Cruz Biotechnology, USA). Sections stained with FITC IgG anti-goat antibody served as negative controls. Sections were mounted with Vectashield medium and were visualized with an Axioscope 2 Plus fluorescence microscope (Carl Zeiss).

2.7. RT-PCR. The popliteal lymph node was homogenized using the TH-01 (OMNI-INC). The total RNA from the lymph node and aortic valve was extracted using the TRIzol reagent according to the manufacturer's protocol. The reverse transcription was performed using 2 μg of the total RNA, 200 U of the reverse transcriptase, 2.5 μL of the 5X RT buffer, 1.8 μL of the 10 mM dNTPs, 0.2 μL of the 10000 U/mL RNasin, and 1.0 μL of the 50 μM oligo dT. The temperature settings for this reaction were 70°C for 5 min, on ice for 2 min, 42°C for 60 min, 70°C for 15 min, and 4°C for the final step. The resulting cDNA was used for real-time PCR as described later. The specific primers were designed using the Primer Express software and synthesized by IDT. Real-time PCR was carried out on a StepOne sequence detection system (Applied Biosystems) using the Power SYBR Green PCR Master Mix (Applied Biosystems). The dissociation curve indicated that only one product was obtained in each reaction. The relative levels of gene expression were determined using the $\Delta\Delta$ cycle threshold method as described by the manufacturer, in which data for each sample is normalized to the β-actin expression and the data are shown as the relative expression (the fold increase over the control). The PCR results were analyzed with the SDS 2.1 software (Applied Biosystems), and the amount of mRNA of each gene of interest was normalized to the amount of the murine β-actin gene. mRNA expression levels were calculated as the fold difference relative to the housekeeping gene by the formula: relative expression = $2^{-(\text{CT [target gene]}-\text{CT }[\beta\text{-actin-1}])}$.

The sequences of the primers used are as follows:

VCAM-1: 5′-CCCCAAGGATCCAGAGATTCA-3′ and 5′-ACTTGACCGTGACCGGCTT-3′;

CD36: 5′GTACAGATTTGTTCTTCCAGCCAAT-3′ and 5′-TCAGTGCAGAAACAATGGTTGTC-3′;

MCP1/CCL2: 5′-AGGAAGATCTCAGTGCAGAG-3′ and 5′-AGTCTTCGGAGTTTGCCTTTG-3′;

β-actin: 5′-CTGCCTGACGGCCAAGTC-3′ and 5′-CAAGAAGGAA GGCTGGAAAAGA-3′;

IL-6: 5′-ACAACCACGGCCTTCCCTACTT3′ and 5′-CACGATTTCCCAGAGAACATGTG-3′;

IFN-γ: 5′-TGGCTCTGCAGGATTTTCATG-3′ and 5′-TCAAGTGGCATAGATGTGGAAGAA-3′;

IL-10: 5′-GGTTGCCAAGCCTTATCGGA-3′ and 5′-ACCTGCTCCACTGCCTTGCT-3′;

IL-4: 5′-ACAGGAGAAGGGACGCCAT-3′ and 5′-GAAGCCCTACAGACGAGCTCA-3′;

LmjF36.5520: 5′-GGCCATCACCACAAACAGAG-3′ and 5-GCTCAGGTCATACAAGGGGA-3′.

2.8. Statistical Analyses. The data were initially analyzed by the Kolmogorov-Smirnov test to check their symmetry and by the Mann-Whitney or Student's t-test using GraphPad Prism, version 5.00, for Windows, GraphPad Software, San Diego, CA, USA. A P value of <0.05 was considered significant.

TABLE 1: Final body weight, food intake, and cecal and hepatic lipids of non-infected (control) and *L. major*-infected (*L. major*) apoE KO mice 6 weeks after the inoculation of 1×10^6 parasites (clone WHO MHOM/IL/80/Friedlin) into footpad.

Parameter	Control ApoE KO	*L. major* ApoE KO
Final body weight (g)	22.18 ± 0.77	20.67 ± 0.7
Food intake (g/week/mouse)	25.10 ± 0.95	24.72 ± 0.85
Liver lipids		
Total lipids (mg/g)	252.0 ± 12.0	172.0 ± 21.0*
Total cholesterol (mg/g)	14.1 ± 1.3	13.2 ± 0.9
Triacylglycerols (mg/g)	49.7 ± 4.4	30.2 ± 4.5*
Cecum lipids		
Total lipids (mg/g)	51.1 ± 8.9	70.0 ± 11
Total cholesterol (mg/g)	2.8 ± 0.3	2.4 ± 0.3
Triacylglycerols (mg/g)	0.97 ± 0.2	0.86 ± 0.21

Control group, $n = 8$–11, and *L. major* group, $n = 10$–13. Results are expressed as the means ± SE. $^*P \leq 0.05$.

3. Results

3.1. L. major Infection in ApoE KO and Wild-Type Control C57BL/6 Mice. Our first aim was to confirm that *L. major* causes a self-limited infection in apoE KO mice similar to that observed in the wild-type control C57BL/6 mice. The results showed that after 6 weeks of infection, although apoE KO mice presented higher levels of the cytokines TNF alpha and IL-10 (Figures 1(a) to 1(d)), these mice controlled parasite load and footpad swelling similarly to C57BL/6 mice (Figures 1(e) and 1(f)). Therefore, only apoE KO animals were used for further experiments.

There were no differences in the food intake between apoE experimental and control groups. As expected, *L. major* infection did not cause a significant weight loss in these animals (Table 1).

3.2. Lipid Profile. L. major infection was associated with increased serum cholesterol due to an increase in both HDL and non-HDL fractions (Figure 2). These alterations in the lipid profile were not due to differences in the hepatic cholesterol content or cecal excretion because the levels of these were similar between groups (Table 1).

L. major infection resulted in a reduction in the blood and hepatic triacylglycerol content compared to the controls (Figure 2(a) and Table 1), highlighting the possible influence of *L. major* on triacylglycerol metabolism. With regard to blood cholesterol, *L. major* infection was associated with increased serum total cholesterol due to an increase in both HDL and non-HDL fractions (Figures 2(b) to 2(d)), highlighting the influence of this parasite also on plasma cholesterol levels.

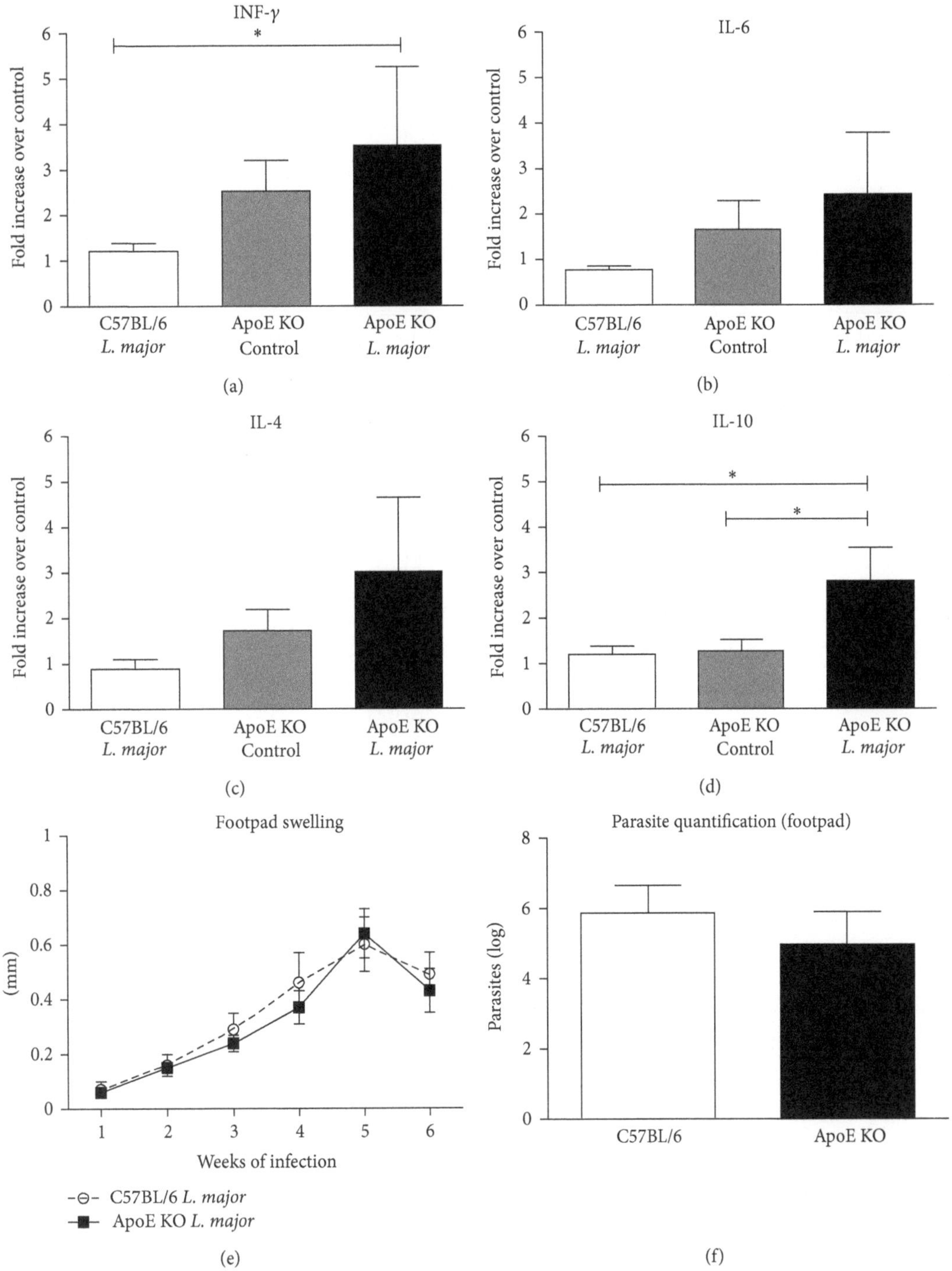

Figure 1: The infection profile of *L. major* in apoE KO and C57BL/6 animals infected with 1×10^6 parasites (clone WHO MHOM/IL/80/Friedlin) into left footpad. (a to d) Cytokine (IL-4, IL-10, TNF-α, and IL-6) mRNA transcripts in the popliteal lymph nodes of apoE KO control, apoE KO *L. major*-infected, and C57BL/6 *L. major*-infected (n = 4/group) mice at the 6th experimental week. Values of average and standard error of cytokine mRNA transcripts in C57BL infected, apoE KO control, and apoE KO infected were, respectively, IL-4 = 0.89 ± 0.20; 1.72 ± 0.46 and 3.01 ± 1.6; IL-10 = 1.2 ± 0.12; 1.28 ± 0.24 and 2.81 ± 0.7; IFNγ = 1.20 + 0.82; 2.53 ± 0.63 and 3.52 + 1.7; IL-6 = 0.78 ± 0.80; 1.65 ± 0.63 and 2.4 ± 1.3. (e) The infection curve of apoE KO and C57BL/6 *L. major* infected mice. The results are expressed as the average of the footpad swelling calculated by the difference between the measures of the infected (left) and control (right) footpads. Number of mice: n = 11 in apoE KO and n = 7 in C57BL/6 groups for each week. (f) Footpad parasite quantification from apoE KO and C57BL/6 mice infected with *L. major* 6 weeks after infection. The results are expressed as the average of the log of the total parasites from apoE KO (n = 11) and C57BL/6 (n = 7) mice. Bars = average and vertical lines = standard error. $^*P < 0.05$.

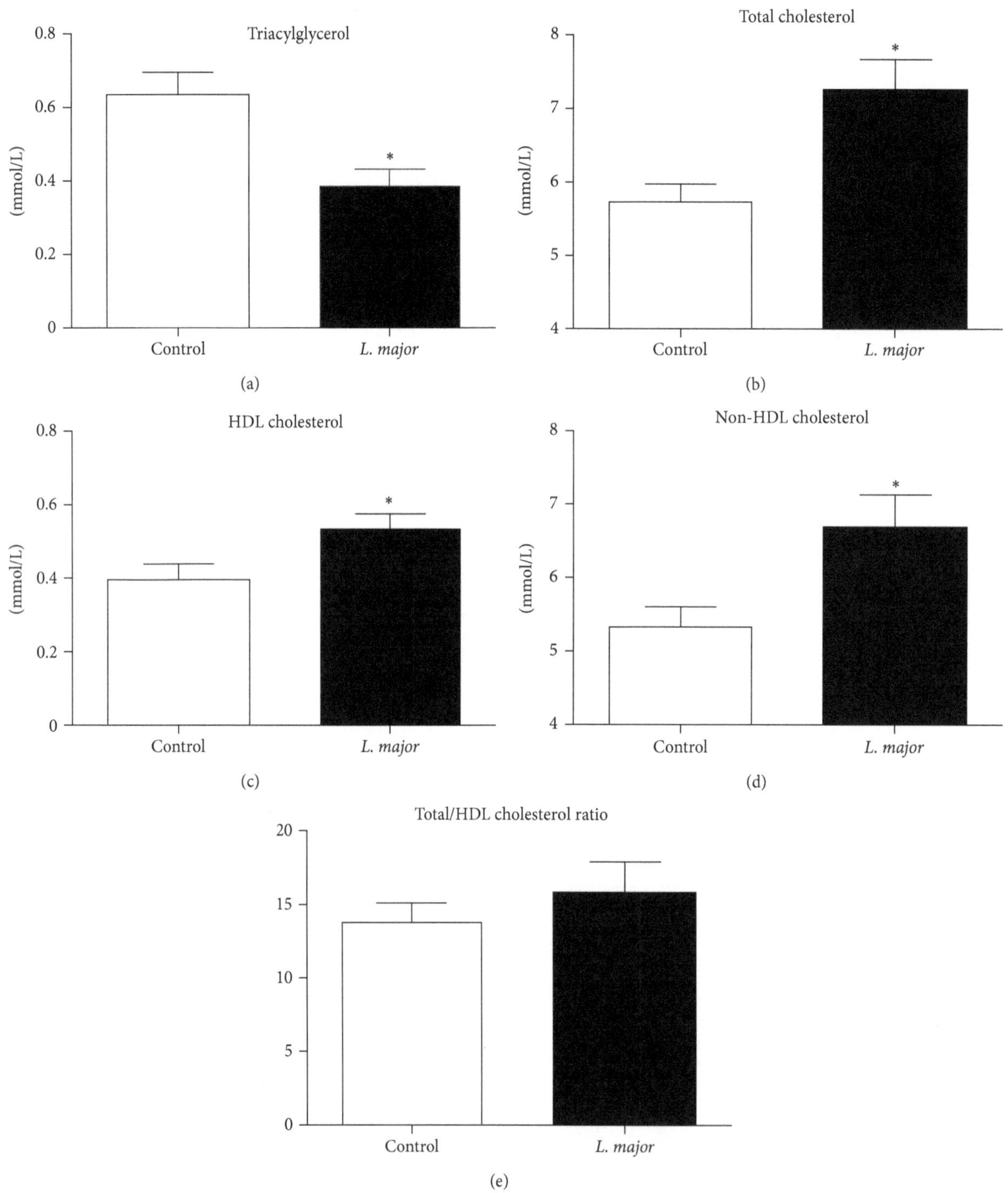

Figure 2: Blood lipid profile of noninfected ($n = 9$) and *L. major*-infected ($n = 12$) apoE KO mice 6 weeks after the inoculation of 1×10^6 parasites (clone WHO MHOM/IL/80/Friedlin) into left footpad. (a) Total triacylglycerols; (b) total cholesterol; (c) high density lipoprotein (HDL) cholesterol; and (d) non-HDL cholesterol (sum of cholesterol in low density (LDL), intermediate density (IDL) lipoproteins, and remnant chylomicron), calculated as the difference between cholesterol and HDL cholesterol. Bars = average and vertical lines = standard error. $^*P < 0.05$.

3.3. Atherosclerotic Lesions. Animals infected with *L. major* presented larger and more developed atherosclerotic lesions when compared to the controls (Figures 3(a), 3(c), and 3(e)). In the control group, atherosclerotic lesions were formed by fatty streaks and several layers of foam cells. On the other hand, in the infected animals, an intense inflammatory infiltrate and necrotic areas with deposition of cholesterol crystals (characteristics of an advanced atherosclerotic lesion) were frequently found (Figures 3(b), 3(d), and 3(f)). The inflammatory infiltrate was composed by cells of the innate immune

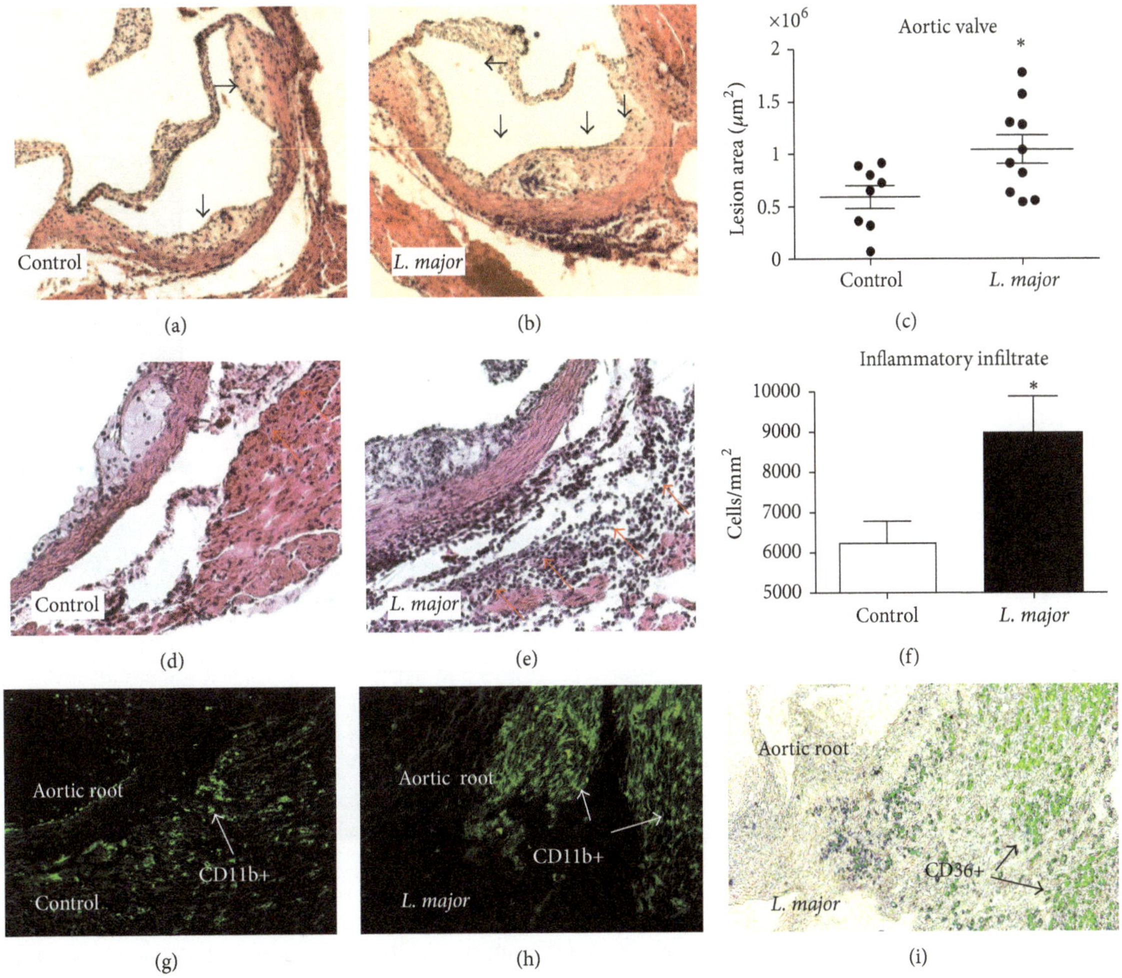

FIGURE 3: Atherosclerotic lesions and inflammatory infiltrate in apoE KO mice infected or noninfected (control) with *L. major* for 6 weeks. (a, b) Histology of the aorta from noninfected (a) and *L. major*-infected (b) apoE KO mice, 6 weeks after infection. (c) Atherosclerosis lesion area in aortic valve of noninfected (Control) and *L. major*-infected apoE KO mice. The results represent the average of the lesion area (μm^2) in the aortic valve of animal from the control ($n = 7$) and the infected groups ($n = 10$), 6 weeks after infection. The major lines represent the means and the minor lines represent the standard error. $^*P = 0.05$. (d, e) Inflammatory infiltrate around the atherosclerotic lesion in aortic valve of non-infected (d) and *L. major*-infected (e) apoE KO mice. (f) Average number of cells/mm^2 of aortic valve of non-infected ($n = 5$) and infected ($n = 5$) apoE KO mice 6 weeks after infection. The bars represent the average and vertical lines represent standard error, $^*P < 0.05$. (g, h) Immunofluorescence: CD11b FITC conjugated positive cells in aortic root of control (g) and *L. major*-infected (h) mice. (i) Anti-CD36 antibody Alexa488 conjugated in aortic valve of *L. major*-infected group. In (a), (b), (d), and (e), the sections were stained with H&E. Image magnification: 20x in (a), (b), (g), and (h) and 100x in (d), (e), and (i).

system, including monocytes and macrophages as suggested by the higher number of CD11b positive cells around the atherosclerotic lesion of infected mice (Figures 3(g) and 3(h)).

3.4. Expression of VCAM-1, MCP1/CCL2, and CD36 in the Aortic Valve. The expression of the adhesion molecule VCAM-1, the monocyte chemotactic protein MCP-1/CCL2, and the scavenger receptor CD36 was also assessed in atherosclerotic lesions.

Confirming the histological data, the results showed that CD36 expression was significantly increased in the *L. major* group ($P = 0.02$). There was a tendency for increased ($P = 0.11$) MCP1/CCL2 expression, and there were no changes in VCAM 1 ($P = 0.67$) expression (Figure 4).

3.5. L. major DNA in Peripheral Tissues. Spleen and liver were tested for the presence of *L. major* DNA. The parasite was not detected in the spleen or liver of mice from both groups, suggesting the absence of viable parasites in these organs (Figure 5).

4. Discussion

To our knowledge, this is the first study investigating the effect of *Leishmania* infection on atherogenesis. A previous study [21] using apoE KO mice analyzed the influence of genetic and high-fat/cholesterol diet-induced dyslipidemia on T cell and dendritic cell (DC) responses to *L. major* infection *in vivo* and, mainly, *in vitro*. Although using the same mouse

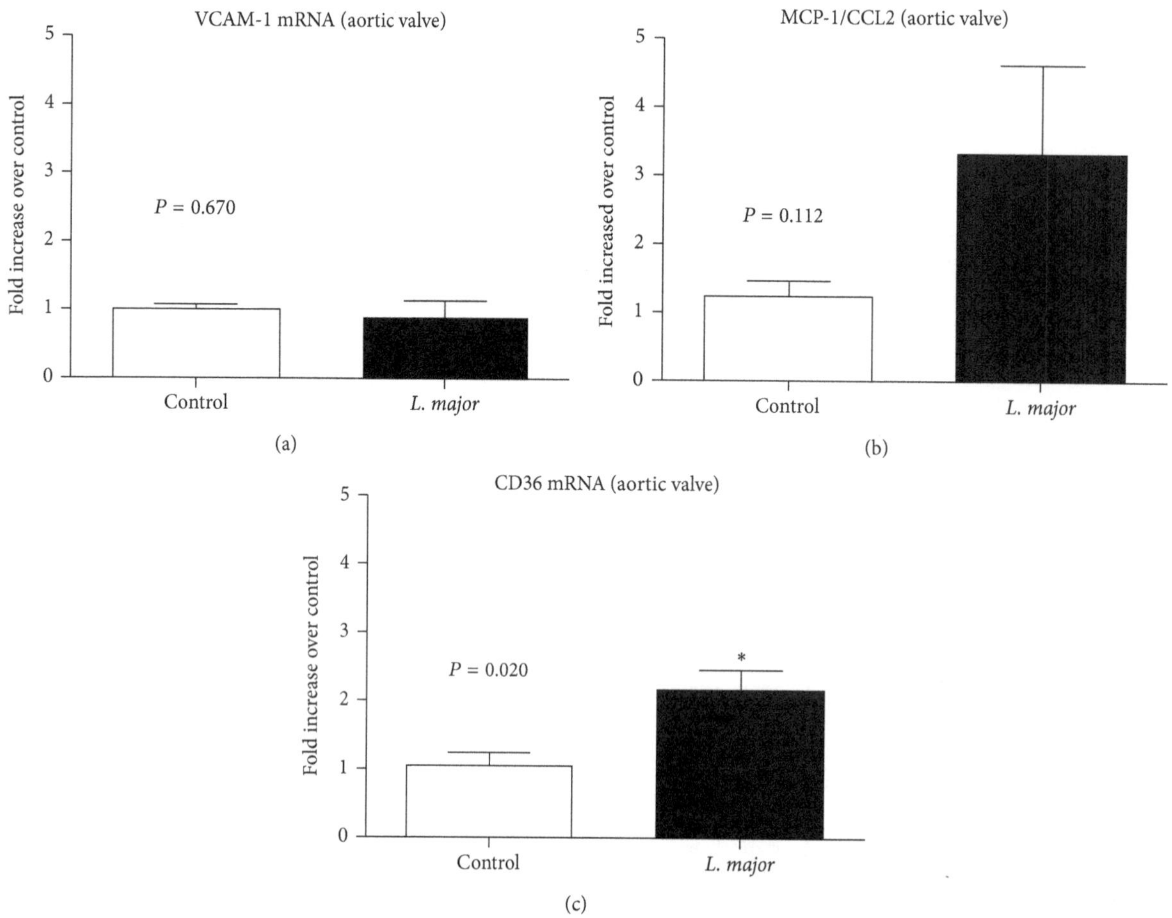

FIGURE 4: Relative increase of (a) VCAM-1, (b) MCP1/CCL2, and (c) CD36RNA expression in the aortic valve of non-infected and infected apoE KO mice, 6 weeks after infection. Bars = average and vertical lines = standard error, $n = 4$/group. $^{*}P < 0.05$. The values of apoE KO control and *L. major* groups were, respectively, VCAM = 1.01 ± 0.07 and 0.89 ± 0.21; CD36 = 1.05 ± 0.19 and 2.16 ± 0.20; MCP-1 = 1.22 ± 0.22 and 2.75 ± 0.83.

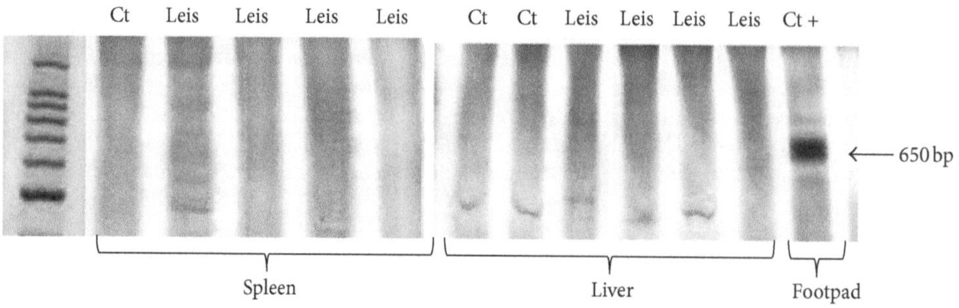

FIGURE 5: PCR amplification of *L. major* DNA in the spleen and liver of non-infected and *L. major*-infected apoE KO mice. First line: molecular weight marker; last line: positive control DNA from an *L. major*-infected footpad. Ct = apoE KO control mice; Leis- apoE KO *L. major*-infected mice.

model used in the present study, the authors did not analyze atherosclerosis development and lipid profile. Moreover, cytokine determinations were done mainly *in vitro*, after parasite antigen restimulation. Finally, the resolution of *L. major* infection in C57BL/6 mice (measured by footpad swelling) started only after 10 weeks of infection while in ours and other studies [22–24] it occurred after 5 weeks of infection.

Our results show that *L. major* infection modifies blood lipid metabolism, resulting in the increase of total cholesterol and its fractions. In addition to the hypercholesterolemia, *L. major* infection also interfered with the metabolism of triacylglycerols, reducing their levels in the blood and liver. Despite the reduction in blood triacylglycerols, we found larger and more advanced atherosclerotic lesions in the aortic valves of infected mice.

Our previous studies showed that *T. gondii*, which induces a strong systemic inflammation, promotes atherogenesis in apoE KO mice [11]. Because *L. major* infection is self-limited in mice, we expected that *L. major* would have little influence on atherosclerosis development compared to *T. gondii* infection. However, our results suggest an important role for *L. major* infection in macrophage activation and atherosclerosis development.

Several mouse strains, including C57BL/6, effectively control *L. major* infection, while others, such as the BALB/c strain, develop progressive damage to the site of infection and systemic disease [25]. Our results indicate that apoE KO animals present the same pattern of resistance to *L. major* infection as that observed in the C57BL/6 animals, as determined by similar degrees of parasite load and footpad swelling. However, the pattern of cytokine expression after 6 weeks of infection shows a strong tendency to be higher in ApoE KO infected mice compared to the ApoE control and the C57BL/6 infected groups. This higher inflammatory status of ApoE KO mice has been previously presented as a consequence of the absence of anti-inflammatory effects of apoE as well as the proinflammatory stimulus of hypercholesterolemia and oxidized lipoproteins [26].

L. major infection leads to hypercholesterolemia associated with a reduction in blood and hepatic triacylglycerols without changes in cholesterol excretion. This pattern of lipid alteration was not found during a *T. gondii* infection [11], which reduces cholesterolemia with no alterations in the level of triacylglycerols in the blood. These different findings reflect the specific metabolic characteristics of each protozoan with regard to their use of host lipids. *T. gondii* is unable to produce cholesterol on its own. Thus, it is dependent on host cholesterol taken from the blood. Additionally, *T. gondii* causes a more severe infection that induces a reduction in food intake and weight loss in the mice. One of the consequences of this is the preferential use of acetyl CoA to supply energy, reducing its availability to the cholesterol synthesis pathway [27]. Both factors contribute (host cholesterol uptake and acetyl-coA redirection) to the reduction of cholesterolemia during a *T. gondii infection. Leishmania*, on the other hand, is able to synthesize its own cholesterol [28] but is dependent on host fatty acids, an important source of energy for amastigotes [29]. It is possible that *L. major* acquires fatty acids from triacylglycerol-rich lipoproteins, particularly IDL, which is the primary lipoprotein in apoE KO mice, resulting in the decrease of circulating triacylglycerol from lipoproteins in infected mice. On the other hand, the reduction of triacylglycerol could be related to the weight loss and a catabolic state. Independently of the cause, the reduction of the blood triacylglycerols stimulates the rapid conversion of the IDL into the more atherogenic, small, and dense LDL [30], which could explain the higher cholesterol and atherogenic fractions in the *L. major* group [31, 32].

L. major infection also stimulated the migration of inflammatory cells to the atherosclerotic lesion site. Aside from the hypercholesterolemia, these results could be explained by the oxidative stress and endothelial dysfunction resulting from inflammation [33], which leads to rapid migration of immune cells to the atherosclerotic lesion, where they accelerate atherogenesis. Moreover, *L. major* infected leukocytes could egress from the footpad tissue or draining lymph node and, following chemotactic stimulus, and migrate to other inflammatory regions such as the atherosclerotic site. Macrophages are connected to the progression of atherosclerosis through the production of inflammatory cytokines, which activate endothelial mediators and prothrombotic factors that are important in the atherosclerosis development. The increased movement of *L. major*-activated leukocytes to the site of atherosclerosis is suggested by the higher inflammatory infiltration and the higher expression of CD36, the major macrophage scavenger receptor for abnormal (oxidized) LDL. The introduction of minimally oxidized LDL into the intimae of arteries causes endothelial activation and release of leukocyte chemotactic factors that attract macrophages and other immune cells, which aggravates the inflammation and enhances plaque formation. In our study, parasite DNA was not found in the spleen or liver, refuting the hypothesis of visceralization.

In conclusion, *L. major* infection, although localized and self-limited in resistant apoE KO mice, has a detrimental effect on the blood lipid profile, increasing the inflammatory cell migration to atherosclerotic lesions and accelerating atherogenesis. The latter is the consequence of the increase of the inflammatory component of atherosclerosis that could be trigged by the parasite-activated macrophages.

Acknowledgments

This work was supported by PRPq/UFMG, *Pró-reitoria de Pesquisa* of *Universidade Federal de Minas Gerais*, CNPq (Conselho Nacional de Desenvolvimento Científico e Tecnológico), and CAPES (CAPES—Coordenação de Aperfeiçoamento de Pessoal de Nível. Superior). The authors are grateful to Maria Helena Alves de Oliveira, who was responsible for the animal facility. This work was conducted at the Universidade Federal de Minas Gerais, Brazil.

References

[1] J. Liese, U. Schleicher, and C. Bogdan, "The innate immune response against Leishmania parasites," *Immunobiology*, vol. 213, no. 3-4, pp. 377–387, 2008.

[2] G. K. Hansson, "Inflammatory mechanisms in atherosclerosis," *Journal of Thrombosis and Haemostasis*, vol. 7, no. 1, pp. 328–331, 2009.

[3] R. Ross, "Atherosclerosis—an inflammatory disease," *The New England Journal of Medicine*, vol. 340, no. 2, pp. 115–126, 1999.

[4] G. K. Hansson and P. Libby, "The immune response in atherosclerosis: a double-edged sword," *Nature Reviews Immunology*, vol. 6, no. 7, pp. 508–519, 2006.

[5] S. Kiechl, G. Egger, M. Mayr et al., "Chronic infections and the risk of carotid atherosclerosis: prospective results from a large population study," *Circulation*, vol. 103, no. 8, pp. 1064–1070, 2001.

[6] G. Noll, "Pathogenesis of atherosclerosis: a possible relation to infection," *Atherosclerosis*, vol. 140, no. 1, pp. S3–S9, 1998.

[7] F. F. Mussa, H. Chai, X. Wang, Q. Yao, A. B. Lumsden, and C. Chen, "Chlamydia pneumoniae and vascular disease: an update," *Journal of Vascular Surgery*, vol. 43, no. 6, pp. 1301–1307, 2006.

[8] L. J. Murray, K. B. Bamford, D. P. J. O'Reilly, E. E. McCrum, and A. E. Evans, "Helicobacter pylori infection: relation with cardiovascular risk factors, ischaemic heart disease, and social class," *British Heart Journal*, vol. 74, no. 5, pp. 497–501, 1995.

[9] M. S. Burnett, S. Durrani, E. Stabile et al., "Murine cytomegalovirus infection increases aortic expression of proatherosclerotic genes," *Circulation*, vol. 109, no. 7, pp. 893–897, 2004.

[10] M. J. Doenhoff, R. G. Stanley, K. Griffiths, and C. L. Jackson, "An anti-atherogenic effect of Schistosoma mansoni infections in mice associated with a parasite-induced lowering of blood total cholesterol," *Parasitology*, vol. 125, no. 5, pp. 415–421, 2002.

[11] L. R. Portugal, L. R. Fernandes, G. C. Cesar et al., "Infection with Toxoplasma gondii increases atherosclerotic lesion in ApoE-deficient mice," *Infection and Immunity*, vol. 72, no. 6, pp. 3571–3576, 2004.

[12] J. H. Meurman, M. Sanz, and S. J. Janket, "Oral health, atherosclerosis, and cardiovascular disease," *Critical Reviews in Oral Biology and Medicine*, vol. 15, no. 6, pp. 403–413, 2004.

[13] H. Zhang, L. M. Wu, and J. Wu, "Cross-talk between apolipoprotein E and cytokines," *Mediators of Inflammation*, vol. 2011, Article ID 949072, 10 pages, 2011.

[14] L. S. Capettini, S. F. Cortes, J. F. Silva, J. I. Alvarez-Leite, and V. S. Lemos, "Decreased production of nNOS-derived hydrogen peroxide contributes to endothelial dysfunction in atherosclerosis," *British Journal of Pharmacology*, vol. 164, no. 6, pp. 1738–1748, 2011.

[15] P. G. Reeves, F. H. Nielsen, and G. C. Fahey, "AIN-93 purified diets for laboratory rodents: final report of the american institute of nutrition ad hoc writing committee on the reformulation of the AIN-76A rodent diet," *The Journal of Nutrition*, vol. 123, no. 11, pp. 1939–1951, 1993.

[16] L. Q. Vieira, M. Goldschmidt, M. Nashleanas, K. Pfeffer, T. Mak, and P. Scott, "Mice lacking the TNF receptor p55 fail to resolve lesions caused by infection with *Leishmania major*, but control parasite replication," *The Journal of Immunology*, vol. 157, no. 2, pp. 827–835, 1996.

[17] S. Fazio, V. R. Babaev, A. B. Murray et al., "Increased atherosclerosis in mice reconstituted with apolipoprotein E null macrophages," *Proceedings of the National Academy of Sciences of the United States of America*, vol. 94, no. 9, pp. 4647–4652, 1997.

[18] J. Folch, M. Lees, and S. G. H. Sloane, "A simple method for the isolation and purification of total lipides from animal tissues," *The Journal of biological chemistry*, vol. 226, no. 1, pp. 497–509, 1957.

[19] B. Paigen, A. Morrow, P. A. Holmes, D. Mitchell, and R. A. Williams, "Quantitative assessment of atherosclerotic lesions in mice," *Atherosclerosis*, vol. 68, no. 3, pp. 231–240, 1987.

[20] G. Anders, C. L. Eisenberger, F. Jonas, and C. L. Greenblatt, "Distinguishing *Leishmania tropica* and *Leishmania major* in the Middle East using the polymerase chain reaction with kinetoplast DNA-specific primers," *Transactions of the Royal Society of Tropical Medicine and Hygiene*, vol. 96, supplement 1, pp. S87–S92, 2002.

[21] A. T. Shamshiev, F. Ampenberger, B. Ernst, L. Rohrer, B. J. Marsland, and M. Kopf, "Dyslipidemia inhibits Toll-like receptor-induced activation of CD8α-negative dendritic cells and protective Th1 type immunity," *Journal of Experimental Medicine*, vol. 204, no. 2, pp. 441–452, 2007.

[22] H. C. Santiago, C. F. Oliveira, L. Santiago et al., "Involvement of the chemokine RANTES (CCL5) in resistance to experimental infection with *Leishmania major*," *Infection and Immunity*, vol. 72, no. 8, pp. 4918–4923, 2004.

[23] C. F. Oliveira, D. Manzoni-de-Almeida, P. S. Mello et al. , "Characterization of chronic cutaneous lesions from TNF-receptor-1-deficient mice infected by *Leishmania major*," *Clinical and Developmental Immunology*, vol. 2012, Article ID 865708, 12 pages, 2012.

[24] F. Benhnini, M. Chenik, D. Laouini, H. Louzir, P. A. Cazenave, and K. Dellagi, "Comparative evaluation of two vaccine candidates against experimental leishmaniasis due to *Leishmania major* infection in four inbred mouse strains," *Clinical and Vaccine Immunology*, vol. 16, no. 11, pp. 1529–1537, 2009.

[25] D. Sacks and N. Noben-Trauth, "The immunology of susceptibility and resistance to *Leishmania major* in mice," *Nature Reviews Immunology*, vol. 2, no. 11, pp. 845–858, 2002.

[26] X. Zhou, G. Paulsson, S. Stemme, and G. K. Hansson, "Hypercholesterolemia is associated with a T helper (Th) 1/Th2 switch of the autoimmune response in atherosclerotic apo E-knockout mice," *Journal of Clinical Investigation*, vol. 101, no. 8, pp. 1717–1725, 1998.

[27] G. R. Jansen, M. E. Zanetti, and C. F. Hutchison, "Stdies on lipogenesis in vivo. Effects of starvation andre-feeding, and studies on cholesterol synthesis," *Biochemical Journal*, vol. 99, no. 2, pp. 333–340, 1966.

[28] M. L. Ginger, M. C. Prescott, D. G. Reynolds, M. L. Chance, and J. L. Goad, "Utilization of leucine and acetate as carbon sources for sterol and fatty acid biosynthesis by old and new world *Leishmania* species, *Endotrypanum monterogeii* and *Trypanosoma cruzi*," *European Journal of Biochemistry*, vol. 267, no. 9, pp. 2555–2566, 2000.

[29] D. T. Hart and G. H. Coombs, "Leishmania mexicana: energy metabolism of amastigotes and promastigotes," *Experimental Parasitology*, vol. 54, no. 3, pp. 397–409, 1982.

[30] M. Rizzo and K. Berneis, "Low-density lipoprotein size and cardiovascular risk assessment," *QJM*, vol. 99, no. 1, pp. 1–14, 2006.

[31] E. Esteve, W. Ricart, and J. M. Fernández-Real, "Dyslipidemia and inflammation: an evolutionary conserved mechanism," *Clinical Nutrition*, vol. 24, no. 1, pp. 16–31, 2005.

[32] C. G. Nieto, R. Barrera, M. A. Habela et al., "Changes in the plasma concentrations of lipids and lipoprotein fractions in dogs infected with *Leishmania infantum*," *Veterinary Parasitology*, vol. 44, no. 3-4, pp. 175–182, 1992.

[33] G. K. Hansson, "Inflammation, atherosclerosis, and coronary artery disease," *The New England Journal of Medicine*, vol. 352, no. 16, pp. 1685–1626, 2005.

16

Cholesterol Metabolism and Weight Reduction in Subjects with Mild Obstructive Sleep Apnoea: A Randomised, Controlled Study

Maarit Hallikainen,[1] Henri Tuomilehto,[2,3] Tarja Martikainen,[4] Esko Vanninen,[5] Juha Seppä,[2] Jouko Kokkarinen,[6] Jukka Randell,[6] and Helena Gylling[1,7]

[1] *Institute of Public Health and Clinical Nutrition, Department of Clinical Nutrition, University of Eastern Finland, P.O. BOX 1627, 70211 Kuopio, Finland*
[2] *Institute of Clinical Medicine, Department of Otorhinolaryngology, Kuopio University Hospital, and University of Eastern Finland, P.O. BOX 1777, 70211 Kuopio, Finland*
[3] *Oivauni Sleep Clinic, Puijonkatu 12 b, 70100 Kuopio, Finland*
[4] *Institute of Clinical Medicine, Department of Medicine, Division of Clinical Nutrition, Kuopio University Hospital, P.O. BOX 1777, 70211 Kuopio, Finland*
[5] *Institute of Clinical Medicine, Clinical Physiology and Nuclear Medicine, Kuopio University Hospital, and University of Eastern Finland, P.O. BOX 1777, 70211 Kuopio, Finland*
[6] *Institute of Clinical Medicine, Respiratory Medicine, Kuopio University Hospital, and University of Eastern Finland, P.O. BOX 1777, 70211 Kuopio, Finland*
[7] *Division of Internal Medicine, Department of Medicine, University of Helsinki, Helsinki, P.O. BOX 700, 00029 HUS, Finland*

Correspondence should be addressed to Maarit Hallikainen; maarit.hallikainen@uef.fi

Academic Editor: Francisco Blanco-Vaca

To evaluate whether parameters of obstructive sleep apnoea (OSA) associate with cholesterol metabolism before and after weight reduction, 42 middle-aged overweight subjects with mild OSA were randomised to intensive lifestyle intervention ($N = 23$) or to control group ($N = 18$) with routine lifestyle counselling only. Cholesterol metabolism was evaluated with serum noncholesterol sterol ratios to cholesterol, surrogate markers of cholesterol absorption (cholestanol and plant sterols) and synthesis (cholestenol, desmosterol, and lathosterol) at baseline and after 1-year intervention. At baseline, arterial oxygen saturation (Sa_{O_2}) was associated with serum campesterol ($P < 0.05$) and inversely with desmosterol ratios ($P < 0.001$) independently of gender, BMI, and homeostasis model assessment index of insulin resistance (HOMA-IR). Apnoea-hypopnoea index (AHI) was not associated with cholesterol metabolism. Weight reduction significantly increased Sa_{O_2} and serum cholestanol and decreased AHI and serum cholestenol ratios. In the groups combined, the changes in AHI were inversely associated with changes of cholestanol and positively with cholestenol ratios independent of gender and the changes of BMI and HOMA-IR ($P < 0.05$). In conclusion, mild OSA seemed to be associated with cholesterol metabolism independent of BMI and HOMA-IR. Weight reduction increased the markers of cholesterol absorption and decreased those of cholesterol synthesis in the overweight subjects with mild OSA.

1. Introduction

Obstructive sleep apnoea (OSA) characterized by repeated episodes of apnoea and hypopnoea during sleep is one of the most common sleep disturbances [1]. OSA is independently associated with hypertension, cardiovascular diseases, metabolic syndrome, insulin resistance, and type 2 diabetes [2–7]. Furthermore, recent epidemiological studies have concluded that OSA is an important risk factor for mortality, particularly due to coronary artery disease [8, 9]. However, the underlying mechanisms explaining these associations are rather complex, and although several possibilities have been proposed, they are not entirely accepted. In general, atherogenesis as well as OSA is considered as slow processes, and the onset is likely to begin years before any symptoms appear. We have earlier demonstrated that even mild OSA is associated with the activation of the proinflammatory system [10]. Furthermore, since elevated LDL cholesterol level is one of the most important risk factors for cardiovascular diseases, the question raises whether OSA has a role in hypercholesterolaemia or in cholesterol metabolism. In some, but not in all studies, OSA has independently associated with increased concentrations of total cholesterol and triglycerides and decreased concentrations of HDL cholesterol [11–14]. The mechanisms of dyslipidaemia in OSA besides obesity are not clearly understood especially for elevated LDL cholesterol level [15], but most likely chronic intermittent hypoxemia (IH), a major component of OSA, may be the primary trigger for a cascade of pathogenetic mechanisms leading to increased triglyceride-rich lipoproteins and reduced HDL cholesterol levels [15]. Regarding cholesterol metabolism there are no clinical studies examining the association between OSA and cholesterol metabolism (i.e., cholesterol synthesis and absorption).

The most important risk factor for OSA is obesity [16]. On the other side, obesity interferes with cholesterol metabolism, so that cholesterol synthesis is upregulated, and cholesterol absorption efficiency is low [17, 18]. Accordingly, it could be assumed that cholesterol metabolism might be disturbed in OSA, but whether it is obesity or OSA that interferes with cholesterol metabolism remains to be evaluated. However, this does not change the fact that 60–90% of all patients with OSA are obese [19] and need to be treated not only for OSA but also other obesity related comorbidities.

It was recently demonstrated that lifestyle intervention with weight reduction reduced both hypopnoea and especially apnoea indices and also other obesity related risk factors for cardiovascular diseases in a vast majority of patients with mild OSA, highlighting the importance of an early lifestyle intervention [20]. Similarly, weight reduction decreases cholesterol synthesis and increases cholesterol absorption in type 2 diabetics [21, 22]. It would be interesting to know whether in subjects with OSA weight reduction alters also cholesterol metabolism, and whether the reduction in apnoea and hypopnoea indices are related to cholesterol metabolism beyond obesity. Therefore, in the present randomised interventional study two main parameters of OSA, that is, apnoea-hypopnoea index (AHI) and arterial oxygen saturation (Sa_{O_2}), were related to those of cholesterol synthesis and absorption at baseline and after one-year weight reduction program in middle-aged overweight subjects with mild OSA. Cholesterol metabolism was evaluated with serum noncholesterol sterols, surrogate markers of cholesterol absorption and synthesis [23].

2. Methods

This study is a substudy of our randomised study originally conducted to determine the effects of changes in lifestyle with weight reduction program designed to prevent the progression of the disease or even cure it in the most prevalent subgroup of OSA, that is, overweight patients with mild OSA. The detailed design of the study was previously reported [20].

2.1. Subjects. The subjects were consecutively recruited from among patients referred to the outpatient clinics of Otorhinolaryngology and Respiratory Medicine of Kuopio University Hospital, Finland, because of a suspicion of OSA. The main study population consisted of 72 subjects who completed the 1-year follow-up [20]. The inclusion criteria were age 18–65 years, overweight (BMI $\geq$ 28 kg/m^2), and mild OSA (AHI 5–15 events/h). The exclusion criteria were active treatment of OSA of any kind, pregnancy, chronic kidney, thyroid, or liver disease. To the present study, an additional inclusion criterion was the availability of both baseline and follow-up measurements, and an additional exclusion criterion was the presence of lipid-lowering medication.

This study was conducted according to the guidelines laid down in the Declaration of Helsinki, and all procedures involving human subjects were approved by the Research Ethics Committee of the Hospital District of Northern Savo (Kuopio, Finland). All subjects gave their written informed consent for the study.

2.2. Intervention. A detailed description of the intervention procedure was previously reported by Tuomilehto et al. [20]. The subjects with mild OSA were randomised to two groups. The subjects in the intervention group were provided with a group-based very low calorie diet (VLCD) of 600–800 kcal/d for 12 weeks, after which they were advised regarding diet and exercise. The lifestyle intervention lasted for 1 year and consisted of 14 visits with the study nutritionist. The subjects in the control group were given standard care consisting of general oral and written information about diet and exercise at baseline and 3-month visits by the study nurse and physician without any specific individualised advice.

2.3. Measurements. Nocturnal cardiorespiratory monitoring by Embletta (Embla, Broomfield, CO, USA) at home was conducted in accordance with accepted guidelines for diagnosing OSA [24]. Apnoea was defined as a cessation (>90%) of airflow for >10 s with oxygen desaturation for ≥4%. Hypopnoea was defined as a reduction (>30%) of airflow for >10 s with oxygen desaturation for ≥4%. AHI was defined as the number of apnoeas and hypopnoeas per hour, and mild OSA was defined as an AHI of 5–15 events/h [24]. Furthermore, mean arterial oxygen saturation (Sa_{O_2}) and time and percentage with arterial oxygen saturation <90% were assessed. The recordings were manually evaluated by two blinded, trained physicians.

Body weight was measured with a digital scale and height using a stadiometer. A trained nurse measured also waist circumference both at the baseline and at the 1-year visit.

Blood samples for biochemical assays were collected from fasting subjects (≥12 h). Serum total and HDL cholesterol, serum triglycerides and plasma glucose were analysed by using automated analyzer system (Konelab 60 Analyzer, ThermoFisher Scientific, Waltham, MA, USA). LDL cholesterol was calculated according to Friedewald equation. Plasma glucose was analysed by using automated analyzer system (Konelab 60 Analyzer, ThermoFisher Scientific, Waltham, MA, USA). Serum insulin was measured by using a fluoroimmunoassay system (Wallac, Perkin-Elmer, Waltham, MA, USA). The homeostasis model assessment index of insulin resistance (HOMA-IR) was calculated as fasting serum insulin concentration × fasting plasma glucose concentration/22.5 [25].

Serum cholesterol, cholesterol precursors reflecting cholesterol synthesis (squalene, cholestenol, lathosterol, and desmosterol), plant sterols (sitosterol and campesterol), and cholestanol reflecting cholesterol absorption [23] were quantified from nonsaponifiable serum material by GLC (Agilent 7890GC System, Agilent Technologies, Wilmington, DE, USA) equipped with a 50 m long Ultra 1 capillary column (5% Phenyl-methyl siloxane) (Agilent Technologies, Wilmington, DE, USA) [26]. Serum values were expressed in terms of 10^2x mmol/mol of cholesterol (called ratio in the text) by dividing the noncholesterol sterol concentrations with the cholesterol value of the same GLC run to eliminate the changing concentrations of lipoproteins (mainly LDL) that transports noncholesterol sterols. Ratios of relative synthesis markers/absorption markers were also calculated reflecting cholesterol metabolism.

2.4. Statistical Analyses. Statistical analyses were performed with SPSS for Windows 14.0 statistics program (SPSS, Chicago, IL, USA).

Normality and homogeneity of variance assumptions were checked before further analyses. Student's t-test was used to compare the baseline values and the changes between the groups. ANOVA for repeated measurements was used to analyse the interaction of time and group and changes over time in between-group comparisons followed by post hoc comparisons with Bonferroni corrections. In between-group comparisons, gender and BMI, were included as ANCOVA. For some variables of interest Pearson or Spearman correlation coefficients were calculated. In addition, to evaluate the effects of gender, BMI and HOMA-IR on associations of parameters of OSA and cholesterol metabolism, a multiple linear regression analysis was used. Variables not normally distributed even after logarithmic transformation, nonhomogenous in variance, or noncontinuous were tested with Mann-Whitney U test or Fisher exact test. A P value of <0.05 was considered statistically significant. The results are given as means ± SEM.

3. Results

3.1. Baseline. A total of 41 subjects (33 men and 8 women) fulfilled the criteria and were included into the statistical analyses. Their mean age was 48.9 ± 1.3 years and BMI 32.5 ± 0.4 kg/m^2. Thirteen subjects had antihypertensive medication, two had thyroxin therapy, and one had oral diabetes medication. Baseline characteristics of the subjects in the control (N = 18) and intervention (N = 23) groups are shown in Table 1. Despite randomisation, the subjects in the intervention group were heavier, and their BMI was higher and waist circumference larger than in the control group. In addition, serum insulin concentration and cholestenol : cholesterol ratio were greater, and HOMA-IR tended to be significantly greater (P = 0.055) compared with controls (Table 2). No other significant differences between the groups were observed.

3.1.1. Baseline Associations. In the whole population, cholesterol synthesis markers were interrelated (e.g., cholestenol versus lathosterol r = 0.572, P < 0.001) as well as the absorption markers (campesterol versus cholestanol r = 0.664, P < 0.001). Cholesterol synthesis markers were inversely associated with the absorption markers (e.g., desmosterol versus cholestanol r = −0.637, P < 0.001) suggesting that cholesterol homeostasis was intact.

The markers of cholesterol synthesis were positively (e.g., desmosterol ratio r = 0.364, P = 0.020) and those of cholesterol absorption inversely (e.g., cholestanol ratio r = −0.376, P = 0.020) associated with BMI. The cholesterol synthesis markers were inversely associated with serum HDL cholesterol concentration (e.g., desmosterol ratio r = −0.502, P = 0.001) and positively with serum triglycerides (e.g., desmosterol ratio r = 0.546, P < 0.001), whereas the associations between the absorption markers and HDL cholesterol (e.g., cholestanol ratio r = 0.316, P = 0.040) and triglycerides (e.g., cholestanol ratio r = −0.343, P = 0.028) were opposite. No associations of the cholesterol synthesis and absorption markers with total and LDL cholesterol were found.

Mean total AHI was not associated with mean arterial oxygen saturation (Sa_{O_2}) or with any other variables, even though AHI tended to be associated with serum cholestenol ratio to cholesterol (r = 0.292, P = 0.064).

Sa_{O_2} was inversely associated with body weight (r = −0.656, P < 0.001) and waist circumference (r = −0.481, P = 0.003) and positively with HDL cholesterol concentration (r = 0.410, P = 0.010). Sa_{O_2} was inversely associated with desmosterol (r = −0.595, P < 0.001) and positively with campesterol ratios to cholesterol (r = 0.381, P = 0.020). In multiple linear regression analysis after adjustment with gender, BMI and HOMA-IR, the associations between Sa_{O_2} and desmosterol and campesterol ratios to cholesterol and desmosterol : campesterol ratio remained significant (Table 3).

3.2. Intervention

3.2.1. Anthropometric Measurements. BMI and waist circumference reduced significantly more in the intervention group compared with the control group (−13.6% versus −2.2% and −10.9% versus −2.2%, resp.) (Table 1) during the follow-up.

3.2.2. Serum Cholesterol, Plasma Glucose, and Serum Insulin. Plasma glucose was similarly reduced in both study groups (P < 0.05), but the reduction was not significant after adjustment with gender and BMI (Table 1). The reduction in serum insulin concentration was greater in the intervention group compared with the controls (−43.6% versus −17.8%, P < 0.05), but the intervention values did not differ between the groups (Table 1). Similarly, the percentage reduction in

TABLE 1: Changes in anthropometric measurements, plasma glucose and serum insulin concentrations, and cardiorespiratory variables during the intervention.

	Control group		Intervention group		P^a	P^b
	Baseline	12 months	Baseline	12 months		
Gender (M/F)	14/4		19/4		0.500	
Age (y)	48.2 ± 2		49.4 ± 1.7		0.667	
Weight (kg)	93.9 ± 2.9	92.2 ± 3.4	103.5 ± 2.2[c]	91.5 ± 2.4[d,e]	<0.001	<0.001
BMI (kg/m^2)	31.4 ± 0.6	30.9 ± 0.9	33.4 ± 0.6[c]	29.5 ± 0.6[d,e]	<0.001	<0.001
Waist circumference (cm)	104.6 ± 2.3	102.9 ± 2.6	112.9 ± 2.1[c]	101.0 ± 2.0[d,e]	<0.001	<0.001
P-Glucose (mmol/L)[(f)]	6.19 ± 0.51	5.57 ± 0.16	5.92 ± 0.19	5.59 ± 0.13	0.528	0.306
S-Insulin (mU/L)	10.18 ± 1.06	8.25 ± 1.05	14.61 ± 1.69[c]	7.16 ± 0.63	0.082	0.105
HOMA-IR	2.66 ± 0.33	2.08 ± 0.28	3.98 ± 0.54	1.80 ± 0.18	0.087	0.103
Total cholesterol (mmol/L)	5.17 ± 0.25	5.21 ± 0.23	4.83 ± 0.11	4.63 ± 0.16	0.246	0.369
LDL cholesterol (mmol/L)	3.13 ± 0.17	3.28 ± 0.17	3.06 ± 0.10	2.88 ± 0.14	0.116	0.226
HDL cholesterol (mmol/L)	1.13 ± 0.10	1.12 ± 0.07	0.98 ± 0.05	1.15 ± 0.06[d]	0.028	0.044
Total triglycerides (mmol/L)[(f)]	1.78 ± 0.24	1.60 ± 0.30	1.73 ± 0.17	1.32 ± 0.12	0.683	0.510
AHI (total)	9.5 ± 0.8	11.2 ± 2.0	9.8 ± 0.6	5.2 ± 1.2[d,(e)]	0.007	0.040
Mean Sa_{O_2}	94.5 ± 0.3	93.9 ± 0.3[d]	94.0 ± 0.3	94.8 ± 0.3[d,e]	<0.001	0.001
Time with Sa_{O_2} < 90%	3.5 ± 0.9	9.2 ± 3.5	6.4 ± 2.2	4.7 ± 2.1[d,e]	0.007	0.004
Percentage time with Sa_{O_2} < 90%	0.9 ± 0.2	2.3 ± 0.9[d]	1.6 ± 0.5	0.8 ± 0.3[d,e]	0.003	0.002

Values shown are means ± SEM.

[a]Group by time interaction analysed with analysis of variance for repeated measurements (GLM). If the baseline differed between groups ($P < 0.06$), it was taken into account as covariance. (Gender Fisher's exact test and age Student's t-test).

[b]Group by time interaction (gender and BMI as covariance).

[c]$P < 0.05$ denotes a significant difference at the baseline between the groups.

[d]$P < 0.05$ denotes a significant difference from the baseline within the groups.

[e]$P < 0.05$ denotes a significant difference at the 12 months between the groups, [(e)]$P > 0.05$ (gender and BMI as covariance).

[f]$P < 0.05$ denotes a significant change over time, [(f)]$P > 0.05$ (gender and BMI as covariance).

HOMA-IR was greater in the intervention group compared with the controls (−46.7% versus −19.5%, $P < 0.05$).

3.2.3. Serum Lipids. Serum total and LDL cholesterol concentrations were not changed during the intervention (Table 1). Serum HDL cholesterol concentration significantly increased in the intervention group, and the percentage increase was greater than in the control group. However, the intervention values did not differ between the groups (Table 1). Serum triglyceride concentration was similarly reduced in both study groups ($P < 0.05$), but the reductions were not significant after adjustment with gender and BMI (Table 1).

3.2.4. Cardiorespiratory Recordings. The mean total AHI at 12 months and the mean percentage change (−49.1% versus +30.9%) during the follow-up significantly differed between the groups (Table 1). However, after adjustment with gender and BMI the mean total AHI only tended to be lower in the intervention group compared with controls ($P = 0.052$). A significant improvement was detected in mean Sa_{O_2} in the intervention group compared with the control group at 12 months (Table 1). In addition, the subjects in the intervention group spent less time with Sa_{O_2} < 90% during their sleep compared with subjects in the control group (Table 1).

3.2.5. Cholesterol Synthesis and Absorption Markers. Of the cholesterol synthesis markers, serum cholestenol ratio to cholesterol was significantly reduced by −18.1% in the intervention group, and the change was significantly different compared with the controls (Table 2). Serum desmosterol and lathosterol ratios to cholesterol similarly reduced in both groups ($P < 0.05$), but the reductions were not significant after adjustment with gender and BMI (Table 2). No changes in serum squalene were found (Table 2).

Of the cholesterol absorption markers, serum cholestanol : cholesterol ratio significantly increased by 11.4% during the follow-up in the intervention group, and the change was significantly different compared with the controls (Table 2). However, the intervention values did not differ between the groups (Table 2). Serum campesterol and sitosterol ratios to cholesterol did not change (Table 2).

The changes in the concentrations of serum cholesterol synthesis and absorption markers were in line with the respective changes in the ratio to cholesterol (data not shown).

TABLE 2: Changes in serum noncholesterol sterols and squalene during the intervention.

	Control group		Intervention group		P^a	P^b
	Baseline	12 months	Baseline	12 months		
Cholesterol (mg/dL)	195.9 ± 9.6	193.9 ± 9.3	181.9 ± 5.2	172.5 ± 5.6	0.219	0.413
Cholesterol synthesis markers						
Squalene : cholesterol	26.5 ± 2.6	24.7 ± 2.7	23.5 ± 1.2	22.1 ± 1.7	0.860	0.408
Cholestenol : cholesterol	15.2 ± 1.4	16.9 ± 1.9	22.3 ± 2.9[c]	18.0 ± 2.9[d,e]	0.025	0.020
Desmosterol : cholesterol[(f)]	66.3 ± 4.5	63.4 ± 5.2	77.8 ± 5.0	65.6 ± 2.8	0.131	0.161
Lathosterol : cholesterol[(f)]	179.4 ± 14	175.1 ± 12.7	208.3 ± 13.0	178.9 ± 14.1	0.126	0.069
Cholesterol absorption markers						
Campesterol : cholesterol	206.1 ± 27.7	208.2 ± 18.3	227.1 ± 24.2	235.1 ± 30.6	0.656	0.670
Sitosterol : cholesterol	108.1 ± 11.6	107.5 ± 7.7	132.5 ± 16.0	136.6 ± 16.1	0.843	0.842
Cholestanol : cholesterol	131.1 ± 5.8	130.6 ± 6.1	121.0 ± 4.6	135.5 ± 6.7[d]	0.002	0.004
Cholesterol metabolism markers						
Squalene : Cholestanol	0.21 ± 0.03	0.20 ± 0.03	0.20 ± 0.01	0.18 ± 0.02	0.293	0.109
Cholestenol : Cholestanol	0.12 ± 0.01	0.14 ± 0.02	0.20 ± 0.03[c]	0.14 ± 0.02[d,e]	0.006	0.006
Desmosterol : Cholestanol	0.54 ± 0.06	0.52 ± 0.06	0.68 ± 0.06	0.52 ± 0.04[d]	0.016	0.029
Lathosterol : Cholestanol	1.42 ± 0.12	1.42 ± 0.13	1.81 ± 0.15	1.45 ± 0.17[d]	0.026	0.017

Values shown are means ± SEM.
[a]Group by time interaction analysed with analysis of variance for repeated measurements (GLM). If the baseline differed between groups ($P < 0.05$), it was taken into account as covariance.
[b]Group by time interaction (gender and BMI as covariance).
[c]$P < 0.05$ denotes a significant difference at the baseline between the groups.
[d]$P < 0.05$ denotes a significant difference from the baseline within the groups.
[e]$P < 0.05$ denotes a significant difference at the 12 months between the groups.
[f]$P < 0.05$ denotes a significant change over time [(f)]$P > 0.05$ (gender and BMI as covariance).

TABLE 3: Associations between serum desmosterol and campesterol ratios to cholesterol and desmosterol : campesterol ratio and Sa_{O_2}*.

	Desmosterol : cholesterol		Campesterol : cholesterol		Desmosterol : campesterol	
	Beta	P value	Beta	P value	Beta	P value
Gender	−0.264	0.062	−0.348	0.094	0.131	0.742
BMI (kg/m^2)	0.047	0.732	−0.033	0.873	0.045	0.802
HOMA-IR	0.524	<0.001	−0.011	0.956	0.247	0.153
Sa_{O_2}	−0.322	0.031	0.604	0.008	−0.584	0.004
R^2	0.623		0.175		0.360	

*Multiple linear regression analysis models (adjustment with gender, BMI, and HOMA-IR).

Serum cholestenol, desmosterol, and lathosterol ratios to cholestanol significantly reduced by −19.6–−25.4% during the follow-up in the intervention group, and the changes significantly differed from controls, but only the intervention values of cholestenol : cholestanol ratio significantly differed compared with controls (Table 2).

3.2.6. Associations during Intervention (Intervention + Control Groups Combined). Figure 1 shows the percentage changes in AHI, Sa_{O_2}, cholestenol, and cholestanol : cholesterol ratios in relation to weight reduction. The greater the weight reduction, the greater the reductions in AHI and serum cholestenol : cholesterol ratio and the increases in Sa_{O_2} and serum cholestanol : cholesterol ratio.

The percentage change of AHI was positively associated with the respective changes of serum synthesis markers (e.g., serum cholestenol : cholesterol ratio, Figure 2(a)) and inversely with the percentage change of serum cholestanol : cholesterol ratio (Figure 2(b)). After adjustment with gender and the percentage changes of BMI and HOMA-IR, the associations between the percentage changes of AHI and cholestanol : cholesterol ratio ($P = 0.004$) and of the cholesterol synthesis markers cholestenol : cholesterol ($P = 0.021$) remained significant. The positive associations between the percentage changes of AHI and cholestenol, desmosterol, and lathosterol ratios to cholestanol ($r = 0.460$–0.519, $P = 0.001$–0.003) remained significant after adjustment with gender and the percentage changes of BMI and HOMA-IR, too. However, the inverse associations

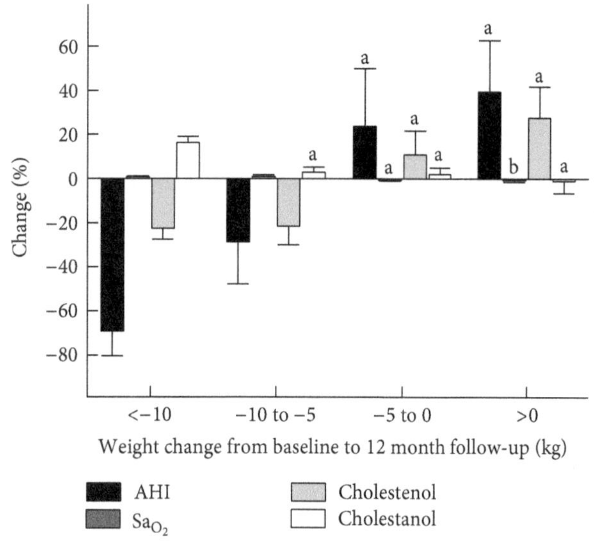

Figure 1: The percentage changes in apnoea-hypopnoea index (AHI), mean oxygen saturation (Sa_{O_2}), and cholestenol and cholestanol : cholesterol ratios (10^2x mmol/mol of cholesterol) in relation to changes in body weight: less than −10 kg, −10 to −5 kg, and −5 to 0 kg and more than 0 kg [a]$P < 0.05$ or less from weight reduction of < −10 kg, [b]$P < 0.05$ or less from weight reduction of −5 to 0 kg.

between the percentage changes of Sa_{O_2} and cholestenol and desmosterol ratios to campesterol ($r = -0.365$–-0.375, $P = 0.024$–0.026) did not remain significant after adjustment with gender and the percentage changes of BMI and HOMA-IR.

4. Discussion

The novel observations of the present study were that mild OSA seems to be associated with cholesterol metabolism independent of BMI and HOMA-IR. Secondly, one-year weight reduction program resulted in changes in cholesterol metabolism. Thirdly, after weight reduction the improvement in OSA was associated with changes in cholesterol metabolism independent of weight and HOMA-IR reductions.

Weight reduction achieved by intensive lifestyle counselling with an initial VLCD program increased Sa_{O_2} and serum cholestanol : cholesterol ratio suggesting that cholesterol absorption was increased. In addition, AHI and serum cholestenol : cholesterol ratio was decreased suggesting that cholesterol synthesis was downregulated. Similar findings regarding cholesterol metabolism were reported in in type 2 diabetics [21, 22]. The present study also demonstrated that all these changes sustained up to 1 year. The negative interrelations of cholesterol synthesis and absorption markers at baseline and after one year (data not shown) suggest that cholesterol homeostasis remained intact irrespective of the intervention.

There is a definite need for further research to better understand the links between OSA and lipid metabolism and to improve the current guidelines of treatment. Thus far, the interventional studies examining the effects of OSA treatment on lipid metabolism have exclusively been conducted with continuous positive airway pressure (CPAP). However, the evidence of the effects of CPAP treatment on dyslipidaemia is limited. In one recent study, CPAP has been demonstrated to reduce postprandial serum triglyceride and total cholesterol concentrations [27] and in another, fasting serum cholesterol, but not triglyceride concentrations [28]. The consensus statement of International Diabetes Federation highly recommends further research on OSA and metabolism in general and particularly intervention studies with emphasis on cardiovascular risk factors, also without using CPAP [29]. The statement concludes that management of OSA should focus initially on weight reduction for the overweight and obese. In general, weight reduction improves serum lipid profile [30]. In the present study, weight reduction did not change serum total and LDL cholesterol concentrations even though it affected cholesterol metabolism.

In animal models, IH was suggested to induce dyslipidaemia by upregulating biosynthesis of VLDL in liver, increasing lipolysis in adipocytes, and inhibiting lipoprotein clearance [31–34]. Recently, in patients with OSA, hepatic expression of stearoyl CoA desaturase, a key enzyme of lipid biosynthesis, has been demonstrated to increase in direct proportion to the severity of nocturnal IH [33]. In addition, overexpression was associated with marked increase in plasma triglyceride and LDL cholesterol concentrations [33]. However, thus far there is no consistent evidence supporting the relationship between OSA and dyslipidaemia in humans [11–14].

Based on animal models, IH was suggested not to affect cholesterol biosynthesis, because there was no effect on the key genes involved in cholesterol biosynthesis [32]. However, we found in the subjects with mild OSA that Sa_{O_2}, one of the key cardiorespiratory variables, was positively associated with cholesterol absorption (serum campesterol : cholesterol ratio) and inversely with cholesterol synthesis (serum desmosterol : cholesterol ratio) at baseline suggesting that the greater Sa_{O_2}, the greater the cholesterol absorption and the lower the cholesterol synthesis. These associations were independent from gender, BMI and HOMA-IR. In addition, although AHI was not significantly associated with cholesterol absorption markers, it tended to be associated positively with cholesterol synthesis markers (cholestenol : cholesterol ratio, $P = 0.062$).

In the whole study population, the greater the weight reduction, the greater the reductions in AHI and serum cholestenol : cholesterol ratio and the increases in Sa_{O_2} and serum cholestanol : cholesterol ratio. In addition, the percentage change of AHI was inversely associated with that of cholesterol absorption marker (cholestanol) and positively with the percentage change of cholesterol synthesis markers. This suggests that the more AHI was improved, the more cholesterol absorption was increased and cholesterol synthesis decreased. The associations between cholestanol and of the cholesterol synthesis marker cholestenol and AHI remained significant after adjustment with gender and the percentage changes of BMI and HOMA-IR. On the contrary, the relationships between the percentage changes of Sa_{O_2}

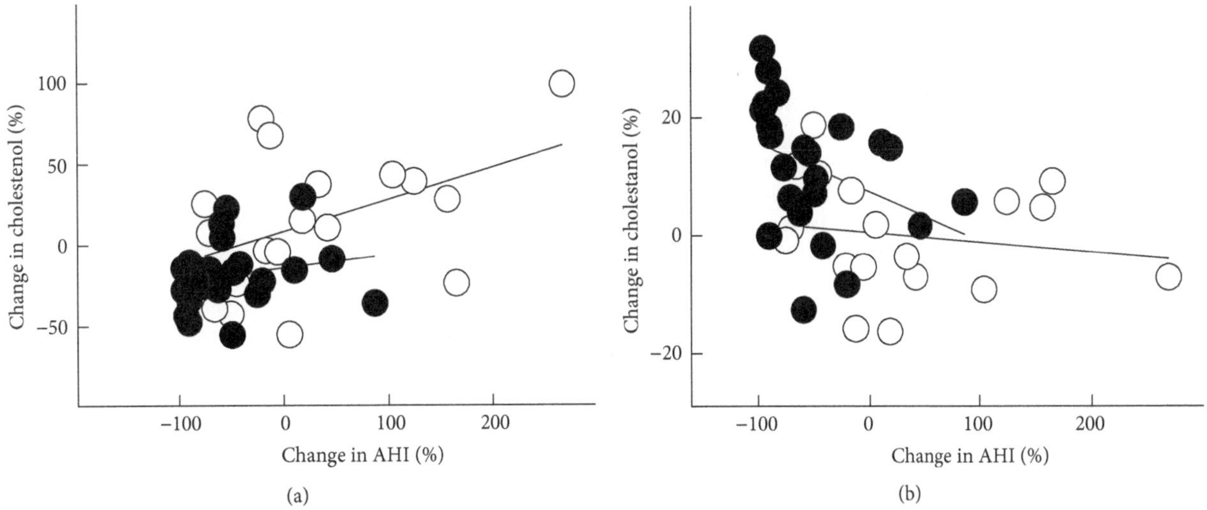

FIGURE 2: The associations between the percentage changes in apnoea-hypopnoea index (AHI) and serum cholestenol ((a), $r = 0.589$, $P < 0.001$, $N = 41$) and cholestanol ratios to cholesterol (10^2 x mmol/mol of cholesterol) ((b), $r = -0.441$, $P = 0.004$, $N = 41$) in the control (○) and intervention (•) groups.

and cholesterol absorption and synthesis markers were to opposite directions than with AHI, but the relationships did not reached statistical significance.

Even mild OSA is associated with increased activation of the inflammatory system and a risk for cardiovascular morbidity, although the risk is more frequently associated with more severe degrees of the disease [8–10]. The exact underlying mechanisms explaining the association between cardiovascular morbidity and OSA are not fully understood, although a multifactorial aetiology is most likely [6]. It is suggested that OSA may accelerate atherosclerosis affecting the key risk factors of atherosclerosis. One of the proposed potential mediators and accelerators of atherosclerosis in OSA is postulated to be dysregulation of lipid metabolism and dyslipidaemia. Cholesterol absorption is low, and cholesterol synthesis is high in obesity [17], insulin resistance [35], and type 2 diabetes even without obesity [36]. In type 2 diabetes, weight reduction increased cholesterol absorption and downregulated cholesterol synthesis simultaneously with improved glucose balance [22]. Therefore, low absorption-high synthesis of cholesterol might be proatherogenic in insulin-resistant situations, possibly frequently present also in OSA. This kind of metabolic profile of cholesterol of insulin resistance is different from that observed in primary hypercholesterolaemia, in which high absorption-low synthesis of cholesterol is associated with unfavorable prognosis during statin treatment in coronary subjects [37]. The present study demonstrates that with weight reduction both OSA and the possibly proatherogenic profile of cholesterol metabolism can be improved. The intriguing question, however, is by which mechanism the variables of OSA and cholesterol metabolism are interrelated beyond obesity. Both at baseline and after the intervention with improved tissue oxygenation the associations between OSA and cholesterol metabolism were similar: better oxygenation is associated with higher absorption and lower synthesis of cholesterol independent of BMI.

Our study population was homogenous consisting only of overweight subjects with mild OSA. Therefore, the results cannot be generalized to all OSA patients, and there exist also some limitations in this study. The sample size per group was relatively small, and it was smaller than in the original study [20], because the subjects using lipid-lowering medication had to be excluded. With larger study population the results, which now tended to be significant, might become significant. Furthermore, the sample size of the present study is similar to those in other recent interventional studies examining lipid metabolisms in OSA patients. Because no stratification in terms of BMI was used in the randomisation, the weight between the groups differed at baseline. Therefore, we adjusted the results for the baseline BMI. Furthermore, because serum insulin concentration and cholestenol : cholesterol ratio were greater and HOMA-IR tended to significantly greater in the intervention group compared with controls at baseline, the baseline values were taken into account as covariance in the analyses of those variables. Regardless of some limitations, the present study is, as far as we know, the first study to examine the associations between OSA and cholesterol metabolism in humans and with and without lifestyle intervention in a randomised settings. Furthermore, this study demonstrated the even mild OSA seemed to be associated with abnormal cholesterol metabolism.

CPAP is considered as a "gold standard" of OSA treatment [38]. However, the adherence of some patients to CPAP treatment is unsatisfactory, particularly in the early stages of the OSA. Based on the recent randomised studies and on the fact that obesity is the most important risk factor for OSA and most OSA patients are obese, weight reduction by lifestyle changes (healthy eating habits, food behaviour therapy if needed and physical activity) should be the first line or at least part of the treatment for all overweight OSA patients. Besides improving OSA, weight reduction seems to improve also other obesity-related disturbances of cardiometabolic syndrome [20, 39].

In conclusion, weight reduction with intensive lifestyle counselling with an initial VLCD program increased the markers of cholesterol absorption and decreased those of cholesterol synthesis in subjects with mild OSA. High Sa_{O_2} seems to be associated with high cholesterol absorption and low Sa_{O_2} with upregulated cholesterol synthesis independent of BMI, HOMA-IR, and gender. Improvement in AHI was associated with increased cholesterol absorption and decreased cholesterol synthesis independent of BMI and HOMA-IR. However, further studies with greater number of subjects are needed to confirm these results.

Conflict of Interests

The authors declare no conflict of interests.

Acknowledgments

The members of Kuopio Sleep Apnoea Group Taina Poutiainen, Grigori Smirnov, Tomi Laitinen, Tiina Lyyra-Laitinen, Matti Uusitupa, Aki Ikonen, Ritva Vanninen, Heimo Viinamäki, Keijo Peuhkurinen, Kari Punnonen, Erkki Soini, and Janne Martikainen are cordially acknowledged. The authors thank also Erja Kinnunen for excellent laboratory work. The study was funded by the Hospital District of Northern Savo. Kuopio University Hospital, the Juho Vainio Foundation, Paavo Nurmi Foundation, and the Finnish Anti-Tuberculosis Foundation have supported the study with grants. The funding sources had no role in study design; collection, analysis, or interpretation of the data; or writing of the report.

References

[1] T. Young, P. E. Peppard, and D. J. Gottlieb, "Epidemiology of obstructive sleep apnea: a population health perspective," *American Journal of Respiratory and Critical Care Medicine*, vol. 165, no. 9, pp. 1217–1239, 2002.

[2] S. R. Coughlin, L. Mawdsley, J. A. Mugarza, P. M. A. Calverley, and J. P. H. Wilding, "Obstructive sleep apnoea is independently associated with an increased prevalence of metabolic syndrome," *European Heart Journal*, vol. 25, no. 9, pp. 735–741, 2004.

[3] F. J. Nieto, T. B. Young, B. K. Lind et al., "Association of sleep-disordered breathing sleep apnea, and hypertension in a large community-based study," *Journal of the American Medical Association*, vol. 283, no. 14, pp. 1829–1836, 2000.

[4] P. E. Peppard, T. Young, M. Palta, and J. Skatrud, "Prospective study of the association between sleep-disordered breathing and hypertension," *The New England Journal of Medicine*, vol. 342, no. 19, pp. 1378–1384, 2000.

[5] E. Shahar, C. W. Whitney, S. Redline et al., "Sleep-disordered breathing and cardiovascular disease: cross-sectional results of the sleep heart health study," *American Journal of Respiratory and Critical Care Medicine*, vol. 163, no. 1, pp. 19–25, 2001.

[6] A. S. M. Shamsuzzaman, B. J. Gersh, and V. K. Somers, "Obstructive sleep apnea: implications for cardiac and vascular disease," *Journal of the American Medical Association*, vol. 290, no. 14, pp. 1906–1914, 2003.

[7] H. Tuomilehto, M. Peltonen, M. Partinen et al., "Sleep-disordered breathing is related to an increased risk for type 2 diabetes in middle-aged men, but not in women -the FIN-D2D survey," *Diabetes, Obesity and Metabolism*, vol. 10, no. 6, pp. 468–475, 2008.

[8] N. M. Punjabi, B. S. Caffo, J. L. Goodwin et al., "Sleep-disordered breathing and mortality: A Prospective Cohort Study," *PLoS Medicine*, vol. 6, no. 8, article e1000132, 2009.

[9] M. Partinen and C. Guilleminault, "Daytime sleepiness and vascular morbidity at seven-year follow-up in obstructive sleep apnea patients," *Chest*, vol. 97, no. 1, pp. 27–32, 1990.

[10] J. Sahlman, K. Miettinen, K. Peuhkurinen et al., "The activation of the inflammatory cytokines in overweight patients with mild obstructive sleep apnoea: sleep apnea and inflammation," *Journal of Sleep Research*, vol. 19, no. 2, pp. 341–348, 2010.

[11] A. B. Newman, F. J. Nieto, U. Guidry et al., "Relation of sleep-disordered breathing to cardiovascular disease risk factors: The Sleep Heart Health Study," *American Journal of Epidemiology*, vol. 154, no. 1, pp. 50–59, 2001.

[12] F. Roche, E. Sforza, V. Pichot et al., "Obstructive sleep apnoea/hypopnea influences high-density lipoprotein cholesterol in the elderly," *Sleep Medicine*, vol. 10, no. 8, pp. 882–886, 2009.

[13] C. Tsioufis, K. Thomopoulos, K. Dimitriadis et al., "The incremental effect of obstructive sleep apnoea syndrome on arterial stiffness in newly diagnosed essential hypertensive subjects," *Journal of Hypertension*, vol. 25, no. 1, pp. 141–146, 2007.

[14] L. F. Drager, L. A. Bortolotto, M. C. Lorenzi, A. C. Figueiredo, E. M. Krieger, and G. Lorenzi-Filho, "Early signs of atherosclerosis in obstructive sleep apnea," *American Journal of Respiratory and Critical Care Medicine*, vol. 172, no. 5, pp. 613–618, 2005.

[15] L. F. Drager, V. Y. Polotsky, and G. Lorenzi-Filho, "Obstructive sleep apnea: an emerging risk factor for atherosclerosis," *Chest*, vol. 140, no. 2, pp. 534–542, 2011.

[16] T. Young, J. Skatrud, and P. E. Peppard, "Risk factors for obstructive sleep apnea in adults," *Journal of the American Medical Association*, vol. 291, no. 16, pp. 2013–2016, 2004.

[17] T. A. Miettinen and H. Gylling, "Cholesterol absorption efficiency and sterol metabolism in obesity," *Atherosclerosis*, vol. 153, no. 1, pp. 241–248, 2000.

[18] H. Gylling, M. Hallikainen, M. Kolehmainen et al., "Cholesterol synthesis prevails over absorption in metabolic syndrome," *Translational Research*, vol. 149, no. 6, pp. 310–316, 2007.

[19] G. Pillar and N. Shehadeh, "Abdominal fat and sleep apnea: the chicken or the egg?" *Diabetes Care*, vol. 31, pp. S303–S309, 2008.

[20] H. P. I. Tuomilehto, J. M. Seppä, M. M. Partinen et al., "Lifestyle intervention with weight reduction: first-line treatment in mild obstructive sleep apnea," *American Journal of Respiratory and Critical Care Medicine*, vol. 179, no. 4, pp. 320–327, 2009.

[21] P. Simonen, H. Gylling, and T. A. Miettinen, "Acute effects of weight reduction on cholesterol metabolism in obese type 2 diabetes," *Clinica Chimica Acta*, vol. 316, no. 1-2, pp. 55–61, 2002.

[22] P. Simonen, H. Gylling, A. N. Howard, and T. A. Miettinen, "Introducing a new component of the metabolic syndrome: low cholesterol absorption," *American Journal of Clinical Nutrition*, vol. 72, no. 1, pp. 82–88, 2000.

[23] T. A. Miettinen, R. S. Tilvis, and Y. A. Kesäniemi, "Serum plant sterols and cholesterol precursors reflect cholesterol absorption and synthesis in volunteers of a randomly selected male population," *American Journal of Epidemiology*, vol. 131, no. 1, pp. 20–31, 1990.

[24] W. W. Flemons, D. Buysse, S. Redline et al., "Sleep-related breathing disorders in adults: recommendations for syndrome definition and measurement techniques in clinical research," *Sleep*, vol. 22, no. 5, pp. 667–689, 1999.

[25] D. R. Matthews, J. P. Hosker, and A. S. Rudenski, "Homeostasis model assessment: Insulin resistance and β-cell function from fasting plasma glucose and insulin concentrations in man," *Diabetologia*, vol. 28, no. 7, pp. 412–419, 1985.

[26] T. A. Miettinen, "Cholesterol metabolism during ketoconazole treatment in man," *Journal of Lipid Research*, vol. 29, no. 1, pp. 43–51, 1988.

[27] C. L. Phillips, B. J. Yee, N. S. Marshall, P. Y. Liu, D. R. Sullivan, and R. R. Grunstein, "Continuous positive airway pressure reduces postprandial lipidemia in obstructive sleep apnea: a randomized, placebo-controlled crossover trial," *American Journal of Respiratory and Critical Care Medicine*, vol. 184, no. 3, pp. 355–361, 2011.

[28] G. V. Robinson, J. C. T. Pepperell, H. C. Segal, R. J. O. Davies, and J. R. Stradling, "Circulating cardiovascular risk factors in obstructive sleep apnoea: data from randomised controlled trials," *Thorax*, vol. 59, no. 9, pp. 777–782, 2004.

[29] J. E. Shaw, N. M. Punjabi, J. P. Wilding, K. G. M. M. Alberti, and P. Z. Zimmet, "Sleep-disordered breathing and type 2 diabetes. A report from the International Diabetes Federation Taskforce on Epidemiology and Prevention," *Diabetes Research and Clinical Practice*, vol. 81, no. 1, pp. 2–12, 2008.

[30] A. M. Dattilo and P. M. Kris-Etherton, "Effects of weight reduction on blood lipids and lipoproteins: a meta- analysis," *American Journal of Clinical Nutrition*, vol. 56, no. 2, pp. 320–328, 1992.

[31] J. Li, V. Savransky, A. Nanayakkara, P. L. Smith, C. P. O'Donnell, and V. Y. Polotsky, "Hyperlipidemia and lipid peroxidation are dependent on the severity of chronic intermittent hypoxia," *Journal of Applied Physiology*, vol. 102, no. 2, pp. 557–563, 2007.

[32] J. Li, L. N. Thorne, N. M. Punjabi et al., "Intermittent hypoxia induces hyperlipidemia in lean mice," *Circulation Research*, vol. 97, no. 7, pp. 698–706, 2005.

[33] V. Savransky, J. Jun, J. Li et al., "Dyslipidemia and atherosclerosis induced by chronic intermittent hypoxia are attenuated by deficiency of stearoyl coenzyme a desaturase," *Circulation Research*, vol. 103, no. 10, pp. 1173–1180, 2008.

[34] L. F. Drager, J. Li, M. K. Shin et al., "Intermittent hypoxia inhibits clearance of triglyceride-rich lipoproteins and inactivates adipose lipoprotein lipase in a mouse model of sleep apnoea," *European Heart Journal*, vol. 19, no. 11, pp. 2167–2174, 2011.

[35] J. Pihlajamäki, H. Gylling, T. A. Miettinen, and M. Laakso, "Insulin resistance is associated with increased cholesterol synthesis and decreased cholesterol absorption in normoglycemic men," *Journal of Lipid Research*, vol. 45, no. 3, pp. 507–512, 2004.

[36] P. P. Simonen, H. K. Gylling, and T. A. Miettinen, "Diabetes contributes to cholesterol metabolism regardless of obesity," *Diabetes Care*, vol. 25, no. 9, pp. 1511–1515, 2002.

[37] T. A. Miettinen, H. Gylling, T. Strandberg, and S. Sarna, "Baseline serum cholestanol as predictor of recurrent coronary events in subgroup of Scandinavian simvastatin survival study," *British Medical Journal*, vol. 316, no. 7138, pp. 1127–1130, 1998.

[38] E. Ballester, J. R. Badia, L. Hernández et al., "Evidence of the effectiveness of continuous positive airway pressure in the treatment of sleep apnea/hypopnea syndrome," *American Journal of Respiratory and Critical Care Medicine*, vol. 159, no. 2, pp. 495–501, 1999.

[39] K. Johansson, E. Hemmingsson, R. Harlid et al., "Longer term effects of very low energy diet on obstructive sleep apnoea in cohort derived from randomised controlled trial: Prospective Observational Follow-up Study," *British Medical Journal*, vol. 342, no. d3017, 2011.

17

Gender Differences Time Trends for Metabolic Syndrome and Its Components among Tehranian Children and Adolescents

Maryam Barzin,[1] Farhad Hosseinpanah,[1] Hamidreza Saber,[1] Parvin Sarbakhsh,[1] Kobra Nakhoda,[2] and Fereidoun Azizi[2]

[1] *Obesity Research Center, Research Institute for Endocrine Science, Shahid Beheshti University of Medical Sciences, 1985717413 Tehran, Iran*
[2] *Endocrine Research Center, Research Institute for Endocrine Science, Shahid Beheshti University of Medical Sciences, 1985717413 Tehran, Iran*

Correspondence should be addressed to Farhad Hosseinpanah, fhospanah@endocrine.ac.ir

Academic Editor: Roya Kelishadi

Aims. To investigate the trend of metabolic syndrome and its components in Tehran children and adolescents during a median followup of 6.6 years. *Methods.* Data from 1999–2001 (phase I), 2002–2005 (phase II), and 2006–2008 (phase III) of the Tehran, Lipid and Glucose Study were analyzed ($n = 5439$; age 6–18 years) for the trend of metabolic syndrome (MetS) and its components. General estimation equation (GEE) models were used to analyze this correlated data. *Results.* The crude prevalence of MetS for boys at baseline was 13.2%, which increased to 16.4% in the third phase. In girls, the prevalence of Mets decreased from 11.8% at baseline to 6% during followup. The odd ratios (OR) of obesity over the whole study period were raised in both sexes. The OR of abdominal obesity increased significantly in boys, but no change was observed in girls. No significant OR was observed in boys, while OR for MetS was shown to have a decreasing trend in girls during the followup. In the three time points, the ORs of MetS decreased significantly in girls but no significant difference was observed in boys. *Conclusion.* Inspite of increasing trend for obesity in both sexes, the trend of MetS decreased in girls and was relatively stable in boys, in Tehranian children, and adolescents.

1. Introduction

The metabolic syndrome (MetS) is defined as a clustering of metabolic risk factors including central obesity, hyperglycemia, dyslipidemia, and hypertension [1]. In recent decades, obesity and metabolic risk factors among children and adolescents have been much focused on several studies showing that increasing obesity and MetS in this population is associated with a number of adverse consequences in adulthood including type 2 diabetes mellitus and coronary heart disease, most likely due to overproduction of inflammatory mediators and insulin resistance [2–4].

While current estimates indicate a 2% to 9% prevalence for MetS in US adolescents [5], 14.1% of Iranian children have MetS based on ATP III criteria resulting from the increasing prevalence of overweight and abdominal obesity among Iranian children and adolescents [6, 7]. Previous studies also demonstrated higher triglyceride and lower HDL-C levels in Iranian adolescents compared to their American counterparts [8, 9]. This increased prevalence would necessitate the need for identifying the time trend of Mets and its components in our population. Although the prevalence and associated risk factors of MetS have been widely studied in recent decades [10–12], much less is known in regard to changes in risk factor status over a longer period of time during childhood and adolescence, particularly in developing countries like Iran.

A few studies have evaluated the tracking of MetS and its components altogether [13–17] and most of them have provided data in support of a stability of MetS and its components in their populations [13, 14, 16]. Other studies have demonstrated an increasing trend in MetS [17] and its individual components [18–21]. In a recent study which used three independent sets of cross-sectional data with limited sample size in Tehranian adolescents, aged 10–19 years, reported an increasing trend for obesity, abdominal obesity [22]. Given the above-mentioned limitations in this study, we aimed to examine the trend of MetS and its components from childhood to adolescence, due a mean of 6.6 years of followup for the first time in Middle East region using general estimation equation (GEE) analysis.

2. Materials and Methods

Subjects in this study were selected from among participants of the Tehran Lipid and Glucose Study (TLGS), a prospective study conducted to determine the risk factors and outcomes for noncommunicable diseases [23]. To summarize, 15,005 people, aged 3 years and over, residents of district-13 of Tehran underwent a baseline examination between February 1999 and August 2001. After this cross-sectional (phase 1), subjects were categorized into the cohort and intervention groups, the latter to be educated for implementation of life-style modifications. We used metabolic and anthropometric data from phases I (1999–2001), II (2002–2005), and III (2006–2008) of the TLGS. For the current study, 5439 participants, 2643 boys and 2797 girls, aged 6–18 years who had participated at least in one of three phases, were enrolled. The study was approved by the institutional ethics committee of the Research Institute for Endocrine Sciences, affiliated to Shahid Beheshti University of Medical Sciences and was conducted in accordance with the principles of the Declaration of Helsinki.

Details of the TLGS protocol and all laboratory procedures have been published elsewhere [10]. Briefly, trained interviewers collected information, using a pretested questionnaire which included demographic data and anthropometric indices. Weight, height, and waist circumference (WC) were measured using standard protocols. Body mass index (BMI) was calculated as weight in kilograms, divided by height in meters squared. A qualified physician measured blood pressure twice with the subject in a seated position after one initial measurement for determining peak inflation level using a standard mercury sphygmomanometer; the mean of two measurements was considered to be the participant's blood pressure. Fasting blood samples for the measurement of glucose and lipid concentrations were drawn after the subjects had fasted overnight. Fasting blood glucose (FBG) was measured on the day of blood collection by the enzymatic colorimetric method using glucose oxidase. Triglyceride (TG) concentrations were measured by commercially available enzymatic reagents (Pars Azmoon, Tehran, Iran) adapted to a Selectra autoanalyzer. High-density lipoprotein cholesterol (HDL-C) was measured after precipitation of the apolipoprotein B-containing lipoproteins with phosphotungstic acid.

2.1. Definitions. We used the definition based on Cook et al. work for definition of the MetS in children and adolescents [24]. This definition is based on criteria analogous to that of the National Cholesterol Education Program Expert Panel on Detection, Evaluation and Treatment of High Blood Cholesterol in Adult Treatment Panel III [1]; it defines MetS as three or more of the following: fasting TG $\geq$ 110 mg/dL; HDL cholesterol <40 mg/dL; WC $\geq$ 90th percentile for age and sex, according to national reference curves [25]; systolic blood pressure (SBP) and/or diastolic blood pressure (DBP) $\geq$90th percentile for sex, age and height, from national reference cut-off points [26]; FBG $\geq$ 100 mg/dL. For the subjects who were aged over 18 years after the followup, we used the criteria for MetS in adults, specified by the Joint Interim Statement (JIS) [27]. Obesity was defined based on the standardized percentile curves of BMI suggested for Iranian children and adolescents as $\geq$95th percentile of BMI for age and sex [6].

2.2. Statistic Analysis. All continuous data are expressed as mean ± SD, and categorical variables are expressed as percentages. Independent t-test was used to compare difference between two sexes within in each phase. The general estimation equation (GEE) use the generalized linear model to estimate more efficient and unbiased analysis of demographic variables, anthropometric indices, and biochemical variables collected in longitudinal, nested, or repeated measures designs [28, 29]. This method relies on independence across subjects to consistently estimate the variance of the proposed estimators even when the assumed working correlation structure is incorrect. Logistic regression analysis was performed using GEE method for binominal variables. Variables were adjusted for age (years), time (phase) and intervention.

All analyses were performed using SPSS for Windows (version 16; SPSS Inc., Chicago, IL, USA), and significance was set at $P < 0.05$.

3. Results

For the current study, we had 3,854, 3,057, and 3,441 observations in phases I, II, and III, respectively. The GEE analysis was performed with 5,439 subjects (2643 boys), aged 6–18 years, who had at least one observation in whole period the study. At baseline, girls had higher mean values for WC ($P = 0.04$), TG ($P = 0.01$), LDL, and cholesterol ($P < 0.001$) but lower SBP and FBS than boys ($P < 0.001$). At the end of followup, all factors were higher in boys, while cholesterol and HDL values were higher in girls ($P = 0.001$, Table 1).

The crude prevalence of obesity increased in both sexes during a median follow-up of 6.6 years. Abdominal obesity increased from 12.3% to 33.1 in phase III in boys, but remained fairly stable in girls. The most frequent component of MetS was low HDL at baseline (39%) that increased up to 47% for boys and 43% for girls in the third phase. High TG was the next most prevalent component that decreased from 35% and 31% at baseline to 21% and 25% in girls and boys, respectively. The prevalence of MetS was 13.2% for boys at baseline that increased to 16.4% in the third phase. In girls, the prevalence of Mets decreased from 11.8% at baseline to 6% during followup (Figure 1).

TABLE 1: Anthropometric and metabolic characteristics of cohort participants by sex in 3 phases.

	Phase I		Phase II		Phase III	
	Boys $N = 1858$	Girls $N = 1995$	Boys $N = 1415$	Girls $N = 1641$	Boys $N = 1592$	Girls $N = 1849$
Age (year)	12.5 ± 3.5	12.6 ± 3.6	14.2 ± 4.53	14.7 ± 4.5	16.0 ± 5.6	16.6 ± 5.4
Weight (kg)	44.7 ± 19.2	42.7 ± 15.56*	53.1 ± 21.8	48.2 ± 16.0*	59.3 ± 23.6	51.4 ± 15.7*
BMI (kg/m^2)	18.9 ± 4.4	19.0 ± 4.5	20.6 ± 5.0	20.6 ± 4.5	22.0 ± 6.3	21.4 ± 4.6*
Overweight (%)	19.7	17.5	28.3	23.7*	34.3	27.2*
Obesity (%)	8.3	6*	11.9	8.4*	13.8	8.9*
WC (cm)	65.0 ± 12.5	65.7 ± 10.8*	73.6 ± 14.6	69.0 ± 11.3*	77.8 ± 15.8	69.2 ± 11.0*
Abdominal obesity (%)	12.3	13.7	26.9	14.3*	33.1	13*
SBP (mmHg)	106.2 ± 12.2	103.6 ± 11.3*	104.0 ± 13.0	98.8 ± 11.3*	104.6 ± 13.2	98.3 ± 11.3*
DBP (mmHg)	71.1 ± 9.5	71.2 ± 9.4	67.2 ± 10.0	67.2 ± 9.4	67.5 ± 10.5	64.7 ± 9.6*
FBG (mg/dL)	88.9 ± 11.3	86.9 ± 8.3*	88.7 ± 11.6	86.2 ± 7.4*	86.9 ± 7.5	84.7 ± 7.0*
TG (mg/dL)	103.7 ± 60. 7	107.9 ± 54.9*	101.6 ± 54.4	99.0 ± 47.7	105.2 ± 61.4	94.6 ± 45.9*
HDL-C (mg/dL)	44.0 ± 10.8	44.0 ± 10.5	40.8 ± 10.3	41.5 ± 10.1	42.8 ± 10.3	45.6 ± 10.4*

Data are presented as mean (SD) or percent.
BMI, body mass index; WC, waist circumference; SBP, systolic blood pressure; DBP, diastolic blood pressure; FBG, fasting blood glucose; TG, triglycerides HDL-C, high density lipoprotein cholesterol. Overweight defined as ≥85th to <95th percentile of BMI for age and sex; obesity defined as ≥95th percentile of BMI for age and sex; abdominal obesity defined as WC ≥ 90th percentile for age and sex.
*$P < 0.001$ (between boys and girls in each phase).

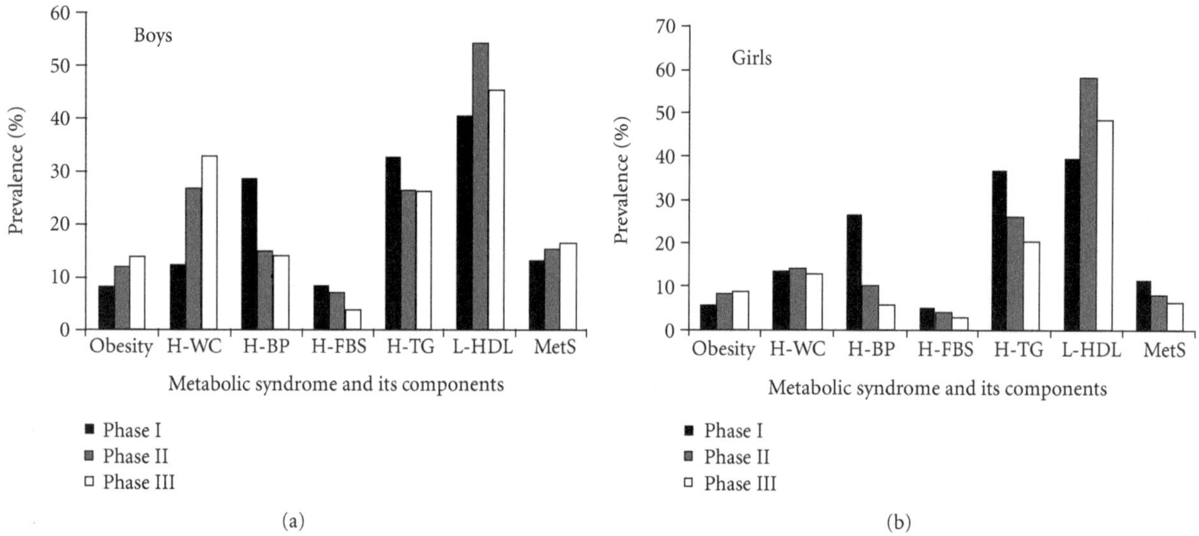

FIGURE 1: Prevalence of metabolic syndrome (MetS) and its components in boys ($n = 2643$) and girls ($n = 2797$). Obesity defined as ≥95th percentile of BMI for age and sex; high waist circumference (H-WC) ≥90th percentile for age and sex, according to national reference curves; high blood pressure (H-BP), SBP and/or DBP ≥90th percentile for sex, age and height, from national reference cut-off points; high fasting blood glucose (H-FBG), fasting glucose ≥100 mg/dL; high triglycerides (H-TG), fasting TG ≥ 110 mg/dL; low HDL cholesterol (L-HDL), HDL < 40 mg/dL.

The odds of obesity over the whole study period were raised in both sexes ($P < 0.01$). While the odds of abdominal obesity increased significantly in boys ($P < 0.001$), whereas no significant change was observed in girls (P = NS). The odds for all other MetS component values declined towards the end of followup, except for HDL in girls. At three time points, the odds of MetS decreased significantly in girls (OR: 0.69 and 0.55 $P < 0.001$ in phases II and III, resp.) but no significant difference was observed in boys (OR: 1.1 and 0.94 P = NS in phases II and III resp., Table 2).

4. Discussion

Using GEE analysis, the results of present study conducted on 5,439 Tehranian children and adolescents, aged 6–18 years, suggest that during a median follow-up of 6.6 years, the trend of obesity increased in both sexes and for abdominal obesity increased almost three folds in boys. In spite of the increasing trend for the above factors, the trend for MetS decreased in girls and remained relatively stable in boys.

The high prevalence of obesity and MetS in childhood and adolescence has been shown to increase the prevalence

TABLE 2: Odd ratios[a] of the incident MetS parameters in phase I, II and III.

Characteristics	phase I	phase II	phase III
Boys			
obesity	1	1.40 (1.16–1.68)*	1.49 (1.19–1.87)*
Abdominal obesity	1	2.28 (1.95–2.67)*	2.61 (2.19–3.12)*
High FBG	1	0.90 (0.69–1.18)	0.47 (0.34–0.64)*
Low HDL-C	1	1.51 (1.32–1.73)*	0.84 (0.73–0.96)*
High TG	1	0.68 (0.58–0.78)*	0.63 (0.54–0.74)*
High BP	1	0.45 (0.37–0.53)*	0.42 (0.34–0.52)*
MetS	1	1.1 (0.90–1.33)	0.94 (0.73–1.22)
Girls			
obesity	1	1.42 (1.14–1.77)*	1.41 (1.07–1.84)*
Abdominal obesity	1	1.08 (0.912–1.28)	0.98 (0.79–1.21)
High FBG	1	0.78 (0.56–1.08)	0.59 (0.42–0.83)*
Low HDL-C	1	1.89 (1.66–2.14)*	1.07 (0.93–1.22)
High TG	1	0.65 (0.67–0.75)*	0.50 (0.43–0.58)*
High BP	1	0.50 (0.43–0.58)*	0.21 (0.16–0.27)*
MetS	1	0.21 (0.16–0.27)*	0.55 (0.41–0.75)*

Obesity, BMI ≥ 95th percentile for age and sex; abdominal obesity, WC ≥ 90th percentile for age and sex; high FBG, FBS ≥ 100 (mg/dL); Low HDL-C, HDL-C < 40 (mg/dL); high TG, TG ≥ 110 (mg/dL); High BP, SBP, and/or DBP ≥90th percentile for sex, age, and height.
[a](95% Confidence interval).
* *P* value <0.05 compare to phase I.

of cardiovascular events in adults [30]. Childhood and adolescent MetS have evolved into a worldwide epidemic, up to 14% in Australian [31] and 11% in Italian children [32]. Findings from previous studies in Iran have revealed a higher prevalence of MetS among Iranian children (9.8% [7]) compared with western (4.2% in US [24]) and Asian countries (1.4% in Japan [33] and 1.8% in Korea [15] 6.6% in China [34]). Several previous epidemiological studies demonstrated different trends for MetS and cardiometabolic risk factors among children and adolescents [13–17], which can be explained by variety in MetS definitions, length of followup, and also specific cultural and ethnical composition of studied population, lifestyle, and public health policies. In the Young Finns Study, a follow-up study of 1769 girls and 1688 boys, aged 3–18 years old, the prevalence of MetS increased with age in boys, and in 9–12 years old age girls [17]. The results from the Quebec family study indicated that indicators of MetS are moderately stable from childhood to adolescence [16]. Based on the Fels longitudinal study, authors concluded that 8 cardiometabolic risk factors associated with the MetS were relatively stable among children and adolescents [13]. On the other hand, results from the Korean NHANES Survey on 4164 subjects, aged 10–19 years, demonstrated a decline in prevalence of MetS, despite an increase in obesity in Korean adolescents [15]. In agreement with the Korean study, despite increasing trend of obesity, we found a decreasing trend of MetS in girls, but it relatively stable in boys mostly as a result of improvement in other MetS components. Similarly, an increasing prevalence of childhood obesity has been reported around the world [35–37]. Rapidly changing dietary practices and a sedentary lifestyle have led to increasing prevalence of childhood obesity (5–19 years) in developing countries recently [38] such as Iran [22]. Moreover, recent systematic reviews and meta-analyses of available randomized trials reported nonsignificant effects of pharmacologic and behavioral treatments for reduction of overweight and obesity in children and adolescents [39, 40]. Regarding above mentioned studies, cardiometabolic risk factors were stable across time besides increasing trend of obesity in children and adolescents.

The decreasing prevalence of cardiometabolic risk factors can be explained by the positive effects of public health interventions in terms of lifestyle behaviors and increased physical activity on unfavorable risk factors. Accordingly, a systematic review has shown that higher physical activity levels were consistently associated with an improved metabolic profile and a reduced risk for MetS and/or insulin resistance in pediatric populations [41]. We speculate that recent changes in physical activity in addition to national health care initiatives in Tehran may have had a positive impact on the prevalence of MetS. We also found some notable differences between genders in the trend of MetS, for which however we do not have an adequate explanation; it could possibly be explained by more focus of public educational programs on girls compared to boys, leading to decreasing trend of MetS in girls.

The strength of our study was the considerable sample size of children and adolescents with a long followup period over which we measured MetS and its components enabling us to assess the time effect of these risk factors in our population using the GEE model for the first time.

However, our study had several limitations. First, our subjects were from a homogeneous population, potentially limiting the generalizability of our results. Second, we did not have data regarding puberty status which have helped us to assess the effects of puberty on MetS, and third, we did not take into account some possible confounders such as physical activity, dietary habits, and socioeconomic status in our analysis.

5. Conclusion

In conclusion, inspite of the increasing trend for obesity in both sexes, the trend for MetS decreased in girls and remained relatively stable in boys in our population. Given the proven association between childhood and adolescence, obesity, and accuracy of cardiovascular events in adulthood, we are not sure that our observations, indicating persistency of excess weight along with reduction of cardiometabolic risk factors can be translated to decrease cardiovascular event rates in future adulthood. Further prospective studies with long-term followup are needed to answer this question.

Conflict of Interests

All the authors declare that there is no conflict of interest that could be perceived as prejudicing the impartiality of the research reported.

Acknowledgments

The authors thank Dr. Kelishadi for her assistance, and Mrs Shiva for language editing of the manuscript. They would like to express their appreciation to the staff of the Endocrine Research Center and especially all of the mothers and children who participated in this study.

References

[1] J. I. Cleeman, "Executive summary of the third report of the National Cholesterol Education Program (NCEP) expert panel on detection, evaluation, and treatment of high blood cholesterol in adults (adult treatment panel III)," *Journal of the American Medical Association*, vol. 285, no. 19, pp. 2486–2497, 2001.

[2] J. A. Morrison, L. A. Friedman, P. Wang, and C. J. Glueck, "Metabolic syndrome in childhood predicts adult metabolic syndrome and type 2 diabetes mellitus 25 to 30 years later," *Journal of Pediatrics*, vol. 152, no. 2, pp. 201–206, 2008.

[3] F. M. Biro and M. Wien, "Childhood obesity and adult morbidities," *American Journal of Clinical Nutrition*, vol. 91, no. 5, pp. 1499S–1505S, 2010.

[4] K. J. Nadeau, D. M. Maahs, S. R. Daniels, and R. H. Eckel, "Childhood obesity and cardiovascular disease: links and prevention strategies," *Nature Reviews Cardiology*, vol. 8, no. 9, pp. 513–525, 2011.

[5] S. Cook, P. Auinger, C. Li, and E. S. Ford, "Metabolic syndrome rates in United States adolescents, from the National Health and Nutrition Examination Survey, 1999–2002," *Journal of Pediatrics*, vol. 152, no. 2, pp. 165–170, 2008.

[6] R. Kelishadi, G. Ardalan, R. Gheiratmand, K. Adeli, A. Delavari, and R. Majdzadeh, "Paediatric metabolic syndrome and associated anthropometric indices: the CASPIAN Study," *Acta Paediatrica*, vol. 95, no. 12, pp. 1625–1634, 2006.

[7] M. Barzin, F. Hosseinpanah, S. Fekri, and F. Azizi, "Predictive value of body mass index and waist circumference for metabolic syndrome in 6-12-year-olds," *Acta Paediatrica*, vol. 100, no. 5, pp. 722–727, 2011.

[8] F. Azizi, M. Rahmani, A. Ghanbarian et al., "Serum lipid levels in an Iranian adults population: Tehran lipid and glucose Study," *European Journal of Epidemiology*, vol. 18, no. 4, pp. 311–319, 2003.

[9] A. Esmaillzadeh, P. Mirmiran, L. Azadbakht, A. Etemadi, and F. Azizi, "High prevalence of the metabolic syndrome in Iranian adolescents," *Obesity*, vol. 14, no. 3, pp. 377–382, 2006.

[10] F. Azizi, P. Salehi, A. Etemadi, and S. Zahedi-Asl, "Prevalence of metabolic syndrome in an urban population: Tehran lipid and glucose Study," *Diabetes Research and Clinical Practice*, vol. 61, no. 1, pp. 29–37, 2003.

[11] R. H. Eckel, K. G. M. M. Alberti, S. M. Grundy, and P. Z. Zimmet, "The metabolic syndrome," *The Lancet*, vol. 375, no. 9710, pp. 181–183, 2010.

[12] E. S. Ford, W. H. Giles, and W. H. Dietz, "Prevalence of the metabolic syndrome among US adults: findings from the third National Health and Nutrition Examination Survey," *Journal of the American Medical Association*, vol. 287, no. 3, pp. 356–359, 2002.

[13] C. Li, E. S. Ford, T. T. K. Huang, S. S. Sun, and E. Goodman, "Patterns of change in cardiometabolic risk factors associated with the metabolic syndrome among children and adolescents: the Fels longitudinal Study," *Journal of Pediatrics*, vol. 155, no. 3, pp. S5.e9–S5.e16, 2009.

[14] J. C. Eisenmann, G. J. Welk, E. E. Wickel, and S. N. Blair, "Stability of variables associated with the metabolic syndrome from adolescence to adulthood: the aerobics center longitudinal Study," *American Journal of Human Biology*, vol. 16, no. 6, pp. 690–696, 2004.

[15] M. J. Park, B. A. Boston, M. Oh, and S. H. Jee, "Prevalence and trends of metabolic syndrome among Korean adolescents: from the Korean NHANES Survey, 1998–2005," *Journal of Pediatrics*, vol. 155, no. 4, pp. 529–534, 2009.

[16] P. T. Katzmarzyk, L. Perusse, R. M. Malina, J. Bergeron, J. P. Despres, and C. Bouchard, "Stability of indicators of the metabolic syndrome from childhood and adolescence to young adulthood: the Quebec Family Study," *Journal of Clinical Epidemiology*, vol. 54, no. 2, pp. 190–195, 2001.

[17] O. T. Raitakari, K. V. K. Porkka, J. S. A. Viikari, T. Ronnemaa, and H. K. Akerblom, "Clustering of risk factors for coronary heart disease in children and adolescents. The cardiovascular risk in young Finns Study," *Acta Paediatrica*, vol. 83, no. 9, pp. 935–940, 1994.

[18] X. Chen and Y. Wang, "Tracking of blood pressure from childhood to adulthood: a systematic review and meta-regression analysis," *Circulation*, vol. 117, no. 25, pp. 3171–3180, 2008.

[19] L. S. Webber, S. R. Srinivasan, W. A. Wattigney, and G. S. Berenson, "Tracking of serum lipids and lipoproteins from childhood to adulthood. The Bogalusa Heart Study," *American Journal of Epidemiology*, vol. 133, no. 9, pp. 884–899, 1991.

[20] R. M. Fuentes, I. L. Notkola, S. Shemeikka, J. Tuomilehto, and A. Nissinen, "Tracking of systolic blood pressure during childhood: a 15-year follow-up population-based family study in eastern Finland," *Journal of Hypertension*, vol. 20, no. 2, pp. 195–202, 2002.

[21] R. M. Fuentes, I. L. Notkola, S. Shemeikka, J. Tuomilehto, and A. Nissinen, "Tracking of body mass index during childhood: a 15-year prospective population-based family study in eastern Finland," *International Journal of Obesity*, vol. 27, no. 6, pp. 716–721, 2003.

[22] F. Hosseini-Esfahani, A. Mousavi Nasl Khameneh, P. Mirmiran, A. Ghanbarian, and F. Azizi, "Trends in risk factors for cardiovascular disease among Iranian adolescents: the tehran lipid and glucose study, 1999–2008," *Journal of Epidemiology*, vol. 21, no. 5, pp. 319–328, 2011.

[23] F. Azizi, A. Ghanbarian, A. A. Momenan et al., "Prevention of non-communicable disease in a population in nutrition transition: Tehran lipid and glucose study phase II," *Trials*, vol. 10, article 5, 2009.

[24] S. Cook, M. Weitzman, P. Auinger, M. Nguyen, and W. H. Dietz, "Prevalence of a metabolic syndrome phenotype in adolescents: Findings from the third National Health and Nutrition Examination Survey, 1988–1994," *Archives of Pediatrics and Adolescent Medicine*, vol. 157, no. 8, pp. 821–827, 2003.

[25] R. Kelishadi, M. M. Gouya, G. Ardalan et al., "First reference curves of waist and hip circumferences in an Asian population of youths: CASPIAN study," *Journal of Tropical Pediatrics*, vol. 53, no. 3, pp. 158–164, 2007.

[26] R. Kelishadi, G. Ardalan, R. Gheiratmand et al., "Blood pressure and its influencing factors in a national representative sample of Iranian children and adolescents: the CASPIAN Study," *European Journal of Cardiovascular Prevention and Rehabilitation*, vol. 13, no. 6, pp. 956–963, 2006.

[27] K. G. M. M. Alberti, R. H. Eckel, S. M. Grundy et al., "Harmonizing the metabolic syndrome: a joint interim statement of the international diabetes federation task force on epidemiology and prevention; National heart, lung, and blood institute; American heart association; World heart federation; International atherosclerosis society; and international association for the study of obesity," *Circulation*, vol. 120, no. 16, pp. 1640–1645, 2009.

[28] S. L. Zeger and K. Y. Liang, "Longitudinal data analysis for discrete and continuous outcomes," *Biometrics*, vol. 42, no. 1, pp. 121–130, 1986.

[29] S. L. Zeger, K. Y. Liang, and P. S. Albert, "Models for longitudinal data: a generalized estimating equation approach," *Biometrics*, vol. 44, no. 4, pp. 1049–1060, 1988.

[30] P. W. Franks, R. L. Hanson, W. C. Knowler, M. L. Sievers, P. H. Bennett, and H. C. Looker, "Childhood obesity, other cardiovascular risk factors, and premature death," *The New England Journal of Medicine*, vol. 362, no. 6, pp. 485–493, 2010.

[31] E. A. C. Sellers, G. R. Singh, and S. M. Sayers, "Large waist but low body mass index: the metabolic syndrome in Australian aboriginal children," *Journal of Pediatrics*, vol. 153, no. 2, pp. 222–227, 2008.

[32] P. Di Bonito, C. Forziato, E. Sanguigno et al., "Prevalence of the metabolic syndrome using ATP-derived definitions and its relation to insulin-resistance in a cohort of Italian outpatient children," *Journal of Endocrinological Investigation*, vol. 33, no. 11, pp. 806–809, 2010.

[33] I. Saito, M. Mori, H. Shibata, H. Hirose, M. Tsujioka, and H. Kawabe, "Prevalence of metabolic syndrome in young men in Japan," *Journal of Atherosclerosis and Thrombosis*, vol. 14, no. 1, pp. 27–30, 2007.

[34] W. Liu, R. Lin, A. Liu, L. Du, and Q. Chen, "Prevalence and association between obesity and metabolic syndrome among Chinese elementary school children: a school-based survey," *BMC Public Health*, vol. 10, article 780, 2010.

[35] C. L. Ogden, K. M. Flegal, M. D. Carroll, and C. L. Johnson, "Prevalence and trends in overweight among US children and adolescents, 1999–2000," *Journal of the American Medical Association*, vol. 288, no. 14, pp. 1728–1732, 2002.

[36] S. Bjornelv, S. Lydersen, J. Holmen, T. I. Lund Nilsen, and T. L. Holmen, "Sex differences in time trends for overweight and obesity in adolescents: the Young-HUNT study," *Scandinavian Journal of Public Health*, vol. 37, no. 8, pp. 881–889, 2009.

[37] M. L. Booth, T. Chey, M. Wake et al., "Change in the prevalence of overweight and obesity among young Australians, 1969–1997," *American Journal of Clinical Nutrition*, vol. 77, no. 1, pp. 29–36, 2003.

[38] N. Gupta, K. Goel, P. Shah, and A. Misra, "Childhood obesity in developing countries: epidemiology, determinants, and prevention," *Endocrine Reviews*, vol. 33, no. 1, pp. 48–70, 2012.

[39] L. McGovern, J. N. Johnson, R. Paulo et al., "Treatment of pediatric obesity: a systematic review and meta-analysis of randomized trials," *Journal of Clinical Endocrinology and Metabolism*, vol. 93, no. 12, pp. 4600–4605, 2008.

[40] C. C. Kamath, K. S. Vickers, A. Ehrlich et al., "Behavioral interventions to prevent childhood obesity: a systematic review and metaanalyses of randomized trials," *Journal of Clinical Endocrinology and Metabolism*, vol. 93, no. 12, pp. 4606–4615, 2008.

[41] B. C. Guinhouya, H. Samouda, D. Zitouni, C. Vilhelm, and H. Hubert, "Evidence of the influence of physical activity on the metabolic syndrome and/or on insulin resistance in pediatric populations: a systematic review," *International Journal of Pediatric Obesity*, vol. 6, no. 5-6, pp. 361–388, 2011.

Effects of Diet, Aerobic Exercise, or Both on Non-HDL-C in Adults: A Meta-Analysis of Randomized Controlled Trials

George A. Kelley and Kristi S. Kelley

Meta-Analytic Research Group, Department of Biostatistics, School of Public Health, Robert C. Byrd Health Sciences Center, West Virginia University, Morgantown, WV 26506-9190, USA

Correspondence should be addressed to George A. Kelley, gkelley@hsc.wvu.edu

Academic Editor: Jan Wouter Jukema

Purpose. To use the meta-analytic approach to examine the effects of diet (D), aerobic exercise (E), or both (DE) on non-high-density lipoprotein cholesterol (non-HDL-C) in adults. *Methods.* Randomized controlled trials in adults ≥18 years of age were included. A mixed-effect model was used to combine effect size (ES) results within each subgroup and to compare subgroups (Q_b). Heterogeneity was examined using the Q and I^2 statistics, and 95% confidence intervals (CI) were also calculated. Statistical significance was set at $P \leq 0.05$, while a trend for statistical significance was set between $P > 0.05$, and ≤ 0.10. *Results.* A statistically significant exercise minus control group decrease in non-HDL-C was found for DE (7 ESs, 389 participants, $\bar{x} = -11.1$ mg/dL, 95% CI = −21.7 to −0.6, $P = 0.04$, $Q = 2.4$, $P = 0.88$, $I^2 = 0\%$), a trend for the D group (7 ESs, 402 participants, $\bar{x} = -8.5$ mg/dL, 95% CI = −18.6 to 1.6, $P = 0.10$, $Q = 0.76$, $P = 0.99$, $I^2 = 0\%$), and no change for the E group (7 ESs, 387 participants, $\bar{x} = 3.0$ mg/dL, 95% CI = −7.1 to 13.1, $P = 0.56$, $Q = 0.78$, $P = 0.99$, $I^2 = 0\%$). Overall, no statistically significant between-group differences were found ($Q_b = 4.1$, $P = 0.12$). *Conclusions.* Diet combined with aerobic exercise may reduce non-HDL-C among adults in some settings.

1. Introduction

Cardiovascular disease is a major public health problem affecting an estimated 82.6 million adults in the United States (USA) [1]. In terms of mortality, heart disease is the leading cause of death in the USA, affecting 616,628 people (25% of all deaths) in 2008 [2]. Not surprisingly, the economic costs associated with cardiovascular disease are also high. In 2008, the annual direct and indirect costs of cardiovascular disease in the USA were estimated to be $297.7 billion [1].

Less than optimal levels of lipids and lipoproteins are a major risk factor for cardiovascular morbidity and mortality in adults [1]. According to recent estimates, 33.6 million USA adults have total cholesterol (TC) levels ≥240 mg/dL, 71.3 million have low-density-lipoprotein cholesterol (LDL-C) levels ≥130 mg/dL and 41.8 million have high-density lipoprotein cholesterol (HDL-C) levels ≤40 mg/dL [1]. Currently, the primary target of lipid-lowering therapy in adults is low-density lipoprotein cholesterol (LDL-C) with non-high-density lipoprotein cholesterol (non-HDL-C) recommended as a secondary target of therapy in adults with triglyceride levels ≥200 mg/dL [3]. However, it has been suggested that non-HDL-C may be a more relevant target for lipid-lowering therapy because it contains all the lipids and lipoproteins considered to be atherogenic (low-density lipoprotein cholesterol, lipoprotein (a), intermediate-density lipoprotein, very-low-density lipoprotein) [4, 5]. Indeed, previous meta-analytic research has shown that non-HDL-C is a better predictor than LDL-C for future cardiovascular risk. For example, Boekholdt et al. found that non-HDL-C was a better predictor than LDL-C for future risk of cardiovascular events in statin-treated patients [6]. In addition, another meta-analysis found that over a 10-year period, a focus on lowering non-HDL-C versus LDL-C would prevent 300,000 more fatal or nonfatal ischemic cardiovascular events [7]. From a practical perspective, the assessment of non-HDL-C versus LDL-C may be preferred because (1) it can be assessed in the nonfasting state,

(2) incurs no additional costs because it is calculated as the difference between TC and HDL-C, and (3) has well-documented benefits [5].

Aerobic exercise and diet are first-line lifestyle interventions recommended for improving lipids and lipoproteins, including LDL-C, in adults [3]. Recently, aggregate data meta-analytic research of randomized controlled trials addressing the effects of diet (D), aerobic exercise (E), or both (DE) on lipids and lipoproteins in adults were reported by the authors [8]. Interventions had to last at least 4 weeks with diet including any type previously considered to improve lipids and lipoproteins in adults (low saturated fat, caloric restriction, etc.) [3]. For both the D and DE groups, statistically significant intervention minus control (C) group improvements were observed for TC, LDL-C, and triglycerides (TG), but not HDL-C. For the E groups, improvements were limited to TG. When between-group comparisons were conducted, reductions in TC and LDL-C were greater in both the D and DE groups versus E group ($P < 0.05$). No other between-group differences were observed. Unfortunately, none of the studies reported data for non-HDL-C, including dispersion data. In this brief paper, we use an existing method for estimating measures of dispersion for non-HDL-C based on data reported for TC and HDL-C [9] in order to conduct a meta-analysis on the effects of D, E, or both on non-HDL-C in adult humans.

2. Methods

2.1. Study Eligibility, Data Sources, Data Extraction, and Risk of Bias Assessment. Study eligibility, data sources, data extraction, and risk of bias assessment have been previously described in detail elsewhere [8]. Briefly, studies in any language were included if they were randomized controlled trials ≥4 weeks that included D, E, DE, and C groups in adults ≥18 years of age and in which mean and dispersion data for TC and HDL-C were available for calculating non-HDL-C. Data sources included searching nine electronic databases, cross-referencing, and expert review. Dual data extraction occurred using predeveloped codebooks. Risk of bias was assessed by both authors, independent of each other, using the Cochrane Risk of Bias Assessment instrument [10].

2.2. Statistical Analysis

2.2.1. Calculation of Treatment Effects from Each Study. The primary outcome for this meta-analysis was treatment effect changes in non-HDL-C. First, each intervention (D, E, DE) and Control (C) group result was calculated as the change outcome difference in TC minus the change outcome difference in HDL-C. Second, the variance for non-HDL-C for each result from each group (D, E, DE, C) was calculated by pooling the variances of the change outcome differences for TC and HDL-C. Third, treatment effect changes in non-HDL-C were calculated as the intervention (D, E, DE) minus the C result. Variances for these changes were calculated by pooling intervention (D, E, DE) and C results [9].

2.2.2. Pooling of Treatment of Effects. A mixed effects model was used to pool non-HDL-C treatment effects (intervention minus control) for each group (D, E, DE) from each study and to compare results across the three groups. This consisted of a random-effects model to combine studies within each group (D, E, DE) and a fixed-effect model to compare results between groups (Q_b). Study-to-study variance (tau-squared) was not assumed to be equal for all subgroups. A z-score alpha value of ≤0.05 (two-tailed) was considered statistically significant while alpha values >0.05 but ≤0.10 were considered as a trend. Precision of treatment effects estimates for non-HDL-C was determined using two-tailed 95% confidence intervals (CIs) based on z. Estimation of treatment effects for non-HDL-C in a new trial was calculated using 95% prediction intervals (PI) [11–13]. Any statistically significant outliers ($P \leq 0.05$) were deleted from the model.

Heterogeneity of results for each group was examined using the Q and I^2 statistics [14, 15]. The alpha value for statistical significance for Q was set at $P \leq 0.10$. For I^2, values of 25% to <50% were considered small, 50% to <75% medium, and ≥75% large [15]. Potential bias due to small-study effects was examined using a funnel plot along with the data imputation approach of Duval and Tweedie [16, 17]. Simple, mixed-effects meta-regression was conducted to examine the effects of age, baseline non-HDL-C, and intervention minus control group changes in body weight on changes in non-HDL-C in each group (D, E, DE). A two-tailed alpha value of ≤0.05 was considered as a statistically significant association while alpha values >0.05 and ≤0.10 were considered as a trend.

All data were analyzed using Comprehensive Meta-Analysis (version 2.2) [18], Microsoft Excel 2007 [19], and SSC-Stat (version 2.18) [20].

3. Results

Six studies representing 788 men and women (D = 207, E = 192, DE = 194, C = 195) from 28 groups (7 groups each for D, E, DE, and C) met all eligibility criteria [21–26] and have been described in detail elsewhere [8]. The baseline between-study range for all groups combined was 34 to 57 years for age ($\bar{x} \pm SD = 46.5 \pm 6.5$ years), 63 to 100 kg for bodyweight ($\bar{x} \pm SD = 80.8 \pm 13.4$ kg), 180 to 254 mg/dL for TC ($\bar{x} \pm SD = 213.6 \pm 22.0$ mg/dL), and 36 to 63 mg/dL for HDL-C ($\bar{x} \pm SD = 48.3 \pm 7.7$ mg/dL).

Baseline values for non-HDL-C are shown in Table 1, group changes in Table 2, and study-level changes in (Figure 1). As can be seen, there was a statistically significant intervention minus control group decrease for non-HDL-C in the DE group, a trend for a statistically significant decrease in the D group, and no statistically significant change in the E group. Nonoverlapping 95% confidence intervals were also observed for the DE group. However, for all groups, the 95% PI for changes in non-HDL-C included zero (0). Changes in non-HDL-C were equivalent to −6.5%, −5.6% and 0.8%, respectively, for DE, D, and E groups. No outliers or heterogeneity were observed. In addition,

Study name	Group by intervention	Statistics for each study		
		Point estimate	Lower limit	Upper limit
Hellenius et al. [21]	G1-Diet	−3.5	−47.4	40.4
Hopewell [22]	G1-Diet	−9.4	−28.1	9.3
Nieman et al. [23]	G1-Diet	−16.2	−41.9	9.5
Stefanick et al. [24] Men	G1-Diet	−8.7	−37.7	20.3
Stefanick et al. [24] Women	G1-Diet	−6.2	−35.2	22.8
Vetro [25]	G1-Diet	−1.4	−26.3	23.5
Wing et al. [26]	G1-Diet	−10.8	−43.7	22.1
	G1-Diet	−8.5	−18.6	1.6
Hellenius et al. [21]	G2-Exercise	−0.8	−37.8	36.2
Hopewell [22]	G2-Exercise	6.8	−15.1	28.7
Nieman et al. [23]	G2-Exercise	2.3	−25.1	29.7
Stefanick et al. [24] Men	G2-Exercise	−2.7	−32.5	27.1
Stefanick et al. [24] Women	G2-Exercise	−6.0	−36.7	24.7
Vetro [25]	G2-Exercise	6.7	−13.1	26.5
Wing et al. [26]	G2-Exercise	5.4	−28.0	38.8
	G2-Exercise	3.0	−7.1	13.1
Hellenius et al. [21]	G3-Diet and Exercise	−12.0	−57.4	33.4
Hopewell [22]	G3-Diet and Exercise	−9.2	−28.5	10.1
Nieman et al. [23]	G3-Diet and Exercise	−21.7	−45.6	2.2
Stefanick et al. [24] Men	G3-Diet and Exercise	−17.3	−46.9	12.3
Stefanick et al. [24] Women	G3-Diet and Exercise	−14.4	−44.0	15.2
Vetro, [25]	G3-Diet and Exercise	6.7	−25.3	38.7
Wing et al. [26]	G3-Diet and Exercise	−2.7	−37.3	31.9
	G3-Diet and Exercise	−11.1	−21.7	−0.6

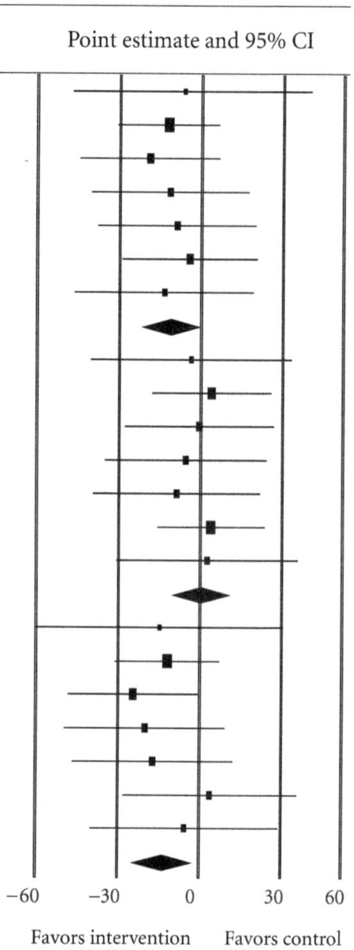

FIGURE 1: Forest plot for intervention minus control group changes in non-HDL-C according to Diet, Exercise and Diet and Exercise interventions. The black squares for each result represent the difference in non-HDL-C in mg/dL while the left and right extremes of the squares represent the corresponding 95% confidence intervals. The middle of the black diamond for the three groups represent the overall mean difference while the left and right extremes of the diamonds represent the corresponding 95% confidence intervals based on a random-effects model. To convert mg/dL to mmol, divide by 38.67.

TABLE 1: Baseline values for non-HDL-C (mg/dL).

Group	Studies#	Groups#	Participants#	$\bar{x} \pm$ SD	Range	Median
Diet	6	7	207	169.0 ± 20.3	136–192	167
Exercise	6	7	192	160.9 ± 29.3	121–192	167
Diet and exercise	6	7	194	168.9 ± 26.4	130–201	162
Control	6	7	195	162.7 ± 24.3	135–192	159

#Number; $\bar{x} \pm$ SD, mean ± standard deviation; to convert from mg/dL to mmol, divide by 38.67.

TABLE 2: Changes in non-HDL-C (mg/dL).

Variable	Studies#	Participants# (I + C)	ES#	$\bar{x}$ (95% CI) (mg/dL)	*P*	*Q*(*P*)	I^2 (%)	95% PI
Diet	6	402	7	−8.5 (−18.6, 1.6)	**0.10****	0.8 (0.99)	0	−21.7, 4.8
Exercise	6	389	7	3.0 (−7.1, 13.1)	0.60	0.8 (0.99)	0	−10.3, 16.3
Diet + Exercise	6	387	7	−11.1 (−21.7, −0.6)	**0.04***	2.4 (0.88)	0	−24.4, 2.1

#Number; ES: effect sizes; $\bar{x}$ (95% CI), mean ± 95% confidence intervals; *P*: alpha value for changes in non-HDL-C; *Q*(*P*): Cochran's *Q* statistic and associated alpha value; I^2 (%): percentage of inconsistency; 95% PI: 95% prediction intervals; I + C: intervention + control; *statistically significant at $P \leq 0.05$; **trend (>0.05 to ≤0.10) for statistical significance; To convert changes in mg/dL to mmol, divide by 38.67.

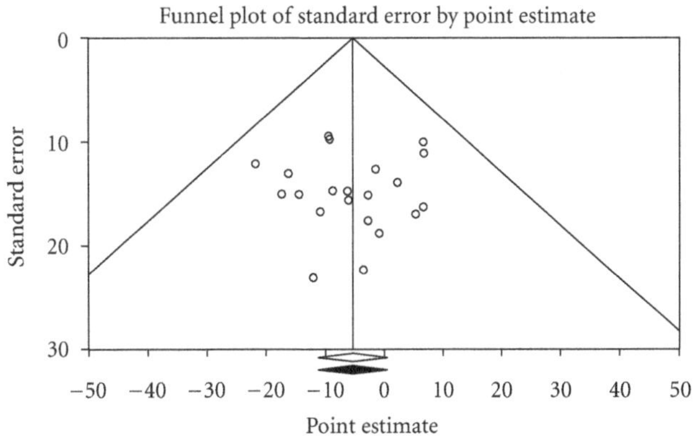

Figure 2: Funnel plot for intervention minus control group changes in non-HDL-C across all results. The x-axis represents changes in non-HDL-C in mg/dL, while the y-axis represents the standard error of the changes in non-HDL-C in mg/dL. The middle of the hollow diamond represents the original overall mean difference, while the left and right extremes of the diamond represent the corresponding 95% confidence intervals based on a random-effects model. The middle of the black solid diamond represents the mean difference in non-HDL-C, adjusted for small-study effects, while the left and right extremes of the diamond represent the corresponding 95% confidence intervals based on a random-effects model. As can be seen by the matching diamonds, no adjustment (imputation) was necessary. To convert mg/dL to mmol, divide by 38.67.

no small-study effects were found as the funnel plot was generally symmetrical and no data points had to be imputed (Figure 2). When between-group changes in non-HDL-C were calculated, no statistically significant difference was observed ($Q_b = 4.2$, $P = 0.13$). No statistically significant or trend for a statistical association was found between changes in non-HDL-C and age, initial non-HDL-C, and changes in bod y weight ($P > 0.10$ for all).

4. Discussion

To the best of the authors' knowledge, this is the first meta-analytic study to examine the effects of D, E, and DE on changes in non-HDL-C in adult humans. The overall findings suggest that DE reduces non-HDL-C in adults, while there was a trend for statistically reductions in the D group. No statistically significant reductions were found for the E group. The observed changes in non-HDL-C for the DE and D groups were almost entirely the result of statistically significant decreases in TC and little or no change in HDL-C [8].

The approximate 7% decrease observed in the DE group may be clinically important. A recent meta-analysis by Robinson et al. found that most lipid-modifying drugs used as monotherapy have an approximate one to one relationship between percent non-HDL-C lowering and reduction in coronary heart disease [27]. Assuming that the same benefits could be achieved as a result of the current interventions, this would result in an approximate 7% reduction in coronary heart disease in the DE groups and an approximate 6% reduction in the D group. The National Cholesterol Education Program currently recommends a target for non-HDL-C, that is, 30 mg/dL higher than the target for LDL-C [3]. Given the current findings, it appears that DE, and possibly D, may contribute to achieving that goal.

No statistically significant associations were found between changes in non-HDL-C and age, initial non-HDL-C and changes in body weight. While these results are interesting, they should be interpreted with caution since studies in a meta-analysis are not randomly assigned to predictors [28]. Therefore, these potential predictors should be tested in large, randomized controlled trials.

While the results of this study suggest that DE, and possibly D, reduce non-HDL-C in adults, they should be interpreted with respect to the following. First, the 95% PI included zero (0) for all groups. This suggests that reductions in non-HDL-C may not occur in every setting. Second, given the small number of studies included as well as missing data, a determination of the optimal diet and dose of aerobic exercise needed to reduce non-HDL-C in adults could not be elucidated. Given the need to determine such, it is suggested that future randomized controlled trials address this issue. Third, because none of the studies reported non-HDL-C, variances were estimated based on the data reported for TC and HDL-C. This could have possibly led to results that are different than if the original variance statistics had been available. Given the former, it is strongly suggested that future studies report non-HDL-C, including the variance statistics for such. Fourth, the results of this study, like most studies, should not be generalized beyond the characteristics of the participants included.

5. Conclusions

Combined diet and aerobic exercise may reduce non-HDL-C among adults in some settings. However, future randomized controlled trials are needed before any final recommendations can be made.

Acknowledgment

This study was supported by Grant R01 HL069802 from the National Institutes of Health, National Heart, Lung, and Blood Institute (G. A. Kelley, Principal Investigator).

References

[1] V. L. Roger, A. S. Go, D. M. Lloyd-Jones et al., "Heart disease and stroke statistics—2012 update: a report from the American Heart Association," *Circulation*, vol. 125, pp. e2–e220, 2012.

[2] M. Heron, "Deaths: leading causes for 2008," *National Vital Statistics Reports*, vol. 60, no. 6, pp. 1–94, 2012.

[3] National Cholesterol Education Program, National Heart Lung and Blood Institute, and National Institutes of Health, "Third report of the National Cholesterol Education Program (NCEP) expert panel on detection, evaluation, and treatment of high blood cholesterol in adults (adult treatment panel III) final report," *Circulation*, vol. 106, pp. 3143–3421, 2002.

[4] R. V. Milani and C. J. Lavie, "Another step forward in refining risk stratification: moving past low-density lipoprotein cholesterol," *Journal of the American College of Cardiology*, vol. 58, no. 5, pp. 464–466, 2011.

[5] J. S. Rana, S. M. Boekholdt, J. J. P. Kastelein, and P. K. Shah, "The role of non-HDL cholesterol in risk stratification for coronary artery disease," *Current Atherosclerosis Reports*, vol. 14, no. 2, pp. 130–134, 2012.

[6] S. M. Boekholdt, B. J. Arsenault, S. Mora et al., "Association of LDL cholesterol, non-HDL cholesterol, and apolipoprotein B levels with risk of cardiovascular events among patients treated with statins: a meta-analysis," *The Journal of the American Medical Association*, vol. 307, no. 12, pp. 1302–1309, 2012.

[7] A. D. Sniderman, K. Williams, J. H. Contois et al., "A meta-analysis of low-density lipoprotein cholesterol, non-high-density lipoprotein cholesterol, and apolipoprotein b as markers of cardiovascular risk," *Circulation*, vol. 4, no. 3, pp. 337–345, 2011.

[8] G. A. Kelley, K. S. Kelley, S. Roberts, and W. Haskell, "Comparison of aerobic exercise, diet or both on lipids and lipoproteins in adults: a meta-analysis of randomized controlled trials," *Clinical Nutrition*, vol. 31, pp. 156–167, 2012.

[9] L. V. Hedges and I. Olkin, *Statistical Methods for Meta-Analysis*, Academic Press, San Diego, Calif, USA, 1985.

[10] J. P. T. Higgins and S. Green, *Cochrane Handbook for Systematic Reviews of Interventions Version 5.1.0*, The Cochrane Collaboration, 2011.

[11] J. P. T. Higgins, S. G. Thompson, and D. J. Spiegelhalter, "A re-evaluation of random-effects meta-analysis," *Journal of the Royal Statistical Society A*, vol. 172, no. 1, pp. 137–159, 2009.

[12] G. A. Kelley and K. S. Kelley, "Impact of progressive resistance training on lipids and lipoproteins in adults: another look at a meta-analysis using prediction intervals," *Preventive Medicine*, vol. 49, no. 6, pp. 473–475, 2009.

[13] P. L. Graham and J. L. Moran, "Robust meta-analytic conclusions mandate the provision of prediction intervals in meta-analysis summaries," *Journal of Clinical Epidemiology*, vol. 65, no. 5, pp. 503–510, 2012.

[14] W. G. Cochran, "The combination of estimates from different experiments," *Biometrics*, vol. 10, pp. 101–129, 1954.

[15] J. P. T. Higgins, S. G. Thompson, J. J. Deeks, and D. G. Altman, "Measuring inconsistency in meta-analyses," *British Medical Journal*, vol. 327, no. 7414, pp. 557–560, 2003.

[16] S. Duval and R. Tweedie, "Trim and fill: a simple funnel-plot-based method of testing and adjusting for publication bias in meta-analysis," *Biometrics*, vol. 56, no. 2, pp. 455–463, 2000.

[17] S. Duval and R. Tweedie, "A Nonparametric "Trim and Fill" method of accounting for publication bias in meta-analysis," *Journal of the American Statistical Association*, vol. 95, no. 449, pp. 89–98, 2000.

[18] Biostat, "Comprehensive meta-analysis. (2.2)," Englewood Cliffs, NJ, USA, 2006.

[19] "Microsoft Excel 2007," Microsoft Corporation, Redmond, Wash, USA, 2007.

[20] Statistical Services Center, "SSC-Stat. (2.18)," University of Reading, Statistical Services Center, UK, 2007.

[21] M. L. Hellenius, U. D. Faire, B. Berglund, A. Hamsten, and I. Krakau, "Diet and exercise are equally effective in reducing risk for cardiovascular disease. Results of a randomized controlled study in men with slightly to moderately raised cardiovascular risk factors," *Atherosclerosis*, vol. 103, no. 1, pp. 81–91, 1993.

[22] R. Hopewell, *The effect of fiber and exercise on weight loss and blood lipids in moderately overweight women [Dissertation]*, West Virginia University, 1989.

[23] D. C. Nieman, D. W. Brock, D. Butterworth, A. C. Utter, and C. C. Nieman, "Reducing diet and/or exercise training decreases the lipid and lipoprotein risk factors of moderately obese women," *Journal of the American College of Nutrition*, vol. 21, no. 4, pp. 344–350, 2002.

[24] M. L. Stefanick, S. Mackey, M. Sheehan, N. Ellsworth, W. L. Haskell, and P. D. Wood, "Effects of diet and exercise in men and postmenopausal women with low levels of HDL cholesterol and high levels of LDL cholesterol," *New England Journal of Medicine*, vol. 339, no. 1, pp. 12–20, 1998.

[25] V. L. Vetro, *The effects of aerobic dance exercise and nutrition intervention on cholesterol levels [M.S. thesis]*, Springfield College, 1990.

[26] R. R. Wing, E. Venditti, J. M. Jakicic, B. A. Polley, and W. Lang, "Lifestyle intervention in overweight individuals with a family history of diabetes," *Diabetes Care*, vol. 21, no. 3, pp. 350–359, 1998.

[27] J. G. Robinson, S. Wang, B. J. Smith, and T. A. Jacobson, "Meta-analysis of the relationship between non-high-density lipoprotein cholesterol reduction and coronary heart disease risk," *Journal of the American College of Cardiology*, vol. 53, no. 4, pp. 316–322, 2009.

[28] J. H. Littell, J. Corcoran, and V. Pillai, *Systematic Reviews and Meta-Analysis*, Oxford University Press, New York, NY, USA, 2008.

The Prevalence of Dyslipidemia in Patients with Spinal Cord Lesion in Thailand

Ratana Vichiansiri, Jittima Saengsuwan, Nuttaset Manimmanakorn, Sirasaporn Patpiya, Arayawichanon Preeda, Kharmwan Samerduen, and Ekasit Poosiripinyo

Department of Physical Medicine and Rehabilitation, Faculty of Medicine, Khon Kaen University, Amphur Muang, Khon Kaen 40002, Thailand

Correspondence should be addressed to Jittima Saengsuwan, sjittima@kku.ac.th

Academic Editor: Gerhard M. Kostner

Objective. To assess the prevalence of dyslipidemia in 90 patients with spinal cord lesion (SCL) of duration greater than 2 years. The study was carried out from November 2007 to September 2008. *Methods.* Clinical history, physical examination, and lipid profiles were recorded and analyzed. Dyslipidemia was assessed using guidelines from the National Cholesterol Education Project Adult Treatment Panel III (ATP III). *Results.* The prevalence of dyslipidemia in at least one lipid parameter was 76.7%. The most frequent finding was low HDL-C (58.9%). Hypertriglyceridemia, hypercholesterolemia and high LDL-C were found in 28.9%, 26.7% and 21.1% of patients, respectively. The factors sex = male and age ≥ 45 years were associated with high LDL-C ($P < 0.05$ and $P < 0.01$). Patients who exercised less than 30 minutes per day had associated hypercholesterolemia ($P < 0.01$), hypertriglyceridemia ($P < 0.01$), and higher LDL-C ($P < 0.05$). Patients with BMI ≥ 23 kg/m^2 had associated hypercholesterolemia and high LDL-C. Age was a significant determinant of high LDL-C. BMI was the most powerful and significant determinant of hypercholesterolemia and high LDL-C. *Conclusion.* SCL patients should have a regular lipid checkup, especially those patients having the following risk factors: males, age ≥ 45 years, BMI ≥ 23 kg/m^2 and exercise duration < 30 minutes per day.

1. Introduction

There has been great improvement in therapeutic care for patients with spinal cord injury (SCI) but patients still have lower-than-normal life expectancy. It has been found that life expectancy of tetraplegia and paraplegia is less than in the normal population [1]. The major established cause of death is cardiovascular disease [2, 3].

Whiteneck [4] reported that cardiovascular disease accounted for nearly half of all deaths in persons with spinal cord injury of duration greater than 30 years. Lee et al. [5] found that the prevalence of asymptomatic coronary artery disease was 63.8% as determined by Thallium-201 myocardial perfusion single-photon emission-computed tomography (T201-SPECT). There are many important risk factors in developing cardiovascular disease such as a decrease in physical activity, obesity, metabolic syndrome, dyslipidemia, impaired glucose tolerance, and decreased cardiovascular fitness [6].

Dyslipidemia is one of the most important risk factors and can be modified for primary prevention in cardiovascular disease. In this study the prevalence of dyslipidemia was determined from ATP III guidelines which were developed from the National Cholesterol Education Program (NCEP) Expert panel on Detection, Evaluation, and Treatment of High Blood Cholesterol in 2001. ATP III sets guidelines for cardiovascular risk evaluation and management [7–9]. It differs from the previous ATP I-II guidelines in the emphasis of primary prevention. The new guidelines decrease the triglyceride (TG) cutoff point for hypertriglyceridemia from ≥200 mg/dL to TG ≥150 mg/dL) increase the HDL cholesterol (HDL-C) cutoff points (HDL-C < 35 to HDL-C < 40 mg/dL), and include metabolic syndrome evaluation [9–11].

Nash and Mendez [12] studied dyslipidemia in 41 paraplegic patients following ATP III guidelines and found that as many as 76% of patients had HDL-C levels less than 40 mg/dL and up to 63.4% need further treatment.

Many studies on the prevalence of dyslipidemia have been conducted in western countries, but data in Asia is still scarce. Since there are many regional differences in genetics, way of life, and diet, the present study was designed to examine the mean lipid level and prevalence of dyslipidemia among spinal cord lesion patients in Thailand.

2. Materials and Methods

2.1. Settings and Subjects. This was a cross-sectional, descriptive study. Participants involved in the study were patients with chronic SCL (duration at least 2 years) either from spinal cord injury of traumatic or nontraumatic cause and intrinsic cord problem such as myelomeningocele who were admitted for urological review to Srinagarind Hospital, located in Khon Kaen in the Northeast of Thailand, from 1 November 2007 to 30 October 2008.

This study included 90 patients (55 men and 35 women) aged 18–80 years. Patients who had a history of diagnosed dyslipidemia, as well as patients who had any condition that could alter lipid profiles were excluded from the study.

The study was conducted in accordance with the 1975 Helsinki Declaration (revised 1983), approved by the Ethics Committee of Khon Kaen University. Written informed consent was obtained from all of the subjects.

2.2. Specimen Collection. Serum samples were collected from subjects in the morning after 10 hours of fasting. Measurements included total cholesterol (TC), triglyceride (TG) and high-density lipoprotein cholesterol (HDL-C). Low-density lipoprotein cholesterol (LDL-C) was calculated by the following equation [13]:

$$\text{LDL-C} = \text{TC} - \left(\text{HDL-C} + \frac{\text{TG}}{5}\right). \tag{1}$$

2.3. NCEP III Guidelines. The classification of dyslipidemia was based on the NCEP III Guidelines. These classify lipid profile as abnormal if, HDL-C is less than 40 mg/dL; TC is more than 200 mg/dL, or TG is more than 150 mg/dL. High LDL-C is classified based on 5 risk factors: age (men $\geq$ 45 years and women $\geq$ 55 years), cigarette smoking, hypertension or currently taking antihypertensive medication, HDL-C level, and family history of premature heart disease. In patients with 1 risk factor, the cutoff point of LDL-C is 160 mg/dL. The cutoff point is 130 mg/dL for patients with 2 or more risk factors. In patients with coronary heart disease (CHD) or CHD risk equivalent, such as diabetes or atherosclerotic disease, the cutoff point of LDL-C is 100 mg/dL.

2.4. Framingham Risk Score. Framingham risk scores were calculated based on the Framingham study [14, 15]. This is widely used to classify people with risk factors into 3 distinct groups (low risk, moderate risk, and high risk), which is based on the observed risk of developing CHD or cardiac cause of death in 5,209 healthy men and women aged 30 to 62 in Framingham, MA, USA. The risks that are accounted for in the calculation are age, gender, TC, HDL-C, cigarette smoking, and systolic blood pressure or the use of antihypertensive drugs. The score calculated is further transformed into a percentage. If the percentage is less than 10%, the classification is low risk; 10–20% will be classified as intermediate risk and greater than 20% will be classified as high risk.

2.5. Statistical Analysis. Statistical analyses were performed on a personal computer using SPSS version 16.0 (SPSS, Inc, Chicago). The results were expressed as means and standard deviations. Chi-squared analyses and Fishers Exact tests were performed to determine factors associated with dyslipidemia and Framingham risk categories. Multiple regression analysis was used to investigate the influences of age, gender, family history of coronary artery disease, smoking, exercise duration, BMI, level of injury, completeness of lesion, duration after injury, and ambulatory level to predict dyslipidemia of any type of lipid.

3. Results

After excluding 6 subjects, data from 90 subjects were analyzed: 62 paraplegics and 28 tetraplegics. Average age was 42.3 (range 18–80 years). Six of the participants were smokers, and 9 regularly consumed alcohol. Five patients had a family history of coronary artery disease.

According to the clinical history, the spinal cord lesion was complete in 51 participants (56.7%). Fifty-five (61.1%) participants were wheelchair users. The average time after spinal cord injury was 5.4 years. Thirteen patients did not exercise (Table 1).

There were 69 participants (76.7%) who had abnormality in at least one lipid profile. In the dyslipidemic group, there were 54 patients (78.3%) who had abnormal lipid profile of more than 1 type, and there were only 15 patients (21.7%) who had dyslipidemia diagnosed from only one profile.

Fifty-three participants (58.4%) had a depressed mean serum HDL-C level, leading to the average level of 39.4 mg/dl as shown in Table 2. TG, LDL-C, and TC were found abnormal in 28.9%, 21.1%, and 26.7% of patients, respectively.

3.1. Factors Associated with Dyslipidemia. Factors that were demonstrated to be associated with dyslipidemia are shown in Table 3. Male sex and age of more than 45 years was associated with high LDL-C ($P < 0.05$ and $P < 0.01$). An average exercise time of less than 30 minutes per day was associated with hypercholesterolemia, hypertriglyceridemia ($P < 0.01$), and higher LDL-C ($P < 0.05$). BMI equal to or greater than 23 kg/m^2 was associated with hypercholesterolemia and high LDL-C.

This study did not demonstrate any significant correlation of the level of injury (tetraplegia or paraplegia), completeness of injury, and duration of injury together with

Table 1: General Characteristics of 90 spinal cord lesion patients (SD: standard deviation).

Characteristics	Value
Number of subjects	90
Age, years, mean (SD)	42.3 (13.7)
Male/Female, *n* (%)	55 (61.1)/35 (38.9)
Family history of coronary artery disease, *n* (%)	5 (5.6)
Duration of injury, years, mean (SD)	5.4 (4.7)
Current smoker, *n* (%)	6 (6.7)
Level, *n* (%)	
Paraplegia	28 (31.1)
Tetraplegia	62 (68.9)
Completeness, *n* (%)	
Complete	51 (56.7)
Incomplete	39 (43.3)
Ambulatory ability, *n* (%)	
Wheelchair	55 (61.1)
Walk	35 (38.9)
Exercise, *n* (%)	
No exercise	13 (14.4)
Exercise	
<30 min/day	41 (45.6)
≥30 min/day	36 (40)

Table 2: Lipid profile values (mean (SD)).

Type	Blood level	
	mg/dL	Range
HDL-C	39.4 (10.4)	23–71
TG	130.5 (86.3)	38–572
LDL-C	111.0 (36.8)	44–196
TC	175.1 (41.3)	87–294

ambulatory level of the patients with dyslipidemia from any type of lipid.

Results of the regression analysis, investigating the influence of subject characteristics and behavioural factors on the lipid profile, are listed in Table 4. Age was a significant determinant of high LDL-C. BMI was the most powerful and significant determinant of hypercholesterolemia and high LDL-C.

3.2. Risks of CHD Based on Framingham Risk Score. Fourteen patients (15.6%) were in the moderate-to-high-risk group for hard CHD or cardiovascular death based on the Framingham risk score. All of them were men and aged more than 45 years. In the moderate-to-high-risk group, there were 71.4% of patients who exercised less than 30 minutes per day; in the low risk group, 57.9% of patients exercised less than 30 minutes per day. There was a higher percentage of patients who smoke in the high-risk group although the difference is not statistically significant. There was no significant difference in association with abdominal circumference, duration of SCL, level of lesion, ambulatory method, and BMI between the low- and high-risk groups (Table 5).

4. Discussion

Individuals with SCI were found to have higher risk of CHD at a younger age. Dyslipidemia is an important modifiable risk factor and with good prevention and control, morbidity, and mortality may be delayed for this group of patients in the future. Using the NCEP (ATP III) Guidelines, this study shows that the prevalence of dyslipidemia is high. Depression of HDL-C level accounted for major abnormalities in lipid profile. This finding was consistent with the study of Nash and Mendez who found abnormality in HDL-C levels in 31 out of 41 participants with paraplegia [12]. This study also correlates with other studies [16–20] which showed that low HDL-C is the most significant lipid alteration after SCI. The low HDL-C may be explained by lower physical activity in the SCI group; previous reports found that sedentary lifestyle leads to an accentuated state of insulin resistance, and this leads to higher triglyceride, uric acid, and lower HDL-C levels [21, 22]. Although immobilization plays a major role in HDL-C levels, other causes of lower HDL-C such as smoking, excessive alcohol intake, and high-fat diet may also contribute to low HDL-C levels [23]. There are many studies that support the proposal that HDL-C helps prevent atherosclerosis through various mechanisms such as antioxidant effects or inhibition of endothelial destruction [24, 25]. An optimum HDL-C level will need to be determined, and effective ways to help improve HDL-C levels, either by medication or exercise, should be found so as to most effectively help this group of patients [26].

A TG level of more than150 mg/dL led to higher overall mortality and incidence of cardiovascular disease. Comparing TG levels from the study of Nash and Mendez [12] to the population in this study, it was found that there was a lower mean TG level, which may have been caused by a difference in genetics, habits, or diet.

There was a difference in the prevalence of low HDL-C and high LDL-C between genders which may have been a result of different sex hormones that influence blood lipid profiles [27, 28].

Age and BMI were shown to be associated with high LDL-C levels, and the results also correlate with a previous study comparing the factors associated with lipid profiles in active and sedentary tetraplegic patients [29]. However, compared to the study of Bauman et al. [20], which determined the effect of residual neurological deficit on lipid profiles in patients with chronic spinal cord injury and found that there was a significant inverse relationship between the degree of neurological deficit and mean serum HDL-C levels, this study did not demonstrate any significant association between level of injury, completeness of injury, or ambulatory level and dyslipidemia. When analyzed in detail, the significance of neurological level may be confounded by the effect of age as the mean age for tetraplegic patients was 38.3 years compared to the higher average age of 44.2 years in paraplegia. This might have a substantial effect considering that age accounted for a significant alteration in lipid level.

Table 3: Factors associated with dyslipidemia classified by each type of lipid.

Factors	Normal	Dyslipidemia	P value
HDL-C			
Male	17/24 (70.8%)	38/66 (57.6%)	0.04
Age ≥ 45 years	6/24 (25%)	25/66 (37.9%)	0.32
BMI ≥ 23 kg/m^2	3/24 (12.5%)	13/66 (19.7%)	0.54
Exercise less than 30 min/day	13/24 (54.2%)	41/66 (62.1%)	0.21
LDL-C			
Male	16/19 (84.2%)	39/71 (54.9%)	0.02
Age ≥ 45 years	13/19 (68.4%)	18/71 (25.4%)	0.000
BMI ≥ 23 kg/m^2	7/19 (36.8%)	9/71 (12.7%)	0.014
Exercise less than 30 min/day	16/19 (84.2%)	38/71 (53.5%)	0.015
TG			
Male	18/26 (69.2%)	37/64 (57.8%)	0.31
Age ≥ 45 years	12/26 (46.2%)	19/64 (29.7%)	0.14
BMI ≥ 23 kg/m^2	7/26 (3.8%)	9/64 (14%)	0.15
Exercise less than 30 min/day	21/26 (81.7%)	33/64 (51.6%)	0.01
TC			
Male	16/24 (66.7%)	39/66 (59%)	0.51
Age ≥ 45 years	12/24 (50%)	19/66 (28.8%)	0.06
BMI ≥ 23 kg/m^2	9/24 (37.5%)	7/66 (10.6%)	0.003
Exercise less than 30 min/day	20/24 (83.3%)	34/66 (51.5%)	0.006

Table 4: Results of multiple logistic regression analysis: effects of age and BMI on TC and LDL-C.

Dependent variables	Independent variables	Crude OR	Adjusted OR	95% CI for adjusted OR	P value
hypercholesterolemia	BMI < 23 kg/ m^2	2.0	1	2.0–57.4	0.006
	≥ 23 kg/m^2	20.7	10.7		
High LDL-C	Age < 45 years	1.0	1	1.3–13.9	0.015
	≥ 45 years	6.4	4.3		
	BMI < 23 kg/m^2	1.0	1.0	1.2–56.7	0.034
	≥ 23 kg/m^2	4.5	8.1		

When comparing the prevalence of dyslipidemia in SCL patients in Thailand with the study of the normal population by Pongchaiyakul et al. [30], the SCL patients showed a significant difference in the prevalence of HDL-C compared to the normal population. The prevalence of hypertriglyceridemia, hypercholesterolemia, and high LDL-C was comparable.

Interestingly, based on the Framingham risk score, all patients with moderate-to-high risk were male and more than 45 years of age; all patients in the high-risk group had low HDL-C levels. BMI and abdominal circumference were not significantly different from the low-risk group. The greater proportion of moderate-to-high-risk patients classified by exercise duration of less than 30 minutes showed a trend for the effect of exercise; lack of significance may be due to the small sample size. Most patients in the moderate-to-high-risk group (78.6%) have a duration of SCL of less than 5 years. This also agrees with the study of Dallmeijer et al., which found lower HDL-C levels within 2 years after SCI [19]. This may imply that physicians should check lipid profiles and estimate the CHD risk even shortly after SCI, especially in men who are more than 45 years of age.

After the lipid screening, the prevalence of SCL patients with at least one lipid abnormality is 76.7%. Seven patients (10.1%) had an indication for lipid-lowering medication based on NCEP III guidelines, and 62 patients (89.9%) were given advice for therapeutic lifestyle modification.

One of the limitations of this work is the cross-sectional nature of the study. We did not follow up with the patients since the onset of SCI so we do not know whether males aged more than 45 years had this risk before injury or not.

In conclusion, the high percentage of dyslipidemia found in SCL patients supports the increased risk of CHD in this group. There is an indication for mandatory annual checking of the lipid profile especially in the high-risk group: those who are male, more than 45 years of age and exercising for less than 30 minutes a day. Moreover, regular followup to advise for activity modification such as eating habits,

Table 5: Factors associated with moderate to high risk based on the Framingham risk score.

Factors	Low risk (<10%)	Moderate/high risk (≥10%)	P-value
Male	41/76 (53.9%)	14/14 (100%)	0.001
Age ≥ 45 years	17/76 (22.3%)	14/14 (100%)	0.000
Tetraplegia	25/76 (32.8%)	3/14 (21.4%)	0.30*
WC ambulation	48/76 (63.2%)	5/14 (35.7%)	0.55
Duration of SCL ≥ 5 years	23/76 (30.3%)	3/14 (21.4%)	0.75*
Cigarette smoking	4/76 (5.3%)	3/14 (21.4%)	0.07*
Abdominal circumference	11/76 (14.5%)	1/14 (7.1%)	0.68*
BMI ≥ 23 kg/m^2	15/76 (7.1%)	1/14 (7.1%)	0.45*
Exercise less than 30 min/day	44/76 (57.9%)	10/14 (71.4%)	0.39

*Fisher's exact test.

exercise, or medication, that is, medical intervention to prevent cardiovascular disease, should be incorporated in the routine clinical followup.

Acknowledgments

The authors wish to thank associate Professor Weerachai Kowsuwan for helpful suggestions and Mr. John Finlay for his assistance with the English language.

References

[1] J. D. Yeo, J. Walsh, S. Rutkowski, R. Soden, M. Craven, and J. Middleton, "Mortality following spinal cord injury," *Spinal Cord*, vol. 36, no. 5, pp. 329–336, 1998.

[2] I. B. Lidal, H. Snekkevik, G. Aamodt, N. Hjeltnes, J. K. Stanghelle, and F. Biering-Sørensen, "Mortality after spinal cord injury in Norway," *Journal of Rehabilitation Medicine*, vol. 39, no. 2, pp. 145–151, 2007.

[3] M. J. DeVivo, J. S. Krause, and D. P. Lammertse, "Recent trends in mortality and causes of death among persons with spinal cord injury," *Archives of Physical Medicine and Rehabilitation*, vol. 80, no. 11, pp. 1411–1419, 1999.

[4] G. G. Whiteneck, "Learning from empirical investigations," in *Perspectives on Aging With Spinal Cord Injury*, G. G. Whiteneck, S. W. Charlifue, K. A. Gerhart, D. P. Lammertese, M. S. Manley, and R. R. Menter, Eds., vol. 32, Demos Publications, New York, NY, USA, 1992.

[5] C. S. Lee, Y. H. Lu, S. T. Lee, C. C. Lin, and H. J. Ding, "Evaluating the prevalence of silent coronary artery disease in asymptomatic patients with spinal cord injury," *International Heart Journal*, vol. 47, no. 3, pp. 325–330, 2006.

[6] J. Myers, M. Lee, and J. Kiratli, "Cardiovascular disease in spinal cord injury: an overview of prevalence, risk, evaluation, and management," *American Journal of Physical Medicine and Rehabilitation*, vol. 86, no. 2, pp. 142–152, 2007.

[7] "Report of the National cholesterol education program expert panel on detection, evaluation, and treatment of high blood cholesterol in adults. The expert panel," *Archives of Internal Medicine*, vol. 148, no. 1, pp. 36–69, 1988.

[8] S. M. Grundy and National Cholesterol Education Program, "National cholesterol education program: Second report of the expert panel on detection, evaluation, and treatment of high blood cholesterol in adults (adult treatment panel II)," *Circulation*, vol. 89, no. 3, pp. 1333–1443, 1994.

[9] National Cholesterol Education Program (NCEP) Expert Panel on Detection, Evaluation, and Treatment of High Blood Cholesterol in Adults (Adult Treatment Panel III), "Third report of the National cholesterol education program (NCEP) expert panel on detection, evaluation, and treatment of high blood cholesterol in adults (Adult treatment panel III) final report," *Circulation*, vol. 106, pp. 3143–3421, 2002.

[10] J. I. Cleeman and Expert Panel on Detection, Evaluation, and Treatment of High Blood Cholesterol in Adults, "Executive summary of the third report of the National cholesterol education program (NCEP) expert panel on detection, evaluation, and treatment of high blood cholesterol in adults (adult treatment panel III)," *The Journal of the American Medical Association*, vol. 285, no. 19, pp. 2486–2497, 2001.

[11] S. M. Grundy, J. I. Cleeman, C. N. Bairey Merz et al., "Implications of recent clinical trials for the National cholesterol education program adult treatment panel III guidelines," *Circulation*, vol. 110, no. 2, pp. 227–239, 2004.

[12] M. S. Nash and A. J. Mendez, "A guideline-driven assessment of need for cardiovascular disease risk intervention in persons with chronic paraplegia," *Archives of Physical Medicine and Rehabilitation*, vol. 88, no. 6, pp. 751–757, 2007.

[13] W. T. Friedewald, R. I. Levy, and D. S. Fredrickson, "Estimation of the concentration of low-density lipoprotein cholesterol in plasma, without use of the preparative ultracentrifuge," *Clinical Chemistry*, vol. 18, no. 6, pp. 499–502, 1972.

[14] K. M. Anderson, P. W. F. Wilson, P. M. Odell, and W. B. Kannel, "An updated coronary risk profile. A statement for health professionals," *Circulation*, vol. 83, no. 1, pp. 356–362, 1991.

[15] R. B. D'Agostino Sr., S. Grundy, L. M. Sullivan, and P. Wilson, "Validation of the Framingham coronary heart disease prediction scores: results of a multiple ethnic groups investigation," *The Journal of the American Medical Association*, vol. 286, no. 2, pp. 180–187, 2001.

[16] W. A. Bauman, A. M. Spungen, Y. G. Zhong, J. L. Rothstein, C. Petry, and S. K. Gordon, "Depressed serum high density lipoprotein cholesterol levels in veterans with spinal cord injury," *Paraplegia*, vol. 30, no. 10, pp. 697–703, 1992.

[17] W. A. Bauman, R. H. Adkins, A. M. Spungen et al., "Is immobilization associated with an abnormal lipoprotein profile? Observations from a diverse cohort," *Spinal Cord*, vol. 37, no. 7, pp. 485–493, 1999.

[18] T. Ozgurtas, R. Alaca, M. Gulec, and T. Kutluay, "Do spinal cord injuries adversely affect serum lipoprotein profiles?" *Military Medicine*, vol. 168, no. 7, pp. 545–547, 2003.

[19] A. J. Dallmeijer, L. H. van der Woude, G. J. van Kamp, and A. P. Hollander, "Changes in lipid, lipoprotein and apolipoprotein profiles in persons with spinal cord injuries during the first 2 years post-injury," *Spinal Cord*, vol. 37, no. 2, pp. 96–102, 1999.

[20] W. A. Bauman, R. H. Adkins, A. M. Spungen, B. J. Kemp, and R. L. Waters, "The effect of residual neurological deficit on serum lipoproteins in individuals with chronic spinal cord injury," *Spinal Cord*, vol. 36, no. 1, pp. 13–17, 1998.
[21] W. A. Bauman and A. M. Spungen, "Disorders of carbohydrate and lipid metabolism in veterans with paraplegia or quadriplegia: a model of premature aging," *Metabolism*, vol. 43, no. 6, pp. 749–756, 1994.
[22] Y. G. Zhong, E. Levy, and W. A. Bauman, "The relationships among serum uric acid, plasma insulin, and serum lipoprotein levels in subjects with spinal cord injury," *Hormone and Metabolic Research*, vol. 27, no. 6, pp. 283–286, 1995.
[23] Y. Hata and K. Nakajima, "Life-style and serum lipids and lipoproteins," *Journal of atherosclerosis and thrombosis*, vol. 7, no. 4, pp. 177–197, 2000.
[24] M. Florentin, E. N. Liberopoulos, A. S. Wierzbicki, and D. P. Mikhailidis, "Multiple actions of high-density lipoprotein," *Current Opinion in Cardiology*, vol. 23, no. 4, pp. 370–378, 2008.
[25] P. Libby, "Managing the risk of atherosclerosis: the role of high-density lipoprotein," *American Journal of Cardiology*, vol. 88, no. 12, pp. 3N–8N, 2001.
[26] M. L. Kashyap, S. Tavintharan, and V. S. Kamanna, "Optimal therapy of low levels of high density lipoprotein-cholesterol," *American Journal of Cardiovascular Drugs*, vol. 3, no. 1, pp. 53–65, 2003.
[27] J. L. Durstine, P. W. Grandjean, P. G. Davis, M. A. Ferguson, N. L. Alderson, and K. D. DuBose, "Blood lipid and lipoprotein adaptations to exercise: a quantitative analysis," *Sports Medicine*, vol. 31, no. 15, pp. 1033–1062, 2001.
[28] A. Schmid, J. Knöebber, S. Vogt et al., "Lipid profiles of persons with paraplegia and tetraplegia: sex differences," *Journal of Spinal Cord Medicine*, vol. 31, no. 3, pp. 285–289, 2008.
[29] A. J. Dallmeijer, M. T. E. Hopman, and L. H. V. van der Woude, "Lipid, lipoprotein, and apolipoprotein profiles in active and sedentary men with tetraplegia," *Archives of Physical Medicine and Rehabilitation*, vol. 78, no. 11, pp. 1173–1176, 1997.
[30] C. Pongchaiyakul, P. Hongsprabhas, V. Pisprasert, and C. Pongchaiyakul, "Rural-urban difference in lipid levels and prevalence of dyslipidemia: a population-based study in Khon Kaen Province, Thailand," *Journal of the Medical Association of Thailand*, vol. 89, no. 11, pp. 1835–1844, 2006.

20

MicroRNA Regulation of Cholesterol Metabolism

Noemi Rotllan and Carlos Fernández-Hernando

Marc and Ruti Bell Vascular Biology and Disease Program, Leon H. Charney Division of Cardiology, Departments of Medicine and Cell Biology, New York University School of Medicine, New York, NY 10016, USA

Correspondence should be addressed to Carlos Fernández-Hernando, carlos.fernandez-hernando@nyumc.org

Academic Editor: Jean Davignon

Disruption of cellular cholesterol balance results in pathologic processes including atherosclerosis, metabolic syndrome, type II diabetes and Alzheimer's disease. Maintenance of cholesterol homeostasis requires constant metabolic adjustment, achieved partly through the fine regulation of the classical transcription factors (e.g., by SREBP and LXR), but also through members of a class of noncoding RNAs termed miRNAs. Some miRNAs have now been identified to be potent post-transcriptional regulators of lipid metabolism genes, including miR-122, miR-33, miR-758, and miR-106b. Different strategies have been developed to modulate miRNA effects for therapeutic purposes. The promise demonstrated by the use of anti-miRs in human preclinical studies, in the case of miR-122, raises the possibility that miR-33, miR-758, and miR-106b may become viable therapeutic targets in future. This review summarizes the evidence for a critical role of some miRNAs in regulating cholesterol metabolism and suggests novel ways to manage dyslipidemias and cardiovascular diseases.

1. Introduction

Cholesterol is the major component of mammalian cells and is essential for diverse cellular functions. Cholesterol levels are maintained through tightly regulated and complex mechanisms. It is well known that insufficient or excessive cellular cholesterol results in a wide range of pathologies, including atherosclerosis, metabolic syndrome, type II diabetes, and Alzheimer's disease (AD) [1–3]. Cholesterol homeostasis has been extensively studied, from the de novo biosynthesis to internalization of exogenous cholesterol, through the efflux of excess cholesterol and finally its elimination through bile. The classical transcription factors that regulate its homeostasis are the sterol response element binding proteins (SREBPs) [4, 5] and the liver X receptors (LXRs) [6, 7].

In addition to the classical transcriptional regulators, a class of noncoding RNAs, termed microRNAs (miRNAs) has emerged as critical regulators of gene expression acting predominantly at the posttranscriptional level. This large family of short (22-nucleotide) noncoding RNA binds to the 3′ untranslated (3′UTR) region of mRNA, thereby repressing gene expression. Thus, they are implicated in the control of many physiological and pathological processes [8–10]. The role of miRNAs in the regulation of lipid metabolism is just beginning to be explored. Several miRNAs have been described to regulate lipid metabolism, including miR-122, miR-33, miR-758, and miR-106b [11–14] (Table 1). Other microRNAs such as miR-370, miR-378/378*, miR-143, miR-27, miR-29a, miR-302a, and miR-335 have also been shown to regulate lipid homeostasis [15–21]. It is also important to highlight that the finding of an exogenous plant microRNA, miR168a, that could bind to the human/mouse low-density lipoprotein receptor adapter protein 1 (LDLRAP1) mRNA, inhibits LDLRAP1 expression in liver and consequently decrease LDL clearance.

This paper addresses recent research and links between miRNAs and their role in regulating cholesterol metabolism and suggests that manipulating their expression *in vivo* may open new avenues for treating dyslipidemias and cardiovascular diseases.

2. Cholesterol Metabolism and Its Regulation

Cholesterol is the precursor of steroid hormones, bile acid, and vitamin D and is required for the maintenance of cell membrane fluidity, membrane formation, cell proliferation

Table 1: MicroRNAs involved in cholesterol metabolism.

miRNA	Target tissue/cell type	Target genes	Biological function	References
miR-122	Primary mouse hepatocytes	*ALDOA* *CS*	Glucose homeostasis Krebs cycle	[22, 23]
miR-33a and miR-33b	Liver and macrophage	*ABCA1; ABCG1; NPC1* *CROT; HADHB; CPT1; SIRT6; PRKAA1* *IRS2*	Cellular cholesterol efflux Fatty acid oxidation Insulin signaling	[12, 24, 25]
miR-758	Human and mouse macrophages and hepatic cell line	*ABCA1*	Cellular cholesterol efflux	[13]
	Human neuroglioma cell line	*SLC38a1; NTM; EPHA7*	Aminoacid synthesis, neurite outgrowing, and neuronal migration	
miR-106b	Mouse neuroblastoma cell line and human hepatocyte	*ABCA1*	Cellular cholesterol efflux and Aβ production	[14]

and embryonic development [26, 27]. An excess of plasma cholesterol leads to its accumulation in the artery wall causing atherosclerosis, the main cause of death in Western societies [28]. Levels of cholesterol are maintained through a tightly regulated and complex mechanism that includes the de novo biosynthesis, internalization of exogenous cholesterol, and efflux of cholesterol excess.

These mechanisms are regulated by transcription factors such as SREBPs and LXRs. SREBPs activate the expression of a variety of genes required for cholesterol, triglycerides, fatty acids, and phospholipid uptake and synthesis. In mammals there are three SREBP isoforms: SREBP1a and SREBP1c encoded by the *Srebp1* gene and SREBP2, encoded by *Srebp2* gene. SREBP1c regulates the transcription of genes involved in fatty acid metabolism, such as fatty acid synthase FASN [5–7]. On the other hand, SREBP2 and SREBP1a activate the transcription of cholesterol-related genes, including 3-hydroxy-3 methylglutaryl coenzyme A reductase (HMGCR), the rate-limiting enzyme that regulates cholesterol biosynthesis, and low-density lipoprotein receptor (LDLr), that scavenges circulating LDL from the bloodstream [5–7].

In addition to SREBPs, the LXRs also contribute to cholesterol and fatty acid homeostasis. LXRs are activated in response to elevated cholesterol levels (oxysterols) and induce the expression of proteins involved in cholesterol absorption, transport, excretion, and efflux, including the ATP binding cassette transporters A1 (ABCA1), G1 (ABCG1) or G5/G8 (ABCG5/G8), and apolipoprotein E (apoE) [29–31].

3. MicroRNAS

miRNAs are small endogenous RNAs approximately 22 nucleotides in length that have emerged as important posttranscriptional regulators of different protein-coding genes. It was first discovered in the nematode *Caenoshabditis elegans*, and since then has been identified in the genomes of most plants, animal, and viruses [8–10, 32].

The miRNAs identified to date are currently curated and annotated at miRBase, hosted by the Sanger Institute as a publicly available repository (http://microrna.sanger.ac.uk/). Experimental approaches using bioinformatic predictions indicates that a single miRNA may simultaneously target more than 100 mRNAs [33]. Similarly, a single mRNA could be regulated by many miRNA. Human miRNAs are predicted to control the activity of 30–60% of all protein-coding genes [32–34]. Thus, their deregulation is closely linked to human diseases, including heart disease and vascular disorders [35–38]. Very interestingly, microvesicles, exosomes, apoptotic bodies, lipoproteins, and large microparticles contain miRNAs. miRNAs are stable in plasma and differential plasma miRNA profiles have been described for many diseases, including fatty liver [39], atherosclerosis [40], and cancer [41–45]. Circulating extracellular miRNAs have enormous potential as novel disease biomarkers. miRNAs could, therefore, be considered like hormones as a possible form of intercellular communication; however, their physiological function and *in vivo* role remains to be definitively established.

4. MicroRNA Biogenesis and Function

The canonical pathway is the classical pathway for the biogenesis of miRNAs. Canonical miRNAs in animals are transcribed in the nucleus by RNA polymerase II, generating a primary long miRNA (pri-miRNA) (Figure 1). These pri-miRNAs are usually hundreds of nucleotides long and contain local hairpin structures. Then, these hairpins are processed sequentially in the nucleus and cytoplasma into a 70-nucleotide hairpin-structure precursor (pre-miRNA) by a multiprotein complex containing a variety of cofactors and two core components, a ribonuclease III (Drosha) and

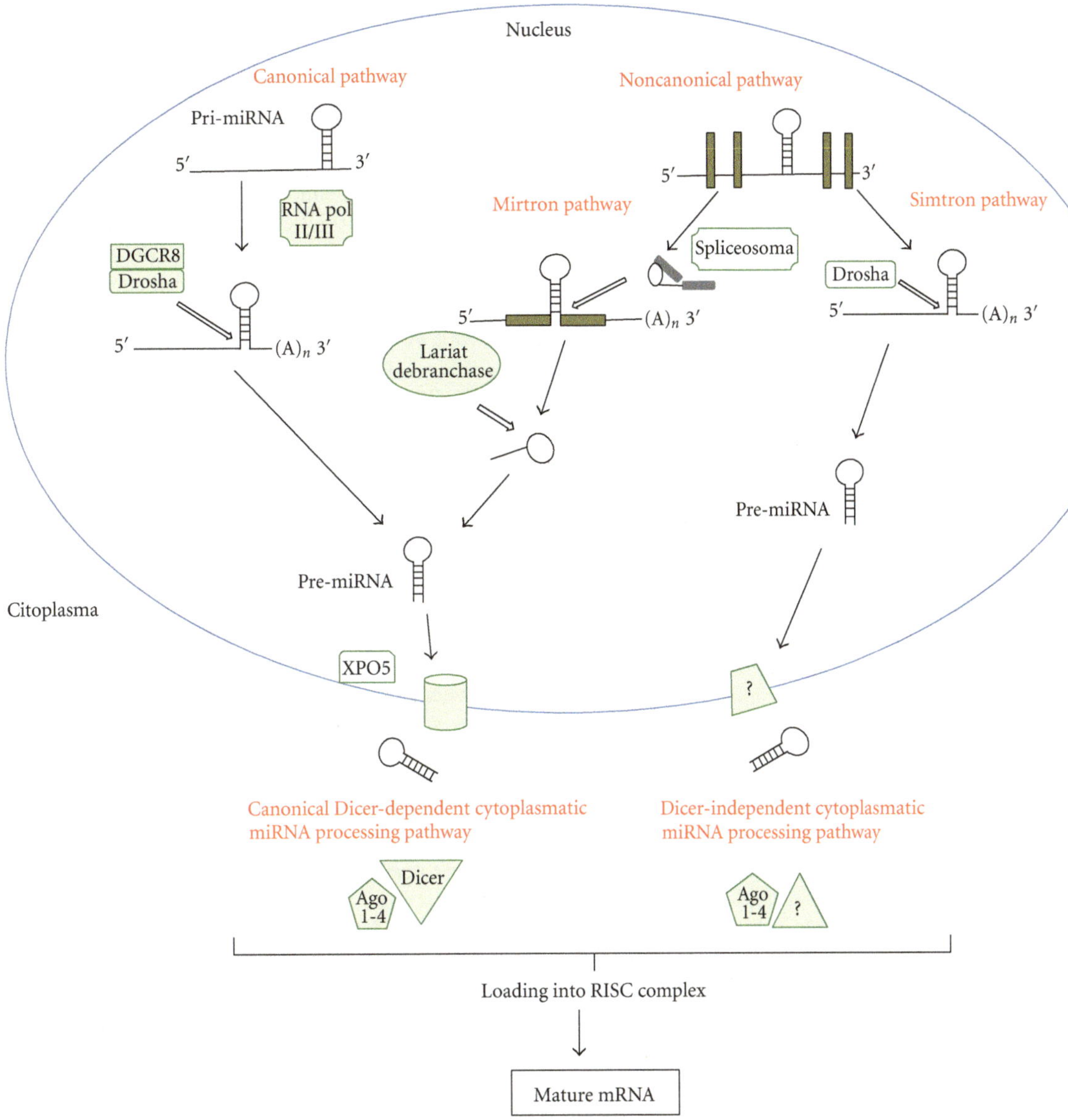

Figure 1: The miRNA biogenesis pathway. MicroRNAs generated by the canonical pathway are transcribed as precursor RNAs from intergenic, intronic, or polycistronic genomic loci by RNA polymerase II (RNA Pol II/III). The primary miRNA (pri-miRNA) transcript forms a stem-loop structure that is processed by the DGCR8/Drosha complex. The pre-miRNA is exported to the cytoplasm by XPO5, where it is processed into a mature miRNA duplex by Dicer. Finally, the mature miRNA enters into the RISC complex in association with an AGO family member. In the noncanonical pathway, mirtrons, a subset of miRNAs derived from introns, are processed by the spliceosome and the debranching enzyme. In addition to mirtrons, another non-canonical pathway called the simtron pathway involves Drosha but not its partner DGCR8 or Dicer. The mature miRNA produced by these different pathways leads to translational repression or degradation of the target mRNA.

a double-stranded RNA-binding domain protein (DGCR8/Pasha). After that, the pre-miRNA is exported to the cytoplasm by Exportin-5 (XPO5). In the cytoplasm, the pre-miRNA is processed into a ~21–23 nt mature miRNA duplex by the endonuclease Dicer. One of the duplex strands is preferentially loaded into the RNA-induced silencing complex (RISC) in association with an Ago family member producing a functional complex that binds to its RNA target. Thus, miRNAs control gene expression by binding to the 3′UTRs of their targets through Watson-Crick base pairing between the target and the 5′-end of the miRNAs, known as the seed sequence (2–8 nt). This interaction typically leads to the translational repression of target mRNAs by either transcript destabilization, translational inhibition, or both. Recent studies have shown that miRNAs can also repress mRNA targets through binding to other regions, including 5′UTRs or protein-coding exons [46–49] and in some cases may even activate translation [48, 50–52]. However, the mechanistic details of protein synthesis inhibition by miRNAs are not well understood. Potential pathways include sequestration from ribosomes (by relocation into P bodies), blockage of translational initiation, translational repression after initiation, and target deadenylation coupled to transcript degradation [53, 54].

In addition to the classical pathway, an alternative, non-canonical pathway for the biogenesis of some intronic miRNAs (mirtrons) has also been reported. Mirtrons are processed from the host gene by the spliceosome, exported from the nucleus by XPO5, cleaved by Dicer and loaded into the RISC complex. Moreover, another alternative miRNA processing pathway has been recently described (the simtron pathway). The simtron (splicing-independent mirtron-like miRNAs) pathway involves Drosha but does not required Drosha's binding partner DGCR8 or the endonuclease, Dicer [55]. Thus, these miRNA are processed in a manner that does not required splicing, the multiprotein complex, Dicer or Ago2 (Figure 1).

To study the microRNAs functions, antisense reagents against miRNAs have been developed as a reverse genetic tool. Synthetic oligonucleotide analogues, including 2′-O-methyl oligonucleotides [56], locked nucleic acids [57], 2′-O-methoxyethyl oligoribonucleotides [20], and morpholinos [58] have been tested. These antisense nucleotide analogues have been used to knock down miRNAs in cultured cells [20, 56, 57], and in live animals including zebrafish [58], *D. melanogaster* [59], and mice [22].

5. Control of Cholesterol Metabolism by MicroRNAs

5.1. Role of MiR-122 in Liver Metabolism. The liver is the major regulator of cholesterol and lipoprotein metabolism. miR-122 is highly expressed in the liver, and it is estimated to account for approximately 70% of all liver miRNA [22, 60]. miR-122 is highly conserved from human to frogs, suggesting an important role for this miRNA that has been under selective pressure throughout evolution [61]. A role for miR-122 in lipid metabolism was revealed in knockdown studies [11, 23]. miR-122 inhibition by antisense oligonucleotides (ASO) in mice resulted in increased hepatic fatty-acid oxidation and a reduced cholesterol synthesis [23]. In addition, miR-122 inhibition reduced total plasma cholesterol by 25–35%, and this was reflected by changes in both the LDL and HDL fractions [23]. Similar effects were observed in African green monkeys treated with miR-122 antagomirs wherein inhibition caused a dose-dependent decrease in plasma cholesterol without any signs of toxicity [11]. Due to the lack of toxicity, miR-122 has become a strong candidate as a therapeutic target in the treatment of hypercholesterolemia in humans. miR-122 inhibition caused a significant decrease of genes involved in cholesterol synthesis including 3-hydroxy-3-methylglutaryl-CoA synthase 1 (HMGCS1), 3-hydroxy-3-methylglutaryl-CoA reductase (HMGCR), 7-dehydrocholesterol reductase (DHCR7), and squalene epoxidase (SQLE) [22]. Conversely, miR-122 overexpression increases the expression of HMGCS1, DHCR7 and SQLE [22]. Importantly, all these genes are not direct targets of miR-122. Therefore, the mechanism by which miR-122 regulates lipid metabolism remains undetermined. This lack of a mechanistic understanding of the effects of miR-122 on cholesterol homeostasis, and the possibilities of other adverse consequences as the decline levels of HDL, both in mice and in nonhuman primates [11, 23, 62], and hepatocellular carcinoma, has also dampened the enthusiasm for the development of miR-122 antisense technologies as a therapeutic approach for long-term management of cholesterol disorders. It is important to take into account that many miR-122 validated targets are involved in glucose homeostasis and the Krebs cycle, including aldolase A (ALDOA) and citrate synthase (CS) [22, 23]. In addition to regulate lipid and glucose metabolism, miR-122 also plays an important role in regulating iron homeostasis [63]. miR-122 inhibition increased the expression of several genes that control systemic iron levels, such as hemochromatosis (Hfe), hemojuvelin (Hjv), bone morphogenetic protein receptor type 1A (Bmpr1a) and Hamp. Interestingly, mice treated with miR-122 antisense oligonucleotides develop systemic iron deficiency, characterized by reduced plasma and liver iron levels, mildly impaired hematopoiesis, and increased extramedullary erythropoiesis in the spleen.

Recently, miR-122 was found to be required for the propagation of hepatitis C virus (HCV). miR-122 binds two positions in the 5′UTR of the HCV genome, and this binding is essential to viral accumulation and propagation infected hepatocytes [64–66]. In a recent study in nonhuman primates, silencing of miR-122 resulted in a sustained reductions in HVC viremia and improvement in liver pathology, with no evidence of viral resistance [66]. Very interestingly, miR-122 inhibition also decreased Bach1 and increased heme oxygenase-1 (HO-1), which is an antioxidant defense and key cytoprotective enzyme repressed by Bach1 [67]. These data suggest that the therapeutic targeting of miR-122 and upregulation of HO-1 may represent a new strategy for anti-HCV intervention and cytoprotection.

5.2. MiR-33: A Key Regulator of Lipid Metabolism. We and others have recently identified *miR-33a* and *miR-33b*, intronic miRNAs located within the *Serbp2* and *Srebp1* genes, respectively [12, 24, 25]. *mir-33a* and *mir-33b* are co-transcribed with their host genes and regulate cholesterol and fatty acid metabolism. miR-33 overexpression strongly represses ABCA1 expression at the RNA and protein level and decreases cellular cholesterol efflux to apolipor protein A-I (ApoA-I), a key step in regulating reverse cholesterol transport (RCT). Conversely, antagonism miR-33 upregulates ABCA1 expression *in vitro* and *in vivo* and promotes cholesterol efflux to ApoA-I. Importantly, *in vivo* inhibition of miR-33 expression leads to a significant increase in plasma HDL levels and the regression of atherosclerosis, thus confirming the physiological effects of miR-33 in regulating lipid metabolism [12, 25, 68, 69].

In addition to ABCA1, two important genes involved in cholesterol metabolism were described as targets of miR-33: ABCG1 which mobilizes cellular free cholesterol to more lipidated HDL particles, and Niemann Pick C1 (NPC1), which transports cholesterol from lysosomes to other cellular compartments. Interestingly, *Abcg1* has two miR-33 binding sites in its 3′UTR that are only present in rodents, suggesting that cellular efflux to mature HDL is differently regulated between species [12, 24]. Another interesting difference between humans and rodents is that the 3′UTR of *Npc1* in humans contains two miR-33 binding sites resulting in a significant repression of NPC1 protein expression, whereas mice only contain one site, which is modestly suppressed by miR-33 [12]. ABCA1 also plays a key role in the biogenesis of HDL in the liver and intestine [31, 70]. To assess whether anti-miRNA-33 therapy increases liver ABCA1 expression and plasma HDL levels, several groups silenced miR-33 expression using a variety of strategies including modified oligonucleotides and antisense oligonucleotides expressed in lentiviral or adenoviral constructs. As expected, mice treated with anti-miR-33 oligonucleotides have a significant increase in liver ABCA1 expression and plasma HDL levels. These results were later confirmed genetically in the miR-33 knockout mice. Although the preclinical studies of miR-33 inhibition in mice are encouraging, extrapolation of these findings to human is complicated by the fact that mice lack miR-33b. Nevertheless, anti-miR-33 therapy in nonhuman primates has demonstrated to be very effective in increasing the levels of HDL and reducing VLDL [71].

miR-33a and miR-33b also target genes involved in the β-oxidation of fatty acids, including carnitine palmitoyltransferase 1A (CPT1A), carnitine O-octanoyltransferase (CROT), hydroxyacyl-CoA dehydrogenase/3-ketoacyl-CoA thiolase/enoyl-CoA hydratase (HADHB), 5′ adenosine monophosphate-activated protein kinase (AMPK), and sirtuin 6 (SIRT6). Moreover, miR-33a and miR-33b also target the insulin receptor substrate 2 (IRS2), an essential component of the insulin-signaling pathway in the liver [72]. In addition to the role of miR-33 in regulating cholesterol and fatty acid metabolism, we have also recently shown that miR-33 regulates cell cycle progression and cellular proliferation [73]. miR-33 negatively regulates cyclin-dependent kinase 6 (CDK6) and cyclin D1 (CCND1), which results in cell cycle arrest in G1 phase. Furthermore, this study also shows that *in vivo* inhibition of miR-33 using antisense oligonucleotides improves liver regeneration after partial hepatectomy [73].

Altogether, these data suggest that the inhibition of miR-33 expression may be a promising strategy to treat atherosclerotic vascular disease, metabolic syndrome, and liver regeneration in chronic liver disease.

5.3. Role of miR-758 and miR 106b in Regulating Cholesterol Homeostasis. miR-758 and miR-106b also regulate post-transcriptional ABCA1 expression [13, 14]. miR-758 was identified performing an unbiased genomewide screen together with a bioinformatic analysis. miR-758 was downregulated by cellular cholesterol content in macrophages and in the liver from mice fed a high-fat diet [13]. Even though the mechanism by which miR-758 expression is regulated remains unclear, these data strongly suggest that the downregulation of miR-758 in cholesterol-loaded cells may cooperate to up-regulate ABCA1 expression to avoid further cholesterol accumulation [10]. Interestingly, miR-758 is highly expressed in brain tissue and human neuronal cell lines. Overexpression of miR-758 in H4 human neuroglioma cells significantly decreases ABCA1 expression. Moreover, several genes involved in amino acid synthesis, including sodium-coupled neutral amino acid transporter 1 (SLC38a1), neurite outgrowth, such as neurotrimin (NTM), and the development of the nervous system, like ephrin type-A receptor 7 (EPHA7) were also downregulated in H4 cells transfected with miR-758 mimics [13].

Genetic studies with Alzheimer disease (AD) mouse models have demonstrated that the deletion of ABCA1 increases $A\beta$ deposition, while overexpression of ABCA1 dramatically reduces $A\beta$ deposition, suggesting a role for ABCA1 in $A\beta$ metabolism [22, 74–76]. Interestingly, miR106b has been recently reported to decrease ABCA1 expression and impair cellular cholesterol efflux in neuronal cells. Moreover, Neuro2a cells transfected with miR-106b dramatically increase levels of secreted $A\beta$ by increasing $A\beta$ production and preventing $A\beta$ clearance [14]. Overall, these findings suggest an important role for miR-758 and miR106b in regulating neurological functions and might have important implications in the pathogenesis of AD through posttranscriptional repression of ABCA1. Interestingly, miR-33 is highly expressed in the brain, and many predicted targets for miR-33 are involved in neurogenesis, such as Sema-3a and netrin-1, and synaptic regulation, including glutamate receptor ionotropic Kainate 2 (GRIK2) and glutamate receptor ionotropic AMPA 3 (AMPA 3).

6. Conclusion

miRNAs represent an elegant layer above transcriptional control for both fine-tuning and dramatically altering activity and output of cell signaling. In addition, miRNAs may serve as points of crosstalk between signaling pathways, by integrating transcriptional inputs or by their functional regulatory output on different pathways. Recently, short interfering RNAs (siRNAs) and miRNAs have gained considerable attention as therapeutic targets. Different strategies have been developed to modulate miRNA effects for therapeutic purposes. Inhibition of miR expression can be achieved using antisense oligonucleotides "antagomirs," or their chemically modified versions, 2′-O-methyl-group(OMe)-modified oligonucleotides and locked nucleic acids (LNAs) "antimiRs", as well as by inhibiting the production of the mature forms via affecting their processing. There is tremendous therapeutic potential for the treatment of cardiovascular diseases, by either overexpression or inhibition of miRNAs. The data summarized in this paper pointed out that anti-miR-33, miR-758 therapy, and miR-106 may be useful for treating dyslipidemia and cardiovascular disorders.

Disclosure

C. Fernández-Hernando has patents on the use of miRNA-33 inhibitors.

Acknowledgments

This work was supported by Grants from the National Institutes of Health R01HL107953 and R01HL106063 (to C. Fernández-Hernando). The authors thank Leigh Goedeke for the editing work and helpful comments on the paper.

References

[1] E. Ikonen, "Mechanisms for cellular cholesterol transport: defects and human disease," *Physiological Reviews*, vol. 86, no. 4, pp. 1237–1261, 2006.

[2] F. R. Maxfield and I. Tabas, "Role of cholesterol and lipid organization in disease," *Nature*, vol. 438, no. 7068, pp. 612–621, 2005.

[3] P. Foley, "Lipids in Alzheimer's disease: a century-old story," *Biochimica et Biophysica Acta*, vol. 1801, no. 8, pp. 750–753, 2010.

[4] P. Tontonoz, J. B. Kim, R. A. Graves, and B. M. Spiegelman, "ADD1: a novel helix-loop-helix transcription factor associated with adipocyte determination and differentiation," *Molecular and Cellular Biology*, vol. 13, no. 8, pp. 4753–4759, 1993.

[5] M. S. Brown and J. L. Goldstein, "The SREBP pathway: regulation of cholesterol metabolism by proteolysis of a membrane-bound transcription factor," *Cell*, vol. 89, no. 3, pp. 331–340, 1997.

[6] D. J. Peet, B. A. Janowski, and D. J. Mangelsdorf, "The LXRs: a new class of oxysterol receptors," *Current Opinion in Genetics and Development*, vol. 8, no. 5, pp. 571–575, 1998.

[7] B. A. Janowski, P. J. Willy, T. R. Devi, J. R. Falck, and D. J. Mangelsdorf, "An oxysterol signalling pathway mediated by the nuclear receptor LXRα," *Nature*, vol. 383, no. 6602, pp. 728–731, 1996.

[8] V. Ambros, "MicroRNA pathways in flies and worms: growth, death, fat, stress, and timing," *Cell*, vol. 113, no. 6, pp. 673–676, 2003.

[9] V. Ambros, "The functions of animal microRNAs," *Nature*, vol. 431, no. 7006, pp. 350–355, 2004.

[10] D. P. Bartel, "MicroRNAs: target recognition and regulatory functions," *Cell*, vol. 136, no. 2, pp. 215–233, 2009.

[11] J. Elmén, M. Lindow, S. Schütz et al., "LNA-mediated microRNA silencing in non-human primates," *Nature*, vol. 452, no. 7189, pp. 896–899, 2008.

[12] K. J. Rayner, Y. Suárez, A. Dávalos et al., "MiR-33 contributes to the regulation of cholesterol homeostasis," *Science*, vol. 328, no. 5985, pp. 1570–1573, 2010.

[13] C. M. Ramirez, A. Davalos, L. Goedeke et al., "MicroRNA-758 regulates cholesterol efflux through posttranscriptional repression of ATP-binding cassette transporter A1," *Arteriosclerosis, Thrombosis, and Vascular Biology*, vol. 31, pp. 2707–2714, 2011.

[14] J. Kim, H. Yoon, C. M. Ramirez et al., "miR-106b impairs cholesterol efflux and increases Abeta levels by repressing ABCA1 expression," *Experimental Neurology*, vol. 235, no. 2, pp. 476–483, 2011.

[15] D. Iliopoulos, K. Drosatos, Y. Hiyama, I. J. Goldberg, and V. I. Zannis, "MicroRNA-370 controls the expression of MicroRNA-122 and Cpt1α and affects lipid metabolism," *Journal of Lipid Research*, vol. 51, no. 6, pp. 1513–1523, 2010.

[16] I. Gerin, G. T. Bommer, C. S. McCoin, K. M. Sousa, V. Krishnan, and O. A. MacDougald, "Roles for miRNA-378/378∗ in adipocyte gene expression and lipogenesis," *American Journal of Physiology*, vol. 299, no. 2, pp. E198–E206, 2010.

[17] Q. Lin, Z. Gao, R. M. Alarcon, J. Ye, and Z. Yun, "A role of miR-27 in the regulation of adipogenesis," *FEBS Journal*, vol. 276, no. 8, pp. 2348–2358, 2009.

[18] N. Nakanishi, Y. Nakagawa, N. Tokushige et al., "The up-regulation of microRNA-335 is associated with lipid metabolism in liver and white adipose tissue of genetically obese mice," *Biochemical and Biophysical Research Communications*, vol. 385, no. 4, pp. 492–496, 2009.

[19] T. Chen, Z. Li, J. Tu et al., "MicroRNA-29a regulates pro-inflammatory cytokine secretion and scavenger receptor expression by targeting LPL in oxLDL-stimulated dendritic cells," *FEBS Letters*, vol. 585, no. 4, pp. 657–663, 2011.

[20] C. Esau, X. Kang, E. Peralta et al., "MicroRNA-143 regulates adipocyte differentiation," *The Journal of Biological Chemistry*, vol. 279, no. 50, pp. 52361–52365, 2004.

[21] M. Hoekstra, R. J. van der Sluis, J. Kuiper, and T. J. C. Van Berkel, "Nonalcoholic fatty liver disease is associated with an altered hepatocyte microRNA profile in LDL receptor knockout mice," *Journal of Nutritional Biochemistry*, vol. 23, no. 6, pp. 622–628, 2012.

[22] J. Krützfeldt, N. Rajewsky, R. Braich et al., "Silencing of microRNAs in vivo with 'antagomirs'," *Nature*, vol. 438, no. 7068, pp. 685–689, 2005.

[23] C. Esau, S. Davis, S. F. Murray et al., "miR-122 regulation of lipid metabolism revealed by in vivo antisense targeting," *Cell Metabolism*, vol. 3, no. 2, pp. 87–98, 2006.

[24] T. J. Marquart, R. M. Allen, D. S. Ory, and A. Baldan, "miR-33 links SREBP-2 induction to repression of sterol transporters," *Proceedings of the National Academy of Sciences of the United States of America*, vol. 107, no. 27, pp. 12228–12232, 2010.

[25] S. H. Najafi, F. Kristo, Y. Li et al., "MicroRNA-33 and the SREBP host genes cooperate to control cholesterol homeostasis," *Science*, vol. 328, no. 5985, pp. 1566–1569, 2010.

[26] C. Fernández, M. D. V. T. Lobo, D. Gómez-Coronado, and M. A. Lasunción, "Cholesterol is essential for mitosis progression and its deficiency induces polyploid cell formation," *Experimental Cell Research*, vol. 300, no. 1, pp. 109–120, 2004.

[27] C. Fernández, M. Martín, D. Gómez-Coronado, and M. A. Lasunción, "Effects of distal cholesterol biosynthesis inhibitors on cell proliferation and cell cycle progression," *Journal of Lipid Research*, vol. 46, no. 5, pp. 920–929, 2005.

[28] C. K. Glass and J. L. Witztum, "Atherosclerosis: The road ahead," *Cell*, vol. 104, no. 4, pp. 503–516, 2001.

[29] N. Zelcer and P. Tontonoz, "Liver X receptors as integrators of metabolic and inflammatory signaling," *Journal of Clinical Investigation*, vol. 116, no. 3, pp. 607–614, 2006.

[30] N. Zelcer, C. Hong, R. Boyadjian, and P. Tontonoz, "LXR regulates cholesterol uptake through idol-dependent ubiquitination of the LDL receptor," *Science*, vol. 325, no. 5936, pp. 100–104, 2009.

[31] A. R. Tall, L. Yvan-Charvet, N. Terasaka, T. Pagler, and N. Wang, "HDL, ABC transporters, and cholesterol efflux: implications for the treatment of atherosclerosis," *Cell Metabolism*, vol. 7, no. 5, pp. 365–375, 2008.

[32] W. Filipowicz, S. N. Bhattacharyya, and N. Sonenberg, "Mechanisms of post-transcriptional regulation by microRNAs: are the answers in sight?" *Nature Reviews Genetics*, vol. 9, no. 2, pp. 102–114, 2008.

[33] R. C. Friedman, K. K. H. Farh, C. B. Burge, and D. P. Bartel, "Most mammalian mRNAs are conserved targets of microRNAs," *Genome Research*, vol. 19, no. 1, pp. 92–105, 2009.

[34] S. Griffiths-Jones, H. K. Saini, S. Van Dongen, and A. J. Enright, "miRBase: tools for microRNA genomics," *Nucleic Acids Research*, vol. 36, no. 1, pp. D154–D158, 2008.

[35] D. Catalucci, P. Gallo, and G. Condorelli, "Advances in molecular genetics, genomics, proteomics, metabolomics, and systems biology: microRNAs in cardiovascular biology and heart disease," *Circulation*, vol. 2, no. 4, pp. 402–408, 2009.

[36] T. C. Chang and J. T. Mendell, "MicroRNAs in vertebrate physiology and human disease," *Annual Review of Genomics and Human Genetics*, vol. 8, pp. 215–239, 2007.

[37] E. Van Rooij, W. S. Marshall, and E. N. Olson, "Toward microRNA-based therapeutics for heart disease: the sense in antisense," *Circulation Research*, vol. 103, no. 9, pp. 919–928, 2008.

[38] I. Alevizos and G. G. Illei, "MicroRNAs as biomarkers in rheumatic diseases," *Nature Reviews Rheumatology*, vol. 6, no. 7, pp. 391–398, 2010.

[39] O. Cheung, P. Puri, C. Eicken et al., "Nonalcoholic steatohepatitis is associated with altered hepatic MicroRNA expression," *Hepatology*, vol. 48, no. 6, pp. 1810–1820, 2008.

[40] S. Fichtlscherer, A. M. Zeiher, and S. Dimmeler, "Circulating microRNAs: biomarkers or mediators of cardiovascular diseases?" *Arteriosclerosis, Thrombosis, and Vascular Biology*, vol. 31, pp. 2383–2390, 2011.

[41] A. M. Friel, C. Corcoran, J. Crown, and L. O'Driscoll, "Relevance of circulating tumor cells, extracellular nucleic acids, and exosomes in breast cancer," *Breast cancer research and treatment*, vol. 123, no. 3, pp. 613–625, 2010.

[42] N. Kosaka, H. Iguchi, and T. Ochiya, "Circulating microRNA in body fluid: a new potential biomarker for cancer diagnosis and prognosis," *Cancer Science*, vol. 101, no. 10, pp. 2087–2092, 2010.

[43] G. Rabinowits, C. Gerçel-Taylor, J. M. Day, D. D. Taylor, and G. H. Kloecker, "Exosomal microRNA: a diagnostic marker for lung cancer," *Clinical Lung Cancer*, vol. 10, no. 1, pp. 42–46, 2009.

[44] R. Rosell, J. Wei, and M. Taron, "Circulating microRNA signatures of tumor-derived exosomes for early diagnosis of non-small-cell lung cancer," *Clinical Lung Cancer*, vol. 10, no. 1, pp. 8–9, 2009.

[45] D. D. Taylor and C. Gercel-Taylor, "MicroRNA signatures of tumor-derived exosomes as diagnostic biomarkers of ovarian cancer," *Gynecologic Oncology*, vol. 110, no. 1, pp. 13–21, 2008.

[46] J. J. Forman and H. A. Coller, "The code within the code: microRNAs target coding regions," *Cell Cycle*, vol. 9, no. 8, pp. 1533–1541, 2010.

[47] J. R. Lytle, T. A. Yario, and J. A. Steitz, "Target mRNAs are repressed as efficiently by microRNA-binding sites in the 5′ UTR as in the 3′ UTR," *Proceedings of the National Academy of Sciences of the United States of America*, vol. 104, no. 23, pp. 9667–9672, 2007.

[48] U. A. Ørom, F. C. Nielsen, and A. H. Lund, "MicroRNA-10a binds the 5′UTR of ribosomal protein mRNAs and enhances their translation," *Molecular Cell*, vol. 30, no. 4, pp. 460–471, 2008.

[49] I. Rigoutsos, "New tricks for animal micrornas: targeting of amino acid coding regions at conserved and nonconserved sites," *Cancer Research*, vol. 69, no. 8, pp. 3245–3248, 2009.

[50] J. I. Henke, D. Goergen, J. Zheng et al., "MicroRNA-122 stimulates translation of hepatitis C virus RNA," *The EMBO Journal*, vol. 27, no. 24, pp. 3300–3310, 2008.

[51] S. Vasudevan, Y. Tong, and J. A. Steitz, "Switching from repression to activation: microRNAs can up-regulate translation," *Science*, vol. 318, no. 5858, pp. 1931–1934, 2007.

[52] S. Vasudevan, Y. Tong, and J. A. Steitz, "Cell cycle control of microRNA-mediated translation regulation," *Cell Cycle*, vol. 7, no. 11, pp. 1545–1549, 2008.

[53] J. Liu, "Control of protein synthesis and mRNA degradation by microRNAs," *Current Opinion in Cell Biology*, vol. 20, no. 2, pp. 214–221, 2008.

[54] R. S. Pillai, S. N. Bhattacharyya, and W. Filipowicz, "Repression of protein synthesis by miRNAs: how many mechanisms?" *Trends in Cell Biology*, vol. 17, no. 3, pp. 118–126, 2007.

[55] M. A. Havens, A. A. Reich, D. M. Duelli, and M. L. Hastings, "Biogenesis of mammalian microRNAs by a non-canonical processing pathway2012," *Nucleic Acids Research*, vol. 40, no. 10, pp. 4626–4640.

[56] G. Hutvágner, M. J. Simard, C. C. Mello, and P. D. Zamore, "Sequence-specific inhibition of small RNA function," *PLoS Biology*, vol. 2, no. 4, p. E98, 2004.

[57] U. A. Ørom, S. Kauppinen, and A. H. Lund, "LNA-modified oligonucleotides mediate specific inhibition of microRNA function," *Gene*, vol. 372, no. 1-2, pp. 137–141, 2006.

[58] A. S. Flynt, N. Li, E. J. Thatcher, L. Solnica-Krezel, and J. G. Patton, "Zebrafish miR-214 modulates Hedgehog signaling to specify muscle cell fate," *Nature Genetics*, vol. 39, no. 2, pp. 259–263, 2007.

[59] A. Boutla, C. Delidakis, and M. Tabler, "Developmental defects by antisense-mediated inactivation of micro-RNAs 2 and 13 in Drosophila and the identification of putative target genes," *Nucleic Acids Research*, vol. 31, no. 17, pp. 4973–4980, 2003.

[60] M. Lagos-Quintana, R. Rauhut, A. Yalcin, J. Meyer, W. Lendeckel, and T. Tuschl, "Identification of tissue-specific MicroRNAs from mouse," *Current Biology*, vol. 12, no. 9, pp. 735–739, 2002.

[61] M. Girard, E. Jacquemin, A. Munnich, S. Lyonnet, and A. Henrion-Caude, "miR-122, a paradigm for the role of microRNAs in the liver," *Journal of Hepatology*, vol. 48, no. 4, pp. 648–656, 2008.

[62] J. Elmén, M. Lindow, A. Silahtaroglu et al., "Antagonism of microRNA-122 in mice by systemically administered LNA-antimiR leads to up-regulation of a large set of predicted target mRNAs in the liver," *Nucleic Acids Research*, vol. 36, no. 4, pp. 1153–1162, 2008.

[63] M. Castoldi, M. V. Spasic, S. Altamura et al., "The liver-specific microRNA miR-122 controls systemic iron homeostasis in mice," *Journal of Clinical Investigation*, vol. 121, no. 4, pp. 1386–1396, 2011.

[64] C. L. Jopling, M. Yi, A. M. Lancaster, S. M. Lemon, and P. Sarnow, "Molecular biology: modulation of hepatitis C virus RNA abundance by a liver-specific MicroRNA," *Science*, vol. 309, no. 5740, pp. 1577–1581, 2005.

[65] C. L. Jopling, S. Schütz, and P. Sarnow, "Position-dependent function for a tandem microRNA miR-122-binding site located in the hepatitis C virus RNA genome," *Cell Host and Microbe*, vol. 4, no. 1, pp. 77–85, 2008.

[66] G. Randall, M. Panis, J. D. Cooper et al., "Cellular cofactors affecting hepatitis C virus infection and replication," *Proceedings of the National Academy of Sciences of the United States of America*, vol. 104, no. 31, pp. 12884–12889, 2007.

[67] Y. Shan, J. Zheng, R. W. Lambrecht, and H. L. Bonkovsky, "Reciprocal effects of micro-RNA-122 on expression of heme oxygenase-1 and hepatitis C virus genes in human hepatocytes," *Gastroenterology*, vol. 133, no. 4, pp. 1166–1174, 2007.

[68] I. Gerin, L. A. Clerbaux, O. Haumont et al., "Expression of miR-33 from an SREBP2 intron inhibits cholesterol export and fatty acid oxidation," *The Journal of Biological Chemistry*, vol. 285, no. 44, pp. 33652–33661, 2010.

[69] T. J. Marquart, R. M. Allen, D. S. Ory, and A. Baldan, "miR-33 links SREBP-2 induction to repression of sterol transporters," *Proceedings of the National Academy of Sciences of the United States of America*, vol. 107, no. 27, pp. 12228–12232, 2010.

[70] T. Plösch, A. Kosters, A. K. Groen, and F. Kuipers, "The ABC of hepatic and intestinal cholesterol transport," *Handbook of experimental pharmacology*, no. 170, pp. 465–482, 2005.

[71] K. J. Rayner, C. C. Esau, F. N. Hussain et al., "Inhibition of miR-33a/b in non-human primates raises plasma HDL and lowers VLDL triglycerides," *Nature*, vol. 478, pp. 404–407, 2011.

[72] A. Dávalos, L. Goedeke, P. Smibert et al., "miR-33a/b contribute to the regulation of fatty acid metabolism and insulin signaling," *Proceedings of the National Academy of Sciences of the United States of America*, vol. 108, no. 22, pp. 9232–9237, 2011.

[73] D. Cirera-Salinas, M. Pauta, R. M. Allen et al., "Mir-33 regulates cell proliferation and cell cycle progression," *Cell Cycle*, vol. 11, no. 5, 2012.

[74] S. E. Wahrle, H. Jiang, M. Parsadanian et al., "Overexpression of ABCA1 reduces amyloid deposition in the PDAPP mouse model of Alzheimer disease," *Journal of Clinical Investigation*, vol. 118, no. 2, pp. 671–682, 2008.

[75] V. Hirsch-Reinshagen, S. Zhou, B. L. Burgess et al., "Deficiency of ABCA1 impairs apolipoprotein E metabolism in brain," *The Journal of Biological Chemistry*, vol. 279, no. 39, pp. 41197–41207, 2004.

[76] R. Koldamova, M. Staufenbiel, and I. Lefterov, "Lack of ABCA1 considerably decreases brain ApoE level and increases amyloid deposition in APP23 mice," *The Journal of Biological Chemistry*, vol. 280, no. 52, pp. 43224–43235, 2005.

Use of Lipid-Lowering Medications and the Likelihood of Achieving Optimal LDL-Cholesterol Goals in Coronary Artery Disease Patients

Dean G. Karalis,[1,2] Brett Victor,[2] Lilian Ahedor,[2] and Longjian Liu[3]

[1] *Cardiology Consultants of Philadelphia, Philadelphia, PA 19107, USA*
[2] *Division of Cardiology, Drexel University College of Medicine, Philadelphia, PA 19107, USA*
[3] *Department of Epidemiology and Biostatistics, Drexel University School of Public Health, Philadelphia, PA 19107, USA*

Correspondence should be addressed to Dean G. Karalis, dean.karalis@drexelmed.edu

Academic Editor: Jan Wouter Jukema

Background. In clinical practice, most coronary artery disease patients are not achieving their recommend LDL-cholesterol goal of <70 mg/dL. Methods. We conducted a retrospective analysis of outpatient electronic health records and the most recent lipid profile, lipid-lowering medications and doses were collected. Results. We identified 9950 coronary artery disease patients. Only 37% on a statin alone achieved an LDL-cholesterol of <70 mg/dL, and most were on moderate-to-high-potency statins. The intensity of statin therapy did not improve LDL-cholesterol goal attainment. Among patients on combination therapy, 41% on statin plus ezetimibe and 46% on statin plus niacin achieved an LDL-cholesterol of <70 mg/dL ($P = 0.01$ and <0.0001 versus statin alone). If patients were switched to a high-potency statin LDL-cholesterol goal attainment of <70 mg/dL would increase to 46% and would increase up to 72% with combination therapy. Conclusions. Most coronary artery disease patients in clinical practice do not attain an LDL-cholesterol of <70 mg/dL, even among patients on high potency statins. The combination of statin plus either ezetimibe or niacin is the most effective regimen to achieve an LDL-cholesterol of <70 mg/dL, however, these drug combinations are used infrequently in clinical practice.

1. Introduction

Coronary artery disease (CAD) is the leading cause of death and disability in both men and women in the United States [1]. Patients with known CAD are considered at high or very high cardiovascular risk and require aggressive modification of all their risk factors [2]. Several major clinical trials with statin therapy in patients with CAD have shown that lowering low-density lipoprotein (LDL) cholesterol can reduce cardiovascular events and the lower the LDL-cholesterol achieved the lower the cardiovascular risk [3–7]. In the Cholesterol Treatment Trialists' (CTT) Collaboration meta-analysis of individual data from over 170,000 patients in 26 randomized trials of statins, coronary mortality was reduced by just over one-fifth per 1.0 mmol/L (or 39 mg/dL) reduction in LDL-cholesterol with no evidence of any threshold within the range of cholesterol studied [8]. In a recent analysis from the JUPITER (Justification for the Use of Statins in Prevention: an Intervention Trial of Evaluating Rosuvastatin) trial, individuals who achieved an LDL-cholesterol of <50 mg/dL had a lower cardiovascular risk than those with higher on-treatment levels of LDL-cholesterol [9].

Based on a wealth of clinical trial evidence, current guidelines now recommend more aggressive LDL-cholesterol targets. Recent guidelines from the United States recommend that an LDL-cholesterol goal of <70 mg/dL is reasonable in high and very high risk patients such as those with CAD [2, 10, 11]. The American Diabetes Association and the American College of Cardiology identify adults with clinical CAD as being at the highest risk and recommend an LDL-cholesterol treatment goal of <70 mg/dL for these patients [12]. The new ESC/EAS Guidelines for the management of dyslipidaemias also recommend an LDL-cholesterol goal of <70 mg/dL for individuals with known cardiovascular disease [13].

Despite current guidelines, several studies have shown that most CAD patients do not achieve their recommended LDL-cholesterol goal of <70 mg/dL. We have previously reported that in clinical practice only about one-third of CAD patients achieve an LDL-cholesterol goal of <70 mg/dL [14]. Other observational studies have shown a similar low rate of attaining an LDL-cholesterol goal of <70 mg/dL in CAD patients [15–17]. There have been a number of barriers identified as to why CAD patients fail to achieve their optimal LDL-cholesterol goals in clinical practice [18]. These include patient noncompliance, physician nonadherence to current guidelines, intolerance to lipid-lowering therapy, and the lack of affordable and effective lipid-lowering medications to allow patients to achieve their more aggressive LDL-cholesterol goals.

The purpose of this study was to evaluate in a real-world setting what lipid-lowering medications are prescribed, the potency of statin therapy and the frequency of combination therapy being used in clinical practice to treat patients with CAD. It was our intention to determine if one barrier to achieving an LDL-cholesterol of <70 mg/dL was the under-utilization of lipid-lowering therapy in CAD patients by physicians in clinical practice.

2. Methods

The study site was Cardiology Consultants of Philadelphia, a large cardiology subspecialty practice in the Philadelphia area. Using an electronic medical record, we identified 23,408 patients with a history of CAD who had been seen in one of our outpatient offices over a 12-month period from September 2008 to September 2009. Patients were excluded if they did not have a complete lipid panel within the electronic medical record flow sheet dated from within the study period or within 6 months of their last office visit. In patients with more than one complete lipid panel, the most recent lipid panel was used. The use of lipid-lowering medications and their doses was noted. We identified 9950 CAD patients who met the study criteria. The study was approved by the Institutional Review Board of Drexel University College of Medicine.

Statin potency was categorized as low, moderate, or high potency. High-potency statins included atorvastatin (40 mg or 80 mg), rosuvastatin (20 mg or 40 mg), or simvastatin 80 mg. Moderate-potency statins included atorvastatin (10 mg or 20 mg), rosuvastatin (10 mg), simvastatin 40 mg, lovastatin 80 mg, or pravastatin 80 mg. All other statin doses were considered as low-potency statins. We used the following assumptions to predict LDL-cholesterol goal attainment if patients were switched to a more potent statin or if another non-statin LDL-cholesterol lowering drug was added to their statin therapy. For each change from a low to moderate potency statin or from a moderate to high potency statin we assumed a 6% additional decrease in LDL-cholesterol. We assumed a 15% additional decrease in LDL-cholesterol when a non-statin LDL-lowering drug was added to a patient on statin therapy alone. Non-statin LDL-lowering drugs included ezetimibe, bile-acid sequestrants or niacin. We assumed a 10% intolerance rate for any change to a more potent statin or for all non-statin LDL-lowering drugs.

For statistical analysis we examined mean differences between two groups using the t-test, and among three groups using analysis of variance, and examined differences in the prevalence of goal attainment across different groups using the chi-square test. All data analyses were conducted using SAS software version 9.2 (SAS Institute Inc., Cary, NC 27513). The level of significance was set at a two-sided P-value of ≤ 0.05.

3. Results

Among the 9950 CAD patients, a total of 5885 patients (59%) were treated with statin therapy alone, 2730 patients (27%) were treated with a statin in combination with another lipid-lowering drug, 389 (4%) were not on a statin but taking another non-statin lipid-lowering drug, and 946 (10%) were on no lipid-lowering therapy (Table 1). Among patients treated with statin therapy alone, 2174 patients (37%) achieved an LDL-cholesterol goal of <70 mg/dL (Table 2). Most patients were on moderate-potency statin therapy (41%), while the number of patients on high- and low-potency statin therapy was similar; 29% and 30%, respectively.

The mean achieved LDL-cholesterol level in the high potency statin group was significantly higher (81.4 mg/dL ± 27.0) when compared to the moderate-potency group (78.7 mg/dL ± 26.7); $P < 0.01$ and to the low-potency group (79.8 mg/dL ± 26.5); $P = 0.02$. Fewer patients on high-potency statins achieved their LDL-cholesterol goal of <70 mg/dL (33%) compared to patients on moderate potency statins (39%); $P < 0.0001$, and to patients on low potency statins (37%); $P < 0.01$. Only 37% of patients taking any dose of atorvastatin or rosuvastatin attained an LDL-cholesterol goal of <70 mg/dL. There was no relationship between increasing statin dose and improved LDL-cholesterol goal attainment (Figure 1).

Patients treated with a combination of statin and niacin were more likely to attain an LDL-cholesterol of <70 mg/dL (46% versus 37%; $P < 0.0001$) compared to patients treated with statin therapy alone as were patients treated with a combination of statin and ezetimibe (41% versus 37%; $P = 0.01$, Figure 2). However, only 9% of patients were treated with a combination of statin and niacin and only 14% of patients were on a combination of statin and ezetimibe. Patients treated with statin and a fibrate did not improve their LDL-cholesterol goal attainment when compared to patients treated with a statin alone (35% versus 37%; $P = 0.23$). The number of patients treated with a bile acid sequestrant or high-dose fish oil in combination with a statin was small; both <1%. Patients on no statin but treated with other lipid lowering drugs were less likely to achieve their LDL-cholesterol goals compared to patients on statin therapy

Table 1: Lipid-lowering medications in the 9950 coronary artery disease patients.

Lipid-lowering medications	Patients
Total number of patients	9950
Statin monotherapy	5885 (59%)
High potency	1692 (17%)
Moderate potency	2398 (24%)
Low potency	1795 (18%)
*Combination therapy**	2730 (27%)
Statin plus ezetimibe	1378 (14%)
Statin plus niacin	866 (9%)
Statin plus fibrate	650 (7%)
Statin plus fish oil	69 (<1%)
Statin plus bile acid sequestrant	43 (<1%)
No statin	1335 (13%)
No statin but other lipid lowering therapy†	389 (4%)
Ezetimibe	179 (2%)
Niacin	113 (1%)
Fibrate	170 (2%)
Fish oil	11 (<1%)
Bile acid sequestrant	37 (<1%)
No lipid-lowering therapy	946 (10%)

*Among patients on a statin plus another lipid-lowering medication, 276 patients were on more than one non-statin lipid-lowering drug.
†Among patients on no statin but another lipid-lowering medication, 121 patients were on more than one nonstatin lipid-lowering drug.

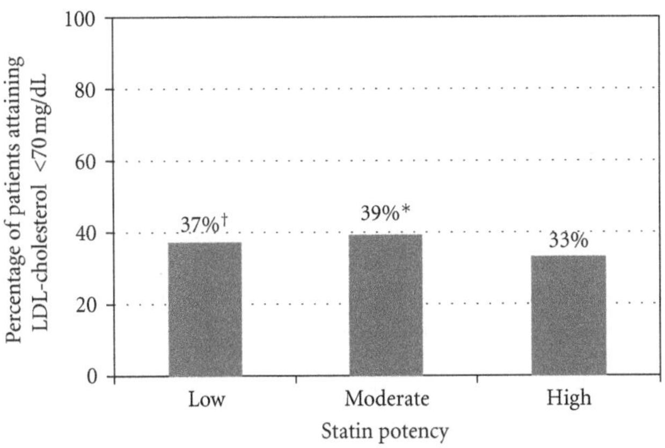

Figure 1: Percentage of patients achieving an LDL-cholesterol of <70 mg/dL based on the potency of their statin therapy. Fewer patients achieved an LDL-cholesterol goal of <70 mg/dL on high-potency statins compared to those on moderate or low-potency statins (*$P < 0.0001$ and †$P < 0.01$ compared to high potency statin therapy).

alone (18% versus 37%; $P < 0.0001$) as were patients on no lipid-lowering therapy (20% versus 37%; $P < 0.0001$).

Among patients taking a statin in combination with another lipid-lowering drug, most were taking only one additional drug (90%), while 10% were taking 2 or more lipid lowering drugs plus statin therapy. Among patients taking other lipid-lowering therapy, but not on a statin, 69% were on only one non-statin drug while 31% were on 2 or more non-statin drugs.

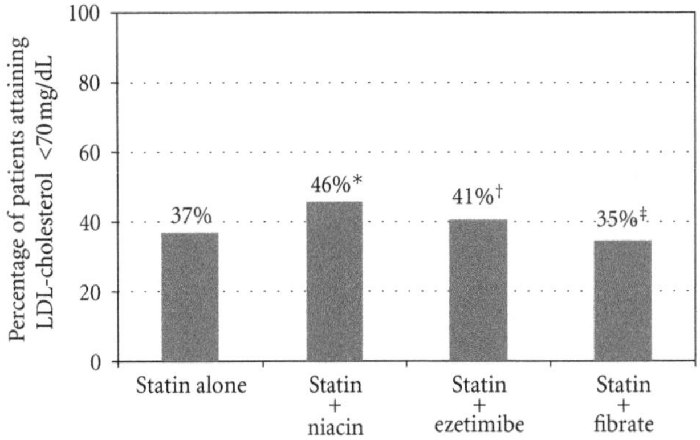

Figure 2: Percentage of patients achieving an LDL-cholesterol of <70 mg/dL on statin therapy alone compared to statin therapy in combination with another lipid-lowering drug. More patients achieved an LDL-cholesterol goal of <70 mg/dL with statin plus niacin (*$P < 0.001$) and with statin plus ezetimibe (†$P = 0.01$) compared with statin therapy alone. The combination of a statin and fibrate did not improve LDL-cholesterol goal attainment compared to statin therapy alone (‡$P = 0.23$).

It was estimated that if statin alone patients who had not attained their LDL-cholesterol goal of <70 mg/dL on a low or moderate potency statin were switched to a high-potency statin, assuming 90% tolerance of high-dose statin therapy, LDL-cholesterol goal attainment of <70 mg/dL would have increased from 37% to 46%; $P < 0.01$. If these patients were started on a non-statin LDL-cholesterol lowering drug instead of switching to a high-potency statin, and again assuming 90% tolerance to their non-statin lipid-lowering therapy, LDL-cholesterol goal attainment of <70 mg/dL would have increased from 37% to 60%; $P < 0.01$. More CAD patients would have achieved an LDL-cholesterol of <70 mg/dL by adding another non-statin LDL-lowering drug as compared to switching to a high-potency statin (60% versus 46%; $P < 0.01$). If all statin-alone patients were on a high-potency statin in combination with another non-statin LDL-cholesterol-lowering drug, LDL-cholesterol goal attainment of <70 mg/dL would have increased to 63%. If all patients were taking a high-potency statin and 2 additional non-statin LDL-cholesterol-lowering drugs, LDL-cholesterol goal attainment of <70 mg/dL would increase further to 72%.

4. Discussion

Our study demonstrates that, among CAD patients treated with statin therapy alone, only about one in three are achieving an LDL-cholesterol goal of <70 mg/dL, despite the fact that most are on moderate-to-high-potency statins. Although previous studies have also shown that few high-risk CAD patients attain an LDL-cholesterol of <70 mg/dL, few studies such as ours have evaluated the attainability of this more aggressive LDL-cholesterol goal as it relates to the choice of lipid lowering therapy. Kauffman and colleagues

TABLE 2: Patients attaining an LDL-cholesterol of <70 mg/dL according to their lipid lowering medications.

Lipid-lowering medications	Patients	LDL (mg/dL)	Patients attaining LDL <70
All Patients	9950	82.0 ± 29.2	3555 (36%)
Statin monotherapy	5885	79.8 ± 26.5	2174 (37%)
High potency	1692	81.4 ± 27.0	559 (33%)
Moderate potency	2398	78.7 ± 26.7	946 (39%)
Low potency	1795	79.8 ± 25.7	669 (37%)
*Combination therapy**	2730		1119 (41%)
Any statin plus ezetimibe	1378	79.0 ± 28.6	559 (41%)
Any statin plus niacin	866	74.1 ± 24.7	396 (46%)
Any statin plus fibrate	650	81.3 ± 27.6	224 (35%)
No statin	1335	99.9 ± 35.7	262 (20%)
No statin but other lipid-lowering therapy†	389		70 (18%)
Ezetimibe	179	107.1 ± 33.1	20 (11%)
Niacin	113	96.3 ± 36.0	23 (20%)
Fibrate	170	94.3 ± 35.1	39 (23%)
No lipid-lowering therapy	946	99.5 ± 35.5	192 (20%)

*Among patients on a statin plus another lipid-lowering drug 276 patients were on more than one non-statin lipid-lowering drug.
†Among patients on no statin but another lipid-lowering drug, 121 patients were on more than one non-statin lipid-lowering drug.
LDL-cholesterol values are expressed as mean ± SD.

[19] found that, among 7427 CAD patients, 43% achieved an LDL-cholesterol goal of <70 mg/dL and similar to our findings, the majority of patients were receiving moderate to high-potency statin monotherapy. In addition, patients taking high-potency statin monotherapy were less likely to attain an LDL-cholesterol goal of <70 mg/dL compared to patients taking less potent statins. We observed the same finding in our study. This paradoxical finding may be explained by the fact that, in clinical practice, managed care plans often mandate the use of a generic statin first and only when patients fail to achieve their desired LDL-cholesterol goal are the use of higher potency nongeneric statins allowed. It is likely that patients with the most difficult to treat lipids are the ones that are treated with the highest doses of the most potent statins, such as atorvastatin or rosuvastatin. However, even if all CAD patients could be switched to a high-potency statin, less than one-half of these high-risk patients would achieve an LDL-cholesterol goal of <70 mg/dL.

Statins remain the cornerstone of LDL-cholesterol lowering, however, in clinical practice, most CAD patients will not be able to achieve an LDL-cholesterol goal of <70 mg/dL without adding another LDL-cholesterol-lowering drug to statin therapy. In our study, as in previously published reports, the number of patients on a statin in combination with another LDL-cholesterol-lowering drug was low despite the evidence for the safety and efficacy of combination lipid-lowering therapy [20–24]. Numerous studies have shown that the combination of a statin plus ezetimibe is superior to statin monotherapy with regards to LDL-cholesterol-lowering and attaining an LDL-cholesterol goal of <70 mg/dL [25–27]. Ezetimibe will lower LDL-cholesterol by an additional 15 to 20% when added to statin therapy. However, few patients in our study were on ezetimibe in combination with a statin. This may be related to the lack of cardiovascular outcome data with ezetimibe in combination with a statin compared to statin therapy alone, as well as to some safety concerns regarding ezetimibe that have been raised from other clinical trials. However, in the recent Study of Heart and Renal Protection (SHARP), cholesterol lowering with a combination of simvastatin and ezetimibe reduced major atherosclerotic events by 17% compared to placebo in a population of chronic kidney disease patients [28]. In addition, there was a significant 25% reduction in nonhemorrhagic stroke and a significant 27% reduction in coronary revascularization in this population without any evidence for excess risk of hepatitis, gallstones, or cancer in ezetimbe-treated patients. This should reassure physicians about the safety and efficacy of ezetimibe and its role in clinical practice in attaining optimal LDL-cholesterol levels in patients who have not achieved their LDL-cholesterol goal despite statin monotherapy.

Although niacin is thought mostly as a high-density lipoprotein (HDL) raising drug, in higher doses niacin will lower LDL-cholesterol by approximately 15 to 20% when added on to statin therapy [29, 30]. As with ezetimibe, niacin was used infrequently in our study in combination with a statin, yet both of these combinations led to significantly greater attainment of an LDL-cholesterol goal of <70 mg/dL than did statin monotherapy. While the negative findings from the AIM-HIGH (Atherothrombosis Intervention in Metabolic Syndrome with Low HDL/High Triglycerides: Impact on Global Health Outcomes) trial [31] may dissuade physicians from using niacin more often in clinical practice, niacin may play a role to lower LDL-cholesterol levels in statin intolerant patients. Niacin may also be beneficial in patients on statin monotherapy who have not achieved their LDL-cholesterol goal especially in the setting of a low HDL-cholesterol or high levels of triglycerides. Bile acid sequestrants also provide additional LDL-cholesterol lowering, however, in our study these drugs were used in less than one percent of our CAD patients.

It must be emphasized that statins are the drug of choice to lower LDL cholesterol in patients with CAD and the addition of another LDL-lowering drug to a statin should only be considered in patients not at their LDL-cholesterol goal on a maximally tolerated dose of statin or for those patients who are statin intolerant. Despite the abundant outcome data for statins in CAD patients, there is no large prospective outcome study that had demonstrated the benefits of combination lipid-lowering therapy over statin therapy alone. However, many CAD patients are unable to achieve their LDL-cholesterol goal even with a high-potency statin and statin intolerance remains a significant problem in real world clinical practice. In large randomized clinical trials with statin therapy, the incidence of myalgias is generally low and approximately 2 to 4% [3–6]. However, data from observational studies have reported a much higher incidence of myalgias from statin therapy. In one study from a large managed care database, 8 to 9% of patents reported myalgias that led to discontinuing their statin therapy [32]. In our study, the number of patients who were not on a statin was high at 13%. Other studies have shown an even higher number of high-risk CAD patients who are not taking a statin. In a recent analysis from a large managed-care claims database in the United States, almost 30% of patients with coronary heart disease or atherosclerotic vascular disease were on no lipid-lowering therapy [33]. Despite the clear benefit in reducing cardiovascular events afforded by statin therapy, many high-risk patients are not treated with statin therapy. This reality plus the finding that many patients on high potency statins still do not achieve an LDL-cholesterol of <70 mg/dL makes achieving optimal LDL-cholesterol goals difficult with statin therapy alone.

In our study, we made assumptions to estimate how many patients already tolerating statin therapy could achieve an LDL-cholesterol goal of <70 mg/dL if they were switched to a high-potency statin in combination with one or two additional non-statin LDL-lowering drugs. We used a liberal estimate of 10% for intolerance to a high-potency statin or to a non-statin LDL-lowering drug. In such a scenario attainment of an LDL-cholesterol goal of <70 mg/dL increased from 46% to 63% when patients on a high-potency statin had one additional non-statin LDL-lowering drug added and to 72% if 2 additional non-statin LDL-lowering drugs were added. In real-world clinical practice physicians need to use combination therapy more often if an LDL-cholesterol goal of <70 mg/dL is to be achieved.

The dilemma that physicians face in clinical practice is that no large cardiovascular outcome study has shown a benefit of combination lipid lowering therapy over statin therapy alone, yet most high-risk patients cannot achieve their recommended LDL-cholesterol goal without combination lipid-lowering therapy. This poses a significant challenge to the practicing clinician since more than one-half of CAD patients will not achieve their LDL-cholesterol goal of <70 mg/dL with statin therapy alone. The AIM-HIGH (Atherothrombosis Intervention in Metabolic Syndrome with Low HDL/High Triglycerides: Impact on Global Health Outcomes) trial [31] randomized 3414 with atherosclerotic cardiovascular disease and low levels of HDL-cholesterol to extended-release niacin, 1500 to 2000 mg a day, or placebo. All patients received simvastatin, 40 to 80 mg a day plus ezetimibe if needed to maintain an LDL-cholesterol of <80 mg/dL. The primary end point was a composite of coronary heart disease death and major cardiovascular events. No clinical benefit was seen with the addition of niacin during a 36-month follow-up period, however, the placebo group was well treated with a mean LDL-cholesterol level of 68 mg/dL by the end of the trial. The ACCORD (Action to Control Cardiovascular Risk in Diabetes) trial [34] randomized 5518 patients with type 2 diabetes to fenofibrate or placebo. All patients were also treated with open label simvastatin. The primary outcome was nonfatal myocardial infarction, stroke, or death from cardiovascular causes and patients were followed for a mean of 4.7 years. By the end of the study, there was no difference in LDL-cholesterol levels between groups and although triglyceride levels were reduced further in the fenofibrate group, the placebo group had normal triglyceride levels by the end of the study. The simvastatin-alone group was well treated with a mean LDL-cholesterol of <80 mg/dL. The combination of fenofibrate and simvastatin did not improve outcomes compared to simvastatin alone. In both the ACCORD and AIM-HIGH trials, the LDL-cholesterol levels in the placebo group were low and these studies do not adequately address the problem of how to treat the patient who is statin intolerant or whose LDL-cholesterol is not a goal despite statin therapy. Ongoing large outcome studies such as the HPS2-THRIVE comparing simvastatin plus niacin and laropiprant to simvastatin alone in CAD patients and IMPROVE-IT comparing the combination of ezitimibe and simvastatin to simvastatin alone in acute coronary syndrome patients will provide important information on the role of combination lipid-lowering therapy in the treatment of CAD patients.

As we await the results of these trials the practicing clinician should use statin therapy as the first choice for LDL-cholesterol-lowering in CAD patients. Other non-statin lipid lowering drugs should be used when the LDL-cholesterol and non-HDL cholesterol are not at goal despite statin therapy or in the statin-intolerant patient. Clinical studies and current guidelines support this recommendation. The SANDS (Stop Atherosclerosis in Native Diabetics Study) trial [35] randomized 499 American Indian men and women over the age of 40 with type 2 diabetes and no prior cardiovascular events to aggressive versus standard treatment for their lipids. The aggressive treatment group had an LDL-cholesterol goal of <70 mg/dL and a non-HDL cholesterol goal of <100 mg/dL while the standard treatment group had an LDL-cholesterol goal of <100 mg/dL and a non-HDL cholesterol goal of <130 mg/dL. Patients were treated with statin therapy and then as needed additional non-statin lipid lowering drugs were added to achieve the specified LDL and non-HDL cholesterol goals. The primary end point was progression of atherosclerosis as measured by common carotid artery intimal medial thickness (IMT). Patients were followed for 3 years. Compared with baseline, IMT regressed in the aggressive group and progressed in the standard group.

The strength of our study is that it represents real clinical practice. However, there are several limitations to our study. Our study was from a single site and only involved patients who were managed by a cardiologist. Our findings may not be generalizable to high-risk patients managed by primary care physicians or to CAD patients in other parts of the country. In addition, we only included patients who had a recent lipid profile in their electronic medical record and since patients without a recent lipid profile are more likely to be undertreated, we may have overestimated the actual number of patients who achieved their LDL-cholesterol goal. However, our findings are similar to other surveys that have reported that few CAD patients achieve optimal LDL-cholesterol levels with statin therapy alone. Furthermore, baseline lipid levels before treatment, specific information as to intolerance to lipid lowering therapy, and why specific patients were not on statin therapy, were not available from the electronic medical record.

5. Conclusions

In conclusion, most CAD patients in real-world clinical practice do not attain an LDL-cholesterol of <70 mg/dL, even among patients on high-potency statins. The number of CAD patients on no statin is high. The combination of statin plus either ezetimibe or niacin is the most effective regimen to achieve an LDL-cholesterol of <70 mg/dL, however, these drug combinations are used infrequently in clinical practice. Statins remain the cornerstone of LDL-cholesterol-lowering in CAD patients, however, physicians need to consider using combination lipid-lowering therapy more often if an LDL-cholesterol goal of <70 mg/dL is to be realized in clinical practice. Finally, there is a need for novel lipid-lowering therapies, especially given the large number of high-risk patients not treated with statin therapy.

References

[1] V. L. Roger, A. S. Go, D. M. Lloyd-Jones et al., "Heart disease and stroke statistics—2011 update: a report from the American Heart Association," *Circulation*, vol. 123, pp. e18–e209, 2011.

[2] S. C. Smith Jr., E. J. Benjamin, R. O. Bonow et al., "AHA/ACCF secondary prevention and risk reduction therapy for patients with coronary and other atherosclerotic vascular disease: 2011 update: a guideline from the American Heart Association and American College of Cardiology Foundation," *Circulation*, vol. 124, pp. 2458–2473, 2011.

[3] Heart Protection Study Collaborative Group, "MRC/BHF heart protection study of cholesterol lowering with simvastatin in 20,536 high-risk individuals: a randomised placebo-controlled trial," *The Lancet*, vol. 360, no. 9326, pp. 7–22, 2002.

[4] C. P. Cannon, E. Braunwald, C. H. McCabe et al., "Intensive versus moderate lipid lowering with statins after acute coronary syndromes," *The New England Journal of Medicine*, vol. 350, no. 15, pp. 1495–1504, 2004.

[5] J. C. LaRosa, S. M. Grundy, D. D. Waters et al., "Intensive lipid lowering with atorvastatin in patients with stable coronary disease," *The New England Journal of Medicine*, vol. 352, no. 14, pp. 1425–1435, 2005.

[6] T. R. Pedersen, O. Faergeman, J. J. P. Kastelein et al., "High-dose atorvastatin versus usual-dose simvastatin for secondary prevention after myocardial infarction: the IDEAL study: a randomized controlled trial," *Journal of the American Medical Association*, vol. 294, no. 19, pp. 2437–2445, 2005.

[7] Study of the Effectiveness of Additional Reductions in Cholesterol and Homocysteine (SEARCH) Collaborative Group, "Intensive lowering of LDL cholesterol with 80 mg versus 20 mg simvastatin daily in 12, 064 survivors of myocardial infarction: a double-blind randomized trial," *The Lancet*, vol. 376, pp. 1658–1669, 2010.

[8] Cholesterol Treatment Trialists' (CTT) Collaboration, "Efficacy and safety of more intensive lowering of LDL cholesterol: a meta-analysis of data from 170,000 participants in 26 randomized trials," *The Lancet*, vol. 376, pp. 1670–1681, 2010.

[9] J. Hsia, J. G. MacFadyen, J. Monyak, and P. M. Ridker, "Cardiovascular event reduction and adverse events among subjects attaining low-density lipoprotein cholesterol <50 mg/dl with rosuvastatin: the JUPITER trial (justification for the use of statins in prevention: an intervention trial evaluating rosuvastatin)," *Journal of the American College of Cardiology*, vol. 57, no. 16, pp. 1666–1675, 2011.

[10] S. M. Grundy, J. I. Cleeman, N. B. Merz et al., "Implications of recent clinical trials for the National Cholesterol Education Program Adult Treatment Panel III guidelines," *Circulation*, vol. 110, no. 2, pp. 227–239, 2004.

[11] L. Mosca, E. J. Benjamin, K. Berra et al., "Effectiveness-based guidelines for the prevention of cardiovascular disease in women-2011 update: a guideline from the American heart association," *Circulation*, vol. 123, pp. 1243–1262.

[12] J. D. Brunzell, M. Davidson, C. D. Furberg et al., "Lipoprotein management in patients with cardiometabolic risk: consensus statement from the American Diabetes Association and the American College of Cardiology Foundation," *Diabetes Care*, vol. 31, no. 4, pp. 811–822, 2008.

[13] A. L. Catapano, J. Chapman, O. Wiklund, and M. R. Taskinen, "The new joint EAS/ESC guidelines for the management of dyslipidaemias," *Atherosclerosis*, vol. 217, no. 1, p. 1, 2011.

[14] D. G. Karalis, R. D. Subramanya, S. E. Hessen, L. Liu, and M. F. Victor, "Achieving optimal lipid goals in patients with coronary artery disease," *American Journal of Cardiology*, vol. 107, no. 6, pp. 886–890, 2011.

[15] H. Ghandehari, S. Kamal-Bahl, and N. D. Wong, "Prevalence and extent of dyslipidemia and recommended lipid levels in US adults with and without cardiovascular comorbidities: the National Health and Nutrition Examination Survey 2003-2004," *American Heart Journal*, vol. 156, no. 1, pp. 112–119, 2008.

[16] M. H. Davidson, K. C. Maki, T. A. Pearson et al., "Results of the National Cholesterol Education (NCEP) program evaluation project utilizing novel T-technology (NEPTUNE) II survey and implications for treatment under the recent NCEP writing group recommendations," *American Journal of Cardiology*, vol. 96, no. 4, pp. 556–563, 2005.

[17] D. D. Waters, C. Brotons, C. W. Chiang et al., "Lipid treatment assessment project 2: a multinational survey to evaluate the proportion of patients achieving low-density lipoprotein cholesterol goals," *Circulation*, vol. 120, no. 1, pp. 28–34, 2009.

[18] L. T. Meade, "Barriers to achieving LDL cholesterol goals," *U.S. Pharmacist*, vol. 32, no. 3, pp. 66–71, 2007.

[19] A. B. Kauffman, K. L. Olson, M. L. Youngblood, E. B. Zadvorny, T. Delate, and J. A. Merenich, "Attainment of low-density lipoprotein cholesterol goals in coronary artery disease," *Journal of Clinical Lipidology*, vol. 4, no. 3, pp. 173–180, 2010.

[20] L. Mosca, N. B. Merz, R. S. Blumenthal et al., "Opportunity for intervention to achieve American Heart Association guidelines for optimal lipid levels in high-risk women in a managed care setting," *Circulation*, vol. 111, no. 4, pp. 488–493, 2005.

[21] A. G. Kennedy, C. D. MacLean, B. Littenberg, P. A. Ades, and R. G. Pinckney, "The challenge of achieving national cholesterol in patients with diabetes," *Diabetes Care*, vol. 28, no. 5, pp. 1029–1034, 2005.

[22] T. A. Stacy and A. Egger, "Results of retrospective chart review to determine improvement in lipid goal attainment in patients treated by high-volume prescribers of lipid-modifying drugs," *Journal of Managed Care Pharmacy*, vol. 12, no. 9, pp. 745–751, 2006.

[23] A. T. Yan, R. T. Yan, M. Tan et al., "Contemporary management of dyslipidemia in high-risk patients: targets still not met," *American Journal of Medicine*, vol. 119, no. 8, pp. 676–683, 2006.

[24] L. Laforest, P. Moulin, T. Souchet et al., "Correlates of LDL-cholesterol goal attainment in patients under lipid lowering therapy," *Atherosclerosis*, vol. 199, no. 2, pp. 368–377, 2008.

[25] E. Stein, S. Stender, P. Mata et al., "Achieving lipoprotein goals in patients at high risk with severe hypercholesterolemia: efficacy and safety of ezetimibe co-administered with atorvastatin," *American Heart Journal*, vol. 148, no. 3, pp. 447–455, 2004.

[26] M. H. Davidson, T. McGarry, R. Bettis et al., "Ezetimibe coadministered with simvastatin in patients with primary hypercholesterolemia," *Journal of the American College of Cardiology*, vol. 40, no. 12, pp. 2125–2134, 2002.

[27] H. S. Friedman, S. Rajagopalan, J. P. Barnes, and H. Roseman, "Combination therapy with Ezetimibe/Simvastatin versus Statin Monotherapy for low-density lipoprotein cholesterol reduction and goal attainment in a real-world clinical setting," *Clinical Therapeutics*, vol. 33, no. 2, pp. 212–224, 2011.

[28] The SHARP Investigators, "The effects of lowering LDL cholesterol with simvastatin plus ezetimibe in patients with chronic kidney disease (study of Heart and Renal Protection): a randomized placebo-controlled trial," *The Lancet*, vol. 377, pp. 2181–2192, 2011.

[29] A. J. Taylor, T. C. Villines, E. J. Stanek et al., "Extended-release niacin or ezetimibe and carotid intima-media thickness," *The New England Journal of Medicine*, vol. 361, no. 22, pp. 2113–2122, 2009.

[30] C. M. Ballantyne, M. H. Davidson, J. McKenney, L. H. Keller, D. R. Bajorunas, and R. H. Karas, "Comparison of the safety and efficacy of a combination tablet of niacin extended release and Simvastatin versus Simvastatin monotherapy in patients with increased Non-HDL cholesterol (from the SEACOAST I study)," *American Journal of Cardiology*, vol. 101, no. 10, pp. 1428–1436, 2008.

[31] The AIM-HIGH Investigators, "Niacin in patients with low HDL cholesterol levels receiving intensive statin therapy," *The New England Journal of Medicine*, vol. 365, pp. 2255–2267, 2011.

[32] G. A. Nichols and C. E. Koro, "Does statin therapy initiation increase the risk for myopathy? An observational study of 32,225 diabetic and nondiabetic patients," *Clinical Therapeutics*, vol. 29, no. 8, pp. 1761–1770, 2007.

[33] J. M. Foody, S. G. Sajjan, X. H. Hu et al., "Loss of early gains in low-density lipoprotein cholesterol goal attainment among high-risk patients," *Journal of Clinical Lipidology*, vol. 4, no. 2, pp. 126–132, 2010.

[34] The ACCORD Study Group, "Effects of combination lipid therapy in type 2 diabetes mellitus," *The New England Journal of Medicine*, vol. 362, pp. 1563–1574, 2010.

[35] B. V. Howard, M. J. Roman, R. B. Devereux et al., "Effect of lower targets for blood pressure and LDL cholesterol on atherosclerosis in diabetes: the SANDS randomized trial," *Journal of the American Medical Association*, vol. 299, no. 14, pp. 1678–1689, 2008.

22

Determinants of Childhood Obesity in Representative Sample of Children in North East of Iran

Fereshteh Baygi,[1] Ahmad Reza Dorosty,[2] Roya Kelishadi,[3] Mostafa Qorbani,[1,4] Hamid Asayesh,[5] Morteza Mansourian,[6] and Kamal Mirkarimi[7]

[1] *Endocrinology and Metabolism Research Center, Tehran University of Medical Sciences, Tehran 1411413137, Iran*
[2] *Department of Nutrition and Biochemistry, Tehran University of Medical Sciences, Tehran, Iran*
[3] *Pediatrics Department, Faculty of Medicine and Child Growth and Development Research Center, Isfahan University of Medical Sciences, Isfahan, Iran*
[4] *Department of Epidemiology and Biostatistics, Tehran University of Medical Sciences, Tehran 1411413137, Iran*
[5] *Faculty of Paramedical, Qom University of Medical Sciences, Qom, Iran*
[6] *Department of Health Education and Promotion, Tehran University of Medical Sciences, Tehran, Iran*
[7] *Department of Health Education and Promotion, Golestan University of Medical Sciences, Gorgan, Iran*

Correspondence should be addressed to Mostafa Qorbani, mqorbani1379@yahoo.com

Academic Editor: Khosrow Adeli

Childhood obesity has become, a global public health problem, and epidemiological studies are important to identify its determinants in different populations. This study aimed to investigate factors associated with obesity in a representative sample of children in Neishabour, Iran. This study was conducted among 1500 randomly selected 6–12-year-old students from urban areas of Neishabour, northeast of Iran. Then, through a case-control study, 114 obese (BMI $\geq$ 95th percentile of Iranian reference) children were selected as the case group and were compared with 102 controls (15th $\leq$ BMI $<$ 85th percentile). Factors suggested to be associated with weight status were investigated, for example, parental obesity, child physical activity levels, socio-economic status (SES), and so forth. The analysis was conducted using univariate and multivariate logistic regression (MLR) in SPSS version 16. In univariate logistic regression model, birth weight, birth order, family extension, TV watching, sleep duration, physical activity, parents' job, parents' education, parental obesity history, and SES were significantly associated with children's obesity. After MLR analysis, physical activity and parental obesity history remained statistically significant in the model. Our findings showed that physical activity and parental obesity history are the most important determinants for childhood obesity in our population. This finding should be considered in implementation of preventive interventions.

1. Introduction

Obesity levels are increasing rapidly in children and youngsters of developed and developing countries [1, 2]. In 1998, the World Health Organization project monitoring of cardiovascular diseases (MONICA) showed that Iran is one of the seven countries with the highest prevalence of childhood obesity [3]. Overweight and obesity among Iranian children are becoming a major public health problem [4]. It is predicted that, by 2020, more than 60% of diseases and their related mortality and morbidity in the developing countries will be due to noncommunicable diseases, for many of which obesity is a potential risk factor [5].

Obesity is a multifactorial consequence. In addition to genetic, metabolic, socioeconomic, and cultural factors, life style habits as unhealthy diet, low physical activity levels, weight and order of birth and other factors like history of breast feeding, as well as the age and type of complementary food are among factors affecting obesity [6]. Therefore, this study was designed to identify probable factors that might affect obesity in a group of Iranian children.

2. Materials and Methods

2.1. Study Design. In this study, 1500 6–12-year-old students were selected via two-stage sampling method from urban areas of Neishabour. Neishabour is a city in the Razavi Khorasan province in northeastern Iran and had a population of 205972 people. On the first stage, 60 primary schools, both public and private, were chosen, and, on the second stage, in each cluster, school children were selected randomly from the class attendance register. It was approved by the ethics committee of Tehran University of Medical Sciences (TUMS). Written informed consent was obtained from parents and oral assent from students.

Then, through a case-control study, 14 obese (body mass index (BMI) ≥ 95th percentile of Iranian reference) children were selected as the case group, and the first nonobese student (15th ≤ BMI < 85th percentile) examined exactly after each obese student, and who was matched by age and sex, was selected as the control. Overall, 102 students were included in the control group.

2.2. Anthropometric Profile. We used the Iranian reference for BMI percentiles [7]. Physical examination was conducted by a trained team of health professionals using calibrated instruments. Height was measured by a stadiometer (Seca, Germany) in a standing position with bare feet (precision 0.5 cm), and body weight was determined with subjects wearing light clothes and no shoes or socks, using an electronic balance. BMI was calculated as weight (kg) divided by height squared (m^2).

2.3. Data Collection. Data were collected by questionnaire via interview with mothers. Interviews were performed by trained health professionals. The questionnaire included mother-reported information about her child regarding the age, sex, birth weight, birth order, number of family household members, duration of breast feeding, age onset of complementary food, TV watching, playing electronic devices, sleep duration, father age, mother age, mother weight, economic status, and parental obesity history. The economic status of family was assessed by having some equipment such as color TV, refrigerators, washing machine, video, computer, video CD, and accessibility to car and private home. In data analysis, economic status was defined as low, moderate, and good based on an average score 3, 4–6, and more than 7, respectively. Physical activity score was evaluated using the modified Beacke et al. questionnaire that was asked from the pupils [8].

2.4. Statistical Analysis. Data were analyzed using the SPSS software version 16.0 (SPSS Inc., Chicago, IL, USA). Quantitative variables are expressed as mean ± standard deviation (SD) and categorical data as percentage. We computed the crude odds ratio (OR) by using logistic regression test to establish the degree of association between various risk factors and childhood obesity. Multiple logistic regression (MLR) model was fitted to data to adjust for the presence of confounding factors. All variables with P value < 0.1 in the univariate analysis were presented to the multiple model by using stepwise method. The results of logistic regression analysis are presented by OR and 95% confidence interval. A P value of less than 0.05 was considered as statistically significant.

3. Results

3.1. Demographic Characteristics. Overall, 216 children consisting of 114 obese and 102 nonobese students were assessed. The mean (SD) of age, weight, height, and BMI of the students were 8.6 ± 1.5 years, 33.4 ± 9.9 kg, 132.3 ± 9.5 cm, and 18.7 ± 3.8 kg/m^2, respectively.

3.2. Determinant Factors. The crude OR_S (univariate analysis) for birth weight, birth order, family extension, duration of breast feeding, age onset of complementary food, TV watching, playing electronic devices, sleep duration, physical activity score, father age, mother age, mother BMI as quantitative variables are shown in Table 1. The estimated crude ORs for birth weight, birth order, family extension, TV watching, playing electronic devices, sleep duration, physical activity score, father age, mother age, and mother BMI were statistically significant.

Associations between qualitative variables and obesity determined by univariate logistic regression model are shown in Table 2. The estimated crude ORs for father job, father education, mother job, mother education, economic status, and parental obesity history were statistically significant. After MLR analysis, at final step, physical activity and parental obesity history remained significant in the model (Table 3).

4. Discussion

This study has demonstrated that parental obesity history and physical activity were the strongest determinants of childhood obesity. These findings are in agreement with some investigations, showing that low physical activity and parental obesity to be the predictors of youngsters obesity [9–11].

The result of Veugelers and Fitzgerald's study showed that, as in other studies, normal-weight children were more physically active and engaged less in sedentary activities [12].

In our study, there was no significant association between mothers' BMI and children obesity, but Sekine and his collogues found that mother's obesity was associated with children's BMI. In addition to genetic susceptibility, this may reflect environmental factors influencing children's body composition because children's food habits and preferences are usually shaped more by mothers than fathers [11].

The controversy between our result and other studies may be because of some factors related to family composition that we did not ask in our study and it may confound our conclusion. Our findings are also consistent with a previous study, which showed that a positive family history of being overweight is one of the most important indicators of the genetic risk for obesity and being overweight [13].

TABLE 1: Association between quantitative variables and obesity in univariate logistic regression model.

Variables	Cases (n = 114) (mean ± SD)	Control (n = 102) (mean ± SD)	Crude OR	95% CI
Birth weight (gr)	3900. 90 ± 846.20	2837.10 ± 671.30	1.00	1.00–1.00
Birth order (n)	1.90 ± 1.20	5.09 ± 13.05	0.62	0.50–0.76
Family extension (n)	4.40 ± 0.97	5.10 ± 1.60	0.63	0.49–0.80
Duration of breast feeding (month)	22.02 ± 9.80	23.76 ± 14.33	0.99	0.97–1.11
Age-onset of complementary food (month)	8.77 ± 17.56	9.63 ± 15.63	1.00	0.98–1.01
TV watching, playing electronic devices (hour)	5.42 ± 1.99	2.77 ± 1.26	2.33	1.87–2.90
Sleep duration (hour)	10.40 ± 0.91	9.76 ± 0.89	2.24	1.60–3.15
Physical activity (score)	2.30 ± 0.37	3.02 ± 0.39	0.01	0.01–0.04
Father age (year)	39.57 ± 5.37	41.71 ± 6.27	0.94	0.90–0.99
Mother age (year)	35.51 ± 5.84	37.50 ± 6.88	0.95	0.91–0.99
Mother BMI (kg/m^2)	26.98 ± 3.99	22.77 ± 3.81	1.40	1.25–1.55

TABLE 2: Association between qualitative variables and obesity in univariate logistic regression model.

Variables	Cases (n = 114) N (%)	Control (n = 102) N (%)	Crude OR	95% CI
Father job				
Jobless	1 (0.90)	4 (4.40)	Ref	
Worker	17 (15.00)	31 (31.60)	2.19	0.23–21.23
Employee	34 (30.10)	40 (40.80)	3.40	0.36–31.89
Other	61 (54.00)	23 (23.50)	10.60	1.13–99.96
Father education				
Illiterate and primary school	23 (20.40)	36 (36.70)	Ref	
Guidance school	16 (14.20)	29 (29.60)	0.86	0.39–1.92
Diploma	24 (21.20)	21 (21.40)	1.78	0.816–3.92
University degrees	50 (44.20)	12 (12.20)	6.52	2.87–14.79
Mother job				
Housewife	55 (48.20)	80 (78.40)	Ref	
Employee	59 (51.80)	22 (21.60)	3.90	2.14–7.09
Mother education				
Illiterate and primary school	35 (30.70)	49 (48.00)	Ref	
Guidance school	12 (10.50)	33 (32.40)	0.51	0.23–1.12
Diploma	12 (10.50)	14 (13.70)	1.20	0.50–2.90
University degrees	55 (48.20)	6 (5.90)	12.80	4.97–33.10
Economic status				
Weak	18 (15.80)	72 (63.20)	Ref	
Moderate	72 (63.20)	57 (55.90)	3.01	1.57–5.78
Good	24 (21.10)	2 (2.00)	28.66	6.12–134.20
Family history of obesity				
Without obesity history	7 (6.10)	76 (74.50)	Ref	
Father side obesity history	24 (21.10)	11 (10.80)	23.68	8.26–67.89
Mother side obesity history	5 (4.40)	13 (12.70)	4.17	1.15–15.16
Both of them	78 (68.40)	2 (2.00)	423.42	85.24–2010.00

We did not document any relationship between SES and obesity, but, in some other studies, investigators observed a gradient whereby children by low SES were more likely to be overweight or obese [12, 14]. This contradiction between our study and others may be related to the homogenous SES of families studied and also because differences in the SES indicators were used. For instance, we asked some questions about having some equipment at home for assessing family income, but other researchers considered direct family income for evaluating economic status [15].

In present study, we did not find any association between the sleep duration and obesity. Some studies demonstrated

Table 3: Association between independent variables and obesity in multiple logistic regression model (last step).

Variables	Adjusted OR	*95% CI
Physical activity (score)	0.23	0.12-0.43
Family history of obesity		
Without obesity history	Ref	
Father side obesity history	47.41	9.87-227.60
Mother side obesity history	2.36	0.39-14.32
Both of them	547.58	45.26-6062.00

*Adjusted for birth weight, birth order, family extension, TV watching, playing electronic devices, sleep duration, physical activity score, father age, mother age, mother BMI, father job, father education, mother job, mother education, economic status, and parental obesity history.

an inverse linear relationship between sleep duration and both mean BMI and obesity [16–18]. Researchers believe that there is association between the secretion of growth hormone and sleeping early at night. Going to sleep early at night increases the secretion of the growth hormone, which activates lipolysis in fat tissues, and obviously sleeping late increases the rate of obesity [19].

But, in our study, no significant association was observed between sleep duration at night and obesity. Maybe in current study, individuals of the case group went to bed later than the controls, and, in order to compensate for the lack of sleep, they slept more during the day instead of being more physically active or exercising.

Our study revealed no significant association between obesity and birth order. It may be related to increasing the knowledge of parents and paying more attention to the nutrition and health care of their children in both case and control groups.

In a meta-analysis carried out by Harder, the duration of breastfeeding was inversely and linearly associated with the risk of overweight. The risk of overweight was reduced by 4 percent for each month of breastfeeding [20]. Investigators think the protective effect of breast milk against obesity is attributed to its special components. Long-chain polyunsaturated fatty acid in breast milk may reduce the risk of obesity in the adulthood. High concentration of these fatty acids in the brain inhibits the production of cytokines and increases insulin receptors in several tissues which improves insulin, and other neurotransmitter functions. The dietary intake is regulated by complex interactions of some neurotransmitters, insulin and its receptors in the brain indicate the necessity of taking these fatty acids in the first year of life [20]. But, in our study, we find no association between obesity and duration of breast feeding and age of beginning complementary foods.

5. Limitation

This study had some limitations, which may have influenced the findings. First, the SES was measured indirectly by asking some relevant questions. Second, family composition was not assessed in this study, and it may be a confounder for some parts of our results. Despite these limitations, this study provides some data on childhood obesity risk factors.

6. Conclusion

Finally, we suggested that a high priority has been given to research strategies to prevent the development of childhood obesity. Also, based on our findings, more physical education classes and providing healthy places for more extracurricular physical activity are strongly recommended, and family education for preventive public health actions should be targeted.

Acknowledgments

The collaboration of the authorities of the Office for Education managers, manager's assistants, teachers and schoolchildren of the primary schools in Neishabour is sincerely appreciated. The study was conducted with the financial support of the School of Public Health, Tehran University of Medical Sciences.

References

[1] A. Y. Li, B. Kaye, C. Rosemary, K. Liang, and M. Stephen, "Parental obesity as a predictor of childhood overweight/obesity in Australian migrant children," *Obesity Research & Clinical Practice*, vol. 2, no. 3, pp. 179–187, 2008.

[2] R. S. Strauss and J. Knight, "Influence of the home environment on the development of obesity in children," *Pediatrics*, vol. 103, no. 6, p. e85, 1999.

[3] R. Kelishadi, M. H. Pour, N. Sarraf-Zadegan et al., "Obesity and associated modifiable environmental factors in Iranian adolescents: Isfahan healthy heart program—heart health promotion from childhood," *Pediatrics International*, vol. 45, no. 4, pp. 435–442, 2003.

[4] A. R. Dorosty, F. Siassi, and J. J. Reilly, "Obesity in Iranian children," *Archives of Disease in Childhood*, vol. 87, no. 5, pp. 388–391, 2002.

[5] B. Caballero, "Obesity in developing countries: biological and ecological factors," *Journal of Nutrition*, vol. 131, pp. 866S–870S, 2001.

[6] P. W. Speiser, M. C. J. Rudolf, H. Anhalt et al., "Consensus statement: childhood obesity," *The Journal of Clinical Endocrinology & Metabolism*, vol. 90, no. 3, pp. 1871–1887, 2005.

[7] M. Hosseini, R. G. Carpenter, K. Mohammad, and M. E. Jones, "Standardized percentile curves of body mass index of Iranian children compared to the US population reference," *International Journal of Obesity and Related Metabolic Disorders*, vol. 23, no. 8, pp. 783–786, 1999.

[8] J. A. Baecke, J. Burema, and J. E. Frijters, "A short questionnaire for the measurement of habitual physical activity in epidemiological studies," *American Journal of Clinical Nutrition*, vol. 36, no. 5, pp. 936–942, 1982.

[9] L. L. Moore, A. S. Di Gao, M. L. Bradlee et al., "Does early physical activity predict body fat change throughout childhood?" *Preventive Medicine*, vol. 37, no. 1, pp. 10–17, 2003.

[10] S. Danielzik, K. Langnäse, M. Mast, C. Spethmann, and M. J. Müller, "Impact of parental BMI on the manifestation

of overweight 5-7 year old children," *European Journal of Nutrition*, vol. 41, no. 3, pp. 132–138, 2002.

[11] M. Sekine, T. Yamagami, S. Hamanishi et al., "Parental obesity, lifestyle factors and obesity in preschool children: results of the toyama birth cohort study," *Journal of Epidemiology*, vol. 12, no. 1, pp. 33–39, 2002.

[12] P. J. Veugelers and A. L. Fitzgerald, "Prevalence of and risk factors for childhood overweight and obesity," *Canadian Medical Association Journal*, vol. 173, no. 6, pp. 607–613, 2005.

[13] R. V. Kries, K. Berthold, T. Sauerwaldet et al., "Breast feeding and obesity: cross sectional study," *British Medical Journal*, vol. 319, pp. 147–150, 1999.

[14] C. Power, H. Graham, P. Dueet et al., "The contribution of childhood and adult socioeconomic position to adult obesity and smoking behavior: an international comparison," *International Journal of Epidemiology*, vol. 34, no. 2, pp. 335–344, 2005.

[15] Y. Wang, "Cross-national comparison of childhood obesity: the epidemic and the relationship between obesity and socioeconomic status," *International Journal of Epidemiology*, vol. 30, no. 5, pp. 1129–1136, 2001.

[16] S. Park, "Association between short sleep duration and obesity among South Korean adolescents," *Western Journal of Nursing Research*, vol. 33, no. 2, pp. 207–223, 2011.

[17] C. N. Hart and E. Jelalian, "Shortened sleep duration is associated with pediatric overweight," *Behavioral Sleep Medicine*, vol. 6, no. 4, pp. 251–267, 2008.

[18] N. S. Marshall, N. Glozier, and R. R. Grunstein, "Is sleep duration related to obesity? A critical review of the epidemiological evidence," *Sleep Medicine Reviews*, vol. 12, no. 4, pp. 289–298, 2008.

[19] N. K. Gupta, W. H. Mueller, W. W. Chan, and J. C. Meininger, "Is obesity associated with poor sleep quality in adolescents?" *American Journal of Human Biology*, vol. 14, no. 6, pp. 762–768, 2002.

[20] U. N. Das, "Is obesity an inflammatory condition?" *Nutrition*, vol. 17, no. 11-12, pp. 953–956, 2001.

23

HDL, Atherosclerosis, and Emerging Therapies

Anouar Hafiane[1] and Jacques Genest[2]

[1] *McGill University, Montreal, QC, Canada H3A 1A1*
[2] *Faculty of Medicine, Center for Innovative Medicine, McGill University Health Center, Royal Victoria Hospital, McGill University, 687 Pine Avenue West, Montreal, QC, Canada H3A 1A1*

Correspondence should be addressed to Jacques Genest; jacques.genest@mcgill.ca

Academic Editor: Francisco Blanco-Vaca

This review aims to provide an overview on the properties of high-density lipoproteins (HDLs) and their cardioprotective effects. Emergent HDL therapies will be presented in the context of the current understanding of HDL function, metabolism, and protective antiatherosclerotic properties. The epidemiological association between levels of HDL-C or its major apolipoprotein (apoA-I) is strong, graded, and coherent across populations. HDL particles mediate cellular cholesterol efflux, have antioxidant properties, and modulate vascular inflammation and vasomotor function and thrombosis. A link of causality has been cast into doubt with Mendelian randomization data suggesting that genes causing HDL-C deficiency are not associated with increased cardiovascular risk, nor are genes associated with increased HDL-C, with a protective effect. Despite encouraging data from small studies, drugs that increase HDL-C levels have not shown an effect on major cardiovascular end-points in large-scale clinical trials. It is likely that the cholesterol mass within HDL particles is a poor biomarker of therapeutic efficacy. In the present review, we will focus on novel therapeutic avenues and potential biomarkers of HDL function. A better understanding of HDL antiatherogenic functions including reverse cholesterol transport, vascular protective and antioxidation effects will allow novel insight on novel, emergent therapies for cardiovascular prevention.

1. Introduction

An increasing body of literature emphasizes the concept that HDL functionality, rather than the absolute cholesterol mass (HDL-C), may be a more accurate indicator for risk of developing atherosclerosis [1]. This hypothesis has led to investigation of HDL as both a biomarker for cardiovascular risk and a therapeutic target to be functionally modulated [2]. Epidemiological studies consistently demonstrate that low plasma level of HDL-C is associated with increased risk of CVD, but this epidemiological association has not translated into evidence that raising HDL-C prevents CVD. Atherosclerosis remains the leading cause of death in developed countries and is a major health concern worldwide. While LDL cholesterol (LDL-C) is clearly established as the major lipoprotein risk factor [3], the residual risk in large-scale clinical trials raises concern that other lipoprotein fractions may be causal in this residual risk. Increasingly, questions have been raised around the hypothesis that raising HDL-C pharmacologically is necessary beneficial. In this regard, after the recent failure of the drugs torcetrapib, dalcetrapib, and niacin [4, 5] that raise HDL-C, attention is focusing on specific HDL subfractions and on biomarkers of HDL function (reflecting its pleiotropic effects) as potential therapeutic targets for cardiovascular protection [6–8]. Such studies have reinforced the need for validated assays of HDL function rather than static measurement of HDL-C. A variety of HDL/apoA-I-based therapies are currently under investigation. This review summarizes the biology of HDL and the importance of reverse cholesterol transport process in lipid-modifying therapy and discusses the novel therapeutic agents to raise HDL.

2. Definition: HDL

HDL is the smallest and densest of plasma lipoproteins. HDL isolated by ultracentrifugation is defined as the lipoprotein with density in the range 1.063–1.21 g/mL. Conventional HDL nomenclatures are based on physical properties such as density [9] or composition [10]. HDL is constituted by a large number of heterogeneous particles differing in size, charge, shape, lipid composition (glycerophospholipids, triglycerides, sphingolipids, cholesterol, and cholesteryl esters), and physiological functions [11].Proteins constitute approximately 50% of HDL protein mass with apoA-I representing approximately 65–70%, with another 12% to 15% being apoA-II. Recent proteomic studies have identified more than 60 different proteins on HDL adding to the biological diversity of this class of lipoproteins [12]. HDL is also highly heterogeneous with regard to its lipidome [7]. Thus, the term HDL applies to a large and heterogeneous group of small (5–70 nm) particles with diverse lipids and proteins [12, 13] that may differ in function [11]. Static mass-based measurement of HDL-C may be an imperfect metric of HDL functionality, particularly in the setting of therapeutic interventions. Proposed definitions of HDL rely on diverse analytical techniques; a unified definition is emerging [7], although consensus is not yet reached [8]. Rosenson et al. [7] proposed a nomenclature based on particle size and density. Other argue that this classification is incomplete and further characterization should be made for HDL of lower density, larger size, and protein components (especially apo E) which may have better discriminant power in the clinical setting [8]. Despite this, the relevance of HDL subfractions to CVD remains ambiguous and lacks standardization and validation [11, 14]. There is a need to refine definitions of HDL to encompass the functional qualities of HDL. It is hoped that the adoption of a uniform nomenclature system for HDL subfractions that integrates several methods will enhance our ability to assess the clinical effects of different compounds that modulate HDL metabolism, function, and structure, and in turn, allow improved cardiovascular risk prediction.

3. Epidemiology of HDL and CVD

Epidemiological studies have shown an inverse relationship between HDL-C levels and CVD risk [15–17]. This negative association is strong, graded, and coherent across population studied and has led to the development of the "HDL-C hypothesis," which proposes that pharmacological intervention to raise HDL-C will reduce cardiovascular risk. However, there is controversial data suggesting that certain patients at high cardiovascular risk have "dysfunctional" HDL despite normal HDL-C levels [16]. Importantly, the association of HDL-C with CVD risk is further confounded by the inverse association of HDL-C with apo B and LDL particles concentrations. Many other variables such as triglycerides, insulin resistance, obesity, and C-reactive protein may bias this association. Despite the data generated from the Emerging Risk Factor Collaboration [17], it may be impossible to take all these factors into account. Indeed in the Multi-Ethnic Study of Atherosclerosis (MESA) in 5,598 volunteer without baseline CHD, Mackey et al. showed that the association of HDL-C and carotid disease was considerably attenuated when taking into account atherogenic lipoproteins [18].

4. Clinical Trials

Fibric acid derivatives (fibrates) are peroxisome proliferator-activated receptor alpha (PPARα) agonists and their major role is to increase lipoprotein lipase; they raise HDL-C modestly, in the range of 10–15%. While early reports of fibrates have shown encouraging results in terms of cardiovascular outcomes,these were performed before the statin era and the results are difficult to interpret in light of the effects of fibrates on LDL-C. Recent studies using fenofibrate in diabetic patients failed to show an effect on cardiovascular outcomes when LDL-C was controlled with statin therapy [19]. A recent meta-analysis of fibrate trials reveals that while fibrates may decrease the risk of nonfatal cardiovascular events and on microvascular disease, their overall effect on cardiovascular mortality is neutral [20]. Statins are widely acknowledged as first-line drugs for the treatment of dyslipidemias and CVD prevention; however, statins may not address residual risk [21]. Significant residual cardiovascular risk remains even after intensive statin therapy and lowering LDL-C to <70 mg/dL [22]. Meta-analysis studies show that reduction of LDL cholesterol by 1 mmol/L reduces risk by about approximately 20–25% and that intensive LDL-C lowering with statins lowers risk by up to 33% [3]. Despite this, HDL-C levels continue to predict risk in statin-treated patients [23, 24]. This has been challenged in clinical trials where LDL-C has reached a very low level [25, 26]. Attempts to decrease cardiovascular risk in statin-treated patients with the CETP inhibitor torcetrapib have failed, despite an increase in HDL-C by 72% [25]. In the ILLUMINATE study [25] adverse events caused by torcetrapib were likely to represent off-target effects of the drug but raised question about the value of raising HDL-C. The dal-OUTCOMES trial using dalcetrapib raised HDL-C by 31 to 40% [27] but had no effects on cardiovascular events. Niacin, used at pharmacological doses (up to 2 gm/day), led to a neutrality of results in terms of cardiovascular outcomes in the AIM-HIGM [4]. The recent failure of the large (>25,000 subjects) HPS2-THRIVE trial with niacin [28] raised questions about the benefits of this therapeutic strategy to raise HDL. The clinical equipoise remains. The failure of torcetrapib and dalcetrapib may be explained by off-target adverse effects and weak CETP inhibition, respectively. AIM-HIGH has been criticized for having a relatively small sample size [29].

5. HDL Genetics

Genes that modulate HDL-C have been characterized by conventional family studies and by genome-wide association studies. Yet not all genetic forms of very low HDL-C and apoA-I are necessarily associated with increased risk of CVD. Tangier disease, in which HDL-C and apoA-I concentrations are virtually undetectable, is not associated with a marked increase of CVD that might be expected from such a dramatic phenotype [1]. Recent Mendelian randomization studies have shown that patients with mutations in the ABCA1 gene (Tangier disease) are not at increased cardiovascular risk in the Copenhagen Heart Study [30] and many mutations within apo AI that cause a very low HDL-C and apo AI are not associated with premature CVD. Thus, genes causing HDL-C deficiency are not necessarily associated with increased cardiovascular risk. Voight et al. recently reported that genes that are associated with an increase in HDL-C (endothelial lipase and CETP) are not associated with decreased cardiovascular risk [31]. Thus, Mendelian randomization experiments have cast into doubt the link of causality between HDL-C and risk of CVD.

6. HDL Functions

6.1. Reverse Cholesterol Transport (RCT). The concept of RCT was first proposed by Glomset [32] in 1968. This concept represents the most widely accepted mechanism underlying the HDL-C hypothesis. Free cholesterol (FC) is toxic to cells. In the endoplasmic reticulum, cholesterol may initiate the unfolded protein response, leading to cell apoptosis [33]. Cellular cholesterol homeostasis is exquisitely maintained and the control of *de novo* synthesis and LDL-receptor-mediated endocytosis remains critical for this process. Cellular cholesterol can also be modulated by efflux. This is mediated via different pathways, which are transporter-independent or depend on the receptor/transporter scavenger receptor class B type I (SR-BI), ATP-binding cassette receptors ABCA1 and ABCG1 (Table 1) (Figures 1 and 2). A measure of HDL-mediated cellular cholesterol efflux from macrophages may provide a novel way to the assessment of CVD risk. It has been shown that cholesterol efflux from macrophages is strongly associated with atherosclerosis and provides better CVD prediction than plasma HDL-C levels [34]. The presence of specific subparticles, especially pre-β HDL, may provide a biomarker for CVD prevention and represent a potential therapeutic target. Thus, identifying biomarkers of HDL quality and function may provide a better discriminant for CVD than HDL-C mass. In turn, these biomarkers can be used to gauge the effects of therapies and be correlated with outcomes. Mechanisms of cholesterol efflux are discussed below.

6.2. Aqueous Diffusion. Aqueous diffusion involves a simple diffusion process in which FC molecules desorb from the plasma membrane, move through the extracellular aqueous space, and are then rapidly incorporated into the surface of HDL particles by gradient diffusion (Figure 2). Our data indicates that approximately 1-2% of cellular cholesterol efflux occurs via this pathway [35]. Aqueous diffusion is the rate limiting step in desorption of FC from the cell membrane into surrounding aqueous phase. This rate is increased by higher phospholipid unsaturation and decreased by higher membrane sphingomyelin content [36] and dependent on the structure and particle size of acceptor particle. Rothblat and Phillips [37] reported recently that larger HDL2 and smaller HDL3 particles are equally effective as acceptors in this efflux mechanism, suggesting that in this pathway the efflux process is not affected by alteration in HDL particle size. The importance of this pathway in maintaining cellular cholesterol homeostasis and preventing atherosclerosis is not clear. A pathway analysis on this protocol using previously published techniques indicated that in mouse peritoneal macrophages 34% of the total efflux was mediated by ABCA1, 20% by SRB1, and 46% by ABCG1 and/or, aqueous diffusion, or undiscovered pathways [38].

6.3. ABCA1. ABCA1 mediates the rate limiting step in HDL biogenesis, namely, the transfer of cellular cholesterol and phospholipids onto lipid-poor apolipoprotein acceptor to form nascent HDL particles. In turn, these particles undergo further lipidation via ABCG1 [39]. ABCA1 mediated cellular cholesterol movement is unidirectional, resulting in net efflux (Figure 2). In this pathway lipid-free apoA-I is the primary acceptor of cholesterol. HDL lipidation of apoA-I by ABCA1 is a complex process and may involve more than a direct interaction with this transporter. The nature of the molecular interactions between apoA-I and ABCA1 continues to generate controversy, and models suggesting a direct protein-protein interaction or indirect association have been proposed. Experimental data supports the concept that apoA-I directly binds to ABCA1 in the process of HDL formation, as shown via cross linking experiments within a distance of $\leq$3 Å [40]. Indeed, cholesterol export function of ABCA1 occurs by a cascade of events involving direct binding of apoA-I to ABCA1, activation of signaling pathways, and solubilization of cholesterol and phospholipids rich membrane domains formed by ABCA1 [41]. This interaction is localized on the cell surface [42] and results in the formation of nascent HDL particles that exhibit size (7–12 nm) and lipid composition heterogeneity, confirming that apoA-I exhibits considerable flexibility and conformational adaptability to its lipid constituents [42, 43]. ApoA-I stabilizes ABCA1 and prevents calpain-mediated degradation [44]. Thus, apoA-I increases the amount of ABCA1 on the plasma membrane and promotes cholesterol transport from intracellular compartments to the plasma membrane and ABCA1 also facilitates mobilization of cholesterol from late endocytic compartment to the cell plasma membrane [45]; the contribution to net efflux via this mechanism is controversial [46]. Many tissues express ABCA1; the liver and intestine are the major organs contributing to plasma HDL-C levels [47, 48]. Other tissues, such as adipocytes have been shown to be important site for HDL formation and lipidation [49]. Recently, an intronic microRNA, located within the SREBF2 gene, suppresses expression of the cholesterol transporter ABCA1 and lowers HDL levels in mouse and human cells [50]. Conversely, mechanisms that inhibit miR-33 increase ABCA1 and circulating HDL levels, suggesting that antagonism of miR-33 may be atheroprotective. Recently, treatment with an antisense oligonucleotide in mice was shown to increase macrophage reverse transport and decrease atherosclerosis [51]. In nonhuman primates, treatment with a miR-33 antisense oligonucleotide was shown to increase HDL-C up to 30% [52]. Strategies to silence miRNA may be a therapeutic in man. The ABCA1 pathway represents an important therapeutic target for the prevention and treatment of CVD (Figure 1, part 6).

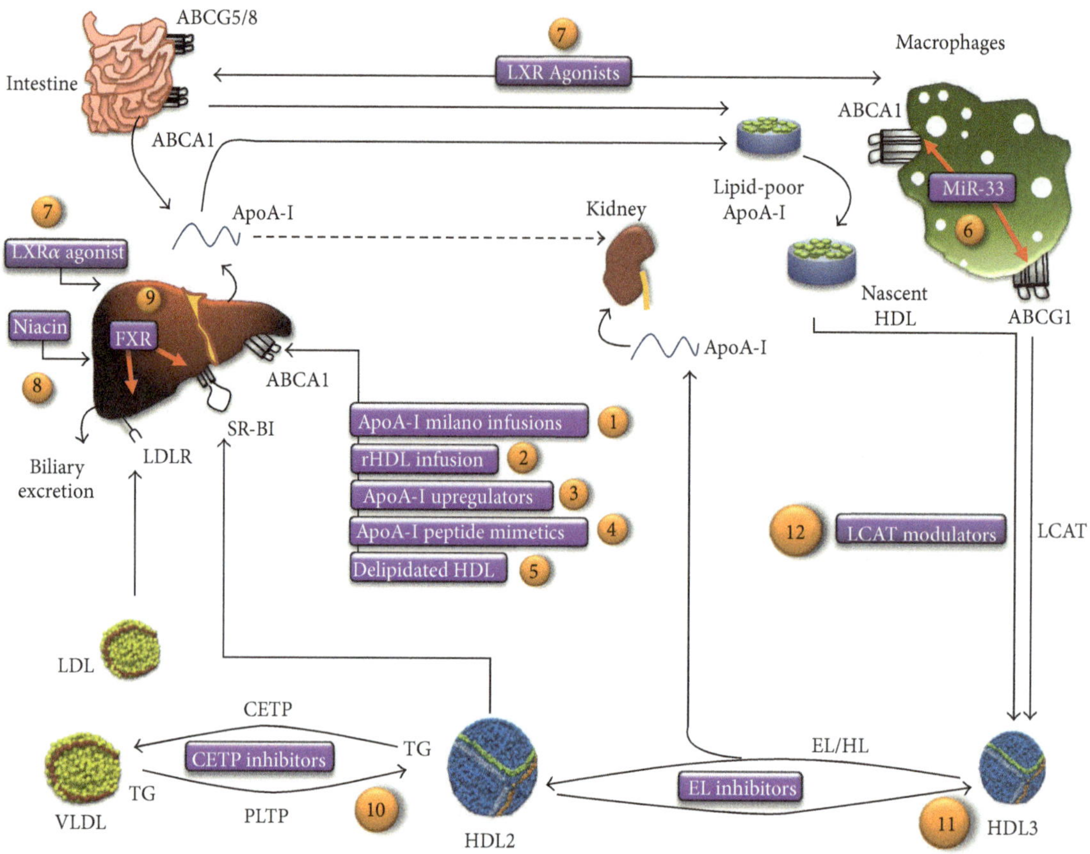

FIGURE 1: Schematic diagram of HDL metabolic pathways and current drugs under development. Numbers in circles refer to Table 2. Pathway influencing HDL cholesterol metabolism, flux, and potential targets of therapeutic interventions. Both liver and intestine synthesize apolipoprotein A-I (ApoA-I) secreted as lipid-poor particles. These particles are lipidated with phospholipids and cholesterol via the hepatocyte ATP-binding cassette A1 (ABCA1) transporter to form nascent HDL. In peripheral tissues these HDL particles obtain free cholesterol via the macrophage ABCA1 and ABCG1 transporters, which are regulated by LXRs and miR-33. Free cholesterol transferred via ABCA1 and ABCG1 onto HDL is esterified by lecithin: cholesterol acyltransferase (LCAT) to form cholesteryl esters (CE). Mature HDL thus formed exchange CE trough cholesteryl ester transfer protein (CETP) onto apoB-containing lipoproteins, (VLDL and LDL) with subsequent uptake in the liver via the low-density lipoprotein receptor (LDLR). PLTP mediates transfer of phospholipid from triglyceride from VLDL into HDL, which promote HDL remodeling. The resulting HDL3 particles can be either taken up by the liver via SB-B1 or modified by hepatic lipase (HL) and endothelial lipase (EL), which hydrolyze HDL phospholipids and triglycerides. Metabolism by EL releases lipid-poor apoA-I, which can be catabolized in kidney. Targets of HDL-directed therapeutic interventions are indicated by red arrow.

TABLE 1: Characteristics of pathways for cholesterol efflux from cells to plasma.

Characteristics	Aqueous diffusion	SR-BI	ABCA1	ABCG1
Energy requirement	Passive	Passive	Active	Active
Cholesterol flux	Bidirectional	Bidirectional	Unidirectional	Unidirectional
Preferred HDL acceptors	HDL2, HDL3	HDL2, HDL3	preβ-HDL Lipid-poor/free apoA-I	HDL2, HDL3

6.4. ABCG1. ABCG1 is a half transporter that homodimerizes to form a full transporter. Unlike ABCA1, lipid-free or lipid-poor apoA-I does not bind to ABCG1 and does not mediate cholesterol efflux. ABCG1-mediated cholesterol efflux requires larger HDL particles and this efflux is unidirectional against a concentration gradient [38] (Figure 2). In macrophages, ABCG1 is an LXR target which was subsequently shown to promote mobilization of intracellular cholesterol [53] to spherical HDL particles; HDL3 particles being the most efficient [54]. In addition to LXR activation, ABCG1 expression can also be induced by agonist of peroxisome proliferator-activated receptor gamma (PPARγ) associated with increased LXR [55]. Regulation of these pathways is complex and recent data shows that miR-33 increases ABCG1 expression *in vivo* [56]. In mouse macrophages, miR-33 targets ABCG1 thereby reducing cholesterol efflux

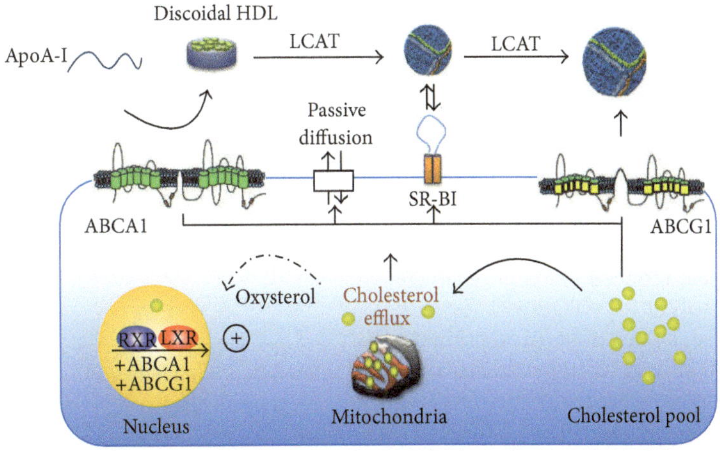

FIGURE 2: HDL biogenesis. Mitochondrial cholesterol transport is rate limiting in the (sterol 27-hydroxylase-) dependent generation of oxysterol ligands for LXR (liver X receptor) transcription factors that regulate the expression of genes encoding proteins in the cholesterol efflux pathway, such as ABC transporters (ATP-binding cassette transporters) ABCA1, and ABCG1. These transporters transfer cholesterol and/or phospholipids across the plasma membrane to (apo) lipoprotein acceptors, generating nascent HDLs (high-density lipoproteins), which can safely transport excess cholesterol through the bloodstream to the liver for excretion in bile. Ligand activation of nuclear LXRs (liver X receptors) (LXRα/β) is pivotal in cellular response to elevated sterol content, triggering cholesterol efflux mechanisms: both synthetic and oxysterol LXR agonists potently upregulate ABCA1 and ABCG1 gene expression. Consequently, elimination of excess cholesterol can be achieved, *in vivo* and *in vitro*, by cellular cholesterol efflux, orchestrated by ABCA1, ABCG1, ABCG4, and passive diffusion along a concentration gradient, and also "acceptor" (apo) lipoproteins, such as apoA-I, and HDLs (high-density lipoproteins). Notably, LXRs form heterodimers with RXRs (retinoic acid receptors) and bound to the nuclear receptor.

to nascent HDL [50, 56]. These data demonstrate that miR-33 deficiency or inhibition raises HDL-C, increases cholesterol efflux from macrophages via ABCA1 and ABCG1, and prevents the progression of atherosclerosis. However, many genes are altered in miR-33-deficient mice, and more experimental data is required to establish miR-33 as a therapeutic modality in humans. Gelissen et al. have characterized two novel isoforms of ABCG1 in human vascular endothelial cells that induce different levels of cholesterol efflux [57]. New insights into coordinated participation of ABCA1 in concert with ABCA1 in promoting cellular cholesterol export to lipid-free/poor apoA-I have evolved; ABCA1 initially donates phospholipids and cholesterol to lipid-poor apoA-I; ABCG1 mediates further cellular efflux onto more mature HDL particles [58]. These transporters thus work synergistically to remove excess cholesterol from cells (particularly macrophages). Murine models of atherosclerosis, using ABCG1-apoE double knock out, showed markedly defective cholesterol efflux and increased macrophage apoptosis [59]. Conversely, overexpression of ABCG1 increased the rate of constant efflux of cholesterol and protected murine tissues from lipid accumulation [60, 61]. The potential importance of ABCG1 in RCT has not been fully established.

6.5. SR-BI. SR-BI is critical in facilitating the delivery of cholesterol from macrophages to the liver. The SR-BI pathway acts as a receptor for large HDL particles (HDL2) and mediates the selective uptake of cholesteryl esters, without incorporation of the holoparticle [36, 54] (Figure 2). SR-B1 also mediates cellular cholesterol efflux onto HDL particles. HDL phospholipids absorb cholesterol that diffuses from the plasma membrane by the interaction between HDL and SR-BI [36, 37]. The relationship of hepatic SR-BI expression to HDL-C levels and atherosclerosis is ambiguous in light of human epidemiologic data. Several studies established a role of SR-BI expressed or inhibited in liver and in bone marrow-derived cells in the protection against atherosclerosis [62, 63]. Carriers of the first reported mutation of SR-BI in humans (*SRB1* P297S) have increased HDL-C levels but reduced capacity for cholesterol efflux from macrophages without increased severity of atherosclerosis [64]. Selective disruption of SR-BI in bone marrow-derived cells, including macrophages, leads to accelerated atherosclerosis indicating a dual role in atherosclerosis lesion development [62]. Mouse SR-BI$^{-/-}$ models exhibit increased HDL-C concentrations, decreased markers of RCT, and increased atherosclerosis [65]. *In vivo* data demonstrated that SR-BI does not promote macrophage RCT as seen with ABCA1 and ABCG1 [66]. The hepatic SR-BI may have an indirect role in atherosclerosis by modulating changes in the composition and structure of HDL particles rather than changes in the HDL pool [65, 67, 68]. A novel blocker of SR-B1, ITX5061 (a molecule initially characterized as p38 mitogen-activated protein kinase (MPK)), increases HDL-C in mice and decreases the formation of early atherosclerosis lesions. In human, SR-BI blockade by ITX5061 increases HDL-C levels without adverse effects on VLDL/LDL cholesterol, although this effect seems to be transient [69]. This data supports the concept that ABCA1, ABCG1, and SR-B1 act cooperatively in the peripheral biogenesis of nascent HDL particles, maturation of HDL, and selective CE uptake by the liver, respectively, completing the RCT in the plasma compartment.

7. Functions of HDL

7.1. Antioxidant. Oxidative modification of lipids, especially fatty acyl residues within phospholipids, leads to free radical formation and cell damage. Products of lipid peroxidation present in oxLDL can induce proinflammatory phenotypes in arterial wall cells, which contribute to endothelial dysfunction and apoptotic cell death, key steps in the initiation and progression of atherosclerosis lesions [70]. HDL prevents LDL from free radical-induced oxidative damage through several mechanisms [71, 72] (Figure 3). Several antioxidant enzymes that are involved in prevention of lipid oxidation or degradation of lipid hydroperoxides, such as LCAT, platelet-activating factor acetylhydrolase, reduced glutathione selenoperoxidase, and paraoxonase 1 (PON 1), are present on HDL. This antioxidative activity of HDL appears to be defective in dyslipidemic patients at high CVD risk [73]. Measuring the antioxidant properties of HDL is cumbersome; novel approaches use indirect measurements of phospholipid oxidation. The HDL oxidant index is an assay based on the chemoluminescence emitted by dichlorofluorescin that quantifies the antioxidation activity of HDL. This assay has been used as a biomarker of HDL functionality in experimental models and in therapeutic interventions in man [74]. Several biomarkers of oxidation potential have been put forth, by measuring the formation of biologically active oxidized phospholipids, by the determination of endothelial superoxide production and NADPH oxidase, or by the measurement of paraoxonase activity [73].

8. Vascular Endothelial Function of HDL

8.1. Anti-Inflammatory. Atherosclerosis is an inflammatory disease. HDL prevents vascular inflammation (Figure 3) through various pathways, in part via modulation of nuclear transcription factor κb- (NF-κb-) activated cell adhesion molecules [71] and via macrophage activation of JAK2/STAT3 interaction with apo AI/ABCA1 complex [75]. *In vitro* studies have demonstrated that HDL inhibits the expression of endothelial adhesion molecules, such as vascular cell adhesion molecule-1 (VCAM-1) and E-selectin [71]. Expression of endothelial adhesion molecules by HDL has also been demonstrated in the aortic endothelium of rabbits *in vivo* [76]. Recently, elegant experiments by Besler et al. have shown that modulation of vascular inflammation by dysfunctional HDL is mediated by upstream regulation of nuclear factor κ-B (nf-κB) [71, 77]. Another anti-inflammatory effect of HDL involves the transport of sphingosine-1-phosphate (S1P) a lipid mediator that has anti-inflammatory actions at low concentrations [78]. In human aortic endothelium and smooth muscle, HDL prevents the expression of IL-8 and monocyte chemoattractant protein (MCP-1) under inflammatory conditions [70], showing that normal HDL is capable of preventing LDL oxidation and the inflammatory response induced by LDL. During inflammation, HDL cargo becomes oxidatively and enzymatically modified, and HDL loses its protective capacity [70]. In the setting of an acute coronary syndrome (ACS), HDL promotes LDL-induced endothelial MCP-1 expression and monocyte adhesion [71]. Moreover,

Table 2: Controversies surrounding the "HDL hypothesis."

HDL and atherosclerosis: pro	The "HDL hypothesis" questioned
Strong biological plausibility for HDL as a therapeutic target	Mendelian Randomization does not support HDL-cholesterol as a causal risk factor
The epidemiological association between HDL-C and CVD is strong and coherent	HDL-C loses its predictive value if LDL-C is low
Animal data is unequivocal: HDL protects against atherosclerosis	The clinical trial data with drugs that raise HDL-C (fibrates, niacin, torcetrapib, and dalcetrapib) is neutral

HDL from these patients reflects a shift to an inflammatory profile which, in turn, might alter the protective effects of HDL on the atherosclerotic plaque [73, 79]. To study the function and the effects of HDL in setting of inflammation, a cell free assay for measuring lipid hyperoxides in plasma was developed to determine the inflammatory properties of HDL [74].

8.2. Vascular Endothelial eNOS. HDL-derived cholesterol has been shown to promote endothelial generation of nitric oxide (NO) *in vitro* and to improve endothelial function and arterial vasoreactivity *in vivo* (Figure 3). Activation of NO production involves HDL binding to SR-BI, which activates the phosphatidylinositol-3-kinase (PI3 K)/Akt signalling pathway and the phosphorylation of endothelial nitric oxide synthase (eNOS) [6]. In previous studies it has been shown that eNOS activation in response to HDL is mediated via Akt-dependent eNOS phosphorylation at Ser1177 [80]. Notably, Besler et al. showed that HDL from patient with CAD, in contrast to HDL from healthy subjects, activates endothelial PKCβII, leading to inhibition of Akt-dependent eNOS activating phosphorylation at Ser1177 and increased phosphorylation of eNOS at Thr495, which inhibits eNOS activity [6]. Experimental studies have consistently demonstrated the capacity of HDL to modify eNOS expression as well as activity to stimulate endothelial NO production *in vitro* and *in vivo* [6, 71, 73]. Several mechanisms have been shown that modulate eNOS and NO production by HDL [71]. The HDL-associated PON-1 has been shown to be an important determinant of the capacity of HDL to stimulate endothelial NO production and to exert NO-dependent endothelial-atheroprotective effects [6]. As observed in patients with CAD, inhibition of HDL-associated PON1 led to the increase of malonaldehyde-(MAD-) lysine adducts in HDL that subsequently activate protein kinase C beta II (PKCβII) via the endothelial LOX-1 receptor [6, 71].

8.3. Antiapoptotic. Cell apoptosis in response to endothelial injury is an important feature in atherosclerosis and is, in part, stimulated in part by oxLDL (Figure 2). It has been

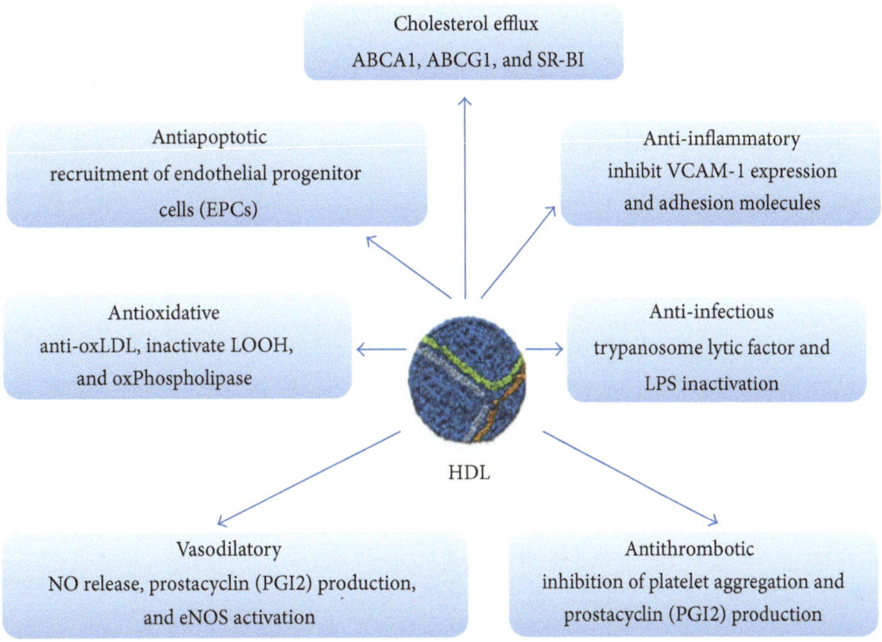

FIGURE 3: Summary of pleiotropic effects of HDL. In addition to their ability to reverse transport cholesterol from peripheral tissues back to the liver, HDLs display pleiotropic effects including antioxidant, antiapoptotic, anti-inflammatory, anti-infectious, and antithrombotic properties that account for their protective action on endothelial cells. Vasodilatation via production of nitric oxide (NO) is also a hallmark of HDL action on those cells.

shown that HDL is able to protect oxLDL-induced apoptosis by blocking intracellular signaling involved in apoptosis [81]. HDL promotes vascular cell migration, proliferation, survival (antiapoptotic), and recruitment of endothelial progenitor cells (EPCs) to sites of vascular injury [17, 82]. Recently, Riwanto et al. demonstrated that HDL from healthy subjects induced expression of the antiapoptotic Bcl-2 protein Bcl-xL from endothelial cells and reduced endothelial cell apoptosis. This effect, however, was lost when HDL from subjects with coronary artery disease was used [77].

8.4. Antithrombotic. HDL may exert antithrombotic activity via inhibition of tissue factor expression, factor X activation, and plasminogen activator inhibitor secretion [83]. HDL blocks the formation of the platelet activator thromboxane A2, and platelet activation factor synthase (Figure 3), thus reducing platelet aggregation [6]. Surrogate measures of HDL antiplatelet and antithrombotic functionality remain underdeveloped, in large part because of the absence of consensus regarding the clinically relevant atheroprotective pathways. Thus, there is strong biological plausibility for targeting HDL-C for the prevention and treatment of CVD. Controversy remains, however, in light of the apparent controversies summarized in Table 2.

8.5. Anti-Infectious (Antitrypanosome). HDL displays anti-infectious activity in the binding and clearance of circulating bacterial lipopolysaccharide (LPS) to the bile and thereby inhibits endotoxins-induced cellular activation, resulting in potent anti-infectious activity (Figure 3). Mechanism of LPS inactivation by HDL is mediated by direct interaction with apo A-I and involves reduced CD14 expression on monocytes as a key step [84]. Apo A-I overexpression in mice diminishes significantly LPS-induced systemic inflammation and multiple organ damage [84]. HDL toxin-neutralizing activity is largely attributed to apo A-I and has been furthermore shown to be effective against enterohemolysin [85] and lipoteichoic acid [84]. More recently, a study demonstrates that apoA-I reduces LPS-induced inflammatory responses, both *in vitro* and *in vivo*, and inhibits the development of atherosclerosis [86]. Furthermore, in cattle, the *Trypanosoma brucei brucei* causes a devastating disease, nagana. In man, HDL prevents trypanosomes from infecting cells by forming a complex with haptoglobin and causing increased permeability to water in *T. brucei brucei*, causing lysis [87].

9. Novel Therapies under Development to Raise HDL-C Levels

Table 3 and Figure 1 summarize selected strategies to increase HDL/apoA-I and describe potential compound under development.

10. CETP Inhibitors (Figure 1, Part 10)

Torcetrapib was the first CETP inhibitor to be used in a large-scale clinical trial. The ILLUMINATE trial failed to show benefit from the drug and the clinical trial was brought to a sudden and unexpected halt because of increased mortality in subjects on torcetrapib. This effect is thought to

TABLE 3: Summary of selected strategies to increase HDL/apoA-I and potential compound under development. Numbers in the right hand column refer to Figure 1.

Pharmacotherapeutic Strategy	Drug	Aim	Figure 1
Recombinant apoA-I Milano/phospholipids	ETC-216	Directly augmenting apoA-I/HDL pool	1
Purified native apoA-I/phospholipids	CSL-111 CSL-112	Directly augmenting apoA-I/HDL pool	2
Upregulators of endogenous apoA-I production	RVX-208	Directly augmenting apoA-I/HDL pool	3
ApoA-I mimetic peptides	D-4F L-4F 6F, 5A ATI-5261	Mimicking apoA-I functionality	4
Autologous Delipidated HDL	Selective HDL delipidated	Directly augmenting apoA-I/HDL pool	5
Gene therapy	miR-33	Modulating HDL levels and cholesterol efflux expression	6
Liver X receptor agonists	LXRα/β agonists LxR-623 T0901317, GW3965 ATI-111	Enhancing RCT & Macrophage cholesterol efflux	7
Niacin receptor agonists	ARI-3037MO	Indirectly augmenting apoA-I and HDL-cholesterol	8
Farnesoid X receptor	FxR-450	Modulate HDL levels	9
Cholesteryl ester transfer inhibitors	Anacetrapib MK-0859Evacetrapib LY248595	Indirectly augmenting apoA-I and HDL-cholesterol	10
Endothelial lipase inhibition	Boronic acid inhibitors Selective sulfonylfuran urea	Increasing HDL-cholesterol	11
LCAT activators	rLCAT ETC-642	Enhancing RCT	12

represent off-targets effects, predominantly on blood pressure control of torcetrapib [25]. A second, weaker CETP inhibitor, dalcetrapib increased HDL-C by 31–40%, without changing LDL-C. The study showed no benefit on cardiovascular outcomes [27]. Two new CETP inhibitors (anacetrapib and evacetrapib) are in phase III clinical trials.

Anacetrapib (MK-0859) (Table 3) raises HDL without affecting blood pressure [88]. The Determining Efficacy and Tolerability (DEFINE) trial randomized 1623 patients with CAD whose statin treatment has achieved LDL < 100 mg/dL to 100 mg of anacetrapib or placebo [89, 90]. Anacetrapib therapy resulted in 138% increase in HDL-C, a 40% reduction in LDL-C, and a 36% decrease in Lp[a] [90]. The off-target effects seen with torcetrapib were not identified [91]. The large REVEAL HPS-3/TIMI-55 trial will test the hypothesis that lipid modification with anacetrapib 100 mg daily reduces the risk of coronary death, myocardial infarction, or coronary revascularization in 30,000 patients with CVD or diabetes on optimal statin treatment with atorvastatin. (ClinicalTrials.gov NCT01252953) The estimated study completion date is 2017 [92].

Evacetrapib is a benzazepine compound (LY248595) and a potent and selective inhibitor of CETP both *in vitro* and *in vivo* (Table 3). Clinical trials with evacetrapib showed substantially increased HDL-C (54–129%) and decreased LDL-C (14–36%) across a dose range of evacetrapib in 398 dyslipidemic patients [93]. In this trial evacetrapib has shown no demonstrable effects on blood pressure or adrenal synthesis of aldosterone or cortisol in preclinical studies. The effects of evacetrapib on cardiovascular outcomes are being examined in the Assessment of Clinical Effects of Cholesteryl Ester Transfer Protein Inhibition with Evacetrapib in Patients at a High-Risk for Vascular Outcomes (ACCELERATE study), enrolling 11,000 patients after ACS [94].

11. Niacin (Figure 1, Part 8)

Niacin (nicotinic acid) is the oldest of the lipid-lowering drugs [95]. The mechanisms by which niacin raises HDL-C remain poorly understood, despite the identification of specific cell receptors (GP109, HM74, and HM74A). Niacin lipid efficacy is independent of both the niacin receptor GPR109A and free fatty acid suppression [91]. Niacin effects involve reducing the synthesis of VLDL in the liver through diaglycerol acyl transferase-2 (DGAT-2) as well as affecting peripheral lipolysis [96]. Niacin was also shown to have pleiotropic effects, such as improving endothelial-protective functions of HDL in patient with type 2 diabetics with low HDL-C levels [73]. In the early lipid-lowering drug therapy the Coronary Drug Prevention project [97], niacin alone was shown to reduce myocardial infarction and stroke in a randomized 3906 patients with previous myocardial infarction. Later, a meta-analysis study of 11 randomized controlled trials, using niacin (none in monotherapy), was shown to significantly reduce major coronary events by 25%, stroke by 26%, and all cardiovascular events by 27% [98]. Two new, large-scale clinical trials examined the role of niacin as an add-on to statin therapy for the secondary prevention of CVD. The Atherothrombosis Intervention in Metabolic Syndrome with Low HDL/High Triglycerides: Impact on Global Health Outcomes (AIM-HIGH) trial randomized 3,414 statin-treated CAD patients with low HDL-C to niacin versus placebo [4]. This trial was stopped prematurely because the lack of benefit on cardiovascular outcomes, despite a 10% increase in HDL-C [99]. The HPS-2/THRIVE (Heart Protection Study-2-Treatment of HDL to Reduce the Incidence of Vascular Events), a study of 25,000 patients at high risk for CVD events [5, 100] examined the effects of niacin and laropiprant on cardiovascular outcomes. After a mean followup of 3 years the combination of niacin/laropiprant therapy added to statin therapy did not reduce CVD risk events compared to statin therapy alone. Further, nonfatal attacks, strokes, or revascularizations were increased in participant who received niacin plus laropiprant. Niacin has many side effects, including hepatotoxicity, hyperglycemia, and flushing [101]. Non-flushing niacin derivatives have been synthesized such as prostaglandin D2 DP1 receptor antagonist-laropiprant. In the phase 3 trials niacin-laropiprant 2 g shows reductions in TG by 23%, 18% in LDL-C, and a 20% increase in HDL-C [102]. Another approach is, ARI-3037MO (Arisaph Pharmaceuticals; Boston, MA, USA) presently in phase I trials [103]. The success of this approach has been put into doubt following AIN-HIGH and HPS2 results (Table 3).

12. Directly Augmenting Apo A-I and ApoA-I/Phospholipid Complexes (Figure 1, Parts 1, 2)

This concept was developed to directly increase HDL, by infusing reconstituted HDL (rHDL) or recombinant HDL particles into the circulation rather than increasing HDL indirectly by modulating HDL metabolism (Table 3). One approach uses recombinant apoA-I_{Milano}. Individuals with apoA-I_{Milano} mutation have low HDL-C levels (10 to 30 mg/dL), and no apparent increased CVD risk [104]. Early studies indicated that recombinant apoA-I_{Milano}, when delivered by intravenous infusion, promotes regression of atherosclerosis lesion to a greater extent than wild type apoA-I as measured by intravascular ultrasound within 5 weeks of treatment [105]. Procedural difficulties complicated the development of ETC-216 (clinical denomination of apoA-I_{Milano}) [106] and no further clinical trials with this formulation have been reported [107]. More recently, it has shown that recombinant HDL apoA-I_{Milano} exerts greater anti-inflammatory and plaque stabilizing properties rather than antisclerotic properties [108]. Another rHDL compound, CSL-111 consists of apoA-I purified from human plasma and complexed with phosphatidylcholine derived from soybean phosphatidylcholine. The first trial of CSL-111 examined the effect of rHDL in the Atherosclerosis Safety and Efficacy (ERASE) trial conducted in 183 patients with ACS [106]. Four weekly infusion of CSL-111 of 4 h each to 111 individuals randomized to the 40 mg/kg proved to be well tolerated and failed to meet its primary end-point. The high dose regimen (80 mg/kg) was discontinued because of abnormal liver transaminase elevations. However, there was no significant change in atheroma volume, as measured by IVUS, compared with the placebo group. Since ERASE, there is one other randomized study investigating the effect of CSL-111 on surrogate cardiovascular marker in patients with ACS [109]. In this trial 29 patients were randomized to single infusion of CSL-111 (80 mg/kg over 4 h) or albumin. An increase of HDL (64%) and a reduction of LDL (23%) notwithstanding human rHDL did not improve vascular function in patients with ACS and there was no significant difference between the two arms suggesting no benefit with a single infusion. CSL-111 and also ECT-216 are currently in phase II trials. A reformulated version of CSL-111, called CSL-112, has been reported in preclinical studies. A phase I safety study has been initiated [110].

13. Delipidated HDL Infusions (Figure 1, Part 5)

Delipidated HDL infusion is a novel approach to raise HDL by intravenous infusion of autologous delipidated HDL [111] (Table 3). Preclinical evaluation of selective delipidated HDL in dyslipidemic monkeys achieved a significant 6.9% reduction in aortic atheroma volume assessed by IVUS [112]. The process involves the selective removal of apoA-I HDL particles, and the delipidation reinfusion of the cholesterol-depleted functional pre-β HDL. In a human trial, 28 patients with ACS received 5 weekly infusions delipidated HDL ($n = 14$) or placebo ($n = 14$). Study results established that selectively increasing preβ-HDL was associated with decreased total atheroma volume by 5.2% from base line [111]. However, it is not clear whether acute regression of atherosclerosis burden will be associated with decreased clinical cardiovascular events. Autologous delipidated HDL infusions did not induce liver toxicity or hypersensitivity reactions. In the study HDL apheresis resulted in hypotension in a third of the participants undergoing the treatment. A delipidation system for human use is now evaluable from lipid Sciences Plasma Delipidation System-2 (PDS-2), which converts αHDL to preβ-like HDL by selectively removing cholesterol from HDL in samples of plasma collected from patients by apheresis.

14. HDL Mimetics

14.1. ApoA-I Mimetic Peptides Drugs (Figure 1, Part 4). ApoA-I mimetics are short synthetic peptides that mimic the amphipathic α-helix of apoA-I.The first apoA-I mimetic peptide consisted of 18 amino acids (compound 18A) [113]. The sequence of 18A (D-W-$_L$-K-A-F-Y-$_D$-K-V-A-E-K-$_L$-K-E-A-F) does not share sequence homology with apoA-I because of the presence of two phenylalanine (F) residues on the hydrophobic face at positions 6 and 18; it is also referred to as 2F. While this sequence has the capacity to assume α-helical configuration in secondary structure and mimics many of the lipid binding properties of apoA-I [114], it failed to decrease diet induced atherosclerosis in mice [115]. Consequently, from 18A structure, additional improved peptides were generated through increasing number of phenylalanine residues on the hydrophobic face (referred to as 2F, 3F, 4F, 5F, 6F, and 7F) [115]. Among the three first peptides, only 4F was highly effective in preventing LDL-induced MCP-1 production by cultured human artery wall cells [115]. Shah and Chyu [116] found that D-4F reduced vein graft atherosclerosis in apoE null mice fed a western diet. Weihrauch et al. [117] gave intraperitoneal injection in a mouse model of systemic sclerosis, deduced that D-4F decreases myocardial inflammation index, improves vascular function, and restored angiogenic potential [118].Optimal physical-chemical properties and biologic activity were found with compound 4F [119]. The apoA-I mimetic peptide 4F showed great promise in a number of animal models and in early human trials [120] leading to a phase I/II study in humans with high risk CVD [118]. In this study, the 4F peptide synthesized from all $_{L}$-amino acids for L-4F was delivered at low doses (0.042–1.43 mg/kg) by intravenous or subcutaneous administration [121]. Very high plasma peptide levels were achieved, but there was no improvement in HDL anti-inflammatory function [121]. On the other hand, data showed that L-4F restores vascular endothelial function in murine models of hypercholesterolemia [122]. In another clinical trial the 4F peptide synthesized from all $_{D}$-amino acids for D-4F was administered orally at higher doses (0.43–7.14 mg/kg). Interestingly, despite very low plasma peptide levels, it has shown significantly improved HDL inflammatory index [118]. In humans with significant cardiovascular risk, a single dose of D-4F was found to improve the inflammatory index of HDL with modest oral bioavailability [119]. In contrast to L-4F, D-4F is poorly degraded in mammals, which led to its prolonged tissue retention time, particularly in liver and kidneys [114]. Despite these differences, the effects of D-4F and L-4F on biomarker and lesion area were similar when administered by subcutaneous injection in cholesterol fed rabbits [119]. In addition, oral D-4F administration in mice can influence several steps in the RCT pathway by increasing plasma LCAT activity, but the effect is likely due to HDL remodelling rather than activation of the enzyme [123]. Recent studies in mice revealed that the site controlling 4F peptide efficiency might be the small intestine even when it is delivered subcutaneously [124, 125]. Interestingly, the dose administered, not the plasma level, was the major determinant of efficiency of the 4F peptide [124]. At high doses, D-4F displayed detergent-like properties and could extract cholesterol from cells independently of ABCA1 [114, 126]. Unfortunately, D-4F may exhibit cytotoxicity through ABCA-1 independent lipid efflux. Furthermore, these mimetics have end-blocking groups (Ac- and NH_2) which can only be added by chemical synthesis. These blocking groups for 4F and for many other apoA-I mimetics stabilize the class A amphipathic helix and dramatically increase efficiency [127].

Recently, peptide 6F—that do not require added chemical groups for efficacy—has been produced in genetically engineered tomatoes. Compound 6F produced by this mean showed anti-inflammatory properties when fed orally to mice, providing a novel approach to orally administered apoA-I mimetic compounds [128]. Of the apoA-I mimetics synthesized to date, both 5F and 6F were able to efficiently inhibit LDL-induced MCP-1 production by cultured human artery wall cells, however, 7F did not [129]. 5A peptide was also effective as rHDL in reducing the expression of VCAM-1 and ICAM-1, and similarly to HDL exerted its effects through ABCA1 *in vivo* and *in vitro* [130] (Table 3).

14.2. ATI-5261 Synthetic Peptide. Native apoA-I is a 243 amino acid protein that contain multiple α-helical repeated in tandem and separated by proline residues. Most of α-helices are 22 amino acids long with a unique secondary structure defined as class A amphipathic α-helix. In this helix, negatively charged amino acid residues are clustered at the center of the polar face and positively charged residues are at the interface between the hydrophilic and hydrophobic faces; α-helices linked via proline are required to support potent biological activity [43]. Studies using the 22-mer amphipathic α-helix of apoA-I have not been able to stimulate ABCA1-dependent cholesterol efflux [131]. Short sequences taken directly from native proteins often cannot typically replicate the biological activity of the parent peptide [132], possibly due to peptide aggregation via nonspecific hydrophobic interactions and decreased solubility in water [133]. Taking these features into account, a 22 amino acids compound (ATI-5261) was synthesized by introducing negatively charged glutamine residues to a segment derived from the C-terminal domain of apoE at positions 14 and 19 together with hydrophobic acids (A, W, F, and L) [133]. This compound lacks tandem helical repeats and exhibits efficient stimulation of cholesterol efflux indicating that the ability to promote cholesterol efflux is not dependent on multiple α-helices as previously thought. ATI-5261 displays high α-helicity as shown by circular dichroism, hydrophobic moment, and increased solubility characteristics [132]. *In vitro*, ATI-5261 exerts its effects through ABCA1 in a fashion similar to that of HDL and successfully enhances cholesterol efflux from macrophages and reduces aortic atherosclerosis by up to 45% after intraperitoneal injection in mice [133]. ATI-526 increases faeces cholesterol transport in mice [133, 134]. The compound presently waits early phase clinical trials.

14.3. Endothelial Lipase Inhibitors (Figure 1, Part 11). EL inhibition may represent potential future therapies to reduce apoA-I catabolism and to increase plasma apoA-I and HDL-C levels (Table 3). Human genetic studies have confirmed that variation of the EL gene is an important determinant of plasma HDL-C level [135]. However, how changes in HDL-C level attributed to EL may affect atherosclerosis is still not clear. Some human studies propose an atherogenic role for EL, with a positive association of plasma level of EL mass and coronary artery calcification [136]. Carrier of EL variants associated with HDL-C levels have been reported to have decreased risk of coronary artery disease [137], but this association has not been observed in other studies [64]. Mendelian randomization data casts doubt on whether genetic variability at the EL gene locus that increases HDL-C protects against cardiovascular diseases [31]. Studies in mice showed that EL overexpression reduces HDL-C and apo A-I levels [36, 138] due to increased renal catabolism. Conversely, gene deletion of EL results in increased HDL-C and apo A-I levels [139]. Although EL inactivation was expected to inhibit atherosclerosis by raising HDL-C, the effect of EL inactivation seems more complex than expected. Deficiency of EL resulted in an accumulation of small dense LDL, a potentially atherogenic mechanism. Brown et al. showed that targeted inactivation of EL increased plasma HDL-C level and inhibited atherosclerosis [140]. On the other hand, Ishida et al. have previously reported that targeted inactivation of EL increased plasma HDL-C level and inhibited atherosclerosis in apoE$^{-/-}$ mice [138]. These findings initiated the synthesis of a library of small molecule inhibitors of EL based on sulfonylurea backbone [141]. Recently, many of new EL inhibitors synthesized from boronic acid were evaluated for potency against both EL and LPL [142]. The enthusiasm for EL inhibitors is somewhat tempered by Mendelian randomization data showing that variabilities at the EL and CETP genes that increase HDL-C are not associated with protection against CVD [143].

14.4. LCAT Modulators (Figure 1, Part 12). Several drug development approaches have recently been started for modulating LCAT activity (Table 3). One strategy is being investigated is the use of engineered recombinant LCAT protein entity (rLCAT) as a replacement therapy in the case of familial LCAT deficiency. Early studies for treatment of atherosclerosis and CVD by raising HDL-C through plasma LCAT enzyme activity were initiated by Zhou et al. in a rabbit model [144]. Data concluded that recombinant LCAT administration may represent a novel approach for the treatment of atherosclerosis and the dyslipidemia associated with low HDL. A preclinical mouse study of human recombinant LCAT (rLCAT) was recently reported [145]. An rLCAT (rLCAT, AlphaCore Pharma, Ann Arbor, MI, USA) was injected into LCAT-null mice and found to reverse the abnormal lipoprotein profile by increasing HDL-C to near normal levels for several days. Intravenous infusion of human rLCAT in rabbits was found to raise HDL-C, to increase fecal secretion of cholesterol, and to reduce atherosclerosis [146]. Another potential alternative to LCAT injection for treatment of human LCAT deficiency was recently reported in which adipocytes transfected with LCAT were transplanted into mice and were found to raise HDL-C [147]. Only one LCAT modulator has reached early clinical development, ETC-642, but little data are available on the outcomes of treatment with this agent [148].

15. Apo A-I Upregulator (Figure 1, Part 3)

15.1. RVX-208. Reservelogix-208 (RVX-208) is a small molecule that increases endogenous synthesis of apoA-I (Table 3). RVX-208 has a molecular weight of roughly 400 Da belonging to the quinazoline family. Recently, in African green monkeys, oral administration of RVX-208 resulted in increased levels of plasma apoA-I and HDL-C [149]. Serum from these animals was shown to mediate enhanced cholesterol efflux from J774 macrophages via the ABCA1, ABCG1, and SR-BI-dependent pathways [149]. Serum from human subjects treated with RVX-208 exhibited increased cholesterol efflux capacity despite a relatively modest increase in HDL-C levels [150]. In a phase II trial, modest changes in HDL-C and apoA-I were reported in 299 statin-treated patients with stable CAD [151]. Two Phase 2b studies are ongoing, one involves 172 statin-treated patients randomized for RVX-208 100 mg or placebo twice daily for 24 weeks [152] and the other phase trial will investigate the effect of RVX-208 on coronary atherosclerosis assessed by intravascular ultrasound [153].

15.2. Synthetic Liver X Receptor (LXR) Agonists (Figure 1, Part 7). Synthetic LXR agonists including LXRα/β are known to induce the transcription of ABCA1 and ABCG1 [53]. As potent activators of the cellular cholesterol efflux, these compounds have been shown to raise HDL-C levels and to reduce atherosclerosis in transgenic mouse models [154]. Thus, LXR agonist's activation may be a promising pharmacologic target for the treatment of dyslipidemia and atherosclerosis (Table 3). Unfortunately, development of first generation LXR compounds has been hampered by their induction of expression of lipogenic genes in the liver, which increase the levels of triglycerides and promote hepatic steatosis [53]. Various synthetically engineered LXR agonists have been developed and tested in animal models (T0901317, LXR-623, GW3965, GW6340, AZ876, and ATI-111). They all show high potency for interacting with LXRα/β receptors, but none of them shows selectivity for ABCA1 and ABCG1 [53, 155–157]. T091317 is a LXR activator, broadly used for research in LXR biology [158, 159]. T091317 consistently decreases atherosclerosis in mice models and induces gene expression of NCP1 and NCP2 in macrophages resulting in enriched cholesterol content in the outer layer of plasma membrane [158]. The LXR agonist LXR-623 is associated with increased expression of ABCA1 and ABCG1 in cells [160], but adverse central nervous system-related effects were noted in more than half of patients, leading to termination of the study [161]. In combination with simvastatin in a rabbit model of advanced atherosclerosis, LXR-623 showed a reduction in the rate of plaque progression [156]. Other agonists (AZ876 and GW3965) were shown to reduce the number of atherosclerotic lesions [159]. The LXR agonist GW6340, an intestine specific LXRα/β agonist, promoted macrophage specific cellular cholesterol efflux and increased intestinal excretion of HDL-derived cholesterol [155]. More recently, a novel synthetic LXR agonist, ATI-111, that is, more potent than T0901317, inhibited atherosclerotic progression and prevented atheromatous plaque formation in mice [157]. It is clear that research on more selective LXR ligands is an active field of experimental pharmacology. A new LXR inverse agonist (SR9238) was designed for nonalcoholic fatty disease to suppress hepatic steatosis [162]. Data from mouse model indicated that this strategy may hold promise in the treatment of liver disease [162].

15.3. Synthetic FXR Agonists (Figure 1, Part 9). The Farnesoid X receptor (FXR) is a bile acid-activated nuclear receptor that plays an important role in the regulation of cholesterol and more specifically HDL homeostasis [163]. Preclinical studies showed that activation of FXR leads to both pro- and antiatherosclerosis and a major metabolic of FXR agonists observed consistently in animal studies was the reduction of plasma HDL [163, 164]. Hambruch et al. showed that FXR agonists induce the hepatic steps of HDL-derived cholesterol excretion into feces in mice and monkeys [164]. For these reasons, FXR agonists have received attention as a potential therapeutic target [165, 166], and different agonists have been generated as a strategy for HDL-C raising therapies. These include GW4064, 6-ECDCA, FXR-450, and PX20606 [163] (Table 3). Both synthetic FXR agonists FXR-450 and PX20606 demonstrated potent plasma cholesterol lowering in mice, whereas GW4064 and 6-ECDCA showed only limited effects [164]. GW4064 as previously demonstrated it has potential cell toxicity and uncertain bioavailability prevents its development for clinical studies [165]. Interestingly, in CETPtg-LDLR($^{-/-}$) mice PX20606 caused highly significant decrease in atherosclerotic plaque size despite the observed HDL-C reduction [164]. Data from normolipidemic monkeys treated with PX20606 significantly and specifically lowered the HDL2 subclass without changing apoA-I levels. In these studies, the basic mechanisms of FXR mediating HDL-C clearance are conserved in mice and monkeys. These observations will support further studies to investigate the potential roles of FXR activation on HDL species.

16. Gene Therapy

Gene therapy or somatic gene transfer for the treatment of severe lipoprotein disorders has been previously attempted, with limited success in homozygous familial hypercholesterolemia [166, 167]. Animal experiments with apoA-I transgenes have yielded beneficial results for the prevention of atherosclerosis [168, 169]. To date, this approach has little application in man. Recently, an adeno-associated virus-based treatment for lipoprotein lipase deficiency of enhanced activity variant of LPL(S447X) alipogene tiparvovec was tested [170, 171]. The LPLS447X variant is found in 20% of Caucasians and is associated with enhanced removal of proatherogenic apoB100-containing particles, including LDL-cholesterol [171], lower plasma TG levels, higher HDL cholesterol concentrations, and lower rates of cardiovascular disease, when compared to the general population. This data provided the rationale for a gene therapy trial in man. Alipogene tiparvovec (AAV1-LPLS447X) therapy in patients with severe hypertriglyceridemia secondary to LPL deficiency and recurrent pancreatitis was performed in 20 subjects. Triglyceride levels fell in 40% of the subjects. Unfortunately, the authors do not report HDL-C levels in these patients. However, this serves as a proof of concept for gene therapy in man. Alipogene tiparvovec was recently discontinued because of unfavorable opinion about its risk-benefit given by the European Medicines Evaluation Agency. Animal data supports novel gene-based approaches to increase HDL-C. A potential mechanism to increase of HDL cholesterol is increasing ABCA1 and ABCG1 expression through the microRNA (inhibition of miR-33 being the most promising candidate to date) (Figure 1, part 6). Overexpression of antisense miR-33 using lentivirus in mice showed a 50% increase in hepatic ABCA1 protein levels and a concomitant 25% increase in plasma HDL levels after 6 days [51]. Marquart et al. showed that injection of an anti-miR-33 oligonucleotide in mice resulted in a substantial increase in ABCA1 expression and HDL levels [172]. Furthermore, it was shown in mice that miR-33 resulted in decreased cholesterol efflux [173] which provide a potentially novel therapeutic approach. These data suggest that miR-33 might be a possible target for the treatment of cardiovascular and metabolic disorders.

17. Concluding Remarks

Potential new therapeutic treatment of atherosclerosis based on HDL biology remains in preclinical steps. Strategies to raise HDL pharmacologically have, so far, not yielded sufficiently positive results to make firm clinical treatment recommendation. The concept that HDL-C is a risk factor (i.e., having a direct, causal role in atherosclerosis) has been challenged (Table 2). It is conceivable that HDL-C may simply be a biomarker of cardiovascular health. Moreover, the recent HSP2-THRIVE and dal-OUTCOMES studies put the HDL-C hypothesis in question. The association between HDL and CVD is more complex than previously thought and is probably mediated by various HDL functions, such as reverse cholesterol transport or anti-inflammatory, antioxidant, and vascular protective properties. It may be possible also that HDL-C level is correlated with other nonmeasured active subfractions that may act directly to reduce and predict CVD risk. To better understand the relation between HDL and atherosclerosis, we should consider developing and measuring better markers of HDL function, rather than the cholesterol mass within HDL particles.

Abbreviations

ABCA1: ATP-binding cassette transporter A1
ABCG1: ATP-binding cassette transporter G1
ApoA-I: Apolipoprotein A-I
ApoB: Apolipoprotein B
ApoE: Apolipoprotein E
CETP: Cholesterol ester transfer protein
CVD: Coronary vascular disease
FC: Free cholesterol
FXR: Farnesoid X-receptor
HDL: High-density lipoprotein
HDL-C: High-density lipoprotein-cholesterol
LCAT: Lecithin-cholesterol acyltransferase
LDL: Low-density lipoprotein

LXR: Liver X-receptor
ox-LDL: Oxidized low-density lipoprotein
RCT: Reverse cholesterol transport
RXR: Retinoid X-receptor
SR-B1: Scavenger-receptor B-I
TG: Triglyceride
UTC: Ultracentrifugation.

Acknowledgments

This work was supported by Grants 15042 and 97752 from the Canadian Institutes of Health Research and by a Grant-in-Aid from the Heart and Stroke Foundation of Canada (Quebec). Anouar Hafiane is supported by a scholarship from the Department of Biochemistry at McGill University.

References

[1] D. J. Rader and E. M. deGoma, "Approach to the patient with extremely low HDL-cholesterol," *The Journal of Clinical Endocrinology & Metabolism*, vol. 97, no. 10, pp. 3399–3407, 2012.

[2] D. J. Rader and A. R. Tall, "The not-so-simple HDL story: is it time to revise the HDL cholesterol hypothesis?" *Nature Medicine*, vol. 18, no. 9, pp. 1344–1346, 2012.

[3] C. Baigent, L. Blackwell, J. Emberson et al., "Efficacy and safety of more intensive lowering of LDL cholesterol: a meta-analysis of data from 170,000 participants in 26 randomised trials," *The Lancet*, vol. 376, no. 9753, pp. 1670–1681, 2010.

[4] W. E. Boden, J. L. Probstfield, T. Anderson et al., "Niacin in patients with low HDL cholesterol levels receiving intensive statin therapy," *New England Journal of Medicine*, vol. 365, no. 24, pp. 2255–2267, 2011.

[5] R. S. Rosenson and A. M. Gotto Jr., "When clinical trials fail to address treatment gaps: the failure of niacin-laropiprant to reduce cardiovascular events," *Current Atherosclerosis Reports*, vol. 15, no. 6, article 332, 2013.

[6] C. Besler, K. Heinrich, L. Rohrer et al., "Mechanisms underlying adverse effects of HDL on eNOS-activating pathways in patients with coronary artery disease," *Journal of Clinical Investigation*, vol. 121, no. 7, pp. 2693–2708, 2011.

[7] R. S. Rosenson, H. B. Brewer Jr., M. J. Chapman et al., "HDL measures, particle heterogeneity, proposed nomenclature, and relation to atherosclerotic cardiovascular events," *Clinical Chemistry*, vol. 57, no. 3, pp. 392–410, 2011.

[8] E. J. Niesor, "Different effects of compounds decreasing cholesteryl ester transfer protein activity on lipoprotein metabolism," *Current Opinion in Lipidology*, vol. 22, no. 4, pp. 288–295, 2011.

[9] O. F. Delalla, H. A. Elliot, and J. W. Gofman, "Ultracentrifugal studies of high density serum lipoproteins in clinically healthy adults," *The American Journal of Physiology*, vol. 179, no. 2, pp. 333–337, 1954.

[10] J. C. Fruchart and J. M. Bard, "Lipoprotein particle measurement: an alternative approach to classification of lipid disorders," *Current Opinion in Lipidology*, vol. 2, no. 6, pp. 362–366, 1991.

[11] L. Camont, M. J. Chapman, and A. Kontush, "Biological activities of HDL subpopulations and their relevance to cardiovascular disease," *Trends in Molecular Medicine*, vol. 17, no. 10, pp. 594–603, 2011.

[12] J. W. Heinecke, "The HDL proteome: a marker—and perhaps mediator—of coronary artery disease," *Journal of Lipid Research*, vol. 50, supplement, pp. S167–S171, 2009.

[13] W. S. Davidson, R. A. G. D. Silva, S. Chantepie, W. R. Lagor, M. J. Chapman, and A. Kontush, "Proteomic analysis of defined hdl subpopulations reveals particle-specific protein clusters: relevance to antioxidative function," *Arteriosclerosis, Thrombosis, and Vascular Biology*, vol. 29, no. 6, pp. 870–876, 2009.

[14] H. R. Superko, L. Pendyala, P. T. Williams, K. M. Momary, S. B. King III, and B. C. Garrett, "High-density lipoprotein subclasses and their relationship to cardiovascular disease," *Journal of Clinical Lipidology*, vol. 6, no. 6, pp. 496–523, 2012.

[15] A. V. Khera and D. J. Rader, "Future therapeutic directions in reverse cholesterol transport," *Current Atherosclerosis Reports*, vol. 12, no. 1, pp. 73–81, 2010.

[16] B. J. Ansell, M. Navab, S. Hama et al., "Inflammatory/antiinflammatory properties of high-density lipoprotein distinguish patients from control subjects better than high-density lipoprotein cholesterol levels and are favorably affected by simvastatin treatment," *Circulation*, vol. 108, no. 22, pp. 2751–2756, 2003.

[17] E. Di Angelantonio, N. Sarwar, P. Perry et al., "Major lipids, apolipoproteins, and risk of vascular disease," *Journal of the American Medical Association*, vol. 302, no. 18, pp. 1993–2000, 2009.

[18] R. H. Mackey, P. Greenland, D. C. Goff Jr., D. Lloyd-Jones, C. T. Sibley, and S. Mora, "High-density lipoprotein cholesterol and particle concentrations, carotid atherosclerosis, and coronary events: MESA (multi-ethnic study of atherosclerosis)," *Journal of the American College of Cardiology*, vol. 60, no. 6, pp. 508–516, 2012.

[19] H. N. Ginsberg, M. B. Elam, L. C. Lovato et al., "Effects of combination lipid therapy in type 2 diabetes mellitus," *New England Journal of Medicine*, vol. 362, no. 17, pp. 1563–1574, 2010.

[20] M. Jun, C. Foote, J. Lv et al., "Effects of fibrates on cardiovascular outcomes: a systematic review and meta-analysis," *The Lancet*, vol. 375, no. 9729, pp. 1875–1884, 2010.

[21] J. C. Fruchart, F. Sacks, M. P. Hermans et al., "The residual risk reduction initiative: a call to action to reduce residual vascular risk in patients with dyslipidemia," *American Journal of Cardiology*, vol. 102, no. 10, supplement, pp. 1K–34K, 2008.

[22] B. J. Arsenault, P. Barter, D. A. DeMicco et al., "TNT Study Investigators. Prediction of cardiovascular events in statin-treated stable coronary patients by lipid and nonlipid biomarkers," *Journal of the American College of Cardiology*, vol. 57, no. 1, pp. 63–69, 2011.

[23] W. A. van der Steeg, I. Holme, S. M. Boekholdt et al., "High-density lipoprotein cholesterol, high-density lipoprotein particle size, and apolipoprotein A-I: significance for cardiovascular risk: the IDEAL and EPIC-Norfolk studies," *Journal of the American College of Cardiology*, vol. 51, no. 6, pp. 634–642, 2008.

[24] P. Barter, "Lessons Learned from the Investigation of Lipid Level Management to Understand its Impact in Atherosclerotic Events (ILLUMINATE) Trial," *American Journal of Cardiology*, vol. 104, no. 10, 2009.

[25] P. J. Barter, M. Caulfield, M. Eriksson et al., "ILLUMINATE Investigators. Effects of torcetrapib in patients at high risk for coronary events," *New England Journal of Medicine*, vol. 357, no. 21, pp. 2109–2122, 2007.

[26] P. M. Ridker, J. Genest, S. M. Boekholdt et al., "HDL cholesterol and residual risk of first cardiovascular events after treatment

with potent statin therapy: an analysis from the JUPITER trial," *The Lancet*, vol. 376, no. 9738, pp. 333–339, 2010.

[27] G. G. Schwartz, A. G. Olsson, M. Abt et al., "dal-OUTCOMES Investigators. Effects of dalcetrapib in patients with a recent acute coronary syndrome," *New England Journal of Medicine*, vol. 367, no. 22, pp. 2089–2099, 2012.

[28] HPS2-THRIVE Collaborative Group, "HPS2-THRIVE randomized placebo-controlled trial in 25 673 high-risk patients of ER niacin/laropiprant: trial design, pre-specified muscle and liver outcomes, and reasons for stopping study treatment," *European Heart Journal*, vol. 34, no. 17, pp. 1279–1291, 2013.

[29] C. Cook and C. Sheets, "Clinical equipoise and personal equipoise: two necessary ingredients for reducing bias in manual therapy trials," *Journal of Manual and Manipulative Therapy*, vol. 19, no. 1, pp. 55–57, 2011.

[30] R. Frikke-Schmidt, B. G. Nordestgaard, P. Schnohr, and A. Tybjærg-Hansen, "Single nucleotide polymorphism in the low-density lipoprotein receptor is associated with a threefold risk of stroke: a case-control and prospective study," *European Heart Journal*, vol. 25, no. 11, pp. 943–951, 2004.

[31] B. F. Voight, G.M. Peloso, M. Orho-Melander et al., "Plasma HDL cholesterol and risk of myocardial infarction: a mendelian randomisation study," *The Lancet*, vol. 380, no. 9841, pp. 572–580, 2012.

[32] J. A. Glomset, "The plasma lecithins:cholesterol acyltransferase reaction," *Journal of Lipid Research*, vol. 9, no. 2, pp. 155–167, 1968.

[33] T. Devries-Seimon, Y. Li, M. Y. Pin et al., "Cholesterol-induced macrophage apoptosis requires ER stress pathways and engagement of the type A scavenger receptor," *Journal of Cell Biology*, vol. 171, no. 1, pp. 61–73, 2005.

[34] A. V. Khera, M. Cuchel, M. De La Llera-Moya et al., "Cholesterol efflux capacity, high-density lipoprotein function, and atherosclerosis," *New England Journal of Medicine*, vol. 364, no. 2, pp. 127–135, 2011.

[35] H. H. Hassan, M. Denis, D. Y. D. Lee et al., "Identification of an ABCA1-dependent phospholipid-rich plasma membrane apolipoprotein A-I binding site for nascent HDL formation: implications for current models of HDL biogenesis," *Journal of Lipid Research*, vol. 48, no. 11, pp. 2428–2442, 2007.

[36] R. S. Rosenson, H. B. Brewer Jr., W. S. Davidson et al., "Cholesterol efflux and atheroprotection: advancing the concept of reverse cholesterol transport," *Circulation*, vol. 125, no. 15, pp. 1905–1919, 2012.

[37] G. H. Rothblat and M. C. Phillips, "High-density lipoprotein heterogeneity and function in reverse cholesterol transport," *Current Opinion in Lipidology*, vol. 21, no. 3, pp. 229–238, 2010.

[38] M. P. Adorni, F. Zimetti, J. T. Billheimer et al., "The roles of different pathways in the release of cholesterol from macrophages," *Journal of Lipid Research*, vol. 48, no. 11, pp. 2453–2462, 2007.

[39] J. F. Oram and A. M. Vaughan, "ABCA1-mediated transport of cellular cholesterol and phospholipids to HBL apolipoproteins," *Current Opinion in Lipidology*, vol. 11, no. 3, pp. 253–260, 2000.

[40] K. Nagao, M. Tomioka, and K. Ueda, "Function and regulation of ABCA1—membrane meso-domain organization and reorganization," *FEBS Journal*, vol. 278, no. 18, pp. 3190–3203, 2011.

[41] Y. Zhao, T. J. C. Van Berkel, and M. Van Eck, "Relative roles of various efflux pathways in net cholesterol efflux from macrophage foam cells in atherosclerotic lesions," *Current Opinion in Lipidology*, vol. 21, no. 5, pp. 441–453, 2010.

[42] M. G. Sorci-Thomas, J. S. Owen, B. Fulp et al., "Nascent high density lipoproteins formed by ABCA1 resemble lipid rafts and are structurally organized by three apoA-I monomers," *Journal of Lipid Research*, vol. 53, no. 9, pp. 1890–1909, 2012.

[43] M. C. Phillips, "New insights into the determination of HDL structure by apolipoproteins," *Journal of Lipid Research*, 2012.

[44] K. Okuhira, M. L. Fitzgerald, N. Tamehiro et al., "Binding of PDZ-RhoGEF to ATP-binding cassette transporter A1 (ABCA1) induces cholesterol efflux through RhoA activation and prevention of transporter degradation," *Journal of Biological Chemistry*, vol. 285, no. 21, pp. 16369–16377, 2010.

[45] E. B. Neufeld, A. T. Remaley, S. J. Demosky et al., "Cellular localization and trafficking of the human ABCA1 transporter," *Journal of Biological Chemistry*, vol. 276, no. 29, pp. 27584–27590, 2001.

[46] G. Kellner-Weibel and M. de la Llera-Moya, "Update on HDL receptors and cellular cholesterol transport," *Current Atherosclerosis Reports*, vol. 13, no. 3, pp. 233–241, 2011.

[47] J. M. Timmins, J. Y. Lee, E. Boudyguina et al., "Targeted inactivation of hepatic Abca1 causes profound hypoalphalipoproteinemia and kidney hypercatabolism of apoA-I," *Journal of Clinical Investigation*, vol. 115, no. 5, pp. 1333–1342, 2005.

[48] L. R. Brunham, J. K. Kruit, J. Iqbal et al., "Intestinal ABCA1 directly contributes to HDL biogenesis in vivo," *Journal of Clinical Investigation*, vol. 116, no. 4, pp. 1052–1062, 2006.

[49] Y. Zhang, F. C. McGillicuddy, C. C. Hinkle et al., "Adipocyte modulation of high-density lipoprotein cholesterol," *Circulation*, vol. 121, no. 11, pp. 1347–1355, 2010.

[50] C. Fernández-Hernando, Y. Suárez, K. J. Rayner, and K. J. Moore, "MicroRNAs in lipid metabolism," *Current Opinion in Lipidology*, vol. 22, no. 2, pp. 86–92, 2011.

[51] K. J. Rayner, F. J. Sheedy, C. C. Esau et al., "Antagonism of miR-33 in mice promotes reverse cholesterol transport and regression of atherosclerosis," *Journal of Clinical Investigation*, vol. 121, no. 7, pp. 2921–2931, 2011.

[52] K. J. Rayner, C. C. Esau, F. N. Hussain et al., "Inhibition of miR-33a/b in non-human primates raises plasma HDL and lowers VLDL triglycerides," *Nature*, vol. 478, no. 7369, pp. 404–407, 2011.

[53] M. H. Oosterveer, A. Grefhorst, A. K. Groen, and F. Kuipers, "The liver X receptor: control of cellular lipid homeostasis and beyond: implications for drug design," *Progress in Lipid Research*, vol. 49, no. 4, pp. 343–352, 2010.

[54] M. De La Llera-Moya, D. Drazul-Schrader, B. F. Asztalos, M. Cuchel, D. J. Rader, and G. H. Rothblat, "The ability to promote efflux via ABCA1 determines the capacity of serum specimens with similar high-density lipoprotein cholesterol to remove cholesterol from macrophages," *Arteriosclerosis, Thrombosis, and Vascular Biology*, vol. 30, no. 4, pp. 796–801, 2010.

[55] T. E. Akiyama, S. Sakai, G. Lambert et al., "Conditional disruption of the peroxisome proliferator-activated receptor γ gene in mice results in lowered expression of ABCA1, ABCG1, and apoE in macrophages and reduced cholesterol efflux," *Molecular and Cellular Biology*, vol. 22, no. 8, pp. 2607–2619, 2002.

[56] K. J. Rayner, Y. Sulrez, A. Dlvalos et al., "MiR-33 contributes to the regulation of cholesterol homeostasis," *Science*, vol. 328, no. 5985, pp. 1570–1573, 2010.

[57] I. C. Gelissen, S. Cartland, A. J. Brown et al., "Expression and stability of two isoforms of ABCG1 in human vascular cells," *Atherosclerosis*, vol. 208, no. 1, pp. 75–82, 2010.

[58] I. D. Kerr, A. J. Haider, and I. C. Gelissen, "The ABCG family of membrane-associated transporters: you don't have to be big to be mighty," *British Journal of Pharmacology*, vol. 164, no. 7, pp. 1767–1779, 2011.

[59] E. J. Tarling, D. D. Bojanic, R. K. Tangirala et al., "Impaired development of atherosclerosis in Abcg1-/- Apoe -/- mice: identification of specific oxysterols that both accumulate in Abcg1-/- Apoe-/- tissues and induce apoptosis," *Arteriosclerosis, Thrombosis, and Vascular Biology*, vol. 30, no. 6, pp. 1174–1180, 2010.

[60] M. A. Kennedy, G. C. Barrera, K. Nakamura et al., "ABCG1 has a critical role in mediating cholesterol efflux to HDL and preventing cellular lipid accumulation," *Cell Metabolism*, vol. 1, no. 2, pp. 121–131, 2005.

[61] L. Yvan-Charvet, N. Wang, and A. R. Tall, "Role of HDL, ABCA1, and ABCG1 transporters in cholesterol efflux and immune responses," *Arteriosclerosis, Thrombosis, and Vascular Biology*, vol. 30, no. 2, pp. 139–143, 2010.

[62] M. Van Eck, I. S. T. Bos, R. B. Hildebrand, B. T. Van Rij, and T. J. C. Van Berkel, "Dual role for scavenger receptor class B, type I on bone marrow-derived cells in atherosclerotic lesion development," *American Journal of Pathology*, vol. 165, no. 3, pp. 785–794, 2004.

[63] E. Demetz, I. Tancevski, K. Duwensee et al., "Inhibition of hepatic scavenger receptor-class B type I by RNA interference decreases atherosclerosis in rabbits," *Atherosclerosis*, vol. 222, no. 2, pp. 360–366, 2012.

[64] M. Vergeer, S. J. A. Korporaal, R. Franssen et al., "Genetic variant of the scavenger receptor BI in humans," *New England Journal of Medicine*, vol. 364, no. 2, pp. 136–145, 2011.

[65] A. Al-Jarallah and B. L. Trigatti, "A role for the scavenger receptor, class B type I in high density lipoprotein dependent activation of cellular signaling pathways," *Biochimica et Biophysica Acta*, vol. 1801, no. 12, pp. 1239–1248, 2010.

[66] X. Wang, H. L. Collins, M. Ranalletta et al., "Macrophage ABCA1 and ABCG1, but not SR-BI, promote macrophage reverse cholesterol transport in vivo," *Journal of Clinical Investigation*, vol. 117, no. 8, pp. 2216–2224, 2007.

[67] R. B. Hildebrand, B. Lammers, I. Meurs et al., "Restoration of high-density lipoprotein levels by cholesteryl ester transfer protein expression in scavenger receptor class B Type i (SR-BI) knockout mice does not normalize pathologies associated with SR-BI deficiency," *Arteriosclerosis, Thrombosis, and Vascular Biology*, vol. 30, no. 7, pp. 1439–1445, 2010.

[68] M. El Bouhassani, S. Gilibert, M. Moreau et al., "Cholesteryl ester transfer protein expression partially attenuates the adverse effects of SR-BI receptor deficiency on cholesterol metabolism and atherosclerosis," *Journal of Biological Chemistry*, vol. 286, no. 19, pp. 17227–17238, 2011.

[69] D. Masson, M. Koseki, M. Ishibashi et al., "Increased HDL cholesterol and ApoA-I in humans and mice treated with a novel SR-BI inhibitor," *Arteriosclerosis, Thrombosis, and Vascular Biology*, vol. 29, no. 12, pp. 2054–2060, 2009.

[70] M. Navab, S. T. Reddy, B. J. Van Lenten, and A. M. Fogelman, "HDL and cardiovascular disease: atherogenic and atheroprotective mechanisms," *Nature Reviews Cardiology*, vol. 8, no. 4, pp. 222–232, 2011.

[71] C. Besler, T. F. Lüscher, and U. Landmesser, "Molecular mechanisms of vascular effects of High-density lipoprotein: alterations in cardiovascular disease," *EMBO Molecular Medicine*, vol. 4, no. 4, pp. 251–268, 2012.

[72] A. Kontush and M. J. Chapman, "Antiatherogenic function of HDL particle subpopulations: focus on antioxidative activities," *Current Opinion in Lipidology*, vol. 21, no. 4, pp. 312–318, 2010.

[73] S. A. Sorrentino, C. Besler, L. Rohrer et al., "Endothelial-vasoprotective effects of high-density lipoprotein are impaired in patients with type 2 diabetes mellitus but are improved after extended-release niacin therapy," *Circulation*, vol. 121, no. 1, pp. 110–122, 2010.

[74] M. Navab, S. Y. Hama, G. P. Hough, G. Subbanagounder, S. T. Reddy, and A. M. Fogelman, "A cell-free assay for detecting HDL that is dysfunctional in preventing the formation of or inactivating oxidized phospholipids," *Journal of Lipid Research*, vol. 42, no. 8, pp. 1308–1317, 2001.

[75] Y. Liu and C. Tang, "Regulation of ABCA1 functions by signaling pathways," *Biochimica et Biophysica Acta*, vol. 1821, no. 3, pp. 522–529, 2012.

[76] S. Patel, B. A. Di Bartolo, S. Nakhla et al., "Anti-inflammatory effects of apolipoprotein A-I in the rabbit," *Atherosclerosis*, vol. 212, no. 2, pp. 392–397, 2010.

[77] M. Riwanto, L. Rohrer, B. Roschitzki et al., "Altered activation of endothelial anti- and proapoptotic pathways by high-density lipoprotein from patients with coronary artery disease: role of high-density lipoprotein-proteome remodeling," *Circulation*, vol. 127, no. 8, pp. 891–904, 2013.

[78] K. Sato and F. Okajima, "Role of sphingosine 1-phosphate in anti-atherogenic actions of high-density lipoprotein," *World Journal of Biological Chemistry*, vol. 1, no. 11, pp. 327–337, 2010.

[79] K. Alwaili, D. Bailey, Z. Awan et al., "The HDL proteome in acute coronary syndromes shifts to an inflammatory profile," *Biochimica et Biophysica Acta*, vol. 1821, no. 3, pp. 405–415, 2012.

[80] C. Mineo, I. S. Yuhanna, M. J. Quon, and P. W. Shaul, "High density lipoprotein-induced endothelial nitric-oxide synthase activation is mediated by Akt and MAP kinases," *Journal of Biological Chemistry*, vol. 278, no. 11, pp. 9142–9149, 2003.

[81] I. Suc, I. Escargueil-Blanc, M. Troly, R. Salvayre, and A. Negre-Salvayre, "HDL and apoA prevent cell death of endothelial cells induced by oxidized LDL," *Arteriosclerosis, Thrombosis, and Vascular Biology*, vol. 17, no. 10, pp. 2158–2166, 1997.

[82] T. Langmann, J. Klucken, M. Reil et al., "Molecular cloning of the human ATP-Binding cassette transporter 1 (hABC1): evidence for sterol-dependent regulation in macrophages," *Biochemical and Biophysical Research Communications*, vol. 257, no. 1, pp. 29–33, 1999.

[83] J. R. Nofer, M. F. Brodde, and B. E. Kehrel, "High-density lipoproteins, platelets and the pathogenesis of atherosclerosis: frontiers in research review: physiological and pathological functions of high-density lipoprotein," *Clinical and Experimental Pharmacology and Physiology*, vol. 37, no. 7, pp. 726–735, 2010.

[84] Y. Li, J. B. Dong, and M. P. Wu, "Human ApoA-I overexpression diminishes LPS-induced systemic inflammation and multiple organ damage in mice," *European Journal of Pharmacology*, vol. 590, no. 1–3, pp. 417–422, 2008.

[85] P. M. S. Figueirêdo, C. F. Catani, and T. Yano, "Serum high-density lipoprotein (HDL) inhibits in vitro enterohemolysin (EHly) activity produced by enteropathogenic Escherichia coli," *FEMS Immunology and Medical Microbiology*, vol. 38, no. 1, pp. 53–57, 2003.

[86] K. Yin, S. L. Tang, X. H. Yu et al., "Apolipoprotein A-I inhibits LPS-induced atherosclerosis in ApoE-/- mice possibly via activated STAT3-mediated upregulation of tristetraprolin," *Acta Pharmacologica Sinica*, 2013.

[87] K. M. Hager and S. L. Hajduk, "Mechanism of resistance of African trypanosomes to cytotoxic human HDL," *Nature*, vol. 385, no. 6619, pp. 823–826, 1997.

[88] R. Krishna, M. S. Anderson, A. J. Bergman et al., "Effect of the cholesteryl ester transfer protein inhibitor, anacetrapib, on lipoproteins in patients with dyslipidaemia and on 24-h ambulatory blood pressure in healthy individuals: two double-blind, randomised placebo-controlled phase I studies," *The Lancet*, vol. 370, no. 9603, pp. 1907–1914, 2007.

[89] M. J. Chapman, W. Le Goff, M. Guerin, and A. Kontush, "Cholesteryl ester transfer protein: at the heart of the action of lipid-modulating therapy with statins, fibrates, niacin, and cholesteryl ester transfer protein inhibitors," *European Heart Journal*, vol. 31, no. 2, pp. 149–164, 2010.

[90] C. P. Cannon, S. Shah, H. M. Dansky et al., "Safety of anacetrapib in patients with or at high risk for coronary heart disease," *New England Journal of Medicine*, vol. 363, no. 25, pp. 2406–2415, 2010.

[91] B. Lauring, A. K. Taggart, J. R. Tata et al., "Niacin lipid efficacy is independent of both the niacin receptor GPR109A and free fatty acid suppression," *Science Translational Medicine*, vol. 4, no. 148, p. 148ra115, 2012.

[92] Clinical trial.gov.REVEAL: Randomized Evaluation of the Effects of Anacetrapib through Lipid-modification, 2010, http://clinicaltrials.gov/ct2/show/NCT01252953.

[93] S. J. Nicholls, H. B. Brewer, J. J. Kastelein et al., "Effects of the CETP inhibitor evacetrapib administered as monotherapy or in combination with statins on HDL and LDL cholesterol: a randomized controlled trial," *Journal of the American Medical Association*, vol. 306, no. 19, pp. 2099–2109, 2011.

[94] http://clinicaltrials.gov/show/NCT01687998.

[95] L. A. Carlson, "Nicotinic acid: the broad-spectrum lipid drug. A 50th anniversary review," *Journal of Internal Medicine*, vol. 258, no. 2, pp. 94–114, 2005.

[96] A. S. Wierzbicki, "Niacin: the only vitamin that reduces cardiovascular events," *International Journal of Clinical Practice*, vol. 65, no. 4, pp. 379–385, 2011.

[97] "Clofibrate and niacin in coronary heart disease," *Journal of the American Medical Association*, vol. 231, no. 4, pp. 360–381, 1975.

[98] E. Bruckert, J. Labreuche, and P. Amarenco, "Meta-analysis of the effect of nicotinic acid alone or in combination on cardiovascular events and atherosclerosis," *Atherosclerosis*, vol. 210, no. 2, pp. 353–361, 2010.

[99] C. P. Cannon, "High-density lipoprotein cholesterol as the Holy Grail," *Journal of the American Medical Association*, vol. 306, no. 19, pp. 2153–2155, 2011.

[100] I. Gouni-Berthold and H. K. Berthold, "The role of Niacin in lipid-lowering treatment: are we aiming too high?" *Current Pharmaceutical Design*, vol. 19, no. 17, pp. 3094–3106, 2013.

[101] H. K. Parson, H. Harati, D. Cooper, and A. I. Vinik, "The role of prostaglandin D2 and the autonomic nervous system on Niacin induced flushing," *Journal of Diabetes*, vol. 5, no. 1, pp. 59–67, 2013.

[102] H. E. Bays, A. Shah, Q. Dong, C. McCrary Sisk, and D. Maccubbin, "Extended-release niacin/laropiprant lipid-altering consistency across patient subgroups," *International Journal of Clinical Practice*, vol. 65, no. 4, pp. 436–445, 2011.

[103] http://www.arisaph.com/newsroom/press.php.

[104] C. R. Sirtori, L. Calabresi, G. Franceschini et al., "Cardiovascular status of carriers of the apolipoprotein A-IMilano mutant: the limone sul garda study," *Circulation*, vol. 103, no. 15, pp. 1949–1954, 2001.

[105] S. E. Nissen, T. Tsunoda, E. M. Tuzcu et al., "Effect of recombinant ApoA-I Milano on coronary atherosclerosis in patients with acute coronary syndromes: a randomized controlled trial," *Journal of the American Medical Association*, vol. 290, no. 17, pp. 2292–2300, 2003.

[106] United States Securities and Exchange Commission filing, 2013, http://www.faqs.org/sec-filings/091224/MEDICINES-CO-DE_8-K.

[107] J. C. Tardif, "Emerging high-density lipoprotein infusion therapies: fulfilling the promise of epidemiology?" *Journal of Clinical Lipidology*, vol. 4, no. 5, pp. 399–404, 2010.

[108] B. Ibanez, C. Giannarelli, G. Cimmino et al., "Recombinant HDL(Milano) exerts greater anti-inflammatory and plaque stabilizing properties than HDL(wild-type)," *Atherosclerosis*, vol. 220, no. 1, pp. 72–77, 2012.

[109] R. Chenevard, D. Hürlimann, L. Spieker et al., "Reconstituted HDL in acute coronary syndromes," *Cardiovascular Therapeutics*, vol. 30, no. 2, pp. e51–e57, 2012.

[110] "A single ascending dose study examining the safety and pharmacokinetic profile of reconstituted high density lipoprotein (CSL112) administered to patients. In: ClinicalTrials.gov. National Library of Medicine," 2012, http://www.clinicaltrials.gov/ct2/show/NCT01499420.

[111] R. Waksman, R. Torguson, K. M. Kent et al., "A first-in-man, randomized, placebo-controlled study to evaluate the safety and feasibility of autologous delipidated high-density lipoprotein plasma infusions in patients with acute coronary syndrome," *Journal of the American College of Cardiology*, vol. 55, no. 24, pp. 2727–2735, 2010.

[112] F. M. Sacks, L. L. Rudel, A. Conner et al., "Selective delipidation of plasma HDL enhances reverse cholesterol transport in vivo," *Journal of Lipid Research*, vol. 50, no. 5, pp. 894–907, 2009.

[113] G. M. Anantharamaiah, J. L. Jones, and C. G. Brouillette, "Studies of synthetic peptide analogs of the amphiphatic helix. Structure of complexes with dimyristoyl phosphatidylcholine," *Journal of Biological Chemistry*, vol. 260, no. 18, pp. 10248–10255, 1985.

[114] J. D. Smith, "Apolipoprotein A-I and its mimetics for the treatment of atherosclerosis," *Current Opinion in Investigational Drugs*, vol. 11, no. 9, pp. 989–996, 2010.

[115] G. Datta, M. Chaddha, S. Hama et al., "Effects of increasing hydrophobicity on the physical-chemical and biological properties of a class A amphipathic helical peptide," *Journal of Lipid Research*, vol. 42, no. 7, pp. 1096–1104, 2001.

[116] P. K. Shah and K. Y. Chyu, "Apolipoprotein A-I mimetic peptides: potential role in atherosclerosis management," *Trends in Cardiovascular Medicine*, vol. 15, no. 8, pp. 291–296, 2005.

[117] D. Weihrauch, H. Xu, Y. Shi et al., "Effects of D-4F on vasodilation, oxidative stress, angiostatin, myocardial inflammation, and angiogenic potential in tight-skin mice," *American Journal of Physiology*, vol. 293, pp. H1432–H1441, 2007.

[118] L. T. Bloedon, R. Dunbar, D. Duffy et al., "Safety, pharmacokinetics, and pharmacodynamics of oral apoA-I mimetic peptide D-4F in high-risk cardiovascular patients," *Journal of Lipid Research*, vol. 49, no. 6, pp. 1344–1352, 2008.

[119] C. B. Sherman, S. J. Peterson, and W. H. Frishman, "Apolipoprotein A-I mimetic peptides: a potential new therapy for the prevention of atherosclerosis," *Cardiology in Review*, vol. 18, no. 3, pp. 141–147, 2010.

[120] M. Navab, I. Shechter, G. M. Anantharamaiah, S. T. Reddy, B. J. Van Lenten, and A. M. Fogelman, "Structure and function

of HDL mimetics," *Arteriosclerosis, Thrombosis, and Vascular Biology*, vol. 30, no. 2, pp. 164–168, 2010.

[121] C. E. Watson, N. Weissbach, L. Kjems et al., "Treatment of patients with cardiovascular disease with L-4F, an apo-A1 mimetic, did not improve select biomarkers of HDL function," *Journal of Lipid Research*, vol. 52, no. 2, pp. 361–373, 2011.

[122] J. Ou, Z. Ou, D. W. Jones et al., "L-4F, an apolipoprotein A-1 mimetic, dramatically improves vasodilation in hypercholesterolemia and sickle cell disease," *Circulation*, vol. 107, no. 18, pp. 2337–2341, 2003.

[123] X. Chen, C. Burton, X. Song et al., "An apoa-I mimetic peptide increases LCAT activity in mice through increasing HDL concentration," *International Journal of Biological Sciences*, vol. 5, no. 5, pp. 489–499, 2009.

[124] M. Navab, S. T. Reddy, G. M. Anantharamaiah et al., "Intestine may be a major site of action for the apoA-I mimetic peptide 4F whether administered subcutaneously or orally," *Journal of Lipid Research*, vol. 52, no. 6, pp. 1200–1210, 2011.

[125] M. Navab, S. T. Reddy, G. M. Anantharamaiah et al., "D-4F-mediated reduction in metabolites of arachidonic and linoleic acids in the small intestine is associated with decreased inflammation in lowdensity lipoprotein receptor-null mice," *Journal of Lipid Research*, vol. 53, pp. 437–445, 2012.

[126] A. T. Remaley, F. Thomas, J. A. Stonik et al., "Synthetic amphipathic helical peptides promote lipid efflux from cells by an ABCA1-dependent and an ABCA1-independent pathway," *Journal of Lipid Research*, vol. 44, no. 4, pp. 828–836, 2003.

[127] G. M. Anantharamaiah, V. K. Mishra, D. W. Garber et al., "Structural requirements for antioxidative and anti-inflammatory properties of apolipoprotein A-I mimetic peptides," *Journal of Lipid Research*, vol. 48, no. 9, pp. 1915–1923, 2007.

[128] A. Chattopadhyay, M. Navab, and G. Hough, "A novel approach to oral ApoA-I mimetic therapy," *Journal of Lipid Research*, vol. 54, no. 4, pp. 995–1010, 2013.

[129] S. Imaizumi, M. Navab, C. Morgantini et al., "Dysfunctional high-density lipoprotein and the potential of apolipoprotein A-1 mimetic peptides to normalize the composition and function of lipoproteins," *Circulation Journal*, vol. 75, no. 7, pp. 1533–1538, 2011.

[130] F. Tabet, A. T. Remaley, A. I. Segaliny et al., "The 5A apolipoprotein A-I mimetic peptide displays antiinflammatory and antioxidant properties in vivo and in vitro," *Arteriosclerosis, Thrombosis, and Vascular Biology*, vol. 30, no. 2, pp. 246–252, 2010.

[131] E. Carballo-Jane, Z. Chen, E. O'Neill et al., "ApoA-I mimetic peptides promote pre-β HDL formation in vivo causing remodeling of HDL and triglyceride accumulation at higher dose," *Bioorganic and Medicinal Chemistry*, vol. 18, no. 24, pp. 8669–8678, 2010.

[132] Y. Zheng, A. B. Patel, V. Narayanaswami, G. L. Hura, B. Hang, and J. K. Bielicki, "HDL mimetic peptide ATI-5261 forms an oligomeric assembly in solution that dissociates to monomers upon dilution," *Biochemistry*, vol. 50, no. 19, pp. 4068–4076, 2011.

[133] J. K. Bielicki, H. Zhang, Y. Cortez et al., "A new HDL mimetic peptide that stimulates cellular cholesterol efflux with high efficiency greatly reduces atherosclerosis in mice," *Journal of Lipid Research*, vol. 51, no. 6, pp. 1496–1503, 2010.

[134] http://circ.ahajournals.org/cgi/content/meeting_abstract/120/18_MeetingAbstracts/S445-a.

[135] A. C. Edmondson, R. J. Brown, S. Kathiresan et al., "Loss-of-function variants in endothelial lipase are a cause of elevated HDL cholesterol in humans," *The Journal of Clinical Investigation*, vol. 119, no. 4, pp. 1042–1050, 2009.

[136] K. O. Badellino, M. L. Wolfe, M. P. Reilly, and D. J. Rader, "Endothelial lipase concentrations are increased in metabolic syndrome and associated with coronary atherosclerosis," *PLoS Medicine*, vol. 3, no. 2, article e22, 2006.

[137] N. P. Tang, L. S. Wang, L. Yang et al., "Protective effect of an endothelial lipase gene variant on coronary artery disease in a Chinese population," *Journal of Lipid Research*, vol. 49, no. 2, pp. 369–375, 2008.

[138] T. Ishida, S. Choi, R. K. Kundu et al., "Endothelial lipase is a major determinant of HDL level," *Journal of Clinical Investigation*, vol. 111, no. 3, pp. 347–355, 2003.

[139] E. M. deGoma and D. J. Rader, "Novel HDL-directed pharmacotherapeutic strategies," *Nature Reviews Cardiology*, vol. 8, no. 5, pp. 266–277, 2011.

[140] R. J. Brown, W. R. Lagor, S. Sankaranaravanan et al., "Impact of combined deficiency of hepatic lipase and endothelial lipase on the metabolism of both high-density lipoproteins and apolipoprotein b-containing lipoproteins," *Circulation Research*, vol. 107, no. 3, pp. 357–364, 2010.

[141] K. B. Goodman, M. J. Bury, M. Cheung et al., "Discovery of potent, selective sulfonylfuran urea endothelial lipase inhibitors," *Bioorganic & Medicinal Chemistry Letters*, vol. 19, no. 1, pp. 27–30, 2009.

[142] D. P. O'Connell, D. F. LeBlanc, D. Cromley, J. Billheimer, D. J. Rader, and W. W. Bachovchin, "Design and synthesis of boronic acid inhibitors of endothelial lipase," *Bioorganic & Medicinal Chemistry Letters*, vol. 22, no. 3, pp. 1397–1401, 2012.

[143] T. M. Teslovich, K. Musunuru, A. V. Smith et al., "Biological, clinical and population relevance of 95 loci for blood lipids," *Nature*, vol. 466, no. 7307, pp. 707–713, 2010.

[144] http://circ.ahajournals.org/cgi/content/meeting_abstract/120/18_MeetingAbstracts/S1175-b.

[145] X. Rousset, B. Vaisman, B. Auerbach et al., "Effect of recombinant human lecithin cholesterol acyltransferase infusion on lipoprotein metabolism in mice," *Journal of Pharmacology and Experimental Therapeutics*, vol. 335, no. 1, pp. 140–148, 2010.

[146] X. Rousset, R. Shamburek, B. Vaisman, M. Amar, and A. T. Remaley, "Lecithin cholesterol acyltransferase: an anti- or pro-atherogenic factor?" *Current Atherosclerosis Reports*, vol. 13, no. 3, pp. 249–256, 2011.

[147] S. Asada, M. Kuroda, Y. Aoyagi et al., "Ceiling culture-derived proliferative adipocytes retain high adipogenic potential suitable for use as a vehicle for gene transduction therapy," *American Journal of Physiology*, vol. 301, no. 1, pp. C181–C185, 2011.

[148] D. J. Rader, "Molecular regulation of HDL metabolism and function: implications for novel therapies," *Journal of Clinical Investigation*, vol. 116, no. 12, pp. 3090–3100, 2006.

[149] D. Bailey, R. Jahagirdar, A. Gordon et al., "RVX-208: a small molecule that increases apolipoprotein A-I and high-density lipoprotein cholesterol in vitro and in vivo," *Journal of the American College of Cardiology*, vol. 55, no. 23, pp. 2580–2589, 2010.

[150] A. Gordon, R. Jahagirdar, J. Johannson et al., "RVX-208 a small molecule that induces apolipoprotein A-I production progresses to phase Ib/IIa clinical trials," in *Proceedings of the American College of Cardiology Scientific Sessions*, Orlando, Fla, USA, 2009.

[151] S. J. Nicholls, A. Gordon, J. Johansson et al., "Efficacy and safety of a novel oral inducer of apolipoprotein A-I synthesis in statin-treated patients with stable coronary artery disease: a randomized controlled trial," *Journal of the American College of Cardiology*, vol. 57, no. 9, pp. 1111–1119, 2011.

[152] S. J. Nicholls, A. Gordon, J. Johansson et al., "ApoA-I induction as a potential cardioprotective strategy: rationale for the SUSTAIN and ASSURE studies," *Cardiovascular Drugs and Therapy*, vol. 26, no. 2, pp. 181–187, 2012.

[153] P. K. Shah, "Atherosclerosis: targeting endogenous apo A-I-a new approach for raising HDL," *Nature Reviews Cardiology*, vol. 8, no. 4, pp. 187–188, 2011.

[154] G. Lo Sasso, S. Murzilli, L. Salvatore et al., "Intestinal specific LXR activation stimulates reverse cholesterol transport and protects from atherosclerosis," *Cell Metabolism*, vol. 12, no. 2, pp. 187–193, 2010.

[155] T. Yasuda, D. Grillot, J. T. Billheimer et al., "Tissue-specific liver X receptor activation promotes macrophage reverse cholesterol transport in vivo," *Arteriosclerosis, Thrombosis, and Vascular Biology*, vol. 30, no. 4, pp. 781–786, 2010.

[156] C. Giannarelli, G. Cimmino, T. M. Connolly et al., "Synergistic effect of liver X receptor activation and simvastatin on plaque regression and stabilization: an magnetic resonance imaging study in a model of advanced atherosclerosis," *European Heart Journal*, vol. 33, no. 2, pp. 264–273, 2012.

[157] D. Peng, R. A. Hiipakka, J. T. Xie et al., "A novel potent synthetic steroidal liver X receptor agonist lowers plasma cholesterol and triglycerides and reduces atherosclerosis in LDLR-/- mice," *British Journal of Pharmacology*, vol. 162, no. 8, pp. 1792–1804, 2011.

[158] E. Rigamonti, L. Helin, S. Lestavel et al., "Liver X receptor activation controls intracellular cholesterol trafficking and esterification in human macrophages," *Circulation Research*, vol. 97, no. 7, pp. 682–689, 2005.

[159] M. N. Bradley, C. Hong, M. Chen et al., "Ligand activation of LXR beta reverses atherosclerosis and cellular cholesterol overload in mice lacking LXR alpha and apoE," *Journal of Clinical Investigation*, vol. 117, no. 8, pp. 2337–2346, 2007.

[160] E. M. Quinet, M. D. Basso, A. R. Halpern et al., "LXR ligand lowers LDL cholesterol in primates, is lipid neutral in hamster, and reduces atherosclerosis in mouse," *Journal of Lipid Research*, vol. 50, no. 12, pp. 2358–2370, 2009.

[161] A. Katz, C. Udata, E. Ott et al., "Safety, pharmacokinetics, and pharmacodynamics of single doses of lxr-623, a novel liver X-receptor agonist, in healthy participants," *Journal of Clinical Pharmacology*, vol. 49, no. 6, pp. 643–649, 2009.

[162] K. Griffett, L. A. Solt, B. E. El-Gendy, T. M. Kamenecka, and T. P. Burris, "A liver-selective LXR inverse agonist that suppresses hepatic steatosis," *ACS Chemical Biology*, vol. 8, no. 3, pp. 559–567, 2012.

[163] A. Mencarelli and S. Fiorucci, "FXR an emerging therapeutic target for the treatment of atherosclerosis," *Journal of Cellular and Molecular Medicine*, vol. 14, no. 1-2, pp. 79–92, 2010.

[164] E. Hambruch, S. Miyazaki-Anzai, U. Hahn et al., "Synthetic farnesoid X receptor agonists induce high-density lipoprotein-mediated transhepatic cholesterol efflux in mice and monkeys and prevent atherosclerosis in cholesteryl ester transfer protein transgenic low-density lipoprotein receptor (-/-) mice," *Journal of Pharmacology and Experimental Therapeutics*, vol. 343, no. 3, pp. 556–567, 2012.

[165] S. Fiorucci, S. Cipriani, F. Baldelli, and A. Mencarelli, "Bile acid-activated receptors in the treatment of dyslipidemia and related disorders," *Progress in Lipid Research*, vol. 49, no. 2, pp. 171–185, 2010.

[166] F. A. Al-Allaf, C. Coutelle, S. N. Waddington, A. L. David, R. Harbottle, and M. Themis, "LDLR-Gene therapy for familial hypercholesterolaemia: problems, progress, and perspectives," *International Archives of Medicine*, vol. 3, no. 1, article 36, 2010.

[167] M. Grossman, D. J. Rader, D. W. M. Muller et al., "A pilot study of ex vivo gene therapy for homozygous familial hypercholesterolaemia," *Nature Medicine*, vol. 1, no. 11, pp. 1148–1154, 1995.

[168] A. S. Plump, C. J. Scott, and J. L. Breslow, "Human apolipoprotein A-I gene expression increases high density lipoprotein and suppresses atherosclerosis in the apolipoprotein E-deficient mouse," *Proceedings of the National Academy of Sciences of the United States of America*, vol. 91, no. 20, pp. 9607–9611, 1994.

[169] N. Maeda, H. Li, D. Lee, P. Oliver, S. H. Quarfordt, and J. Osada, "Targeted disruption of the apolipoprotein C-III gene in mice results in hypotriglyceridemia and protection from postprandial hypertriglyceridemia," *Journal of Biological Chemistry*, vol. 269, no. 38, pp. 23610–23616, 1994.

[170] D. Gaudet, J. de Wal, K. Tremblay et al., "Review of the clinical development of alipogene tiparvovec gene therapy for lipoprotein lipase deficiency," *Atherosclerosis Supplements*, vol. 11, no. 1, pp. 55–60, 2010.

[171] D. Gaudet, J. Méthot, S. Déry et al., "Efficacy and long-term safety of alipogene tiparvovec (AAV1-LPL(S447X)) gene therapy for lipoprotein lipase deficiency: an open-label trial," *Gene Therapy*, vol. 20, no. 4, pp. 361–369, 2013.

[172] T. J. Marquart, R. M. Allen, D. S. Ory, and A. Baldán, "miR-33 links SREBP-2 induction to repression of sterol transporters," *Proceedings of the National Academy of Sciences of the United States of America*, vol. 107, pp. 12228–12232, 2010.

[173] T. Horie, K. Ono, M. Horiguchi et al., "MicroRNA-33 encoded by an intron of sterol regulatory element-binding protein 2 (Srebp2) regulates HDL in vivo," *Proceedings of the National Academy of Sciences of the United States of America*, vol. 107, no. 40, pp. 17321–17326, 2010.

24

Improving Total-Cholesterol/HDL-Cholesterol Ratio Results in an Endothelial Dysfunction Recovery in Peripheral Artery Disease Patients

Silvia Bleda, Joaquín de Haro, César Varela, Leticia Esparza, Javier Rodriguez, and Francisco Acin

Vascular Surgery and Angiology Department, Hospital Universitario Getafe, Ctra Toledo Km 12,500, 28905 Madrid, Spain

Correspondence should be addressed to Silvia Bleda, silbleik@yahoo.es

Academic Editor: Jan Wouter Jukema

Aims. To evaluate the effects of variations of total-cholesterol/HDL-cholesterol ratio and the effects of the atorvastatin on endothelial function in peripheral artery disease (PAD). *Material and Methods.* A prospective, randomised controlled study was carried out in 150 PAD patients. Patients randomized to the control group ($n = 75$) were treated with antiplatelet drugs, angiotensin-converting-enzyme inhibitors and cardiovascular-risk-factor control. Experimental group ($n = 75$) also received treatment with atorvastatin for a month. It was determined baseline nitrite plasma levels and total-cholesterol/HDL-cholesterol ratio and after one month of treatment in both groups. It was also analysed the correlation between the gradient of nitrite levels and the differential of total-cholesterol/HDL ratio in treatment group. *Results.* After a month, a reduction in nitrite levels was detected in treatment group ($11.88 \pm 7.8\,\mu$M versus $5.7 \pm 1.8\,\mu$M, $P < 0.0001$). It was shown a higher decrease in nitrite plasma levels in the atorvastatin group finding lower levels assessments ($5.7 \pm 1.8\,\mu$M versus $13.1 \pm 9.1\,\mu$M, resp., $P < 0.001$). A significant reduction in total-cholesterol/HDL-cholesterol ratio was observed in statin group after treatment ($P < 0.0001$). A strong correlation was found between the gradient of nitrite levels and the differential of total-cholesterol/HDL-cholesterol ratio in atorvastatin group ($r = 0.7$; $P < 0.001$). *Conclusions.* Improvement of nitrite levels are associated with decreased total cholesterol/HDL ratio values in PAD patients treated with atorvastatin.

1. Introduction

Peripheral arterial disease (PAD), the clinical manifestation of atherosclerosis in the lower limbs, is caused by a systemic chronic inflammatory state that affects the entire vascular system [1, 2]. Endothelial damage plays a crucial role in the etiopathogenia of this disease [3].

Endothelial dysfunction is considered to be an early event of atherosclerosis, preceding evidence of atherosclerotic plaques on angiography or ultrasound scan. Such endothelial dysfunction has been attributed to an impairment in nitric oxide (NO) bioactivity, and an increase in the formation of reactive oxygen species (ROS) [4]. NO has several antiatherosclerot-ic effects, such as inhibition of monocyte migration, inhibition of smooth muscle cell proliferation, and inhibition of platelet aggregation [2–4].

Nitrites are the product of the oxidation of the NO derived from the endothelium. Under physiological conditions, 70%–90% of the nitrites in plasma stem from endothelial nitric oxide synthase (eNOS) activity. Patients with PAD have been shown to have increased plasma nitrite levels from the early stages of the disease though this condition is unrelated to the severity of PAD [3].

In turn, hypercholesterolemia is an independent well-established risk factor for the development of atherosclerosis [5]. Previous studies have demonstrated that hypercholesterolemia is associated with endothelial dysfunction [6–8]. It is known to reduce endothelial function either by decreasing the synthesis and release of endothelium-derived relaxing factors or by inactivating NO after its release from endothelial cells by its reactions with superoxide radicals [9].

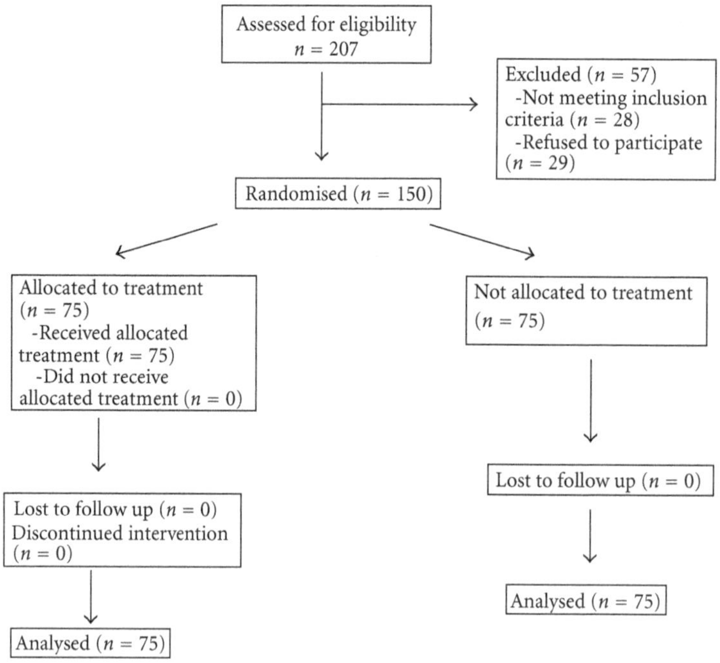

FIGURE 1: Method of randomization and allocation concealment.

Meanwhile, high-density lipoprotein (HDL) has anti-atherosclerotic effects, including augmentation of ability of reverse cholesterol transport, anti-inflammatory activity, inhibition of low-density lipoprotein (LDL) cholesterol oxidation, endothelial cell apoptosis, platelet aggregation, expression of cellular adhesion molecules, and re-endo-vascularization [10, 11].

Plasma HDL levels have been inversely related to the incidence of atherothrombotic disease [12, 13]. Part of its atheroprotective effect has been associated to its role in preserving endothelial function [14, 15]. In fact, several studies have suggested that a decrease in total-cholesterol/HDL-cholesterol ratio is linked to a reduction in the risk of morbidity and mortality in cardiovascular diseases [16–18].

There is some evidence that cholesterol-lowering therapy improves endothelium-dependent vasodilation in patients with normal lipid profile [19, 20]. However, there is little information regarding the effects of changes in total-cholesterol/HDL-cholesterol ratio per se on endothelium function in subjects with PAD.

The purpose of this study was to evaluate the effects of variations of total-cholesterol/HDL-cholesterol ratio on endothelial function indirectly determined by means of measurement of nitrite plasma levels in subjects with PAD. We evaluated the effects of the 3-hydroxy-3-methyl-glutaryl-CoA reductase (HMG-CoA reductase) inhibitor atorvastatin on endothelial function in these subjects.

2. Material and Methods

A prospective, experimental, randomised controlled, and translational study was carried out. There were sequentially included and randomized 150 PAD patients with Fontaine stage II at the time of diagnosis, confirmed by means of haemodynamic study (Doppler) and treadmill stress tests. All the patients included have not undergone previous revascularization procedure and were not received treatment with statins or contraindications for their use. We also excluded all patients with coexistence of chronic inflammatory diseases or steroidal medication.

The target patients who met the inclusion criteria were recruited and assessed in a screening visit at the outpatient clinic of the Angiology and Vascular Surgery Department of the Getafe University Hospital. When the criteria were met, and after signing the informed consent form, the patients were randomly allocated in a 1 : 1 ratio to the experimental intervention arm or the control group (Figure 1). A computer-generated random number sequence was used for randomization. The sequence was concealed until the study arm was assigned. There were three independent vascular surgeons investigators: one who recruited and evaluated the potential target patient in the screening visit and recorded cardiovascular risk factors, treatment, and general condition at the inclusion and after a month of the inclusion, blinded to the arm to which the patients were randomized; one who generated the allocation sequence; another who enrolled participants and assigned them to one of the study groups. Patients in the control group ($n = 75$) were prescribed treatment with aspirin 100 mg or clopidogrel 75 mg daily, if aspirin intolerant, angiotensin-converting-enzyme (ACE) inhibitors, and cardiovascular-risk-factors control. All patients in the experimental group ($n = 75$) also received atorvastatin 40 mg daily for a month.

Cardiovascular risk factors, treatment, and general condition were recorded on inclusion and after a month of treatment with statin. Ankle brachial index (ABI) was measured at rest as per the standard technique in the dorsalis pedis and posterior tibial arteries of both lower limbs [21]. Blood tests were performed at baseline and after one month of treatment with statin, which included basic clinical chemistry (glycemia, renal function, electrolytes, etc.) and lipid profile. Patients with plasma total cholesterol greater than 6.5 mmol L^{-1}, LDL cholesterol greater than 3.2 mmol L^{-1} or triglycerides greater than 2.25 mmol L^{-1}, or those on lipid-lowering treatment were considered to have dyslipidaemia [22]. Patients were considered to be hypertensive if they presented with systolic blood pressure greater than 140 mmHg and/or diastolic pressure greater than 90 mmHg and/or were on antihypertensive treatment for at least 1 year prior to inclusion in the study [23]. Patients were considered diabetic if they presented with baseline blood sugar greater than 120 g dL^{-1} or if they required treatment with hypoglycaemics [24]. Chronic renal failure was defined as serum creatinine greater than 1.5 mg dL^{-1} [25].

For the determination of plasma nitrite levels, the subjects came to the study having fasted for at least 12 hours and without having taken their usual medication during that period. Blood was drawn from an antecubital vein and centrifuged for 10 min at 800 g, with plasma then being stored at −4°C. Plasma nitrite concentrations were determined by colourimetric assay based on the Griess reaction [26]. This is a chemical reaction which uses sulfanilamide and N-(1-naphthyl) ethylenediamine dihydrochloride (NED) under acidic conditions (phosphoric acid). The system can detect NO_2^- in a variety of biological and experimental fluids, the limit of detection being 2.5 mM (125 pmol). Each sample was analysed in triplicate, taking the mean of the three determinations. The blood tests were repeated in a control group of 10 patients to assess the reproducibility of the test, the coefficient of variation being less than 5%.

Cholesterol and triglyceride levels were measured by enzymatic techniques [27, 28]. HDL cholesterol was measured after precipitation of apoB-containing lipoproteins with polyanions [29] and VLDL cholesterol after separation of VLDL ($d < 1.006\,g \cdot mL^{-1}$) by ultracentrifugation [30]. The LDL cholesterol was calculated by subtracting VLDL and HDL cholesterol from total cholesterol.

The laboratory data were determined anonymously, so that the results would not be biased.

This study was approved by the Ethical Committee of Getafe University Hospital.

2.1. Statistical Analysis. The sample size necessary to obtain significant differences with 80% of statistical power and an alpha error of 0.5 was calculated on the basis of previous studies which analysed NO levels in plasma in patients of similar condition [2, 3]. This sample size needed was estimated as 45 patients. Student's t-test was used for the end-points variables with normal distribution analysis and the Mann-Whitney U-test for those in which the distribution was not normal. The Kolmogorov-Smirnov and Shapiro-Wilk tests were used for the analysis of normality. The χ^2-test was used for categorical variables and the Spearman' s-test for the correlation between continuous variables. The data were expressed as mean ± standard deviation (SD) and the categorical as percentages. Statistical significance was assumed for P value <0.05.

Table 1: Demographic data and treatment.

	Treatment group N (75) (%)	Control group N (75) (%)	P
Age	71.4 ± 10.8	70.51 ± 9.7	n.s
Male	65 (87)	62 (82.6)	n.s
Hypertension	55 (73.3)	57 (76)	n.s
DM	30 (40)	33 (44)	n.s
Current smoking	41 (55)	39 (52)	n.s
Ex smoker	26 (35)	32 (42.6)	n.s
AMI	10 (14)	8 (10.6)	n.s
Dyslipidaemia	18 (25)	12 (16)	n.s
CVA	5 (6.6)	6 (8)	n.s
Antiplatelet treatment	65 (86.6)	69 (92)	n.s
ACE inhibitors	35 (46.7)	30 (40)	n.s
ARA-II	10 (13.3)	8 (10.6)	n.s
B-blocker	11 (14.6)	12 (16)	n.s
Nitrites	5 (6.7)	3 (4)	n.s
CA antagonists	15 (20)	17 (22.6)	n.s

DM: diabetes mellitus; AMI: acute myocardial infarction; CVA: cerebrovascular accident.

3. Results

207 patients were consecutively assessed for inclusion in the study. Twenty-eight were excluded for not meeting inclusion criteria. Twenty-nine refused to participate, after we had explained in detail the conditions of the study and the hard recommendation of meeting the follow-up visits established per protocol. 150 patients with Fontaine stage II PAD were recruited and randomly assigned to each group, treatment ($n = 75$), and control ($n = 75$). The patient demographics features and current treatment are described in Table 1. Thus, there were no patient dropouts during the study. All 150 patients included completed the study protocol and were analysed for the primary outcome. No major adverse reactions to the treatment with statin were recorded.

After one month of treatment with statin, a significant reduction in plasma nitrite levels was detected in treatment group patients (11.88 ± 7.8 μM versus 5.7 ± 1.8 μM, $P < 0.0001$) and in the comparison between treatment and control groups (5.7 ± 1.8 μM versus 13.1 ± 9.1 μM, resp., $P < 0.001$). No changes were found in the nitrite levels in the control group patients over the course of the study (12.5 ± 5.1 μM versus 13.1 ± 9.1 μM, $P = 0.83$) (Figure 2).

A significant reduction in plasma levels of total cholesterol, LDL cholesterol, total-cholesterol/HDL-cholesterol ratio, and total triglycerides was observed in treatment group (Table 2).

We defined differential of total-cholesterol/HDL-cholesterol ratio in treatment group as the difference between total-cholesterol/HDL-cholesterol ratio baseline value and total-cholesterol/HDL-cholesterol ratio 1st month treatment value. As well as differential of nitrite plasma levels

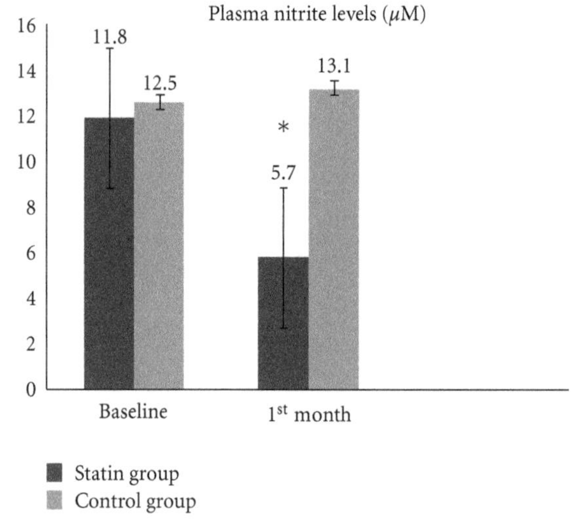

FIGURE 2: Comparison of plasma nitrite levels (μM) at baseline and after a month of atorvastatin therapy ($^{*}P < 0.05$ on comparison baseline versus a month treatment). There were no statistical differences between the control group data.

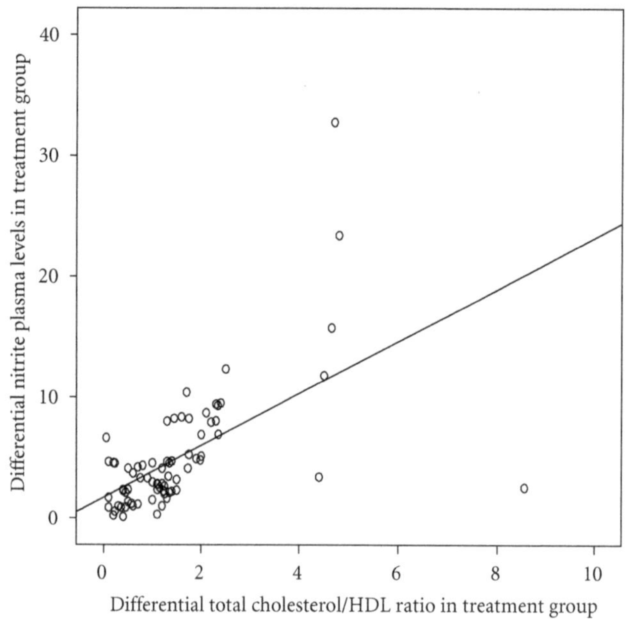

FIGURE 3: Positive Spearman's correlation between differential total cholesterol/HDL ratio and differential nitrite plasma levels in treatment group ($r = 0.7$, $P < 0.001$).

TABLE 2: Initial lipid-profile values and values after 1 month of treatment with atorvastatin.

	Mean ± DS	P
Total CHOL baseline	5.4 ± 1.3 mmol L^{-1}	0.0001
Total CHOL after treatment	3.8 ± 0.1 mmol L^{-1}	
LDL-CHOL baseline	$3.4 \pm 1.$ mmol L^{-1}	0.0001
LDL-CHOL after treatment	1.8 ± 0.6 mmol L^{-1}	
HDL-CHOL baseline	1.3 ± 0.3 mmol L^{-1}	0.12
HDL-CHOL after treatment	1.4 ± 0.4 mmol L^{-1}	
CHOL/HDL baseline	4 ± 0.9 mmol L^{-1}	0.0001
CHOL/HDL after treatment	2.7 ± 0.6 mmol L^{-1}	
TGC baseline	1.3 ± 0.5 mmol L^{-1}	0.024
TGC after treatment	1.1 ± 0.4 mmol L^{-1}	
TGC/HDL baseline	2.3 ± 1.3 mmol L^{-1}	0.113
TGC/HDL after treatment	2 ± 1.2 mmol L^{-1}	

in treatment group as the difference between nitrite basal levels and nitrite levels after one month of treatment with atorvastatin. A strong positive Spearman's correlation was found between the differential of nitrite levels in plasma and the differential of total-cholesterol/HDL-cholesterol ratio on atorvastatin group (rs 0.7; $P < 0.001$) (Figure 3).

4. Discussion

The current study evaluated and analysed in vivo, the effects of the HMG-coA reductase inhibitors upon variations of NO bioavailability and variations in plasma levels of total-cholesterol/HDL-cholesterol ratio, in patients with PAD. Our data revealed that decrease in total-cholesterol/HDL-cholesterol ratio was correlated with reduction of nitrite levels in patients with PAD and atorvastatin treatment.

Hypercholesterolemia is a well-established risk factor for atherosclerosis, in particular by decreasing the availability of nitric oxide [31]. Oxidative stress is known to contribute to atherogenesis, and, during this process, lipid peroxidation takes place in lipoproteins as well as in arterial macrophages [32]. The result is a drop in the bioavailability of endothelial NO, a reduction in the effective lumen of the vessel, and an increase in sensitivity to acetylcholine-induced vasoconstriction.

Several lines of evidence indicate that HDL has beneficial antiatherosclerotic effects [10, 11]. HDL acts as a reverse cholesterol transporter by removing excess cellular cholesterol to the liver, resulting in protection against atherosclerosis. This is the predominant antiatherosclerotic effect of HDL. However, HDL has multifactorial effects to protect vascular function. Thus, HDL activates endothelial NO synthase by enhancing Akt and MAP kinases leading to an increase in NO, suppresses endothelial cell apoptosis by activation of the Akt pathway and inhibition of caspase 3 and 9, inhibits the oxidation of LDLs, limits inflammation processes, stimulates prostacyclin production, and upregulates cyclooxygenase-2 expression leading to anticoagulation and vasodilation [10, 11]. Therefore, under a low HDL cholesterol condition, atherosclerotic processes develop progressively, resulting in cardiovascular impairment.

Previous studies related to the effects of atorvastatin therapy on lipid profile and oxidative stress revealed that atorvastatin therapy decreased the levels of oxidative stress [33]. An improvement on endothelial function has been described in patients diagnosed of PAD treated with atorvastatin at the beginning of the treatment. Nevertheless, this effect was not maintained at long term [34]. Different mechanisms by which atorvastatin improves endothelial function have been postulated. It is well known that statins augment endothelium-dependent vasodilation through an increase in NO bioavailability and decrease in oxidative stress and inflammation [35, 36]. In the present study, we have observed that four-week treatment with the HMG-CoA reductase inhibitor atorvastatin in patients with PAD decreased total-cholesterol/HDL-cholesterol ratio, and this is associated with the improvement on endothelial function provoked at the beginning of the statin treatment. According the results of this study, it could be hypothesized that a possible mechanism by which atorvastatin improves endothelial function is by its decreasing Total-cholesterol/HDL-cholesterol ratio effect.

Nevertheless, recent studies have shown that atorvastatin has more beneficial effects on endothelial function than other statins at similar lipid reduction [37]. However, the conclusions from other studies remain inconsistent [38] contributing to certain controversy.

Anyway, Sugiura et al. have previously described an inverse correlation between total-cholesterol/HDL-cholesterol ratio and endothelial function by flow-mediated dilatation [39]. Our data support their results through variations of nitrite plasma levels. In addition, these findings underline the importance of plasma total-cholesterol/HDL-cholesterol values as a risk factor of endothelial dysfunction in PAD patients. It is noteworthy that the correlation between nitrite levels and total-cholesterol/HDL-cholesterol found in the current study was mainly determined by increasing levels of HDL after atorvastatin treatment.

The limitations of this study include the fact that nitrite levels are influenced by endogenous and exogenous factors such as dietary nitrates, the inhalation of atmospheric NO, its formation in the salivary glands, and renal function. Although it is not possible to exclude these factors, these data are in line with observations from earlier studies. While dealing with plasma nitrites and not other nitrates may seem to be a limitation, it is known that over 70%–90% of all plasma nitrites originate from eNOS activity [40].

5. Conclusions

The present study demonstrated that improvement of nitrite plasma levels, a marker of endothelial function, is associated with decreased total cholesterol/HDL ratio values in patients with PAD treated with atorvastatin. In the early stages of PAD, the impact of total-cholesterol/HDL-cholesterol ratio may relate to endothelial damage.

References

[1] R. Ross, "Atherosclerosis—an inflammatory disease," *The New England Journal of Medicine*, vol. 340, no. 2, pp. 115–126, 1999.

[2] J. De Haro, F. Acín, A. López-Quintana et al., "Direct assotiation between C-reactive protein serum levels and endothelial dysfunction in patients with claudication," *European Journal of Vascular and Endovascular Surgery*, vol. 35, pp. 480–486, 2008.

[3] J. De Haro, E. Martínez-Aguilar, A. Florez, C. Varela, S. Bleda, and F. Acin, "Nitric oxide: link between endothelial dysfunction and inflammation in patients with peripheral arterial disease of the lower limbs," *Interactive Cardiovascular and Thoracic Surgery*, vol. 9, no. 1, pp. 107–112, 2009.

[4] L. J. Ignarro, G. Cirino, A. Casini, and C. Napoli, "Nitric oxide as a signaling molecule in the vascular system: an overview," *Journal of Cardiovascular Pharmacology*, vol. 34, no. 6, pp. 879–886, 1999.

[5] A. Zulli, D. L. Hare, B. F. Buxton, and M. J. Black, "High dietary methionine plus cholesterol exacerbates atherosclerosis formation in the left main coronary artery of rabbits," *Atherosclerosis*, vol. 176, no. 1, pp. 83–89, 2004.

[6] M. A. Creager, J. P. Cooke, M. E. Mendelsohn et al., "Impaired vasodilation of forearm resistance vessels in hypercholesterolemic humans," *Journal of Clinical Investigation*, vol. 86, no. 1, pp. 228–234, 1990.

[7] M. J. Mullen, R. K. Kharbanda, J. Cross et al., "Heterogenous nature of flow-mediated dilatation in human conduit arteries in vivo: relevance to endothelial dysfunction in hypercholesterolemia," *Circulation Research*, vol. 88, no. 2, pp. 145–151, 2001.

[8] A. M. Zeiher, H. Drexler, B. Saurbier, and H. Just, "Endothelium-mediated coronary blood flow modulation in humans: effects of age, atherosclerosis, hypercholesterolemia, and hypertension," *Journal of Clinical Investigation*, vol. 92, no. 2, pp. 652–662, 1993.

[9] R. H. Böger, "Association of asymmetric dimethylarginine and endothelial dysfunction," *Clinical Chemistry and Laboratory Medicine*, vol. 41, no. 11, pp. 1467–1472, 2003.

[10] B. J. Ansell, K. E. Watson, A. M. Fogelman, M. Navab, and G. C. Fonarow, "High-density lipoprotein function: recent advances," *Journal of the American College of Cardiology*, vol. 46, no. 10, pp. 1792–1798, 2005.

[11] J. Davignon, "Beneficial cardiovascular pleiotropic effects of statins," *Circulation*, vol. 109, supplement 1, no. 23, pp. III39–III43, 2004.

[12] D. J. Gordon and B. M. Rifkind, "High-density lipoprotein—the clinical implications of recent studies," *The New England Journal of Medicine*, vol. 321, no. 19, pp. 1311–1316, 1989.

[13] G. Assmann and A. M. Gotto, "HDL cholesterol and protective factors in atherosclerosis," *Circulation*, vol. 109, supplement 1, no. 23, pp. III8–III14, 2004.

[14] X. P. Li, S. P. Zhao, X. Y. Zhang, L. Liu, M. Gao, and Q. C. Zhou, "Protective effect of high density lipoprotein on endothelium-dependent vasodilatation," *International Journal of Cardiology*, vol. 73, no. 3, pp. 231–236, 2000.

[15] J. T. Kuvin, A. R. Patel, M. Sidhu et al., "Relation between high-density lipoprotein cholesterol and peripheral vasomotor function," *American Journal of Cardiology*, vol. 92, no. 3, pp. 275–279, 2003.

[16] K. K. Ray, C. P. Cannon, R. Cairns, D. A. Morrow, P. M. Ridker, and E. Braunwald, "Prognostic utility of ApoB/AI, total cholesterol/HDL, Non-HDL cholesterol, or hs-CRP as predictors of clinical risk in patients receiving statin therapy after acute coronary syndromes results from PROVE IT-TIMI 22," *Arteriosclerosis, Thrombosis, and Vascular Biology*, vol. 29, no. 3, pp. 423–430, 2009.

[17] U. Keil, A. D. Liese, H. W. Hense et al., "Classical risk factors and their impact on incident non-fatal and fatal myocardial infarction and all-cause mortality in southern Germany," *European Heart Journal*, vol. 19, no. 8, pp. 1197–1207, 1998.

[18] J. T. Real, F. J. Chaves, I. Martínez-Usó, A. B. García-García, J. F. Ascaso, and R. Carmena, "Importance of HDL cholesterol

levels and the total/HDL cholesterol ratio as a risk factor for coronary heart disease in molecularly defined heterozygous familial hypercholesterolaemia," *European Heart Journal*, vol. 22, no. 6, pp. 465–471, 2001.

[19] M. Myoishi, H. Hao, T. Minamino et al., "Increased endoplasmic reticulum stress in atherosclerotic plaques associated with acute coronary syndrome," *Circulation*, vol. 116, no. 11, pp. 1226–1233, 2007.

[20] N. Wang, D. L. Silver, P. Costet, and A. R. Tall, "Specific binding of ApoA-I, enhanced cholesterol efflux, and altered plasma membrane morphology in cells expressing ABC1," *Journal of Biological Chemistry*, vol. 275, no. 42, pp. 33053–33058, 2000.

[21] A. B. Newman, L. Shemanski, T. A. Manolio et al., "Ankle-arm index as a predictor of cardiovascular disease and mortality in the Cardiovascular Health study," *Arteriosclerosis, Thrombosis, and Vascular Biology*, vol. 19, no. 3, pp. 538–545, 1999.

[22] National Heart, Lung, and Blood Institute, "Third report of the national cholesterol education program (NCEP) expert panel on detection, evaluation, and treatment of high blood cholesterol in adults (adult treatment panel III, or ATPIII)," 2006, http://www.nhlbi.nih.gov/guidelines/cholesterol/atglance.htm.

[23] P. Verdecchia and F. Angeli, "The seventh report of the joint national committee on the prevention, detection, evaluation and treatment of high blood pressure: the weapons are ready," *Revista Espanola de Cardiologia*, vol. 56, no. 9, pp. 843–847, 2003.

[24] Expert Committee on the Diagnosis and Classification of Diabetes Mellitus, "Report of the expert committee on the diagnosis and classification of diabetes mellitus," *Diabetes Care*, vol. 24, supplement 1, pp. 5–20, 2001.

[25] R. Ferrer and J. Hernández Jara, "Chronic renal insufficiency. I: definition, clinical course stages, progression mechanisms, etiology, and diagnostic criteria," *Nefrologia*, vol. 21, pp. 18–20, 2001.

[26] P. Kleinbongard, T. Rassaf, A. Dejam, S. Kerber, and M. Kelm, "Griess method for nitrite measurement of aqueous and protein-containing samples," *Methods in Enzymology*, vol. 359, pp. 158–168, 2002.

[27] C. C. Allain, L. S. Poon, and C. S. G. Chan, "Enzymatic determination of total serum cholesterol," *Clinical Chemistry*, vol. 20, no. 4, pp. 470–475, 1974.

[28] H. F. ter Welle, T. Baartscheer, and J. W. Fiolet, "Influence of free glycerol on enzymic evaluation of triglycerides," *Clinical Chemistry*, vol. 30, no. 6, pp. 1102–1103, 1984.

[29] M. Burstein, H. R. Scholnick, and R. Morfin, "Rapid method for the isolation of lipoproteins from human serum by precipitation with polyanions," *Journal of Lipid Research*, vol. 11, no. 6, pp. 583–595, 1970.

[30] R. J. Havel, H. J. Eder, and J. H. Bragdon, "The distribution and chemical composition of ultracentrifugally separated lipoproteins in human serum," *The Journal of clinical investigation*, vol. 34, no. 9, pp. 1345–1353, 1955.

[31] C. Rasmusen, L. Cynober, and R. Couderc, "Arginine and statins: relationship between the nitric oxide pathway and the atherosclerosis development," *Annales de Biologie Clinique*, vol. 63, no. 5, pp. 443–455, 2005.

[32] M. Rosenblat, T. Hayek, K. Hussein, and M. Aviram, "Decreased macrophage paraoxonase 2 expression in patients with hypercholesterolemia is the result of their increased cellular cholesterol content: effect of atorvastatin therapy," *Arteriosclerosis, Thrombosis, and Vascular Biology*, vol. 24, no. 1, pp. 175–180, 2004.

[33] M. Harangi, I. Seres, Z. Varga et al., "Atorvastatin effect on high-density lipoprotein-associated paraoxonase activity and oxidative DNA damage," *European Journal of Clinical Pharmacology*, vol. 60, no. 10, pp. 685–691, 2004.

[34] S. Bleda, J. de Haro, A. Florez, C. Varela, L. Esparza, and F. Acin, "Long-term pleiotropic effect of statins upon nitric oxide and C-reactive protein levels in patients with peripheral arterial disease," *Heart Asia*, vol. 3, pp. 130–134, 2011.

[35] Y. Kureishi, Z. Luo, I. Shiojima et al., "The HMG-CoA reductase inhibitor simvastatin activates the protein kinase Akt and promotes angiogenesis in normocholesterolemic animals," *Nature Medicine*, vol. 6, no. 9, pp. 1004–1010, 2000.

[36] Y. Rikitake and J. K. Liao, "Rho GTPases, statins, and nitric oxide," *Circulation Research*, vol. 97, no. 12, pp. 1232–1235, 2005.

[37] M. K. Reriani, S. M. Dunlay, B. Gupta et al., "Effects of statins on coronary and peripheral endothelial function in humans: a systematic review and meta-analysis of randomized controlled trials," *European Journal of Cardiovascular Prevention and Rehabilitation*, vol. 18, no. 5, pp. 704–716, 2011.

[38] J. R. Murrow, S. Sher, S. Ali et al., "The differential effect of statins on oxidative stress and endothelial function: atorvastatin versus pravastatin," *Journal of Clinical Lipidology*, vol. 6, no. 1, pp. 42–49, 2012.

[39] T. Sugiura, Y. Dohi, S. Yamashita et al., "Impact of lipid profile and high blood pressure on endothelial damage," *Journal of Clinical Lipidology*, vol. 5, no. 6, pp. 460–466, 2011.

[40] P. Kleinbongard, A. Dejam, T. Lauer et al., "Plasma nitrite reflects constitutive nitric oxide synthase activity in mammals," *Free Radical Biology and Medicine*, vol. 35, no. 7, pp. 790–796, 2003.

Relationship of Lifestyle Medical Advice and Non-HDL Cholesterol Control of a Nationally Representative US Sample with Hypercholesterolemia by Race/Ethnicity

Joan Anne Vaccaro[1] and Fatma G. Huffman[2]

[1] *Department of Dietetics and Nutrition, MMC AHC 1-450, Florida International University, Miami, FL 33199, USA*
[2] *Department of Dietetics and Nutrition, MMC AHC 1-435, Florida International University, Miami, FL 33199, USA*

Correspondence should be addressed to Fatma G. Huffman, huffmanf@fiu.edu

Academic Editor: Gloria L. Vega

Objective. The main purpose of this study was to evaluate the associations of lifestyle medical advice and non-HDL cholesterol control of a nationally representative US sample of adults with hypercholesterolemia by race/ethnicity. *Methods*. Data were collected by appending sociodemographic, anthropometric, and laboratory data from two cycles of the National Health and Nutrition Survey (2007-2008 and 2009-2010). This study acquired data from male and female adults aged ≥ 20 years ($N = 11,577$), classified as either Mexican American (MA), ($n = 2173$), other Hispanic (OH) ($n = 1298$), Black non-Hispanic (BNH) ($n = 2349$), or White non-Hispanic (WNH) ($n = 5737$). *Results*. Minorities were more likely to report having received dietary, weight management, and exercise recommendations by healthcare professionals than WNH, adjusting for confounders. Approximately 80% of those receiving medical advice followed the recommendation, regardless of race/ethnicity. Of those who received medical advice, reporting "currently controlling or losing weight" was associated with lower non-HDL cholesterol. BNH who reported "currently controlling or losing weight" had higher non-HDL cholesterol than WNH who reported following the advice. *Conclusion*. The results suggest that current methods of communicating lifestyle advice may not be adequate across race/ethnicity and that a change in perspective and delivery of medical recommendations for persons with hypercholesterolemia is needed.

1. Introduction

Cholesterol, the functional unit of numerous, essential hormones and steroids in the human body, circulates in blood. Even though cholesterol is necessary for body function, elevated levels can result in atherosclerosis and cardiovascular disease. Levels of serum cholesterol less than 200 mg/dL are considered in the healthy, normal range; borderline cholesterol is 200–239 mg/dL; elevated blood cholesterol, 240 mg/dL or above, is classified as high cholesterol [1]. Primary goals of therapy and treatment are focused on low-density lipoprotein cholesterol (LDL-C) < 100 mg/dL, where 130 mg/dL is considered borderline high [1]. Despite the decrease in LDL-C since the 1960s, hypercholesterolemia, a key risk factor of atherosclerosis and coronary heart disease, currently affects nearly half of the US adult population [2]. Hypercholesterolemia is a metabolic disorder characterized by high levels of serum cholesterol, particularly LDL-C. For treatment purposes, hypercholesterolemia individually diagnosed based on high LDL-C and concurrence of other cardiovascular disease risk factors such as smoking, hypertension, diabetes, and a family history of premature coronary heart disease [3]. The recommended treatment of hypercholesterolemia involves weight loss, dietary and physical activity changes, and a possible medical regime. Prescription of LDL-C lowering medications should be reserved for aggressive treatment when LDL-C levels do not respond to dietary modifications and increased exercise [3, 4]. The side effects of statins, a commonly prescribed cholesterol-lowing medication, may outweigh their benefit for otherwise healthy adults [4].

A diagnosis of hypercholesterolemia and consequent treatment is only possible for adults who had adequate medical care, which included blood collection for a lipid panel. Among a nationally representative sample of US adults in 2005-2006, aged 20 years or older, only three-quarters reported ever having their cholesterol checked with lower reports for Mexican Americans and non-Hispanic Blacks as compared to non-Hispanic Whites [2]. Minorities have been reported to have less access and quality of health care for cholesterol screening and treatment [5]. Even when treated for hypercholesterolemia, a lower percent of minorities were prescribed dietary and exercise counseling, based on a representative US sample of approximately 27 million adults, aged ≥20 years, from a medical registry [5].

Because the initial treatment of hypercholesterolemia involves dietary and physical activity changes, it is imperative that the diagnosed individuals recall having received these lifestyle medical recommendations. Therefore, the aim of this study was to examine a US representative sample of adults for the years 2007–2010 and to investigate the following (1) the likelihood of lifestyle medical advice received differing by race/ethnicity for those adults who had their cholesterol checked; (2) percents of adults given and following medical advice; (3) the association of non-HDL cholesterol with reporting following lifestyle medical advice.

2. Materials and Methods

2.1. Data Collection. All data used for this study were approved by the research ethics board and publically available from appended 2-year cycles of datasets from the National Health and Nutrition Examination Survey (NHANES) 2007-2008 and 2009-2010 [6]. NHANES uses a complex, multistage, probability sample design to obtain representative samples of the noninstitutionalized, civilian US population [6]. This study acquired data from male and female adults aged ≥20 years ($N = 11,577$). The final sample size for participants with hypercholesterolemia and measurements of total and/or non-HDL cholesterol was 3325 (MA = 505; OH = 362; BNH = 614; WNH = 1844).

2.2. Major Variables. Hypercholesterolemia was considered an affirmative answer to "ever told by a doctor or other health care professional that you had a high blood cholesterol level". Non-HDL cholesterol was constructed by subtracting HDL-C from total cholesterol. *Cholesterol control* (yes/no) was constructed as a binary variable with non-HDL cholesterol <130 mg/dL considered adequate control versus ≥130 mg/dL as inadequate control. The number of participants with this cutoff was chosen based on the National Cholesterol Education Program's (NCEP-ATP III) guideline of 130 mg/dL for persons with >20% cardiovascular disease risk [1] and the American Association of Clinical Endocrinologists' (AACE) guidelines of non-HDL cholesterol as 30 mg/dL above the goal (<100 mg/dL) for LDL-C [7]. *Medical advice* (yes, no) for weight, diet, and exercise were the major independent variables and phrased as follows: to lower your blood cholesterol have you ever been told by your doctor or other health professional to: (1) eat fewer high-fat or high-cholesterol foods? (2) control weight or lose weight? (3) increase physical activity or exercise?

2.3. Adjustment Variables. Comorbidities of hypercholesterolemia used in the analysis were coronary heart disease, diabetes, and hypertension. Coronary heart disease was defined as an affirmative response to the question, "Has a doctor or other health professional ever told you that you had coronary heart disease?" Diabetes was considered an affirmative answer to the question, "Has a doctor or other health care professional told you that you had diabetes or sugar diabetes?" Having hypertension was defined as a systolic blood pressure ≥140 mm Hg, a diastolic blood pressure ≥90 mm Hg (using the average of first two readings), or taking hypertension medication [8].

Obesity was estimated using the proxy measurement of body mass index (BMI) and was calculated from measured weight and height (kg/m^2) and was categorized based on the National Institutes of Health's recommended levels: normal weight (<24.9 kg/m^2); overweight (24.9–29.9 kg/m^2); obese I (30.0–34.4 kg/m^2); obese II or more (≥35 kg/m^2) [9]. A binary variable was created for current cigarette use versus not currently smoking. Education was assessed as < high school; high school diploma or general equivalency diploma; > high school. Health insurance was defined as having any coverage within the past 12 months (yes/no).

2.4. Statistical Analysis. Chi-square tests were performed to determine hypercholesterolemia and medical advice by ethnicity. Logistic regression analyses were conducted for non-HDL cholesterol control as the outcome variable. Reduced models included race/ethnicity adjusted for age and gender. Fully adjusted models included the covariates of the simple models along with: currently smoking, BMI, education, health insurance, and lipid-lowering medication. In addition, hypertension, diabetes, and coronary heart disease were added to test medical advice received by race/ethnicity. Adjusted sample weights were used to account for unequal probabilities of selection and nonresponse in the multistage stratified cluster sampling design used in NHANES in order to achieve unbiased national estimates. The sample weights used were based on the data file with the smallest sample size, the Mobile Examination Center (MEC), and were computed using the average of the 2-year sample weights for each cycle, as per guidelines set by NHANES [10]. Data analysis was conducted with complex module, IBM-SPSS version 19. The Wald F statistic was used to determine model significance for logistic regression analysis [11]. For the chi-squared test, significance was based on the adjusted F statistic, a variant of the second-order Rao Scott adjusted chi-square statistic used for analyses with sample weights, where $df1 + df2 = 33$ (total degrees of freedom).

3. Results

Key risk factors associated with hypercholesterolemia are shown in Table 1. There were significant differences in major

Table 1: Major hypercholesterolemia risk factors of the study population by race/ethnicity.

Variable	MA	OH	BNH	WNH	*P* value
Cholesterol checked (yes)	51.2 (1.6)[a]	60.5 (2.2)[b]	69.7 (1.3)[c]	78.5 (0.9)[d]	<.001
Inadequate non-HDL-C (≥130 mg/dL)	25.8 (2.0)[a]	22.1 (2.5)[a]	33.1 (2.1)[b]	30.6 (1.1)[b]	.008
High cholesterol (≥200 mg/dL)	45.9 (1.4)[a]	42.1 (2.2)[a,b]	39.7 (1.3)[b]	44.5 (0.9)[a,b]	.019
Lipid-lowering medications (yes)	50.7 (3.4)[−]	44.1 (3.4)[−]	51.7 (1.8)[−]	54.7 (1.6)[−]	.129
Age (years)	51.2 (1.2)[a]	52.3 (1.1)[a,b]	53.8 (0.5)[b]	57.4 (0.3)[c]	<.001
Education: <HS	51.5 (1.6)[a]	37.7 (2.4)[b]	26.1 (1.7)[c]	13.8 (1.4)[d]	<.001
No health insurance	52.2 (1.9)[a]	36.3 (3.1)[b]	26.0 (1.4)[c]	13.7 (0.7)[d]	<.001
Current smoker	11.4 (1.1)[a]	14.5 (1.8)[a]	21.7 (1.7)[b]	19.1 (1.2)[b]	<.001
BMI 30–34.9 (kg/m^2) obesity I	22.5 (1.6)[a]	18.6 (1.4)[b,c]	21.6 (1.3)[a,c]	18.5 (0.6)[b]	<.001
BMI ≥ 35(kg/m^2) obesity II	18.0 (0.8)[a]	17.0 (1.3)[a]	26.1 (1.2)[b]	16.2 (0.6)[a]	<.001
HTN (yes)	19.2 (1.4)[a]	21.1 (1.6)[a]	38.7 (1.3)[b]	31.8 (1.0)[c]	<.001
Diabetes (yes)	8.4 (0.8)[a]	8.5 (0.8)[a]	13.5 (0.8)[b]	7.6 (0.6)[c]	<.001
CHD (yes)	1.8 (0.3)[a]	1.4 (0.3)[a]	1.6 (0.2)[a]	3.7 (0.2)[b]	<.001

MA: Mexican American; OH: other Hispanic, not Mexican; BNH: Black non-Hispanic; WNH: White non-Hispanic; non-HDL-C: non-HDL cholesterol (total cholesterol minus HDL-C); BMI: body mass index; HTN: hypertension; CHD: coronary heart disease.

The data represent the weighted percent and standard error [% (SE)]. Significance is based on the adjusted *F*, a variant of the second-order Rao-Scott adjusted chi-square statistic and its degrees of freedom. Each superscript letter denotes a subset of race/ethnicity categories whose column proportions do not differ significantly from each other at the 0.05 level for each row (variable). Significant differences between each group were measured by complex logistic regression analyses across race/ethnicity separately for each dependent binary variable. Age was tested by complex general linear models, recoding ethnicity to measure differences between groups.

sociodemographics, body mass index, morbidities, and having cholesterol checks among race/ethnicity. WNH had the highest prevalence of reporting having their cholesterol checked followed by BNH, OH, and MA. For those with hypercholesterolemia, coronary heart disease was higher in WNH than other race/ethnicity categories. BNH, followed by WNH, had higher prevalence of hypertension as compared to Hispanics. BNH had a higher prevalence of obesity II [BMI ≥ 35(kg/m^2)] and diabetes than other groups. A lower percent of minorities were covered by health insurance with MA having the least coverage.

The likelihood of receiving medical advice by race/ethnicity is shown in Table 2. Compared to WNH, MA and BNH were more likely to be given advice to eat fewer high-fat or –cholesterol foods. MA and OH were more likely to be told to lose or control their weight as compared to WNH. All Hispanics and BNH were more likely to be told to increase physical activity or exercise as compared to WNH.

The percent of adults with hypercholesterolemia who reported affirmatively that they were given diet, weight, and exercise medical advice to reduce their cholesterol levels and who reported affirmatively now following the advice is shown in Table 3. Despite the fact that weight management and increasing physical activity are vital recommendations for individuals with hypercholesterolemia, approximately 40% and 30%, respectively, reported not receiving advice for these lifestyle behaviors. The majority of the participants (approximately 80%), who reported having received medical advice, followed the corresponding recommendations.

Participants who responded affirmatively to being given medical advice for hypercholesterolemia were included in a chi-squared test of whether they followed each recommendation (yes/no) across non-HDL-C control (<130 mg/dL, yes/≥130 mg/dL, no) (Table 3). Reporting now eating fewer fatty foods ($P = .002$) and now losing weight ($P = .005$) were significantly associated with the corresponding recommendation. Cholesterol control (non-HDL-C < 130 mg/dL) was found for approximately two-thirds of those who reported eating fewer fatty foods (67.5%, SE = 1.2%). Similarly, of those participants who reported now controlling or losing weight, 67.3% (SE = 1.4%) had cholesterol control (non-HDL-C < 130 mg/dL).

Reporting following medical recommendations for diet and physical activity (yes/no) and non-HDL cholesterol (continuous) was tested by a complex general linear model. The model was significant; however, of the behaviors only "now controlling or losing weight" was significant (data not shown). Reduced and full models were constructed for reporting "controlling or losing weight" by race/ethnicity (Table 4). Lower non-HDL cholesterol levels were associated with an affirmative report of "now controlling or losing weight" for the reduced model (adjusted only for age and gender ($P = .001$)). For the fully adjusted model, which included, BMI, health insurance, education, currently smoking, and lipid-lowering medication(s), the 2-way interaction "controlling or losing weight" by race/ethnicity was significant ($P = .014$) and the main effect (controlling or losing weight) was no longer significant ($P = .998$); however race/ethnicity remained significant ($P < .001$). BNH who reported "controlling or losing weight" had significantly higher non-HDL cholesterol as compared to WNH ($P = .003$).

Use of lipid-lowering medications did not negate the association of losing weight with non-HDL cholesterol as a continuous variable; however, for logistic regression models lipid-lowering medications did negate the likelihood of having cholesterol control (non-HDL cholesterol < 130 mg/dL); albeit the results were marginal [OR = 1.49 (1.18, 1.76),

Table 2: Odds ratios for receiving medical advice by race/ethnicity.

Dependent variable	Independent	Model 1	Model 2	Model 3
Told to eat less fat	MA	1.48 (1.09, 2.04)	1.59 (1.14, 2.20)	1.60 (1.14, 2.26)
	OH	1.10 (0.81, 1.48)	1.13 (0.82, 1.56)	1.15 (0.82, 1.60)
	BNH	1.70 (1.36, 2.12)	1.59 (1.37, 1.99)	1.49 (1.19, 1.86)
	WNH	1.00	1.00	1.00
Told to control or lose weight	MA	1.54 (1.12, 2.12)	1.58 (1.12, 2.21)	1.55 (1.07, 2.25)
	OH	1.75 (1.33, 2.31)	1.77 (1.32, 2.39)	1.75 (1.26, 2.41)
	BNH	1.37 (1.11, 1.70)	1.38 (1.11, 1.71)	1.21 (0.95, 1.54)
	WNH	1.00	1.00	1.00
Told to exercise	MA	1.65 (2.23, 2.22)	1.64 (1.21, 2.23)	1.64 (1.20, 2.26)
	OH	1.56 (1.20, 2.04)	1.56 (1.19, 2.06)	1.54 (1.15, 2.07)
	BNH	1.71 (1.41, 2.08)	1.51 (1.24, 1.85)	1.35 (1.09, 1.68)
	WNH	1.00	1.00	1.00

Model 1: adjusted for age and gender (and BMI for "told to control or lose weight").
Model 2: adjusted for age, gender, BMI, current smoker, education, and health insurance.
Model 3: adjusted for age, gender, BMI, current smoker, education, health insurance, coronary heart disease, diabetes, and hypertension.

Table 3: Percent of adults given and following medical advice.

Given the recommendation to lower serum cholesterol	Percent given the advice who are following the recommendation	SE
Told to eat less high-fat or high-cholesterol foods 81.8% (yes)	82.8 (80.7, 84.7)	1.0
Told to control weight or lose weight 59.4% (yes)	84.0 (81.3, 86.3)	1.2
Told to increase physical activity or exercise 69.9% (yes)	78.0 (75.4, 80.3)	1.2

Results are given as [mean (95% CI) SE].

with independents: race, gender, age, BMI, health insurance, education, and smoking; OR = 1.18 (0.93, 1.49) with the same independents and the additional covariate, lipid-lowering medications] (data not shown).

4. Discussion

In a nationally representative population of adults with hypercholesterolemia, we found discrepancies in medical advice for diet, weight management, and exercise by race/ethnicity. Reporting having received medical advice was associated with performing the recommended behavior; yet, over one-third of adults across race/ethnicity with hypercholesterolemia reported not receiving dietary, weight management, or exercise recommendations by either their physician or other health care professional. Moreover, there were differences by race/ethnicity in reporting having received these lifestyle recommendations. These results suggest confounders such as patient-provider relationships and health beliefs, which may vary by race/ethnicity and may also influence interpretation of advice and resulting health outcomes.

African Americans, as compared to WNH with comparable healthcare coverage, were found to have a poorer quality of patient-provider relationships as well as poorer control of cholesterol, in a national, multicentered prospective study of patients with diabetes [12]. In the current study, BNH who reported "controlling or losing weight" had significantly higher non-HDL cholesterol as compared to WNH. This disparity may be the result of differences in perceived vulnerability or susceptibility by race/ethnicity. In this case, BNH may not perceive danger of cardiac events until their cholesterol level in a higher range than their WNH counterparts.

The Agency for Health Care Research and Quality (AHRQ) [13] calculated 70% disparity (worsening or no improvement) between minorities and WNH with respect to quality of care change in five years (from 2003 to 2008). In contrast to the findings of Willson et al. [5], minorities were more likely to receive medical advice than WNH in our analysis; however, patient-provider relationships were not assessed and may have confounded the results. It has been suggested that physicians who positively engage minority patients may either be members of a minority group or have had experiences dealing with minority patient's health barriers and may be acting in an attempt to reduce health disparities [14]. Piette et al. [15] found that African Americans and Spanish-speaking patients as well as patients with a lower education reported having better communication with their physicians than patients of other race/ethnicities. Conversely, African American patients reported poorer patient-physician communication as compared to Whites with the same healthcare coverage in a national multicenter prospective study [12]. The investigators found that health outcomes and disease control had been positively associated with the quality of patient-physician communication, as measured by the patients' trust and report of physicians listening, explaining, showing respect, and spending time [12].

TABLE 4: Effect of reporting "now controlling or losing weight" on non-HDL cholesterol of those participants who were told to "control or reduce weight" by race/ethnicity.

Independent variables	Model 1		Model 2	
	B (95% CI)	SE	B (95% CI)	SE
Now controlling or losing weight (yes)	−8.9 (−13, −4.5)	2.2*	−4.4 (−8.4, −1.3)	1.8
MA	2.2 (−5.8, 10.2)	3.9	−1.1 (−9.1, 6.8)	3.9
OH	−2.9 (−12, 6.5)	4.7	−3.8 (−12, 4.6)	4.1
BNH	−16 (−22, −11)	2.8*	−18 (24, 11)	3.2*
Lose wt by MA	0.70 (−9.9, 11)	5.2	0.66 (−8.2, 9,5)	4.3
Lose wt by OH	9.7 (−0.32, 19)	4.9	5.0 (−4.0, 14)	4.4
Lose wt by BNH	15 (6.8, 23)	4.1*	14 (5.2, 22)	4.2*
Model summary	$R^2 = 0.063$ $F(9, 24) = 41.0, P < 0.001$		$R^2 = 0.21$ $F(17, 16) = 58.7, P < 0.001$	

Non-HDL cholesterol: non-high-density lipoprotein cholesterol; MA: Mexican American; OH: other Hispanic; BNH: Black, non-Hispanic; wt: weight. Model 1 was adjusted for gender and age. Model 2 included body mass index, health insurance, education, currently smoking, and taking cholesterol-lowering medication(s) along with the adjustments of Model 1. White non-Hispanic (WNH) is the reference group for race/ethnicity. Significance ($P < 0.05$) is denoted by (∗).

In the current study, there were no differences in LDL-C managing behaviors among race/ethnicity for adults with hypercholesterolemia given lifestyle medical advice. Instead, being given medical recommendations was associated with making the changes. These findings support the benefit of secondary prevention measures of diet and exercise recommendations by medical professionals. Several studies found racial/ethnic differences in therapeutic lifestyle changes for patients with chronic disease. BeLue et al. [16] reported different patterns of diet-exercise behavior (fruit and vegetable intake, fat intake and exercise) by race/gender groups for Black and White adults with hypercholesterolemia. Oster et al. [17] reported that Blacks and Hispanics were less likely to monitor their diet than WNH with diabetes in a national managed care organization. Moreover, for patients with diabetes, Blacks were less likely to exercise as compared to Whites [17, 18].

Weight loss, but not reducing fatty foods nor increasing physical activity, was associated with lower non-HDL cholesterol in our study. Several meta-analyses of dietary interventions for cardiovascular risk reduction have reported modest effects in cholesterol reduction [19–21]. Albeit, even modest reductions in serum cholesterol, about 10%, have been associated with a 50% decrease in the incidence of coronary heart disease for age 40 and 20% for age 70 for approximately 500,000 men in a meta-analysis of cohort studies [22].

In order for serum non-HDL cholesterol management to be effective, several precursors are necessary: (1) access to quality medical care that provides a diagnosis of hypercholesterolemia; (2) a culturally appropriate, nondiscriminatory environment that encourages continuation of healthcare utilization; and, (3) effective patient-provider relationships that involve patients in their treatment plans and empower them to follow disease-specific recommendations. Barriers for receiving and interpreting medical advice may differ by race/ethnicity. Based on a national survey of healthcare quality, African Americans, Hispanics, and Asians reported more perceived healthcare provider discrimination than WNH [23]. Poorer health status was associated with perceived healthcare discrimination more frequently in minorities than WNH [23]. There is inconclusive evidence regarding differences in patient-provider communication among the Hispanic subgroups. Although access to healthcare varies among Hispanic groups [24], the differences in access were not related to the quality of communication between the patient and their healthcare provider [25].

Receiving advice may not be interpreted equally across patients and may be a confounder in serum non-HDL cholesterol control. In particular, the interpretation of the medical recommendation to "eat fewer high-fat or high-cholesterol foods" may not be consistent among patients and may vary by race/ethnicity. Since people usually eat *ad libitum* (until they are satisfied), they are likely to exchange one food for another, rather than to reduce total calories [26]. In an effort to reduce "fatty foods," patients may substitute any combination of the following: refined carbohydrates (such as white flour or white rice), unrefined grains (such as whole oats, wheat, or brown rice), or healthy fats (such as nuts, seeds, avocados, and mono- and poly-unsaturated oils) for "fatty foods." The range of actions resulting in the interpretation of this dietary advice may have been a confounder in non-HDL cholesterol control.

Numerous prospective studies of both primary and secondary preventive measures to reduce the prevalence of hypercholesterolemia suggest that these efforts may prove to be beneficial by reducing its prevalence in the US. Healthy adults followed for 27 years were 26% and 30% less likely to develop hypercholesterolemia that maintained or increased their fitness level, respectively, compared to those who lost fitness levels [27]. Secondary prevention, aimed at non-HDL cholesterol control for those with hypercholesterolemia, also entails medical recommendations for diet, weight, and physical activity; yet, research regarding the efficacy of advice with behavior changes and health outcomes for persons with hypercholesterolemia is limited.

Our results should be interpreted with respect to the study strengths and limitations. A major strength of this study was the use of a large, nationally representative dataset. Another strength of this study was the use of non-HDL cholesterol as both a binary and continuous variable to measure cholesterol control as opposed to total cholesterol. The use of non-HDL cholesterol <130 mg/dL as adequate control may not be a suitable goal for all persons with hypercholesterolemia. The AACE guidelines are that goals for non-HDL cholesterol be set at 30 mg/dL above the target for LDL-C [7]. Although a target of non-HDL cholesterol <130 mg/dL is recommended for most patients, guidelines for lipid goals for patients at risk for coronary artery disease vary by physician and should be set as 30 mg/dL above the patient's LDL-C goals [7]. Several limitations were noted. The category "Others" was not used due to a small sample size. Data concerning having serum cholesterol checked and being given medical advice to manage hypercholesterolemia were self-reported and may contain some inaccuracies. Moreover, bias by race/ethnicity, age, gender, or other characteristics are possible due to recall differences among people.

5. Conclusions

The findings of this study indicate a lack of congruence in following medical advice and achieving adequate non-HDL cholesterol control by race/ethnicity. These results suggest that current methods of communicating lifestyle advice may not be adequate across ethnicity/race and that a change in perspective and delivery of medical recommendations for persons with hypercholesterolemia is needed. Evaluation of patient-provider communication with cholesterol management across race/ethnicity may be necessary to develop effective dietary and physical activity intervention strategies. The results of our study may inform healthcare professionals of the need to develop client-centered treatment plans with clear, individualized goals for diet, weight management, and physical activity.

Conflict of Interests

The authors declare that they have no conflict of interests.

References

[1] National Cholesterol Education Program, ATP III. US Department of Health and Human Services, Public Health Service National Institutes of Health National Heart, Lung, and Blood Institute. NIH Publication No. 01-3305, 2012 http://www.nhlbi.nih.gov/guidelines/cholesterol.

[2] E. S. Ford, C. Li, W. S. Pearson, G. Zhao, and A. H. Mokdad, "Trends in hypercholesterolemia, treatment and control among United States adults," *International Journal of Cardiology*, vol. 140, no. 2, pp. 226–235, 2010.

[3] "Third Report of the National Cholesterol Education Program (NCEP) Expert Panel on Detection, Evaluation, and Treatment of High Blood Cholesterol in Adults (Adult Treatment Panel III) final report," *Circulation*, vol. 106, no. 25, pp. 3143–3421, 2002.

[4] R. F. Redberg and M. H. Katz, "Healthy men should not take statins," *JAMA*, vol. 307, no. 14, pp. 1491–1492, 2012.

[5] M. N. Willson, J. J. Neumiller, D. A. Sclar, L. M. Robison, and T. L. Skaer, "Ethnicity/Race, use of pharmacotherapy, scope of physician-ordered cholesterol screening, and provision of diet/nutrition or exercise counseling during us office-based visits by patients with hyperlipidemia," *American Journal of Cardiovascular Drugs*, vol. 10, no. 2, pp. 105–108, 2010.

[6] National Health and Nutrition Examination Survey, Questionnaires, datasets and related documentation, http://www.cdc.gov/nchs/nhanes/nhanes_questionnaires.htm.

[7] P. S. Jellinger, D. A. Smith, A. E. Mehta et al., "American association of clinical endocrinologists' guidelines for management of dyslipidemia and prevention of atherosclerosis," *Endocrine Practice*, vol. 18, supplement 1, pp. 1–78, 2012.

[8] A. V. Chobanian, G. L. Bakris, H. R. Black et al., "Seventh report of the Joint National Committee on Prevention, Detection, Evaluation, and Treatment of High Blood Pressure," *Hypertension*, vol. 42, no. 6, pp. 1206–1252, 2003, http://www.nhlbi.nih.gov/guidelines/hypertension/index.htm.

[9] National Institutes of Health, National Heart, Lung and Blood Institute. NHLBI Obesity education initiative expert panel on the identification, evaluation, and treatment of overweight and obesity in adult. NIH publication 00 4084, October 2000.

[10] National Center for Health Statistics (NCHS): Center for Disease Control and Prevention. National Health and Nutrition Examination Survey (NHANES), *Analytical and Reporting Guidelines*, Hyattsville, Md, USA, 2006, http://www.cdc.gov/nchs/nhanes/nhanes2003-2004/analytical_guidelines.htm.

[11] R. N. Forthofer, E. S. Lee, and M. Hernandez, *Contingency Table Analysis. Biostatistics: A Guide to Design, Analysis and Discovery*, Academic Press, Elsevier, Burlington, Mass, USA, 2nd edition, 2007.

[12] Center for Disease Control and Prevention (CDC), "Translating Research into Action for Diabetes, (TRIAD) fact sheet," Program Announcement Number 04005 and 98086 from the Centers for Disease Control and Prevention (CDC) Division of Diabetes Translation and the National Institute of Diabetes and Digestive and Kidney Diseases (NIDDK), 2009, http://www.cdc.gov/diabetes/projects/pdfs/TRIAD_fact_sheet.pdf.

[13] Agency for Healthcare Research and Quality, *2008 National Healthcare Disparities Report (NHDR)*, Agency for Healthcare Research and Quality, Rockville, Md, USA, 2009.

[14] S. K. Vanderbilt, M. K. Wynia, M. Gadon, and G. C. Alexander, "A qualitative study of physicians' engagement in reducing healthcare disparities," *Journal of the National Medical Association*, vol. 99, no. 12, pp. 1315–1322, 2007.

[15] J. D. Piette, D. Schillinger, M. B. Potter, and M. Heisler, "Dimensions of patient-provider communication and diabetes self-care in an ethnically diverse population," *Journal of General Internal Medicine*, vol. 18, no. 8, pp. 624–633, 2003.

[16] R. BeLue, S. T. Lanza, and M. K. Figaro, "Lifestyle therapy changes and hypercholesterolemia: identifying risk groups in a community sample of blacks and whites," *Ethnicity and Disease*, vol. 19, no. 2, pp. 142–147, 2009.

[17] N. V. Oster, V. Welch, L. Schild, J. A. Gazmararian, K. Rask, and C. Spettell, "Differences in self-management behaviors and use of preventive services among diabetes management enrollees by race and ethnicity," *Disease Management*, vol. 9, no. 3, pp. 167–175, 2006.

[18] C. Nwasuruba, M. Khan, and L. E. Egede, "Racial/ethnic differences in multiple self-care behaviors in adults with diabetes," *Journal of General Internal Medicine*, vol. 22, no. 1, pp. 115–120, 2007.

[19] E. Brunner, I. White, M. Thorogood, A. Bristow, D. Curle, and M. Marmot, "Can dietary interventions change diet and

cardiovascular risk factors? A meta-analysis of randomized controlled trials," *American Journal of Public Health*, vol. 87, no. 9, pp. 1415–1422, 1997.

[20] E. J. Brunner, K. Rees, K. Ward, M. Burke, and M. Thorogood, "Dietary advice for reducing cardiovascular risk," *Cochrane Database of Systematic Reviews*, no. 4, Article ID CD002128, 2007.

[21] J. L. Tang, J. M. Armitage, T. Lancaster, C. A. Silagy, G. H. Fowler, and H. A. W. Neil, "Systematic review of dietary intervention trials to lower blood total cholesterol in free-living subjects," *BMJ*, vol. 316, no. 7139, pp. 1213–1219, 1998.

[22] M. R. Law, N. J. Wald, and S. G. Thompson, "By how much and how quickly does reduction in serum cholesterol concentration lower risk of ischaemic heart disease?" *BMJ*, vol. 308, no. 6925, pp. 367–372, 1994.

[23] C. Lee, S. L. Ayers, and J. J. Kronenfeld, "The association between perceived provider discrimination, healthcare utilization and health status in racial and ethnic minorities," *Ethnicity and Disease*, vol. 19, no. 3, pp. 330–337, 2009.

[24] A. Jerant, R. Arellanes, and P. Franks, "Health status among us hispanics: ethnic variation, nativity, and language moderation," *Medical Care*, vol. 46, no. 7, pp. 709–717, 2008.

[25] L. S. Wallace, J. E. Devoe, E. S. Rogers, J. Protheroe, G. Rowlands, and G. E. Fryer Jr., "Digging deeper: quality of patient-provider communication across Hispanic subgroups," *BMC Health Services Research*, vol. 9, article 240, 2009.

[26] J. Scholl, "Traditional dietary recommendations for the prevention of cardiovascular disease: do they meet the needs of our patients?" *Cholesterol*, vol. 2012, Article ID 367898, 9 pages, 2012.

[27] D.-C. Lee, X. Sui, T. S. Church, C. J. Lavie, A. S. Jackson, and S. N. Blair, "Changes in fitness and fatness on the development of cardiovascular disease risk factors: hypertension, metabolic syndrome, and hypercholesterolemia," *Journal of the American College of Cardiology*, vol. 59, no. 7, pp. 665–672, 2012.

Permissions

The contributors of this book come from diverse backgrounds, making this book a truly international effort. This book will bring forth new frontiers with its revolutionizing research information and detailed analysis of the nascent developments around the world.

We would like to thank all the contributing authors for lending their expertise to make the book truly unique. They have played a crucial role in the development of this book. Without their invaluable contributions this book wouldn't have been possible. They have made vital efforts to compile up to date information on the varied aspects of this subject to make this book a valuable addition to the collection of many professionals and students.

This book was conceptualized with the vision of imparting up-to-date information and advanced data in this field. To ensure the same, a matchless editorial board was set up. Every individual on the board went through rigorous rounds of assessment to prove their worth. After which they invested a large part of their time researching and compiling the most relevant data for our readers. Conferences and sessions were held from time to time between the editorial board and the contributing authors to present the data in the most comprehensible form. The editorial team has worked tirelessly to provide valuable and valid information to help people across the globe.

Every chapter published in this book has been scrutinized by our experts. Their significance has been extensively debated. The topics covered herein carry significant findings which will fuel the growth of the discipline. They may even be implemented as practical applications or may be referred to as a beginning point for another development. Chapters in this book were first published by Hindawi Publishing Corporation; hereby published with permission under the Creative Commons Attribution License or equivalent.

The editorial board has been involved in producing this book since its inception. They have spent rigorous hours researching and exploring the diverse topics which have resulted in the successful publishing of this book. They have passed on their knowledge of decades through this book. To expedite this challenging task, the publisher supported the team at every step. A small team of assistant editors was also appointed to further simplify the editing procedure and attain best results for the readers.

Our editorial team has been hand-picked from every corner of the world. Their multi-ethnicity adds dynamic inputs to the discussions which result in innovative outcomes. These outcomes are then further discussed with the researchers and contributors who give their valuable feedback and opinion regarding the same. The feedback is then collaborated with the researches and they are edited in a comprehensive manner to aid the understanding of the subject.

Apart from the editorial board, the designing team has also invested a significant amount of their time in understanding the subject and creating the most relevant covers. They scrutinized every image to scout for the most suitable representation of the subject and create an appropriate cover for the book.

The publishing team has been involved in this book since its early stages. They were actively engaged in every process, be it collecting the data, connecting with the contributors or procuring relevant information. The team has been an ardent support to the editorial, designing and production team. Their endless efforts to recruit the best for this project, has resulted in the accomplishment of this book. They are a veteran in the field of academics and their pool of knowledge is as vast as their experience in printing. Their expertise and guidance has proved useful at every step. Their uncompromising quality standards have made this book an exceptional effort. Their encouragement from time to time has been an inspiration for everyone.

The publisher and the editorial board hope that this book will prove to be a valuable piece of knowledge for researchers, students, practitioners and scholars across the globe.

List of Contributors

Mojgan Gharipour, Nizal Sarrafzadegan and Mohammad Talaie
Isfahan Cardiovascular Research Centre, Isfahan Cardiovascular Research Institute, Isfahan University of Medical Sciences, Isfahan, Iran

Masoumeh Sadeghi
Rehabilitation Research Center, Isfahan Cardiovascular Research Institute, Isfahan University of Medical Sciences, P.O. Box 81465-1148, Isfahan, Iran

Elham Andalib
Hypertension Research Centre, Isfahan Cardiovascular Research Institute, Isfahan University of Medical Sciences, Isfahan, Iran

Davood Shafie and Esmaiel Aghababaie
Cardiology Department, School of Medicine, Isfahan University of Medical Sciences, Isfahan, Iran

Gerda-Maria Haas
Arteriosklerose-Praventions-Institut, 81477 Munchen, Germany

Thomas Bertsch
Institute of Clinical Chemistry, Klinikum Nurnberg, 90419 Nurnberg, Germany

Peter Schwandt
Arteriosklerose-Praventions-Institut, 81477 Munchen, Germany
Ludwig-Maximilians-Universitat Munchen, 80539 Munchen, Germany

Matthias Orth
Institut fur Laboratoriumsmedizin, Vinzenz von Paul Kliniken gGmbH, Adlerstraβe 7, Postfach 103163, 70199 Stuttgart, Germany

Stefano Bellosta
Dipartimento di Scienze Farmacologiche e Biomolecolari, Facolt`a di Farmacia, Universita di Milano, Via Balzaretti 9, 20133 Milano, Italy

Agostino Di Ciaula
Division of Internal Medicine Hospital of Bisceglie, 76011 Bisceglie, Italy

David Q.-H. Wang
Saint Louis University School of Medicine, Division of Gastroenterology and Hepatology, Department of Internal Medicine, Edward Doisy Research Center, St. Louis, MO 63104, USA

Leonilde Bonfrate
Clinica Medica "A. Murri", Department of Biomedical Sciences & Human Oncology, University "Aldo Moro" of Bari Medical School, 70124 Bari, Italy

Piero Portincasa
Clinica Medica "A. Murri", Department of Biomedical Sciences & Human Oncology, University "Aldo Moro" of Bari Medical School, 70124 Bari, Italy
European Society for Clinical Investigation (ESCI), 3584 CJ Utrecht, The Netherlands

Johannes Scholl
Prevention First, 65385 Ruedesheim, Germany

Lawrence Baruch
James J. Peters VA Medical Center, Bronx, NY 10468, USA
Mt. Sinai School of Medicine, NY, USA

Valerie J. Chiong
James J. Peters VA Medical Center, Bronx, NY 10468, USA

Sanjay Agarwal
Confluence Health, Moses Lake, WA 98837, USA

Bhanu Gupta
St. Luke's Hospital, University of Missouri, Kansas City, MO 64111, USA

Marieke Boekel and Iris Kindt
Foundation for the Identification of Persons with Inherited Hypercholesterolemia (StOEH), Amsterdam, The Netherlands

Roeland Huijgen, Joep C. Defesche and John J. P. Kastelein
Department of Vascular Medicine, Academic Medical Center (AMC), 1105 AZ Amsterdam, The Netherlands

Peter de Knijff and Kristiaan J. van der Gaag
Department of Human Genetics, Forensic Laboratory for DNA Research, Leiden, The Netherlands

Olarewaju M. Oluba and Leye J. Babatola
Department of Biochemistry, College of Natural Science, Joseph Ayo Babalola University, Ikeji-Arakeji, Osun, Nigeria

Augustine O. Olusola
Department of Biochemistry, Faculty of Science, Adekunle Ajasin University, Akungba Akoko, Ondo, Nigeria

George O. Eidangbe
Department of Medical Biochemistry, College of Medicine, Ambrose Alli University, Ekpoma, Nigeria

E. Chukwu Onyeneke
Department of Biochemistry, Faculty of Life Sciences, University of Benin, Benin, Nigeria

Ji Sun Baek, Longhou Fang, Andrew C. Li and Yury I. Miller
Department of Medicine, University of California, San Diego, La Jolla, CA 92093, USA

Vijay V. Kakkar
Department of Molecular Immunology, Thrombosis Research Institute, Narayana Hrudayalaya Hospital, 258/A, Bommasandra Industrial Area, Bangalore 560099, India
Scientific Chairman, Thrombosis Research Institute, London, UK

Sonia Samson and Lakshmi Mundkur
Department of Molecular Immunology, Thrombosis Research Institute, Narayana Hrudayalaya Hospital, 258/A, Bommasandra Industrial Area, Bangalore 560099, India

Dimitrios Papandreou
2nd Department of Pediatrics, School of Medicine and Ahepa General Hospital, Aristotle University of Thessaloniki, Street Kiriakidi 1, 54636 Thessaloniki, Greece
Department of Life and Health Sciences, University of Nicosia, Makedonitissas Avenue, 1700 Nicosia, Cyprus

Zaharoula Karabouta and Israel Rousso
2nd Department of Pediatrics, School of Medicine and Ahepa General Hospital, Aristotle University of Thessaloniki, Street Kiriakidi 1, 54636 Thessaloniki, Greece

Anna L. Newton, Lynae J. Hanks, Elizabeth Williams, Michelle Davis and Krista Casazza
Department of Nutrition Sciences, University of Alabama at Birmingham, 1675 University Boulevard, WEBB 439 Birmingham, AL 35294-3360, USA

Ambika P. Ashraf
Division of Pediatric Endocrinology, Department of Medicine, University of Alabama at Birmingham, Birmingham, AL 35294-3360, USA

Remco Franssen, Sander I. van Leuven and Erik S. G. Stroes
Department of Vascular Medicine, Academic Medical Center Amsterdam, 1105 AZ Amsterdam, The Netherlands

Alinda W. M. Schimmel
Department of Experimental Vascular Medicine, Academic Medical Center Amsterdam, 1105 AZ Amsterdam, The Netherlands

Simone C. S. Wolfkamp
Department of Gastroenterology, Tytgat Institute for Liver and Intestinal Research, Academic Medical Center Amsterdam, 1105 AZ Amsterdam, The Netherlands

Jennifer B. Christian
GlaxoSmithKline, Clinical Effectiveness & Safety, 5 Moore Drive, B.3116, Durham, NC 27709-3398, USA

Geesje M. Dallinga-Thie
Department of Vascular Medicine, Academic Medical Center Amsterdam, 1105 AZ Amsterdam, The Netherlands
Department of Experimental Vascular Medicine, Academic Medical Center Amsterdam, 1105 AZ Amsterdam, The Netherlands

Eric J. Olson
GlaxoSmithKline, Heart Failure DPU, Medicines Discovery and Development, King of Prussia, PA 19406, USA

Jeffery K. Allen
GlaxoSmithKline, Worldwide Epidemiology, Durham, NC 27709, USA

Kimberly A. Lowe
Exponent Health Sciences, Bellevue, WA 98004, USA

Luciana R. Fernandes, Ana Cecília C. Ribeiro, Marcela Segatto, Luís Felipe F. F. Santos, Luciane R. Portugal and Jacqueline I. A. Leite
Departamento de Bioqu´ımica e Imunologia, Universidade Federal Minas Gerais, 31270-901 Belo Horizonte, MG, Brazil

Joana Amaral
Centro Universitario, Av. Prof. Mario Werneck, 1685-Estoril, 30455-610 Belo Horizonte, MG, Brazil

Maarit Hallikainen
Institute of Public Health and Clinical Nutrition, Department of Clinical Nutrition, University of Eastern Finland, P.O. BOX 1627, 70211 Kuopio, Finland

Henri Tuomilehto
Institute of Clinical Medicine, Department of Otorhinolaryngology, Kuopio University Hospital and University of Eastern Finland, P.O. BOX 1777, 70211 Kuopio, Finland
Oivauni Sleep Clinic, Puijonkatu 12 b, 70100 Kuopio, Finland

Juha Seppä
Institute of Clinical Medicine, Department of Otorhinolaryngology, Kuopio University Hospital and University of Eastern Finland, P.O. BOX 1777, 70211 Kuopio, Finland

Tarja Martikainen
Institute of Clinical Medicine, Department of Medicine, Division of Clinical Nutrition, Kuopio University Hospital, P.O. BOX 1777, 70211 Kuopio, Finland

Esko Vanninen
Institute of Clinical Medicine, Clinical Physiology and Nuclear Medicine, Kuopio University Hospital and University of Eastern Finland, P.O. BOX 1777, 70211 Kuopio, Finland

Jouko Kokkarinen and Jukka Randell
Institute of Clinical Medicine, Respiratory Medicine, Kuopio University Hospital and University of Eastern Finland, P.O. BOX 1777, 70211 Kuopio, Finland

Helena Gylling
Institute of Public Health and Clinical Nutrition, Department of Clinical Nutrition, University of Eastern Finland, P.O. BOX 1627, 70211 Kuopio, Finland
Division of Internal Medicine, Department of Medicine, University of Helsinki, Helsinki, P.O. BOX 700, 00029 HUS, Finland

Maryam Barzin, Farhad Hosseinpanah, Hamidreza Saber and Parvin Sarbakhsh
Obesity Research Center, Research Institute for Endocrine Science, Shahid Beheshti University of Medical Sciences, 1985717413 Tehran, Iran

Kobra Nakhoda and Fereidoun Azizi
Endocrine Research Center, Research Institute for Endocrine Science, Shahid Beheshti University of Medical Sciences, 1985717413 Tehran, Iran

George A. Kelley and Kristi S. Kelley
Meta-Analytic Research Group, Department of Biostatistics, School of Public Health, Robert C. Byrd Health Sciences Center, West Virginia University, Morgantown, WV 26506-9190, USA

Ratana Vichiansiri, Jittima Saengsuwan, Nuttaset Manimmanakorn, Sirasaporn Patpiya, Arayawichanon Preeda, Kharmwan Samerduen and Ekasit Poosiripinyo
Department of Physical Medicine and Rehabilitation, Faculty of Medicine, Khon Kaen University, Amphur Muang, Khon Kaen 40002, Thailand

Noemi Rotllan and Carlos Fernandez-Hernando
Marc and Ruti Bell Vascular Biology and Disease Program, Leon H. Charney Division of Cardiology, Departments of Medicine and Cell Biology, New York University School of Medicine, New York, NY 10016, USA

Dean G. Karalis
Cardiology Consultants of Philadelphia, Philadelphia, PA 19107, USA
Division of Cardiology, Drexel University College of Medicine, Philadelphia, PA 19107, USA

Brett Victor and Lilian Ahedor
Division of Cardiology, Drexel University College of Medicine, Philadelphia, PA 19107, USA

Longjian Liu
Department of Epidemiology and Biostatistics, Drexel University School of Public Health, Philadelphia, PA 19107, USA

Fereshteh Baygi
Endocrinology and Metabolism Research Center, Tehran University of Medical Sciences, Tehran 1411413137, Iran

Ahmad Reza Dorosty
Department of Nutrition and Biochemistry, Tehran University of Medical Sciences, Tehran, Iran

Roya Kelishadi
Pediatrics Department, Faculty of Medicine and Child Growth and Development Research Center,
Isfahan University of Medical Sciences, Isfahan, Iran

Mostafa Qorbani
Endocrinology and Metabolism Research Center, Tehran University of Medical Sciences, Tehran 1411413137, Iran
Department of Epidemiology and Biostatistics, Tehran University of Medical Sciences, Tehran 1411413137, Iran

Hamid Asayesh
Faculty of Paramedical, Qom University of Medical Sciences, Qom, Iran

Morteza Mansourian
Department of Health Education and Promotion, Tehran University of Medical Sciences, Tehran, Iran

Kamal Mirkarimi
Department of Health Education and Promotion, Golestan University of Medical Sciences, Gorgan, Iran

Anouar Hafiane
McGill University, Montreal, QC, Canada

Jacques Genest
Faculty of Medicine, Center for Innovative Medicine, McGill University Health Center, Royal Victoria Hospital, McGill University, 687 Pine AvenueWest, Montreal, QC, Canada

Silvia Bleda, Joaquın de Haro, Cesar Varela, Leticia Esparza, Javier Rodriguez and Francisco Acin
Vascular Surgery and Angiology Department, Hospital Universitario Getafe, Ctra Toledo Km 12,500, 28905 Madrid, Spain

Joan Anne Vaccaro
Department of Dietetics and Nutrition, MMC AHC 1-450, Florida International University, Miami, FL 33199, USA

Fatma G. Huffman
Department of Dietetics and Nutrition, MMC AHC 1-435, Florida International University, Miami, FL 33199, USA